Ocular Angiogenesis

Jonathan Stone • *CNS Stability and Degeneration Group, Research School of Biological Science, Australian National University, Canberra, Australia*
Kanji Takahashi • *Department of Ophthalmology, Kansai Medical University, Moriguchi, Osaka, Japan*
Takashi Tokoro • *Department of Ophthalmology, Tokyo Medical and Dental University, Japan*
Joyce Tombran-Tink • *Division of Pharmaceutical Sciences, University of Missouri-Kansas City, Kansas City, MO, and Department of Ophthalmology and Visual Science, Yale University School of Medicine, New Haven, CT*
James C. Tsai • *Edward S. Harkness Eye Institute, Department of Ophthalmology, Columbia University College of Physicians and Surgeons, New York, NY*
Olga V. Volpert • *Department of Urology, Northwestern University Feinberg School of Medicine, Chicago, IL*
Steven M. Wolchok • *Department of Ophthalmology, Emory University School of Medicine, Atlanta, GA*
Sarah X. Zhang • *Department of Medicine, Department of Cell Biology, The University of Oklahoma Health Sciences Center, Oklahoma City, OK*
Ari Ziskind • *Department of Ophthalomology, Tygerberg Hospital, Tygerberg, South Africa*

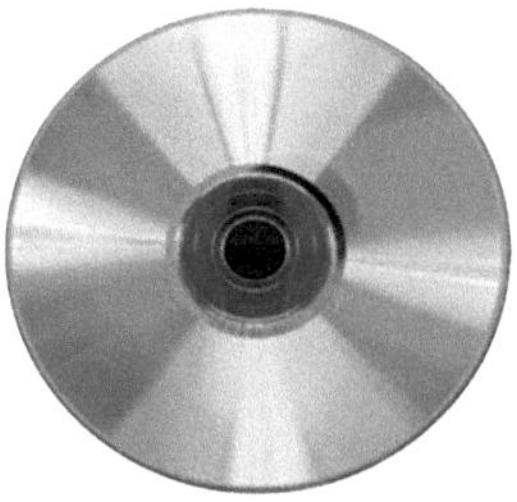

Companion CD

Color versions of illustrations listed here may be found on the Companion CD attached to the inside back cover. The image files are organized into folders by chapter number and are viewable in most Web browsers. The number following "f" at the end of the file name identifies the corresponding figure in the text. The CD is compatible with both Mac and PC operating systems.

Chapter 1	Figs. 1–6, 10, and 11
Chapter 2	Fig. 1
Chapter 3	Figs. 1–8
Chapter 4	Figs. 1–5
Chapter 5	Figs. 1–6 and 8
Chapter 6	Figs. 1–5
Chapter 7	Figs. 1 and 2
Chapter 8	Figs. 1 and 2
Chapter 12	Fig. 1
Chapter 13	Figs. 1 and 3
Chapter 14	Figs. 1–3
Chapter 15	Figs. 1 and 3
Chapter 17	Figs. 1A, 2A–C, and 3–5
Chapter 18	Figs. 1–3, 5–11, 13, and 14,
Chapter 19	Figs. 2–4 and 6–8
Chapter 21	Fig. 1–7
Chapter 22	Fig. 2

I
ANGIOGENIC DISEASES

1
Age-Related Macular Degeneration

Curtis L. Hagedorn, MD and Ron A. Adelman, MD, MPH

CONTENTS

INTRODUCTION

Age-related macular degeneration (AMD) is the leading cause of blindness in people 60 years of age or older in the Western Hemisphere *(1)*. There are approx 15 million people affected by AMD in the United States, as AMD affects approx 18% of Americans between the ages of 65 and 74 yr and 30% of those aged 75 yr and older *(2)*. The diagnosis of AMD is based on visual dysfunction and characteristic macular findings *(3)*. AMD has been classified into neovascular (wet or exudative) and nonneovascular (dry) types. Neovascular AMD is less common but far more devastating than the dry type. The Beaver Dam Study demonstrated a prevalence of neovascular AMD that is approximately one-tenth the prevalence of the dry type *(2)*. The most severe form of dry AMD is geographic atrophy, which accounts for 12 to 21% of legal blindness caused by AMD, while the neovascular form accounts for the balance *(4–6)*. Neovascular AMD affects approx 1 million Americans, and each year about 200,000 new cases are diagnosed. Without treatment, most of these patients with neovascular AMD will progress to visual acuity of 20/200 or worse within 2 yr *(7,8)*. Even though there is clearly an association with advancing age, identifying other factors that put a patient at risk for development and progression of AMD has proven to be a difficult challenge. Several studies have demonstrated an increased risk with cigarette smoking *(9–14)*, and the Rotterdam Study showed a dose–response relationship between smoking and AMD *(9)*. There are conflicting reports on the association between AMD and

From: *Ophthalmology: Ocular Angiogenesis: Diseases, Mechanisms, and Therapeutics*
Edited by: J. Tombran-Tink and C. J. Barnstable © Humana Press Inc., Totowa, NJ

diabetes, cardiovascular disease, hypercholesterolemia, hypertension, alcohol use, obesity, aspirin use, and estrogen use *(15,16)*. Diet may play a role. The type and amount of dietary fat intake may modify risk of progression of AMD, and intake of fish, fruit, nuts, and green leafy vegetables may be protective *(17–19)*. Antioxidant intake has been proven to be beneficial in certain patients with AMD *(20)*. Recently, there has been much interest and investigation into the role of genetic influences on AMD. Studies have demonstrated an increased risk of AMD if a first-degree family member is affected. Approximately 20% of AMD patients have a positive family history, and monozygotic twins demonstrate higher levels of concordance *(21–28)*.

PATHOLOGY

Dry AMD is characterized by irregularities in the retinal pigment epithelium (RPE) and Bruch's membrane. Hard drusen have been demonstrated to represent either lipid accumulation in RPE cells or deposits of hyaline material in Bruch's membrane *(29,30)*. Soft drusen are composed of three histopathological types: RPE detachments with diffuse basal linear deposits, RPE detachments with diffuse basal laminar deposits, and focal accumulation of basal linear deposits *(29,30)*. Basal linear deposits are located within the inner collagenous zone of Bruch's membrane and consist of lipid-rich material and collagen, whereas basal laminar deposits are located between the plasma membrane and basement membrane of the RPE and are primarily made of collagen *(31)*. Focal pigment changes in AMD may be referred to as nongeographic atrophy. The fundus appearance is one of pigment mottling and areas of hypopigmentation and hyperpigmentation. Histopathology has shown these areas to be atrophic RPE overlying diffuse basal linear and basal laminar deposits *(30)*. Geographic atrophy is the advanced form of dry AMD. Histopathology demonstrates thinning of the neurosensory retina over atrophic choriocapillaris and RPE *(32)*. Changes in Bruch's membrane caused by accumulation of extracellular debris and deposition of drusen can predispose the membrane to breaks and impair transport and diffusion functions. Decreased permeability to water-soluble proteins from the plasma, as well as impaired transport of RPE waste products from the retina, can lead to a state of oxidative stress *(33)*. This oxidative stress possibly leads to formation of factors stimulating growth of choroidal neovascularization (CNV). Several studies of CNV have demonstrated RPE production of such angiogenic factors, including vascular endothelial growth factor (VEGF) and basic fibroblast growth factor (bFGF) *(34–36)*. Breaks in weakened Bruch's membrane are likely mediated by chemical factors, and enzymatic digestion and chronic inflammation may play a role in Bruch's membrane breakdown *(37–39)*. CNV can lead to subretinal and sub-RPE bleeding with fluid accumulation and eventual formation of fibrovascular and fibroglial tissue and disciform scarring.

CLINICAL EXAM

Dry AMD

Dry AMD is diagnosed when the characteristic fundus findings of drusen, RPE irregularities, and geographic atrophy are found in the appropriate clinical setting (*see* Fig. 1). By definition, dry AMD does not include CNV. Many classifications of drusen size

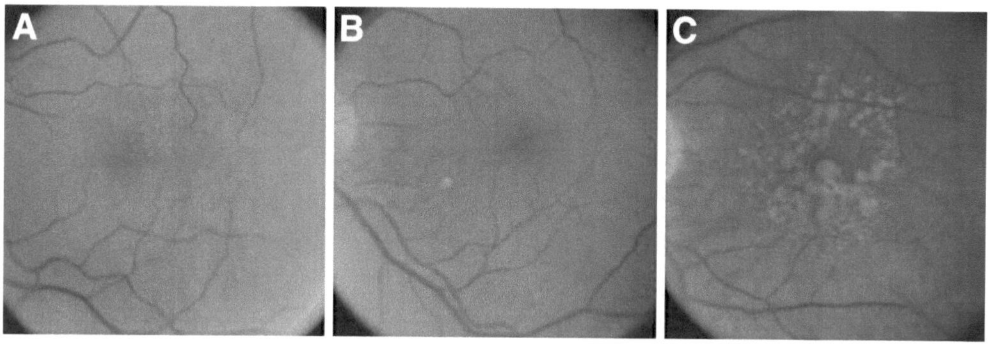

Fig. 1. Funduscopic appearance of drusen. **(A)** Few medium-sized drusen. **(B)** Large drusen. **(C)** Many medium and large drusen with confluence. (Courtesy of the Age-Related Eye Disease Study Research Group [AREDS].) *See* color version on companion CD.

have been utilized, but it is generally accepted that drusen are considered small if less than 63 μm, intermediate if 63 to 124 μm, and large if 125 μm or greater *(3)*. Certain retinal changes are more predictive of future vision loss. Increasing size, increasing number, and confluence of drusen confer a greater risk of neovascular AMD *(40)*. Soft drusen have been shown to confer an increased risk of development of geographic atrophy *(41)* and CNV *(41,42)*. The Macular Photocoagulation Study (MPS) examined the fellow eye of patients with unilateral CNV and AMD in a masked randomized prospective clinical trial. The MPS reported 46% of eyes with large drusen developed CNV compared to 10% of eyes without such drusen after 5 yr of follow-up *(43)*. Geographic atrophy is the most severe form of dry AMD. Geographic atrophy is responsible for approx 12 to 21% of the cases of legal blindness from AMD *(4–6)*. Clinically, geographic atrophy appears as areas of atrophic retina, often with visualization of underlying large caliber choroidal blood vessels (*see* Fig. 2).

Neovascular AMD

The majority of patients who suffer severe vision loss from AMD manifest the neovascular form of the disease. CNV can lead to subretinal fluid, subretinal hemorrhage, RPE detachments, and eventual disciform scarring. Patients with CNV from AMD usually complain of relatively acute vision loss or metamorphopsia. Clinically, patients may have a gray-green subretinal lesion with associated subretinal fluid, subretinal hemorrhage, sub-RPE hemorrhage, intraretinal bleeding, subretinal fibrosis, or retinal edema (*see* Figs. 3–5).

RELATED DISEASES

Retinal Angiomatous Proliferation

Retinal angiomatous proliferation (RAP) has been described as a subcategory of AMD and is characterized by angiomatous proliferation that originates in the retina and then progresses deep, sometimes communicating with choroidal vasculature. Clinically, RAP can present as intraretinal or subretinal hemorrhage and fluid. Appearance on fluorescein angiography (FA), indocyanine green angiography (ICG), and optical coherence tomography (OCT) is usually diagnostic *(44)* and includes focal retinal

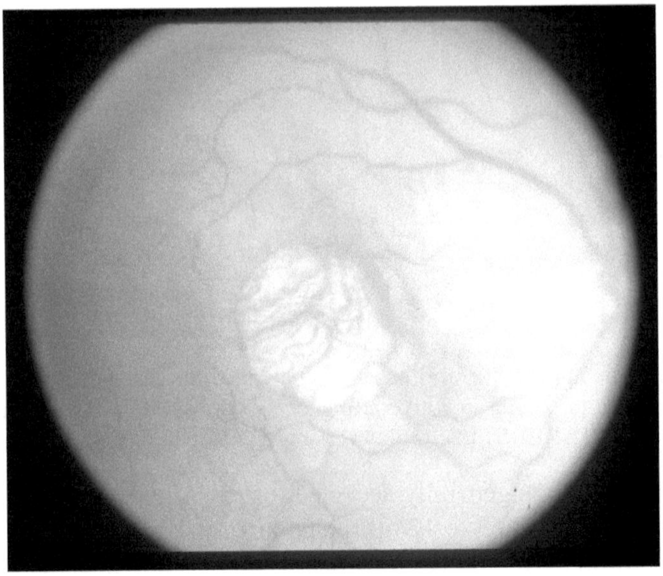

Fig. 2. Geographic atrophy in a patient with dry AMD. (Courtesy of the Age-Related Eye Disease Study Research Group [AREDS].) *See* color version on companion CD.

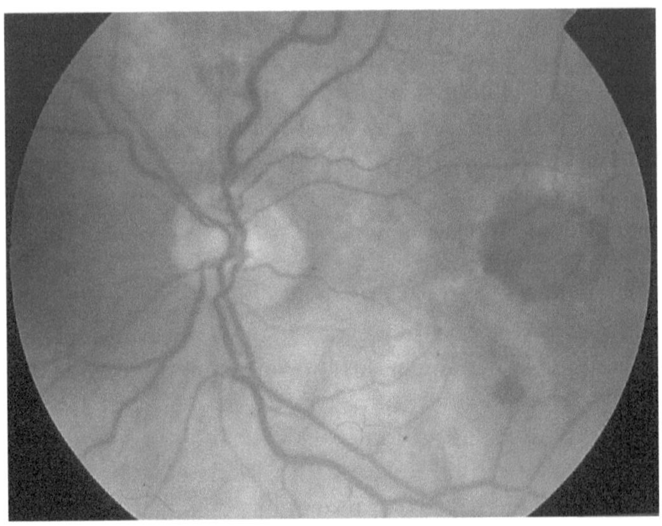

Fig. 3. Neovascular age-related macular degeneration with subretinal hemorrhage from a choroidal neovascularization. *See* color version on companion CD.

hyperfluorescence with an indistinct border on FA, focal intense hyperfluorescence on ICG, and irregular reflectance on OCT at the site of intraretinal neovascularization. RAP may progress and eventually connect with the choroidal vasculature, forming a retinal–choroidal vascular anastomosis and frank CNV. It is important to distinguish RAP from AMD with primary CNV, as the treatment options may be different. Yannuzzi et al. *(44)* have suggested that a classification system be used for RAP, as different stages may be amenable to different treatments. Thermal laser may be beneficial for focal intraretinal neovascularization, whereas vascularized retinal pigment epithelial

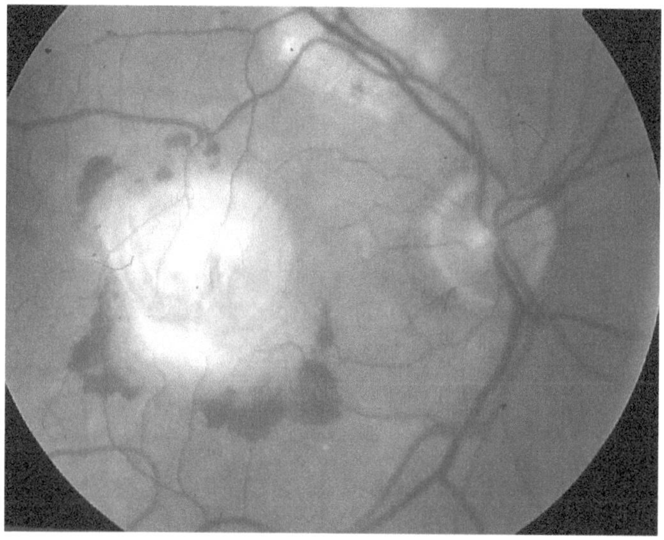

Fig. 4. Disciform scar with adjacent subretinal hemorrhage. *See* color version on companion CD.

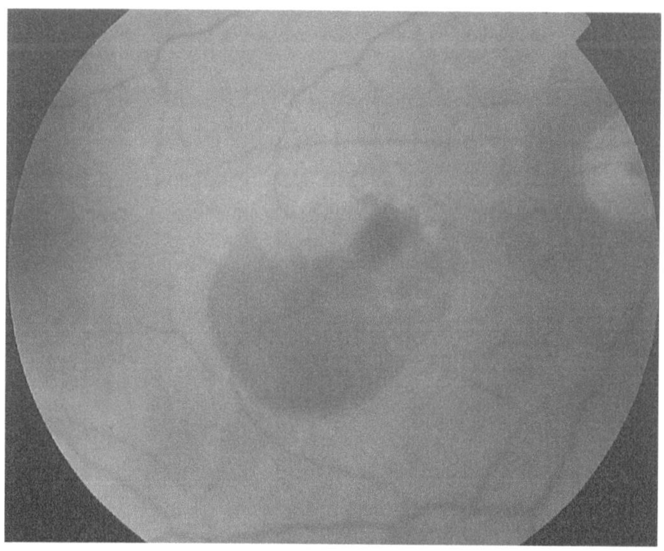

Fig. 5. Large submacular hemorrhage from choroidal neovascularization. *See* color version on companion CD.

detachments with retinal–choroidal vascular anastomosis may be most amenable to injection of an angiostatic agent. Currently, photodynamic therapy (PDT) with verteporfin, with or without intravitreal triamcinolone acetate, is a commonly used treatment. Surgical treatment may also be considered, and a procedure using specific surgical lysis of the feeding arteriole and draining venule of a RAP lesion has been described *(45)*.

Polypoidal Choroidal Vasculopathy

Polypoidal choroidal vasculopathy (PCV) is thought to arise from aneurismal dilations in the inner choroid that may be venular *(46,47)*. These lesions may expand, leak,

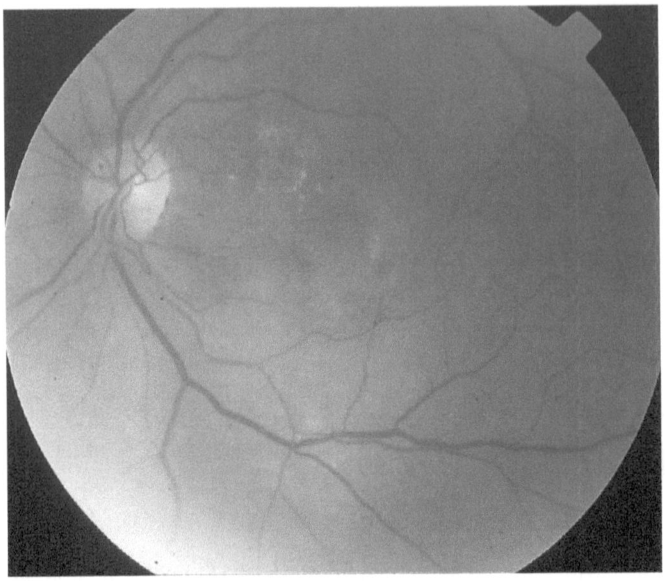

Fig. 6. Funduscopic appearance of polypoidal choroidal vasculopathy. *See* color version on companion CD.

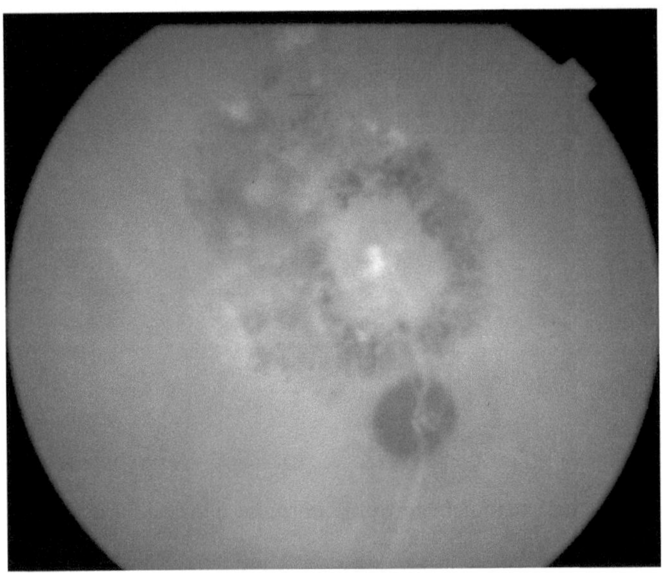

Fig. 7. Indocyanine green (ICG) angiogram of a patient with PCV. Note the sacular pattern of ICG fluorescence.

and bleed. PCV usually presents as dilated choroidal vessels in orange-colored polypoidal lesions in the macula and peripapillary area (*see* Fig. 6). Associated subretinal bleeding and fluid can be seen. ICG is diagnostic and demonstrates saccular dilations of the choroidal vasculature that may be more numerous and far-reaching than that seen clinically *(48,49)* (*see* Fig. 7). Treatment is not well established, and differentiation from CNV is critical *(48)*.

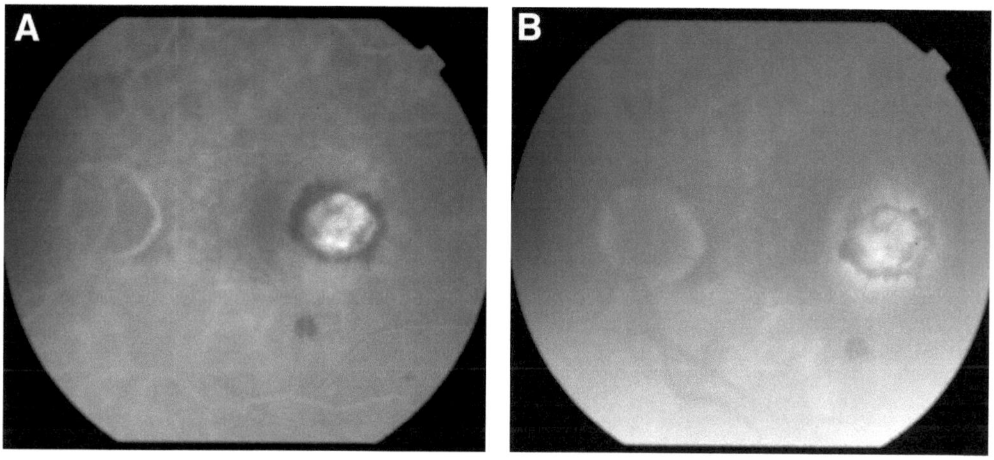

Fig. 8. Fluorescein angiography of predominantly classic choroidal neovascularization in age-related macular degeneration. (**A**) Early phase demonstrates hyperfluorescence. (**B**) Lesion demonstrates leakage in the late phase.

DIAGNOSTIC TESTING

Angiography

FA is useful for evaluation of advanced forms of AMD. Drusen generally hyperfluoresce early and either fade or stain in the later stages of angiography, and RPE degeneration demonstrates diffuse hyperfluorescence with areas of blockage corresponding to pigment clumping *(50)*. Areas of RPE loss demonstrate transmission of choroidal fluorescence (window defects), whereas geographic atrophy may sometimes demonstrate staining characteristics owing to the increased visibility of the scleral tissue staining *(50)*. Unlike neovascular AMD, dry AMD does not demonstrate signs of leakage on FA. FA is critical in evaluation of CNV. It is important to distinguish between classic and occult components of a CNV. A classic CNV demonstrates an area of early (usually within 1 min) hyperfluorescence that leaks and becomes brightly hyperfluorescent in the late phase (usually 5 to 10 min) (*see* Fig. 8). An occult CNV has two possible fluorescence patterns. It may consist of a fibrovascular pigment epithelial detachment that demonstrates a stippled pattern on FA (*see* Fig. 9), or it may consist of late leakage of an unknown source. Areas obscured angiographically due to such elements as subretinal blood or a retinal pigment epithelium detachment are considered part of the nonclassic CNV complex. ICG can be helpful in evaluating these obscured components, as its high protein binding provides better visualization of choroidal vasculature.

Optical Coherence Tomography

Optical coherence tomography was introduced in the 1990s; currently, the third-generation machine is commercially available. Ultrafast high-resolution OCT has been developed and will be available in the future *(51)*. OCT works on the principle of interferometry, measuring differences in light reflections from ocular tissues, and provides a cross-sectional image of retinal layers *(52,53)*. OCT provides excellent analysis of the vitreoretinal interface and has become a standard diagnostic test for conditions such as macular hole and vitreomacular traction syndrome. OCT can also provide valuable information in AMD *(54)*.

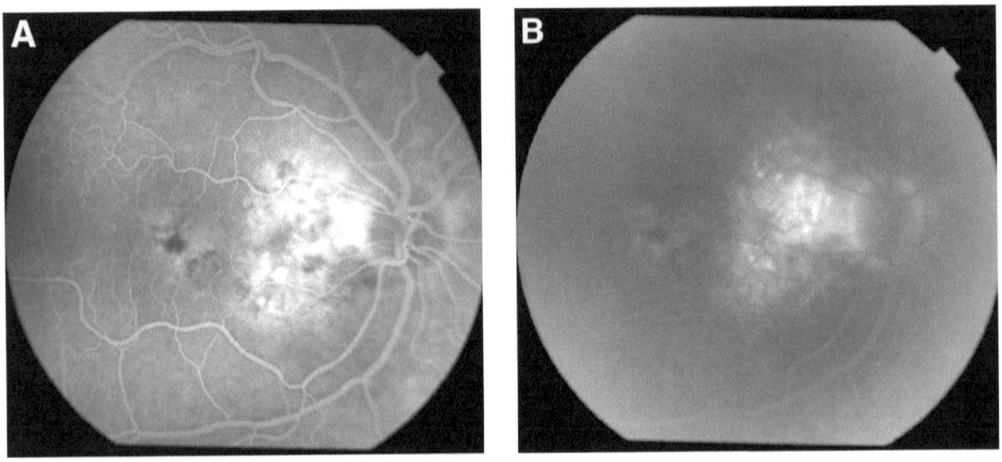

Fig. 9. Fluorescein angiography of an occult choroidal neovascularization in age-related macular degeneration. **(A)** Early phase demonstrates a stippled pattern of hyperfluorescence. **(B)** Lesion leaks in the late phase.

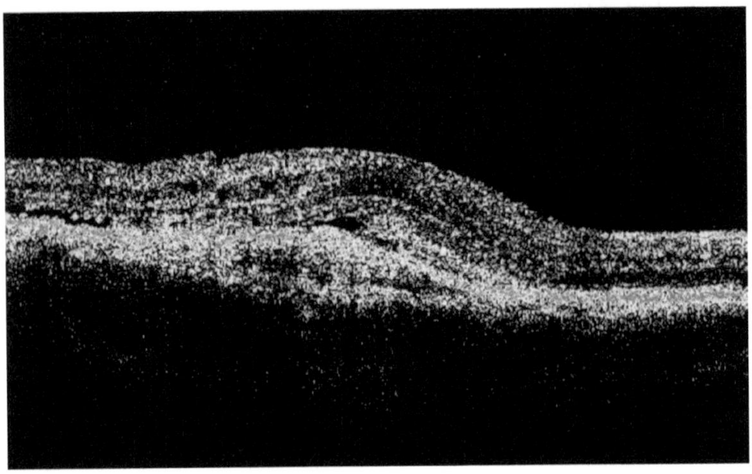

Fig. 10. Optical coherence tomography of a choroidal neovascularization in age-related macular degeneration. Retinal pigment epithelium layer is thickened and overlying retina is edematous. *See* color version on companion CD.

Drusen can be visualized as elevations of the highly reflective RPE layer, and CNV appears as thickening of the RPE and retin (*see* Fig. 10). Although FA is currently the standard for diagnosis of CNV in AMD, recent reports indicate a possible role for OCT in follow-up for determination of subsequent treatment in these lesions, as changes in retinal edema and RPE elevations are readily quantifiable with OCT *(55,56)* (*see* Fig. 11). OCT may also be valuable in differentiating conditions such as retinal RAP from CNV *(44)*.

MANAGEMENT

Dry AMD

Until recently, there was no proven treatment for dry AMD. Patients were simply given Amsler grids to monitor vision changes, and were instructed to return immediately if any

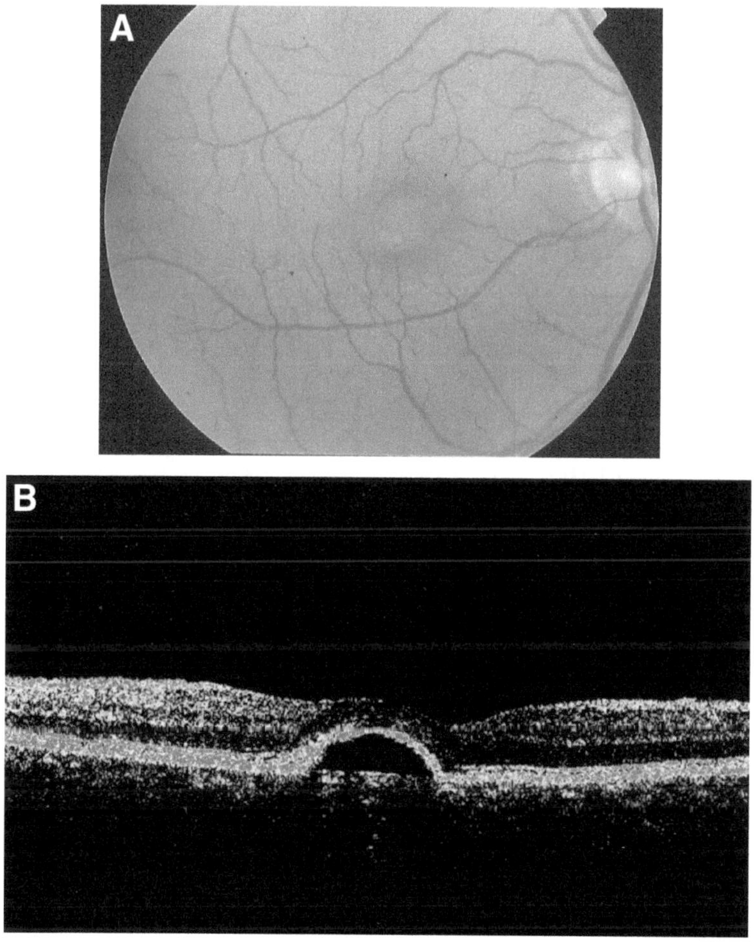

Fig. 11. Retinal pigment epithelium (RPE) detachment in age-related macular degeneration. (**A**) Fundus photograph demonstrates sub-RPE fluid in the macula. (**B**) Optical coherence tomography confirms diagnosis of RPE detachment. *See* color version on companion CD.

abrupt change should occur, as this could represent a conversion to the neovascular form of the disease, which may require treatment. Today, in addition to home monitoring, patients may use antioxidants and zinc to slow progression of AMD. The Age-Related Eye Disease Study Research Group (AREDS) conducted a large randomized masked multicenter clinical trial that demonstrated a combination of vitamin C, vitamin E, beta carotene, zinc, and copper was beneficial in slowing the course of AMD in patients with moderate to severe AMD *(20)*. This study demonstrated a 25% reduction in risk of moderate vision loss over 5 yr in patients with AMD consisting of extensive intermediate-sized drusen, one large druse, noncentral geographic atrophy, or advanced AMD by taking 500 mg of vitamin C, 400 international units (IU) of vitamin E, 15 mg of beta carotene, 80 mg of zinc oxide, and 2 mg of cupric oxide. Cigarette smoking is considered a contraindication to taking these medicines, as studies have demonstrated an increased risk of lung cancer and mortality in patients on high doses of beta carotene *(57,58)*. Recent reports suggest that human retinal carotenoids lutein and zeaxanthin (found in green leafy vegetables) may reduce risk of geographic atrophy and neovascular AMD in patients at risk *(19)*. Consumption of fish, which is high in omega-3 long-chain polyunsaturated fatty acids (LCPUFAs), may also decrease risk of neovascular AMD *(19)*. Currently, a trial is planned to further evaluate the effect of these micronutrients on the progression of AMD in patients at risk. Some studies have demonstrated regression of drusen with low-intensity macular laser *(59–61)*, and the Complications of AMD Prevention Trial (CAPT) is investigating whether this laser treatment can reduce the incidence of severe vision loss in eyes with high-risk drusen. Anecortave acetate, a synthetic steroid without glucocorticoid activity, is currently being evaluated for prevention of vision loss in the Anecortave Acetate Risk Reduction Trial (AART). This study is evaluating the effect of posterior juxtascleral delivery of this medicine in patients with high-risk dry AMD.

Neovascular AMD

Treatment of CNV remains an extremely active area of research. In 1986, the Macular Photocoagulation Study (MPS) *(7,8)* began investigating the effect of laser photocoagulation on macular CNV. These studies demonstrated laser photocoagulation treatment to be beneficial for CNV, but outcomes after treatment of subfoveal lesions were suboptimal. For initial subfoveal CNV treatment, few eyes had visual acuity better than 20/200 at 4 yr. Laser photocoagulation works by a thermal mechanism. Laser light is absorbed by the RPE and choroids, and this is converted into heat. Studies have shown that CNV may not be completely ablated by the laser, but may actually become enveloped by RPE fibrous tissue and proliferation of RPE cells, which may aid in absorption of subretinal fluid and limit spread of CNV *(62–65)*. Transpupillary thermotherapy (TTT) using a diode laser has also been utilized for treatment of CNV in AMD. The longer wavelength of laser light has the theoretical advantage of deeper chorioretinal treatment with relative sparing of the inner retinal layers and may pass through subretinal hemorrhage. Pilot studies have shown encouraging results *(66,67)*, and currently a well-designed study is under way evaluating TTT for CNV smaller than 3.0 mm (TTT4CNV). Recent reports from this study demonstrate that it is relatively safe in eyes without concomitant glaucoma, but the efficacy of TTT is questionable *(68)*. In April 2000, the US Food and Drug Administration approved the use of verteporfin (Visudyne®) for use in PDT for CNV in AMD. This approval was based on the Treatment of Age-Related Macular Degeneration with Photodynamic Therapy (TAP) study *(69)*. This study demonstrated a statistically significant visual benefit for patients with subfoveal predominantly classic CNV at the 1- and 2-yr marks. The Verteporfin in Photodynamic Therapy (VIP) study demonstrated a benefit in patients with select subfoveal occult CNV at the 2-yr mark *(70)*. Recently, multiple linear regression models of the aforementioned studies have demonstrated lesion size may actually be more important than type when evaluating the benefit of PDT. Treatment of occult and minimally classic CNV may have similar success to that of predominantly classic CNV if the lesion was equal to or less than 4 disk areas and demonstrated evidence of recent progression *(71)*. Recent progression was defined as subretinal hemorrhage associated with CNV, or loss of visual acuity of at least 5 letters within 3 mo, or growth of the CNV of at least 10% in the greatest linear dimension within 3 mo.

Verteporfin is a benzoporphyrin derivative monoacid ring A. It is a photosensitizer synthesized from protoporphyrin and is activated by a low-intensity laser light of 689 nm

(72,73). In the excited state, verteporfin generates singlet oxygen, which is thought to be responsible for cell death with PDT *(74)*. Verteporfin concentrates in neovascular endothelium as it is preferentially taken up by cells with high levels of low-density lipoprotein receptors *(75,76)*. PDT with verteporfin may destroy neovascular tissue while sparing normal tissue *(77–84)*. Although PDT with verteporfin has been shown to be better than placebo for select cases, the need for multiple treatments, the high cost, and the rarity of visual improvement with this therapy *(85)* has led medical researchers to continue the search for a better treatment for CNV in AMD.

Intravitreal and periocular injections of medicine have also been used to treat CNV. Intravitreal triamcinolone acetonide has been widely used in the management of CNV. A randomized, double-masked, placebo-controlled study by Gillies et al. *(86)* using a single dose of 4 mg of intravitreal triamcinolone acetonide demonstrated no effect on the loss of visual acuity during the first year; however, the size of the CNV in treated eyes was significantly smaller at 3 mo. A study by Jonas et al. *(87)* evaluating the effect of 25 mg of intravitreal triamcinolone acetonide found significant improvement in visual acuity. Highest visual acuity was demonstrated in the 1- to 3-mo postoperative period followed by loss of effect at 4 to 5 mo. Six of 71 eyes were injected a second time, and half of these experienced another improvement in visual acuity. Both these studies also demonstrated an increased risk of developing mild to moderate elevation of intraocular pressure with intravitreal injection of triamcinolone acetonide. Combining this injection with PDT/verteporfin may be synergistic. A recent study by Spaide et al. *(88)* evaluated the effect of PDT with verteporfin immediately followed by intravitreal injection of triamcinolone acetonide in patients with AMD and CNV without restriction to type (predominantly classic, minimally classic, and occult included). This pilot study demonstrated the potential benefit of this treatment as first-line therapy. Periocular delivery of steroid medications has also been advocated. Although this is not as direct a delivery method, the risks of introducing a needle into the vitreous cavity are avoided—namely, endophthalmitis, vitreous hemorrhage, retinal detachment, and unintended penetration of intraocular structures. As mentioned previously, anecortave acetate is a synthetic angiostatic steroid without glucocorticoid activity. This medicine has been evaluated in a multicenter randomized trial using juxtascleral delivery for treatment of subfoveal choroidal neovascularization in AMD. The study tested 3-, 15-, and 30-mg doses administered every 6 mo. At 1 yr, the 15-mg dose was found to stabilize vision and decrease rates of severe vision loss compared to placebo *(89)*. The beneficial effect of synthetic steroids may involve improvement in the blood-retinal barrier and downregulation of VEGF *(90)*. Recently there has been much interest in antiangiogenesis molecules for CNV. Studies of surgically excised and experimentally induced CNV have demonstrated high levels of VEGF, transforming growth factor β (TGF-β), and bFGF *(91–101)*. These molecules are thought to play a role in the development of CNV. Ranibizumab (Lucentis™) is a recombinant humanized antibody fragment that binds to and inactivates all VEGF isoforms. Intravitreal injection of this molecule is currently being investigated as a treatment for CNV in AMD. Preliminary results indicate that ranibizumab is well tolerated after 1 yr of injections, and phase III results are encouraging *(102)*. Pegaptnib sodium (Macugen®) is a chemically synthesized anti-VEGF aptamer with high affinity and specificity for VEGF isomer 165. Reports from phase III trials suggest that intravitreal injection of pegaptnib every 6 wk improves visual outcomes compared to placebo and is relatively safe in patients with CNV from AMD *(103)*. Submacular surgery is another option for treatment of CNV in AMD. The Submacular Surgery Trial (SST) is a multicenter randomized trial evaluating this surgical option for CNV from AMD, ocular histoplasmosis, and idiopathic causes. Recently published study results demonstrate no benefit in regard to improvement or stabilization of visual acuity in studied patients with AMD, but there may be a role for this procedure in select cases of predominantly hemorrhagic CNV in AMD *(104,105)*.

Another surgical option is macular translocation. The concept is to actually move the macula from diseased RPE and reposition it eccentrically onto a healthier area of RPE. Options include limited macular translocation (LMT) and macular translocation with 360-degree retinotomy (MT360). The LMT technique involves preplacement of scleral sutures for imbrication, vitrectomy, injection of subretinal fluid to detach temporal retina, creation of choroid/scleral folding by tying the preplaced sutures, and gas bubble placement with positioning to optimize translocation *(106)*. Select cases may benefit from this procedure *(107–109)*. The MT360 technique involves performing a vitrectomy, creation of total retinal detachment, 360-degree retinotomy, removal of submacular CNV and blood, and rotation of the retina with reattachment *(110)*. Recent studies have shown some success with MT360 *(111–113)*, but no controlled randomized studies have been performed. Macular translocation procedures have many reported complications including retinal detachment, proliferative vitreoretinopathy, macular hole, epiretinal membrane, strabismus, subretinal perfluorocarbon, choroidal hemorrhage, and hypotony. MT360 inevitably causes cyclovertical strabismus, necessitating additional surgery on the extraocular muscles, whereas LMT may be less likely to yield this problem *(114)*. Various procedures have been attempted to address the problem of massive subretinal hemorrhage in CNV in AMD. Pneumatic displacement with or without tissue plasminogen activator (tPA), and submacular surgery with or without tPA have all been attempted with varying results *(115)*.

Low-vision aids and consultation are critical elements in the total vision care of a patient with visual disability from AMD. AMD patients report higher rates of depression and poorer quality of life than an age-matched population *(116–118)*. Low-vision therapy consists of a wide array of services including low-vision evaluation, training to maximize residual vision, optical aids, and education. Optical aids such as magnifiers, telescopes, closed-circuit television, and high-contrast household identifiers are a few of the items in the low-vision armamentarium. Low-vision therapy has demonstrated improvement in functional status and quality of life in patients with low vision from AMD *(119)*.

FUTURE TREATMENTS

As scientists continue the search for new and better treatments for CNV in AMD, several new developments hold promise, and may one day become viable treatment options for patients with this blinding disease. Pigment epithelium-derived factor (PEDF) is an endogenous molecule involved in angiogenesis *(120,121)*. Although it is generally accepted that PEDF is an anti-VEGF molecule, there remains some controversy as to the precise role this molecule plays in CNV in AMD *(122–125)*. Preliminary phase I data using PEDF gene vector therapy were recently presented *(126)*, and this modality may be safe in humans.

Directly replacing diseased tissue is also an extremely active area of current research. Some researchers have been successful in transplanting autologous RPE in humans, but visual results have been in large part unimpressive *(127,128)*. Stem cell transplantation is in early stages, but may hold great potential *(129,130)*. Retinal prosthetic devices with incident light-induced electronic stimulation have become a reality in recent years *(131)*. Visual function has been demonstrated in humans using subretinal implants *(132)* and epiretinal implants *(133,134)*. Although most of the studied patients have been blind from retinitis pigmentosa, the prosthesis has also been used and visual function demonstrated in patients with advanced AMD *(134)*.

SUMMARY

AMD is a significant public health problem and the leading cause of legal blindness in the industrialized world. Dry AMD is the most common form, but neovascular AMD is the most debilitating type, as subretinal bleeding and scarring can lead to catastrophic rapid visual loss. AMD may progress to advanced forms such as geographic atrophy or neovascular AMD, and studies have demonstrated specific risk factors such as smoking, diet, heredity, and type and size of drusen to be predictive of such progression. Diagnosis is based on clinical exam and angiographic testing. FA and ICG provide important information as to the type and extent of retinal lesions, and OCT may be a valuable tool for follow-up. It is important to differentiate AMD with CNV from similar diseases such as RAP or PCV, as treatment, prognosis, and follow-up differ. Intense research regarding treatment and prevention of AMD has provided antioxidants, zinc, laser, PDT, intravitreal and periocular injections of angiostatic agents, and surgery as possible options for treatment of AMD. There are promising preliminary data regarding gene therapy, retinal prosthetic devices, and retinal tissue transplants. The search continues for better treatments for this debilitating disease.

REFERENCES

1. Klein R, Klein BE, Jensen SC, Meuer SM. The five-year incidence and progression of age-related maculopathy: the Beaver Dam Eye Study. Ophthalmology 1997;104:7–21.
2. Klein R, Klein BE, Linton KL. Prevalence of age-related maculopathy: the Beaver Dam Eye Study. Ophthalmology 1992;99:933–943.
3. Bird AC, Bressler NM, Bressler SB, et al. An international classification and grading system for age-related maculopathy and age-related macular degeneration. Surv Ophthalmol 1995;39:367–374.
4. Leibowitz HM, Krueger DE, Maunder LU, et al. The Framingham Eye Study Monograph: VI. Macular degeneration. Surv Ophthalmol 1980;24:428–457.
5. Hyman LG, Lilienfeld AM, Ferris FL, Fine SL. Senile macular degeneration: a case control study. Am J Epidemiol 1983;118:213–227.
6. Ferris FL, Fine SL, Hyman L. Age-related macular degeneration and blindness due to neovascular maculopathy. Arch Ophthalmol 1984;102:1640–1642.
7. Macular Photocoagulation Study Group. Laser photocoagulation of subfoveal neovascular lesions in age-related macular degeneration. Results of a randomized clinical trial. Macular Photocoagulation Study Group. Arch Ophthalmol 1991;109:1220–1231.

8. Macular Photocoagulation Study Group. Laser photocoagulation of subfoveal neovascular lesions of age-related macular degeneration. Updated findings from two clinical trials. Macular Photocoagulation Study Group. Arch Ophthalmol 1993;111:1200–1209.
9. Vingerling JR, Hofman A, Grobbee DE, de Jong PT. Age-related macular degeneration and smoking: the Rotterdam Study. Arch Ophthalmol 1996;114:1193–1196.
10. Paetkau ME, Boyd TA, Grace M, Bach-Mills J, Winshop B. Senile disciform macular degeneration and smoking. Can J Ophthalmol 1978;13:67–71.
11. Seddon JM, Willett WC, Speizer FE, Hankinson SE. A prospective study of cigarette smoking and age-related macular degeneration in women. JAMA 1996;276:1141–1146.
12. Christen WG, Glynn RJ, Manson JE, Ajani UA, Buring JE. A prospective study of cigarette smoking and risk of age-related macular degeneration in men. JAMA 1996;276:1147–1151.
13. Mitchell P, Wang JJ, Smith W, Leeder SR. Smoking and the 5-year incidence of age-related maculopathy: the Blue Mountains Eye Study. Arch Ophthalmol 2002;120:1357–1363.
14. Klein R, Klein BE, Tomany SC, Moss SE. Ten-year incidence of age-related maculopathy and smoking and drinking: the Beaver Dam Eye Study. Am J Epidemiol 2002;156:589–598.
15. Klein R, Klein BE, Tomany SC, Cruickshanks KJ. The association of cardiovascular disease with the long-term incidence of age-related maculopathy: the Beaver Dam Eye study. Ophthalmology 2003;110:1273–1280.
16. Snow KK, Seddon JM. Do age-related macular degeneration and cardiovascular disease share common antecedents? Ophthalmic Epidemiol 1999:6:125–143.
17. Seddon JM, Cote J, Rosner B. Progression of age-related macular degeneration: association with dietary fat, transunsaturated fat, nuts, and fish intake. Arch Ophthalmol 2003;121: 1728–1737.
18. Cho E, Seddon JM, Rosner B, Willett WC. Hankinson SE. Prospective study of intake of fruits, vegetables, vitamins, and carotenoids and risk of age-related maculopathy. Arch Ophthalmol 2004;122:883–892.
19. Chew EY. Age-Related Eye Disease Study Research Group. Micronutrient supplementation. Presented at AAO meeting, Subspecialty Day, New Orleans, 2004.
20. The AREDS Research Group. A randomized, placebocontrolled, clinical trial of high-dose supplementation with vitamins C and E, beta carotene, and zinc for age-related macular degeneration and vision loss—AREDS Report No 8. Arch Ophthalmol 2001;119:1417–1436.
21. Heiba IM, Elston RC, Klein BE, Klein R. Sibling correlations and segregation analysis of age-related maculopathy: the Beaver Dam Eye Study. Genet Epidemiol 1994;11:51–67.
22. Seddon JM, Ajani UA, Mitchell BD. Familial aggregation of age-related maculopathy. Am J Ophthalmol 1997;123:199–206.
23. Klaver CCW, Wolfs RCW, Assink JJM, et al. Genetic risk of age related maculopathy. Population-based Familial Aggregation Study. Arch Ophthalmol 1998;116:1646–1651.
24. Klein M, Maudlin W, Stoumbos V. Heredity and age-related macular degeneration: observations in monozygotic twins. Arch Ophthalmol 1994;112:932–937.
25. Meyers S, Green T, Gutman F. A twin study of age-related macular degeneration. Am J Ophthalmol 1995;120:757–766.
26. Seddon J, Samelson I, Page W, Neale M. Twin study of macular degeneration: methodology and application to genetic epidemiology studies. Invest Ophthalmol Vis Sci 1997;38:S676.
27. Tuo J, Bojanowski CM, Chan CC. Genetic factors of age-related macular degeneration. Prog Retinal Eye Res 2004;23:229–249.
28. Abecasis GR, Yashar BM, Zhao Y, et al. Age-related macular degeneration: a high-resolution genome scan for susceptibility loci in a population enriched for late-stage disease. Am J Hum Genet 2004;74:482–494.
29. Green WR, Enger C. Age-related macular degeneration histopathologic studies: the 1992 Lorenz E. Zimmerman Lecture. Ophthalmology 1993;100:1519–1535.

30. Bressler NM, Silva JC, Bressler SB, et al. Clinicopathologic correlation of drusen and retinal pigment epithelial abnormalities in age-related macular degeneration. Retina 1994;14:130–142.
31. Sarks SH. Aging and degeneration in the macular region: a clinicopathological study. Br J Ophthalmol 1976;60:324–341.
32. Green WR, Key SN. Senile macular degeneration: a histopathologic study. Trans Am Ophthalmol Soc 1977;75:180–254.
33. Zarbin MA. Current concepts in the pathogenesis of age-related macular degeneration. Arch Ophthalmol 2004;122:598–614.
34. Lopez PF, Sippy BD, Lambert HM, Thach AB, Hinton DR. Transdifferentiated retinal pigment epithelial cells are immunoreactive for vascular endothelial growth factor in surgically excised age-related macular degeneration–related choroidal neovascular membranes. Invest Ophthalmol Vis Sci 1996;37:855–868.
35. Frank RN. Growth factors in age-related macular degeneration: pathogenic therapeutic implications. Ophthalmic Res 1997;29:341–353.
36. Kvanta A, Algvere P, Berglin L, Seregard S. Subfoveal fibrovascular membranes in age-related macular degeneration express vascular endothelial growth factor. Invest Ophthalmol Vis Sci 1996;37:1929–1934.
37. Ernst E, Hammerschmidt DE, Bagge U, Matrai A, Dormandy JA. Leukocytes and the risk of ischemic diseases. JAMA 1987;257:2318–2324.
38. Hageman GS, Luthert PJ, Chong NHV, et al. An integrated hypothesis that considers drusen as biomarkers of immune-mediated processes at the RPE-Bruch's membrane interface in aging and age-related macular degeneration. Prog Ret Eye Res 2001;20:705–732.
39. Oh H, Takagi H, Takagi C, et al. The potential angiogenic role of macrophages in the formation of choroidal neovascular membranes. Invest Ophthalmol Vis Sci 1999;40:1891–1898.
40. Abdelsalam A, Del Priore L, Zarbin MA. Drusen in age-related macular degeneration: pathogenesis, natural course, and laser photocoagulation-induced regression. Surv Ophthalmol 1999;44:1–29.
41. Klein R, Klein BEK, Jensen SC, Meuer SM. The 5-year incidence and progression of age-related maculopathy: the Beaver Dam Eye Study. Ophthalmology 1997;104:7–21.
42. Bressler SB, Maguire MG, Bressler NM, Fine SL. The Macular Photocoagulation Study Group: relationship of drusen and abnormalities of the retinal pigment epithelium to the prognosis of neovascular macular degeneration. Arch Ophthalmol 1990;108:1442–1447.
43. Maguire MG, Bressler SB, Bressler NM, et al. for the Macular Photocoagulation Study Group. Risk factors for choroidal neovascularization in the second eye of patients with juxtafoveal or subfoveal choroidal neovascularization secondary to age-related macular degeneration. Arch Ophthalmol 1997;115:741–747.
44. Yannuzzi LA, Negrao S, Iida T, et al. Retinal angiomatous proliferation in agerelated macular degeneration. Retina 2001;21:416–434.
45. Borrillo JL, Sivalingam A, Martidis A, et al. Surgical ablation of retinal angiomatous proliferation. Arch Ophthalmol 2003;121:558–561.
46. Lafaut BA, Aisenbrey S, van den Broecke C. Polypoidal choroidal vasculopathy pattern in age-related macular degeneration. Retina 2000;20:650–654.
47. Okubo A, Sameshima M, Uemara A. Clinicopathological correlation of polypoidal choroidal vasculopathy revealed by ultrastructural study. Br J Ophthalmol 2002;86:1093–1098.
48. Ciardella AP, Donsoff IM, Huang SJ, Costa DL, Yannuzzi LA. Polypoidal choroidal vasculopathy. Surv Ophthalmol 2004;49:25–37.
49. Spaide RF, Yannuzzi LA, Slakter JS. Indocyanine green videoangiography of idiopathic polypoidal choroidal vasculopathy. Retina 1995;15:100–110.
50. Bressler SB, Rosberger DF. Nonneovascular (nonexudative) age-related macular degeneration. In: Guyer DR, Yannuzzi LA, Chang S, Shields JA, Green WR, eds. Retina-Vitreous-Macula Vol 1. W.B. Saunders Co., Philadelphia: 1999;79–93.

51. Duker JS. OCT, fourth generation and beyond. Presented at AAO meeting, Subspecialty Day, New Orleans, 2004.
52. Hee MR, Izatt JA, Swanson EA, et al. Optical coherence tomography of the human retina. Arch Ophthalmol 1995;113:325–332.
53. Chauhan DS, Marshall J. The interpretation of optical coherence tomography images of the retina. Invest Ophthalmol Vis Sci 1999;40:2332–2342.
54. Hee MR, Baumal CR, Puliafito CA, et al. Optical coherence tomography of age related macular degeneration and choroidal neovascularization. Ophthalmology 1996;103: 1260–1270.
55. Costa RA, Farah ME, Cardillo JA, Belfort R Jr. Photodynamic therapy with indocyanine green for occult subfoveal choroidal neovascularization caused by age-related macular degeneration. Curr Eye Res 2001;23:271–275.
56. Rogers AH, Martidis A, Greenberg PB, Puliafito CA. Optical coherence tomography findings following photodynamic therapy of choroidal neovascularization. Am J Ophthalmol 2002;134:566–576.
57. The Alpha-Tocopherol, Beta Carotene Cancer Prevention Study Group. The effect of vitamin E and beta carotene on the incidence of lung cancer and other cancers in male smokers. N Engl J Med 1994;330:1029–1035.
58. Omenn GS, Goodman GE, Thornquist M, et al. Effects of combination of beta-carotene and vitamin A on lung cancer and cardiovascular disease. N Engl J Med 1996;334:1150–1155.
59. Ho AC, Maguire MG, Yoken J, et al. Laser-induced drusen reduction improves visual function at 1 year. Ophthalmology 1999;106:1367–1374.
60. Olk RJ, Friberg TR, Stickney KL, et al. Therapeutic benefits of infrared (810-nm) diode laser macular grid photocoagulation in prophylactic treatment of nonexudative age-related macular degeneration: two-year results of a randomized pilot study. Ophthalmology 1999;106:2082–2090.
61. Rodanant N, Friberg TR, Cheng L, et al. Predictors of drusen reduction after subthreshold infrared (810 nm) diode laser macular grid photocoagulation for nonexudative age-related macular degeneration. Am J Ophthalmol 2002;134:577–585.
62. Green WR. Clinicopathologic studies of treated choroidal neovascular membranes. A review and report of two cases. Retina 1991;11:328–356.
63. Miller H, Miller B, Ryan SJ. Correlation of choroidal subretinal neovascularization with fluorescein angiography. Am J Ophthalmol 1985;99:263–271.
64. Miller H, Miller B, Ryan SJ. Newly formed subretinal vessels. Fine structure and fluorescein leakage. Invest Ophthalmol Vis Sci 1986;27:204–213.
65. Miller H, Miller B, Ryan SJ. The role of the retinal pigment epithelium in the involution of subretinal neovascularization. Invest Ophthalmol Vis Sci 1986;27:1644–1652.
66. Thach AB, Sipperley JO, Dugel PU, et al. Large-spot size transpupillary thermotherapy for the treatment of occult choroidal neovascularization associated with age-related macular degeneration. Arch Ophthalmol 2003;121:817–820.
67. Algvere PV, Libert C, Lindgarde G, et al. Transpupillary thermotherapy of predominantly occult choroidal neovascularization in age-related macular degeneration with 12 months follow-up. Acta Ophthalmol Scand 2003;81:110–117.
68. Reichel E. Transpupillary Thermotherapy. The TTT4CNV Clinical Trial. Presented at AAO meeting, Subspecialty Day, New Orleans, 2004.
69. Treatment of Age-related Macular Degeneration with Photodynamic Therapy (TAP) Study Group. Photodynamic therapy of subfoveal choroidal neovascularization in age-related macular degeneration with verteporfin: two-year results of 2 randomized clinical trials—TAP report no. 2. Arch Ophthalmol 2001;119:198–207.
70. Verteporfin in Photodynamic Therapy (VIP) Study Group. Verteporfin therapy of subfoveal choroidal neovascularization in age-related macular degeneration: two-year results of a

randomized clinical trial including lesions with occult with no classic choroidal neovascularization—Verteporfin in Photodynamic Therapy report 2. Am J Ophthalmol 2001;131: 541–560.
71. Blinder KJ, Bradley S, Bressler NM, et al. Effect of lesion size, visual acuity, and lesion composition on visual acuity change with and without verteporfin therapy for choroidal neovascularization secondary to age-related macular degeneration: TAP and VIP report no. 1. Am J Ophthalmol 2003;136:407–418.
72. Richter AM, Waterfield E, Jain AK, et al. In vitro evaluation of phototoxic properties of four structurally related benzonamic porphyrin derivatives. Photochem Photobiol 1990;52:495–500.
73. Aveline B, Hasan T, Redmond RW. Photophysical and photo-sensitizing properties of benzoporphyrin derivative monoacid ring A (BPD-MA). Photochem Photobiol 1994;59: 328–335.
74. Richter AM, Waterfield E, Jain AK, et al. Photosensitising potency of structural analogues of benzoporphyrin derivative (BPD) in a mouse tumour model. Br J Cancer 1991;63:87–93.
75. Allison BA, Pritchard PH, Levy JG. Evidence for low-density lipoprotein receptor-mediated uptake of benzoporphyrin derivative. Br J Cancer 1994;69:833–839.
76. Schmidt-Erfurth U, Hasan T, Schomacker K, et al. In vivo uptake of liposomal benzoporphyrin derivative and photothrombosis in experimental corneal neovascularization. Lasers Surg Med 1995;17:178–188.
77. Michels S, Schmidt-Erfurth U. Sequence of early vascular events after photodynamic therapy. Invest Ophthalmol Vis Sci 2003;44:2147–2154.
78. Schnurrbusch UE, Welt K, Horn L-C, et al. Histological findings of surgically excised choroidal neovascular membranes after photodynamic therapy. Br J Ophthalmol 2001; 85:1086–1091.
79. Ghazi NG, Jabbour NM, De La Cruz ZC, et al. Clinicopathologic studies of age-related macular degeneration with classic subfoveal choroidal neovascularization treated with photodynamic therapy. Retina 2001;21:478–486.
80. Schmidt-Erfurth U, Laqua H, Schlotzer-Schrehard U, et al. Histopathological changes following photodynamic therapy in human eyes. Arch Ophthalmol 2002;120:835–844.
81. Schlötzer-Schrehardt U, Viestenz A, Naumann GOH, et al. Dose-related structural effects of photodynamic therapy on choroidal and retinal structures of human eyes. Graefes Arch Clin Exp Ophthalmol 2002;240:748–757.
82. Schmidt-Erfurth U, Miller J, Sickenberg M, et al. Photodynamic therapy of subfoveal choroidal neovascularization: clinical and angiographic examples. Graefes Arch Clin Exp Ophthalmol 1998;236:365–374.
83. Miller JW, Schmidt-Erfurth U, Sickenberg M, et al. Photodynamic therapy with verteporfin for choroidal neovascularization by age-related macular degeneration: results of a single treatment in a phase I and 2 study. Arch Ophthalmol 1999;117:1161–1173.
84. Chen JC, Marinier JA, Kergoat H, et al. Choroidal blood flow in verteporfin treatment of age related macular degeneration. Invest Ophthalmol Vis Sci 2002;43:E586.
85. Sternberg P, Lewis H. Photodynamic therapy for age-related macular degeneration: a candid appraisal. Am J Ophthalmol 2004;137:483–485.
86. Gillies MC, Simpson JM, Luo W, et al. A randomized clinical trial of a single dose of intravitreal triamcinolone acetonide for neovascular age-related macular degeneration: one-year results. Arch Ophthalmol 2003;121:667–673.
87. Jonas JB, Kreissig I, Hugger P, et al. Intravitreal triamcinolone acetonide for exudative age related macular degeneration. Br J Ophthalmol 2003,87:462–468.
88. Spaide RF, Sorenson J, Maranan L. Combined photodynamic therapy with verteporfin and intravitreal triamcinolone acetonide for choroidal neovascularization. Ophthalmology 2003;110:1517–1525.

89. The Anecortave Acetate Clinical Study Group. Anecortave acetate as monotherapy for treatment of subfoveal neovascularization in age-related macular degeneration: twelve-month clinical outcomes. Ophthalmology 2003;110:2372–2383.
90. Penfold PL, Wen L, Madigan MC, et al. Triamcinolone acetonide modulates permeability and intercellular adhesion molecule-1 (ICAM-1) expression of the ECV304 cell line: implications for macular degeneration. Clin Exp Immunol 2000;121:458–465.
91. Kvanta A, Algvere PV, Berglin L, et al. Subfoveal fibrovascular membranes in age-related macular degeneration express vascular endothelial growth factor. Invest Ophthalmol Vis Sci 1996;37:1929–1934.
92. Reddy VM, Zamore RL, Kaplan HJ. Distribution of growth factors in subfoveal fibrovascular membranes in age-related macular degeneration and presumed ocular histoplasmosis syndrome. Am J Ophthalmol 1995;120:291–301.
93. Amin R, Puklin JE, Frank RN. Growth factor localization in choroidal neovascular membranes of age-related macular degeneration. Invest Ophthalmol Vis Sci 1994;35:3178–3188.
94. Lopez PF, Sippy BD, Lamber HM, et al. Transdifferentiated retinal pigment epithelial cells are immunoreactive for vascular endothelial growth factor in surgically excised age-related macular degeneration-related choroidal neovascular membranes. Invest Ophthalmol Vis Sci 1996;37:855–868.
95. Yi X, Ogata N, Komada M, et al. Vascular endothelial growth factor expression in choroidal neovascularization in rats. Graefes Arch Clin Exp Ophthalmol 1997;235:313–319.
96. Wada M, Ogata N, Otsuji T, et al. Expression of vascular endothelial growth factor and its receptor (KDR/flk-1) mRNA in experimental choroidal neovascularization. Curr Eye Res 1999;18:201–213.
97. Ogata N, Yamamoto C, Miyashiro M, et al. Expression of transforming growth factor-b mRNA in experimental choroidal neovascularizarion. Curr Eye Res 1997;16:9–18.
98. Amin RH, Frank RN, Eliot D, et al. Vascular endothelial growth factor (VEGF) and basic fibroblast growth factor (bFGF) immunoreactivity in human choroidal neovascular membranes. Invest Opthalmol Vis Sci 1995;36:S2565.
99. Ogata N, Matsushima M, Takada Y, et al. Expression of basic fibroblast growth factor mRNA in developing choroidal neovascularization. Curr Eye Res 1996;15:1008–1018.
100. Matsushima M, Ogata N, Takada Y, et al. Expression of fibroblast growth factor receptor 1 in experimental choroidal neovascularization with in situ hybridization. Jpn J Ophthalmol 1996;40:329–338.
101. Frank RN, Amin RH, Eliott D, et al. Basic fibroblast growth factor and vascular endothelial growth factor are present in epiretinal and choroidal neovascular membranes. Am J Ophthalmol 1996;122:393–403.
102. Heier JS. Anti-VEGF: Genentech–Ranibizumab. Presented at AAO meeting, Subspecialty Day, New Orleans, 2004.
103. Schwartz SD. Anti-VEGF: Eyetech–Macugen. Presented at AAO meeting, Subspecialty Day, New Orleans, 2004.
104. Submacular Surgery Trials (SST) Research Group. Surgery for subfoveal choroidal neovascularization in age-related macular degeneration: ophthalmic findings. SST Report No. 11. Ophthalmology 2004;111:1967–1980.
105. Submacular Surgery Trials (SST) Research Group. Surgery for Hemorrhagic choroidal neovascular lesions of age-related macular degeneraton: ophthalmic findings. SST Report No. 13. Ophthalmology 2004;111:1993–2006.
106. de Juan E Jr, Loewenstein A, Bressler NM, Alexander J. Translocation of the retina for management of subfoveal choroidal neovascularization, II: a preliminary report in humans. Am J Ophthalmol 1998;125:635–646.
107. Fujii GY, de Juan E Jr, Pieramici DJ, et al. Inferior limited macular translocation for subfoveal choroidal neovascularization secondary to age-related macular degeneration: 1-year visual outcome and recurrence report. Am J Ophthalmol 2002;134:69–74.

108. Pawlak D, Glacet-Bernard A, Papp M, Roquet W, Coscas G, Soubrane G. Limited macular translocation compared with photodynamic therapy in the management of subfoveal choroidal neovascularization in age-related macular degeneration. Am Ophthalmol 2004;137:880–887.
109. Fujii GY, de Juan E Jr, Humayun MS, Chang TS. Limited macular translocation for the management of subfoveal choroidal neovascularization after photodynamic therapy. Am J Ophthalmol 2003;135:109–112.
110. Machemer R, Steinhorst UH. Retinal separation, retinotomy, and macular relocation: II. A surgical approach for age-related macular degeneration. Graefes Arch Clin Exp Ophthalmol 1993;231:635–641.
111. Lai JC, Lapolice DJ, Stinnett SS, et al. Visual outcomes following macular translocation with 360-degree peripheral retinectomy. Arch Ophthalmol 2002,120:1317–1324.
112. Park CH, Toth CA. Macular translocation surgery with 360-degree peripheral retinectomy following ocular photodynamic therapy of choroidal neovascularization. Am J Ophthalmol 2003;136:830–835.
113. Aisenbrey S, Lafaut BA, Szurman P, et al. Macular translocation with 360 degrees retinotomy for exudative age-related macular degeneration. Arch Ophthalmol 2002;120: 451–459.
114. Ohtsuki H, Shiraga F, Morizane Y, Furuse T, Takasu I, Hasebe S. Transposition of the anterior superior oblique insertion as a treatment for excyclotorsion induced from limited macular translocation. Am Ophthalmol 2004;137:125–134.
115. Tennant MT, Borrillo JL, Regillo CD. Management of submacular hemorrhage. Ophthalmol Clin N Am 2002;15:445–452.
116. Brody BL, Gamst AC, Williams RA, et al. Depression, visual acuity, comorbidity, and disability associated with age-related macular degeneration. Ophthalmology 2001;108: 1893–1901.
117. Williams RA, Brody BL, Thomas RG, et al. The psychosocial impact of macular degeneration. Arch Ophthalmol 1998;116:514–520.
118. Rovner B, Casten R. Neuroticism predicts depression and disability in age-related macular degeneration. J Am Geriat Soc 2001;49:1097–1100.
119. Scott IU, Smiddy WE, Schiffman J, Feuer WJ, Pappas CJ. Quality of life of low-vision patients and the impact of low-vision services. Am Ophthalmol 1999;128:54–62.
120. Barnstable CJ, Tombran-Tink J. Neuroprotective and antiangiogenic actions of PEDF in the eye: molecular targets and therapeutic potential. Prog Retin Eye Res 2004;23:561–577.
121. Tombran-Tink J, Lara N, Apricio SE, et al. Retinoic acid and dexamethasone regulate the expression of PEDF in retinal and endothelial cells. Exper Eye Res 2004;78:945–955.
122. Matsuoka M, Ogata N, Otsuji T, Nishimura T, Takahashi K, Matsumura M. Expression of pigment epithelium derived factor and vascular endothelial growth factor in choroidal neovascular membranes and polypoidal choroidal vasculopathy. Br J Ophthalmol 2004;88:809–815.
123. Duh EJ, Yang HS, Haller JA, et al. Vitreous levels of pigment epithelium-derived factor and vascular endothelial growth factor: implications for ocular angiogenesis. Am J Ophthalmol 2004;137:668–674.
124. Ogata N, Wada M, Otsuji T, Jo N, Tombran-Tink J, Matsumura M. Expression of pigment epithelium-derived factor in normal adult rat eye and experimental choroidal neovascularization. Invest Ophthalmol Vis Sci 2002;43:1168–1175.
125. Ohno-Matsui K, Morita I, Tombran-Tink J, et al. Novel mechanism for age-related macular degeneration: an equilibrium shift between the angiogenesis factors VEGF and PEDF. Cell Physiol 2001;189:323–333.
126. Holz ER. AdPEDF.I ID Gene vector therapy (GenVec) for AMD, AdPEDF therapy for subfoveal choroidal neovascularization: preliminary phase I results. Presented at AAO meeting, Subspecialty Day, New Orleans, 2004.

127. Del Priore LV, Kaplan HJ, Tezel TH, Hayashi N, Berger AS, Green WR. Retinal pigment epithelial cell transplantation after subfoveal membranectomy in age-related macular degeneration: clinicopathologic correlation. Am J Ophthalmol 2001;131:472–480.
128. Binder S, Stolba U, Krebs I, et al. Transplantation of autologous retinal pigment epithelium in eyes with foveal neovascularization resulting from age-related macular degeneration: a pilot study. Am J Ophthalmol 2002;133:215–225.
129. Schraermeyer U, Thumann G, Luther T, et al. Subretinally transplanted embryonic stem cells rescue photoreceptor cells from degeneration in the RCS rats. Cell Transplant 2001;10:673–680.
130. Caballero S, Sengupta N, Crafoord S, et al. The many possible roles of stem cells in age-related macular degeneration. Graefes Arch Clin Exper Ophthalmol 2004;242:85–90.
131. Margalit E, Maia M, Weiland JD, et al. Retinal prosthesis for the blind. Surv Ophthalmol 2002;47:335–356.
132. Chow AY, Chow VY, Packo KH, Pollack JS, Peyman GA, Schuchard R. The artificial silicon retina microchip for the treatment of vision loss from retinitis pigmentosa. Arch Ophthalmol 2004;122:460–469.
133. Humayun MS, Weiland JD, Fujii GY, et al. Visual perception in a blind subject with a chronic microelectronic retinal prosthesis. Vis Res 2003;43:2573–2581.
134. Humayun MS, de Juan E Jr. Artificial vision. Eye 1998;12:605–607.

2
Endogenous Angiogenic Inhibitors in Diabetic Retinopathy

Jian-Xing Ma, MD, PhD and **Sarah X. Zhang**, MD

CONTENTS

DIABETIC RETINOPATHY

Introduction

Diabetes mellitus is a metabolic disorder of multiple etiologies characterized by chronic hyperglycemia with disturbances of carbohydrate, fat, and protein metabolism resulting from defects in insulin secretion (type 1), insulin action (type 2), or both. Diabetes is a devastating disease as it causes long-term damage, dysfunction, and failure of various organs, such as the eye, kidney, brain, and peripheral nerves. Among these systemic complications, diabetic retinopathy (DR) is one of the most troublesome problems as it is a major cause of blindness. Almost 100% of type 1 diabetic patients and more than 60% of type 2 diabetic patients develop DR during the first two decades of diabetes *(1)*. Great efforts have been made in the past decades to prevent or delay the onset of DR, as well as to prevent vision loss in diabetic patients. Intensive glycemic and blood pressure control, as established by the Diabetes Control and Complications Trial (DCCT) and the Early Treatment Diabetic Retinopathy Study (ETDRS), can decrease the incidence and delay the progression of DR *(2–7)*. Timely laser photocoagulation therapy can prevent the vision loss in a large proportion of patients with severe DR *(8–12)*. However, laser therapy is associated with common adverse effects and high costs. Currently, there is no effective drug treatment for DR and thus, DR remains a leading cause of blindness in the industrialized countries.

There are two common pathological features in DR responsible for vision loss in diabetic patients: diabetic macular edema (DME) and retinal neovascularization (NV). The exact mechanisms underlying the pathogenesis of these changes in DR are largely

From: *Ophthalmology: Ocular Angiogenesis: Diseases, Mechanisms, and Therapeutics*
Edited by: J. Tombran-Tink and C. J. Barnstable © Humana Press Inc., Totowa, NJ

unclear. Accumulating evidence has shown that increases of angiogenic stimulators (e.g., vascular endothelial growth factor [VEGF]) and decreases of angiogenic inhibitors (e.g., pigment epithelium-derived factor [PEDF]) under diabetic milieu lead to a disturbed balance of angiogenesis regulation and subsequently result in DME and retinal NV *(13–19)*. In recent years, a number of endogenous angiogenic inhibitors have been identified *(19–27)*. Some of these inhibitors have been implicated in the pathogenesis of DR *(14,17,18,28,29)*. This chapter will review the recent progress in the research of DR, with a focus on the association of endogenous angiogenic inhibitors with DR and their therapeutic potential in the treatment of DME and retinal NV.

Epidemiology

Diabetes is a common disease in the developed countries and is becoming a major problem throughout the world. The latest WHO Global Burden of Disease estimates the worldwide burden of diabetes in adults was around 173 million in the year 2002 *(30)*. The incidence of diabetes has risen dramatically in the past decades, and a twofold or more increase is expected to occur in the next decades *(30)*. The rising prevalence of diabetes causes a consequent increase of long-term diabetic complications, such as retinopathy, nephropathy, and neuropathy, which set considerable impacts on both the patients and society.

According to the American Diabetes Association (ADA) report, DR is the most frequent cause of blindness in American working-age populations (20–70 yr), with 12,000 to 24,000 diabetics losing their sight each year as a result of DR *(31)*. According to the Eye Diseases Prevalence Research Group, the estimated crude prevalence rates for retinopathy and vision-threatening retinopathy are 40.3% and 8.2%, respectively, in US adult diabetic patients *(32,33)*. The estimated US general population prevalence rates for retinopathy and vision-threatening retinopathy are 3.4% (4.1 million) and 0.75% (899,000) *(32,33)*. Apart from the high prevalence of these complications, their severity presents further problems: 50% of all patients with untreated proliferative retinopathy will lose their sight within 5 yr *(34)*. Moreover, 3.6% of patients with type 1 diabetes, and 1.6% of those with type 2 diabetes, are estimated to be blind *(35)*. With the increasing diabetes rate, DR-related blindness will become more common in the future, unless some breakthrough occurs in basic and clinical diabetic research.

Genetic Factors in DR

Although the development of retinopathy in diabetic patients is largely related to the duration of diabetes, the severity of hyperglycemia, and the existence of hypertension and hyperlipidemia, a high incidence of DR occurs in some patient groups with good systemic conditions, whereas some other individuals remain free of retinopathy inspite of poor glycemic control and long duration of diabetes. Epidemiological study has demonstrated ethnic differences in the prevalence of diabetes and DR. In the United States, African Americans and Hispanics have a higher prevalence of diabetes at approx 25%, compared with 6.2% in the general population *(36–39)*. On average, Hispanic/Latino Americans are 1.9 times more likely to have diabetes than non-Hispanic whites of similar age *(36,37)*. As to the incidence of DR, some small sample size studies have shown that African American individuals are significantly more likely to develop retinopathy than Caucasian American individuals (50% in African Americans vs 19% in Caucasian Americans with type 2 diabetes), and the African American individuals may have higher rates of proliferative diabetic retinopathy *(40)*. In the study of DCCT, familial clustering of severe, vision-threatening forms of DR was observed *(41)*. These data suggest genetic influences are operating in the development and progression of DR as well as in diabetes.

Experimental diabetes studies have also provided evidence supporting the genetic variations in susceptibility to DR. Our group demonstrated that pigmented Brown Norway (BN) rats are more susceptible to hypoxia-induced retinal NV than the albino Sprague-Dawley (SD) rats *(42)*. In the hypoxic retina of BN rats, the level of VEGF, a major angiogenic factor, is significantly increased, whereas the level of PEDF, a potent endogenous angiogenic inhibitor, is substantially decreased, when compared with that in age-matched normal controls. These changes resulted in a significant increase of the VEGF to PEDF ratio. However, these changes are substantially smaller in SD rats after the same treatment. In the streptozotocin (STZ)-induced type 1 diabetes model, diabetic BN rats develop more severe and longer duration of vascular hyperpermeability in the retina, compared with diabetic SD rats with similar hyperglycemic levels (unpublished data). These studies indicate that genetic factors contribute to the different susceptibilities to DR.

A variety of candidate genes have been investigated in diabetic patients as well as in animal models, but few of them have displayed strong associations with DR *(43–47)*. Human lymphocyte antigen (HLA) is one of the earliest genetic factors studied for its association with DR *(45–48)*. However, no consistent result has been obtained so far from large-sized samples of different populations. Recently, HLA-DR7 was reported to be associated with the protection of proliferative retinopathy in type 2 diabetic patients in Mexicans *(49)*. However, another study conducted in Turkey demonstrated that the HLA-DR7 frequency is significantly higher in diabetic patients with proliferative retinopathy than in nonproliferative cases *(50)*. These controversial data suggest that the influence of genetic factors on the development of DR may be complicated, depending on how much influence derives from other risk factors, such as environmental factors and the systemic conditions of the patients examined.

The DR-associated genes identified so far are mainly involved in distinct metabolic and functional pathways known to be affected in diabetes, such as aldose reductase pathway, glucose transporters, cell communication and the extracellular matrix, endothelins, and nitric oxide synthases *(51)*. Different polymorphisms in the same genes can confer either protection against DR or predisposition to the development of DR *(52)*. Recently, two distinct polymorphisms in the genes coding for intracellular adhesion molecule-1 (ICAM-1) and transforming growth factor (TGF)-β have been found as risk factors for retinopathy *(53,54)*. They may be associated with the leukocyte activation and adhesion to the retinal vascular endothelium, which contribute to the development of vascular leakage and capillary closure in DR. However, their genetic effects as risk factors of DR need to be evaluated in large-size α samples. It is also yet to be revealed how the genetic alterations lead to pathological phenotypes of DR.

Pathophysiology and Clinical Features

Prolonged hyperglycemia is the primary and key factor that gives rise to all abnormalities in DR *(55)*. High concentrations of blood glucose lead to changes in cell metabolism, including the polyol pathway activation, diacylglycerol-protein kinase C pathway activation, stimulation of cell oxidative stress, and changes in macromolecule structure and function via the formation of advanced glycation endproducts (AGE) *(55)*. Further, these biochemical changes result in the dysfunction of vascular cells, including the pericytes and vascular endothelial cells. Activated endothelial cells release proangiogenic growth factors and cytokines, which cause cascade changes of other retinal cell types. The impaired antithrombotic function of endothelial cells, the interactions between leukocytes and endothelial cells, the vasoconstriction caused by overproduced endothelin, and the reduced function of vasodilating factors (prostacyclin, nitric oxide) cause the thrombosis and closure of retinal capillaries, resulting in the failure of retinal vascular function and regional hypoxia in the retina.

There are several common pathological changes in DR: the appearance of microaneurysms, increased vascular permeability, capillary occlusion, and retinal NV *(55)*. The earliest histological change in DR is the loss of pericytes. The loss of pericytes and subsequent dilation of capillaries can cause microaneurysm, which is the earliest visible lesion of DR in clinic. Under ophthalmoscopy, microaneurysm appears as a red dot with various diameters from 15 to 60 μm. Although the pathogenesis of microaneurysm is unclear, the increase of microaneurysms has been shown to associate with the progression of retinopathy. The increased vascular permeability resulting from the breakdown of the blood–retinal barrier (BRB) allows the leakage of plasma macromolecules and the fluid into the retina and results in microexudates, infiltrating protein, lipid exudates and most severely, DME. The appearance of DME represents a more advanced stage of DR and can cause significant impairment of central vision.

The occlusion of capillaries often gives rise to focal retinal ischemia and hypoxia. The local hypoxia then induces the overexpression of angiogenic stimulators and decreases the levels of endogenous angiogenic inhibitors in the retina to stimulate new blood vessel formation to improve oxygenation in the retinal tissue. These new vessels cross over both the normal arteries and the normal veins of the retina, showing a sign of their unregulated growth. At advanced stages, new vessels can grow into the vitreous body, resulting in preretinal NV. The abnormal structure of new blood vessels can lead to leakage of plasma proteins and hemorrhage into the retina or vitreous and consequently compromise vision. Some of the new vessels grow with the fibril tissue to form fibrovascular complexes and cause tractional retinal detachment, further exacerbating vision impairment.

Clinically, DR is classified into two stages: nonproliferative DR (NPDR) and proliferative DR (PDR). At the stage of NPDR, the lesions are within the retina and include microaneurysms, small "dot and blot" hemorrhages, "splinter" hemorrhages, intraretinal microvascular abnormalities (IRMAs), and "cotton wool" spots. At the stage of PDR, in addition to the changes in NPDR, NV develops along the surface of the retina or extends into the vitreous cavity.

DME, RETINAL NV, AND VEGF

Breakdown of the Blood–Retinal Barrier and DME

DME can occur at any stage of DR. However, the incidence of DME is closely correlated with the severity of DR. The incidences of DME are 40% and 71% for patients with NPDR and PDR, respectively. As DME directly affects the function of the macula, it often results in significant vision impairment. DME is the single greatest cause of vision loss in diabetic patients *(56–59)*. Approximately 20% of DME patients with type 1 diabetes and 50% of those with type 2 diabetes have visual acuity worse than 20/40. This level of vision loss limits or prevents daily activities such as driving and reading.

Diabetic patients also have significantly higher incidence of cystoid macular edema (CME) secondary to cataract surgery *(60)*. As diabetic patients have increased risks of developing cataract, and many need cataract surgery, CME is a common clinical complication in diabetic patients.

The current treatments for DME are far from satisfactory. Intensive glucose control, as demonstrated by the DCCT, decreased the incidence of DME by 23%, when compared with standard, conventional glucose control *(6,61)*. The ETDRS demonstrated that treatment of DME by focal laser photocoagulation is beneficial for reducing the rate of moderate visual loss by only 50%, and the rate of visual improvement is low *(62,63)*. Furthermore, the laser burns that result from such focal laser treatment in patients treated in the ETDRS have been shown to increase the atrophy of the retinal pigment epithelium (RPE) with the progressive enlargement of the initial focal scars of laser photocoagulation *(10–12,64)*. This may lead to visual loss with central scotomas and a decrease in color vision.

The breakdown of the BRB and subsequent increase in vascular permeability are believed to play a major role in the development of DME. Vascular leakage caused by the breakdown of the BRB is an early and common pathological change in DR and some other ocular disorders *(65–67)*. At early stages of DR, it is found that the increase of retinal vascular permeability precedes the appearance of clinical retinopathy *(68,69)*.

The BRB plays an important role in maintaining normal physiological functions of the retina. The BRB is composed of two spatially distinct barriers limiting the flow of macromolecules and fluid into the retina: the inner barrier is the vascular endothelium, mainly residing at the tight junction between adjacent endothelial cells; the outer barrier is the tight junction between the RPE cells *(60)*. The tight junction between endothelial cells contains an assembly of unique proteins such as occludin, claudins, and zonula occludens (ZO)-1, ZO-2, and ZO-3. The structural interactions between these proteins constitute the tight junctions and limit the fluid flow *(70)*.

Impaired inner BRB has been found to play a major role in the evolution of DME and DR *(71,72)*. In the diabetic animal model, the early BRB breakdown is localized to the retinal venules and capillaries of the superficial retinal vasculature *(73)*. Later, the BRB interruption progresses from the superficial layer to the deep capillary bed *(74)*. The decreased expression, redistribution, and changed phosphorylation of some of the tight junction proteins, such as occludin, can result in disorganization of the tight junction proteins in the vascular endothelium which is considered responsible for the breakdown of the inner BRB *(74–76)*.

Recent studies have shown that unbalanced expression of angiogenic factors and angiogenic inhibitors plays an important role in the development of DME *(77,78)*, and thus represents a new target for pharmacological intervention of DME.

Retinal NV and PDR

Retinal NV is another central feature of DR and a major cause of blindness in diabetic patients. The appearance of NV represents the progression of the disease from NPDR to the advanced stage—PDR. In severe NPDR, the extensive area of capillary closure caused by the dropout of pericytes and the loss of endothelial cells result in local retinal hypoxia, which in turn stimulates the release of angiogenic factors and cause retinal NV to alleviate local ischemia. However, these newly formed blood vessels are malformed with fragile basement membrane, deficient tight junction between endothelial cells, and lack of pericytes. The walls of the new vessels are weak and may break, resulting in hemorrhage into the vitreous and compromised vision.

In the more advanced stages of PDR, the new vessels accompanied by fibrous tissue grow from the anterior retinal surface into the vitreous cavity, forming the fibrovascular membrane, which can pull the retina away from the underlying choroid. This can cause tractional retinal detachment and result in blindness if untreated. In many cases, retinal NV coexists with DME or macular ischemia caused by capillary nonperfusion, leading to more severe condition of vision impairment.

A major obstacle in studying PDR is the lack of ideal animal models. All diabetic rodent models examined so far do not develop typical NV identical to that in PDR patients *(79)*. The STZ-diabetic rat model is a commonly used type 1 diabetes model. This model develops some NPDR features such as pericyte loss, increased retinal vascular permeability, and so on, but does not develop retinal NV, even after long durations of severe hyperglycemia *(80)*. Transgenic mice overexpressing VEGF in the retina have displayed intraretinal NV, but lack preretinal NV *(81,82)*. Galactose-fed dogs can develop some retinal vascular changes similar to human DR, including appearance of microaneurysms and acellular capillary beds associated with nonperfusion areas. Some galactose-fed dogs even develop some PDR-like features, such as appearance of fibrovascular membrane on the retinal surface and on the posterior hyaloid membrane, after several years of galactose diet *(79,83–85)*. However, this model is not practical for the large-scale research, as it is associated with high costs and long experimental durations. Most commonly used model for PDR is oxygen-induced retinopathy (OIR) in newborn rats or mice. This model has also been established in cats and dogs *(86,87)*. Although this is not a diabetic model, the OIR model indeed develops most of the human features of PDR, such as increased vascular permeability, microaneurysm, nonperfusion area, preretinal and intraretinal NV, and hemorrhage. Therefore, OIR is commonly accepted as a model for PDR studies. It is noteworthy that this model has species difference and strain difference in terms of severity of NV and vascular hyperpermeability, even in the same species *(42)*. As mentioned above, BN rats have shown significantly more severe and longer duration of retinal NV and vascular leakage than SD rats after the same high oxygen exposure. Therefore, the strain of rat or mouse used for this model should be brought into the consideration, when results from different groups are compared.

VEGF in DME and Retinal NV

In the past two decades, extensive studies have been conducted to understand the role of growth factors in the development of DR. VEGF, basic fibroblast growth factor (bFGF), insulin-like growth factor (IGF)-1, endothelin (ET), and a number of other angiogenic factors have been implicated in DR *(88–91)*. Among these angiogenic factors, VEGF is believed to play a key role in the development of DME and retinal NV *(71,88,92)*. VEGF is a homodimeric glycoprotein composed of four isoforms resulting from alternative RNA splicing *(93)*. It is a potent angiogenic stimulator with endothelial cell-specific mitogenic activity and plays a crucial role in both normal and pathological angiogenesis *(88,94)*. VEGF is also referred to as vascular permeability factor (VPF), based on its ability to induce vascular hyperpermeability *(94–96)*. It has a potent activity in increasing vascular permeability, with an efficacy 5000-fold higher than that of histamine *(97)*. VEGF is produced by multiple cell types in the retina, including the RPE, pericytes, endothelial cells, glial cells, Müller cells, and ganglion cells *(98–100)*. Among them, Müller cells and RPE are believed to be the major source of VEGF in the retina, and endothelial cells to be the primary target of VEGF *(99,101)*. VEGF exerts its bioactivities through two known VEGF receptors, Flt-1 and Flk-1/KDR, which are expressed predominantly in endothelial cells, and to a lesser extent on monocytes and macrophages *(102,103)*. The binding of VEGF to its receptors initiates a signal transduction cascade mediating vascular permeability and endothelial cell proliferation and migration.

It has become evident from both diabetic patients and diabetic animal models that VEGF levels are increased in the retina with DR. The earlier studies demonstrated that VEGF levels are significantly elevated in the vitreous and the retina from patients with PDR, compared with those with NPDR, and are correlated with the severity of DR *(98,104–108)*. Laser photocoagulation decreased vitreous VEGF levels by 75% in patients with PDR *(109)*, suggesting that the development and regression of retinal NV is closely associated with VEGF levels in the retina. In addition, significantly elevated VEGF levels in the aqueous humor were also reported in diabetic patients with macular edema and correlated with the severity of DME *(108)*.

VEGF overexpression was also confirmed in animal models of DR. In early stages of STZ-diabetic rats, significant increases of retinal VEGF mRNA levels have been found to correlate with retinal vascular permeability *(110)*. This early BRB breakdown can be successfully prevented by VEGF $TrapA_{40}$, a soluble VEGF receptor Flt/F_c chimera *(73)*. These coincided increases of retinal VEGF level and the BRB breakdown were also observed in the relative long-term diabetic animal model *(71)*.

In the OIR model, retinal VEGF levels are significantly elevated, which correlate with the retinal NV progression. The VEGF levels decline to the normal level when the regression of NV occurs *(14)*. The contribution of VEGF to the formation of retinal NV is also supported by observation that intravitreal injection of VEGF successfully induces iris NV in monkey eyes *(111,112)*. Repeated injections of VEGF can cause severe iris NV and neovascular glaucoma, mimicking the condition of neovascular glaucoma that occurs in the very advanced stage of PDR *(111–113)*.

These previous observations all support that overproduction of VEGF is the major cause of DME as well as retinal NV in diabetes *(88–114)*.

ENDOGENOUS ANGIOGENIC INHIBITORS AND THEIR IMPLICATION IN DR

Angiogenesis is normally regulated by two counterbalancing systems: angiogenic stimulators (e.g., VEGF) and angiogenic inhibitors (e.g., PEDF) (Fig. 1). It is the delicate

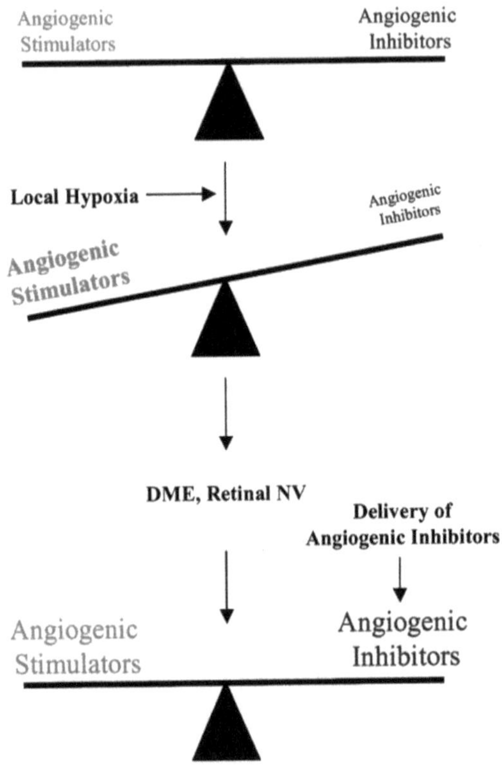

Fig. 1. Significance of the balance between angiogenic stimulators and inhibitors in diabetic retinopathy. Angiogenesis and vascular permeability are normally regulated by the balance between angiogenic stimulators such as vascular endothelial growth factor and angiogenic inhibitors such as pigment epithelium-derived factor. Under diabetic conditions, the retina overproduces angiogenic stimulators and decreases the expression of angiogenic inhibitors. The disturbed balance results in vascular hyperpermeability and diabetic macular edema (DME) and retinal neovascularization (NV). Administration of angiogenic inhibitors can restore the balance and has therapeutic potential in the treatment of diabetic retinopathy. *See* color version on companion CD.

balance between angiogenic stimulators and inhibitors that determine where and when new blood vessels are formed. In the adult retina, the angiogenic inhibitors are predominant in the balance to maintain the quiescent status of retinal vasculature. Our recent studies demonstrate that the disruption of the balance plays an essential role in the development of a variety of neovascular diseases, such as cancer and PDR *(14,115–117)*. In these pathological conditions, the ratio of angiogenic stimulators to inhibitors increases, which breaks the dormancy of angiogenesis and consequently, results in abnormal retinal NV (Fig. 1). Therefore, restoration of the balance by either increase of angiogenic inhibitors or decrease of angiogenic stimulators, or both, should lead to the quiescence of angiogenesis, which may become an important strategy in the prevention and treatment of PDR and other neovascular diseases.

The hypothesis that naturally occurring inhibitors of angiogenesis exist and play important roles in the regulation of angiogenesis was initially proposed by Judah Folkman *(115)*. As early as 1977, evidence has been documented that inhibitors of angiogenesis exist in the vitreous fluid *(119)*. These inhibitors may be responsible for maintaining the avascular status of the vitreous body *(120,121)*. The first endogenous angiogenic inhibitor was isolated in 1994 and named angiostatin, which was later identified in the human vitreous *(25)*. In recent years, nearly 30 angiogenic inhibitors have been identified in a variety of tissues *(20)*. They are classified into five major groups in a recent review *(20)*: (1) endothelial cell specific inhibitors such as angiostatin, endostatin, antithrombin III, plasminogen kringle 5 (K5) and plasminogen kringle 1–5 (K1–5); (2) avascular tissue-derived inhibitors such as kallistatin or kallikrein-binding protein (KBP) and PEDF; (3) antiangiogenic cytokines such as interferon-α, interleukin (IL)-12, interferon-γ, and IL-18; (4) angiogenic factor antagonists, including soluble fibroblast growth factor receptor (FGFR)-1, soluble VEGF receptor (VEGFR)-1 and angiopoietin-2; and (5) the other angiogenic inhibitors such as thrombospondin (TSP)-1, tissue inhibitors of metalloproteinases (TIMPs), maspin, canstatin, and tumstatin *(20)*. Among these inhibitors, 16 have been identified in the eye, and nine of them have been shown as active antiangiogenic factors in the retina, including angiostatin, endostatin, K5, kallistatin, PEDF, interferon-α, interferon-γ, soluble VEGFR-1, and angiopoietin-2.

In contrast to the extensive studies of angiogenic inhibitors in cancer research since 1994, the implication of angiogenic inhibitors in DR was not established until 2001. Our observation that retinal PEDF levels correlate negatively with retinal NV in the OIR model first demonstrated that the VEGF–PEDF ratio in the retina is correlated with the progression of retinal NV *(14)*. Therefore, we proposed that the disturbed balance between angiogenic stimulators and inhibitors is responsible for the development and progression of PDR. Since then, several other angiogenic inhibitors have been implicated in PDR in animal models and in diabetic patients and have displayed therapeutic potential for the treatment of PDR *(122,123)*. Here, we will briefly summarize recent progresses about the implication of angiogenic inhibitors in DR.

Angiostatin

Angiostatin is a proteolytic fragment (kringle 1–4) of plasminogen *(25)*. It exists naturally in significant amounts in the circulation of patients with primary tumors *(20)*. Angiostatin was shown to be a potent angiogenic inhibitor, which blocks NV and suppresses tumor growth and metastases *(25)*. It specifically inhibits proliferation and induces apoptosis in vascular endothelial cells *(124)*. Later evidence has suggested that decreased angiostatin levels in the vitreous may play a role in the development of PDR *(29)*. Moreover, recombinant angiostatin has been shown to block retinal NV in the OIR model *(125)*. Delivery of a recombinant virus expressing angiostatin has been found to suppress laser-induced choroidal neovascularization *(126)*. Systemic and intravitreal injections of angiostatin before the appearance of retinal NV resulted in significantly fewer preretinal vascular cells in the OIR model, suggesting a preventive effect *(127)*. In normal neonatal mice, however, angiostatin does not affect any physiological development of retinal vasculature or the normal development of animals, suggesting no or low toxicities to normal vasculature at the dose and duration of angiostatin administration *(127)*. Recently, we have shown that angiostatin also reduces vascular leakage in the retina of both the OIR and STZ-diabetic rat models, suggesting that decreased angiostatin in the vitreous and retina may also contribute to the development of DME *(128)*.

PEDF

PEDF is a 50-kDa glycoprotein originally identified in conditioned media of cultured fetal human retinal RPE cells by Tombran-Tink and Johnson *(129)*. In 1999, Dawson et al. first reported that PEDF is a potent inhibitor of endothelial cell proliferation and migration, even more potent than the well-studied antiangiogenic factor angiostatin *(19)*. This finding suggests that PEDF is a bifunctional protein and thus has opened a new era for PEDF study.

PEDF is believed to be the major endogenous angiogenic inhibitor in the eye. A number of studies have been documented in the past few years to reveal the role of PEDF in retinal angiogenic diseases. Our group reported that PEDF levels in the retina are significantly decreased in OIR rats, and the decrease is correlated with the progression of retinal NV *(14)*. Laser treatment, which is known as the only effective therapy for retinal NV in PDR, increases the PEDF level in the rat retina and also in cultured RPE cells *(130)*. The PEDF gene knockout results in abnormal vessel density in the retina and prostate *(131)*. The correlation between decreased PEDF levels and DR was later confirmed in human patients *(132,133)*. PEDF levels in the vitreous and aqueous humor have been found significantly lower in patients with PDR than those from nondiabetic eyes *(28,132)*. Furthermore, in diabetic patients with no or very mild retinopathy, the decreased PEDF level in the aqueous humor predicts the progression of DR *(134)*.

The implication of PEDF levels in PDR is also supported by several therapeutic approaches using PEDF. Systemic delivery of a low dose of PEDF successfully inhibited retinal NV in OIR mice by inducing endothelial cell apoptosis *(135)*. Intraocular delivery of PEDF by a viral vector caused regression of retinal NV in VEGF transgenic and OIR mouse models *(136,137)*. Recently, PEDF has also been shown to reduce VEGF-induced vascular leakage, implying its involvement in the regulation of vascular permeability and DME *(138)*. All these studies suggest that PEDF is a crucial inhibitor of retinal NV and DME and has therapeutic potential in the treatment of PDR.

Endostatin

Endostatin is a 20-kDa C-terminal fragment of collagen XVIII, initially purified from conditioned media of murine hemangioendothelioma cells as an angiogenic inhibitor based on its ability to inhibit the proliferation of bovine vascular endothelial cells in vitro and potently inhibit angiogenesis and tumor growth in vivo *(26)*. Although the function of endostatin in the eye and in the retina has not been well studied as that in tumors, solid evidence indicates that endostatin has an important function in the ocular system. Deficient endostatin production in the collagen XVIII gene knockout mouse causes delayed regression of blood vessels in the vitreous and abnormal outgrowth of retinal vessels, suggesting that collagen XVIII/endostatin is important for normal ocular blood vessel formation *(123)*.

Endostatin levels in the vitreous and aqueous humor are decreased in patients with DR and negatively correlated with the severity of retinopathy and the VEGF levels *(122,139)*. Funatsu et al. *(13)* demonstrated that the diabetic patients with low endostatin levels and high VEGF levels in the vitreous have a significantly higher risk of progression of PDR after vitreous surgery than those with high endostatin levels and low VEGF levels. These studies suggest that endostatin may be used as a marker to predict the outcome of surgery treatment in diabetic patients.

Endostatin has also been shown to be a promising antiangiogenic agent in the treatment of ocular neovascularization and DR. Intravenous injection of adenoviral vectors containing sig-mEndo transgene increased the serum level of endostatin and inhibited laser-induced choroidal neovascularization *(140)*. The effect of endostatin on retinal NV was demonstrated by adeno-associated virus (AAV)-mediated delivery of endostatin to the eye in the OIR mouse model *(141)*. Recently, delivery of endostatin into the eyes of VEGF transgenic mice using two different viral systems demonstrated that endostatin not only significantly reduced VEGF-induced retinal vascular hyperpermeability, but also inhibited retinal NV and retinal detachment *(142)*.

K5

K5 is a proteolytic fragment of plasminogen, consisting of 80 amino acids *(143,144)*. Based on in vitro assays, K5 has a more potent antiangiogenic activity than angiostatin *(145)*. Although K5 levels in the retina and vitreous have not been examined in DR patients or animals models, a single intravitreal injection of K5 has been shown to prevent the formation of retinal NV in the OIR rat model *(24)*. Moreover, injection of K5 after the partial formation of retinal NV has been shown to stop the progression of retinal NV *(24)*. However, the injection of K5 does not decrease preexisting preretinal vessels or retinal vasculature in normal retina *(24)*. These results, in consistence with the in vitro studies, suggest that K5 is angiostatic. Recently, we have shown that K5 also reduces vascular leakage in the retina of the OIR and STZ-diabetic models *(146)*. This effect is independent of the K5-induced inhibition of retinal NV. More importantly, the effect of K5 on vascular permeability can be achieved at doses substantially lower than that required for its antiangiogenic activity *(146)*.

Kallistatin

Kallistatin was originally identified from rat serum as a specific inhibitor of tissue kallikrein, a serine proteinase that cleaves kininogen to generate bioactive kinins. Kallistatin is a glycoprotein of 425 amino acids and 58 kDa in the human *(147,148)*. Kallistatin specifically binds to tissue kallikrein, forming a SDS-stable complex *(149,150)*, and thus, is also named KBP. It inhibits kallikrein activity in vitro and in transgenic mice overexpressing kallikrein *(147,151)*.

Kallistatin shares significant sequence homology with other serine proteinase inhibitors (serpins) such as α1-antitrypsin, suggesting that it belongs to the serpin superfamily *(148)*. It also shares significant sequence homology with antithrombin III and PEDF, which are both potent angiogenic inhibitors. Our earlier studies showed that kallistatin levels are significantly reduced in the vitreous from patients with PDR and in the retina of STZ-diabetic rats, suggesting that it is implicated in DR *(152,153)*. Lately, we have shown that kallistatin is a specific inhibitor of endothelial cells and VEGF *(23)*; it inhibits cell proliferation and induces apoptosis in endothelial cells. Moreover, kallistatin inhibits retinal NV and reduces vascular leakage in the retina of the OIR model *(23)*. These vascular activities of kallistatin are independent of its interactions with the kallikrein-kinin system *(23)*. As kallistatin is an angiogenic inhibitor present in the retina and vitreous at high levels, decreased kallistatin levels in the vitreous of patients with PDR may contribute to the development of DME and retinal NV.

Mechanism for Vascular Activity of Angiogenic Inhibitors

In contrast to the significance of these angiogenic inhibitors in DR and their therapeutic potential, little is clear about the mechanisms underlying their vascular activities. Angiostatin is among the most studied angiogenic inhibitors in terms of the mechanism of action. An earlier study reported that angiostatin binds to ATP synthase on the surface of human umbilical vein endothelial cells (HUVEC). This binding was speculated to mediate the inhibitory effect of angiostatin on endothelial cell proliferation and migration *(154)*. However, the ATP synthase-binding mechanism has not been confirmed by other groups. Angiostatin has also been found to inhibit the VEGF- and bFGF-induced activation of the p42/p44 MAP kinase *(155)*. As VEGF- and bFGF-induced angiogenesis is mediated, in part, through the MAP kinase pathway, blocking the activation of MAP kinase has been suggested to be a possible mechanism responsible for the antiangiogenic activity of angiostatin *(156,157)*.

Recent evidence has shown that angiostatin binds to integrins on the surface of endothelial cells. Using blocking antibodies, Tarui and coworkers demonstrated that $\alpha_v\beta_3$ is a predominant receptor for angiostatin on endothelial cells *(158)*. The binding of angiostatin with integrins on the surface of endothelial cells does not induce stress fiber formation, implying that the antiangiogenic activity of angiostatin may be through interfering with the $\alpha_v\beta_3$-mediated signaling in endothelial cells *(158)*. Similarly, endostatin and tumstatin have also been shown to bind to integrins *(159)*. Tumstatin binds with $\alpha_v\beta_3$ integrin in a vitronectin/fibronectin/RGD cyclic peptide-independent manner. This binding may mediate the inhibition of endothelial cells proliferation and induction of apoptosis. Endostatin competes with fibronectin/RGD cyclic peptide for binding with $\alpha_5\beta_3$ integrin, and this interaction with integrin has been suggested to mediate the endostatin-induced inhibition of endothelial cell migration *(159)*.

Recently, interactions between angiogenic stimulators and angiogenic inhibitors have been revealed and may represent a mechanism for the vascular activities of angiogenic inhibitors. Gao and Ma *(117)* demonstrated that K5 downregulates the expression of endogenous VEGF while up-regulating endogenous PEDF in vascular cells and in the retina of OIR rats, suggesting autocrine or paracrine regulations of VEGF and PEDF expression. These regulations can restore the balance between endogenous angiogenic stimulators and angiogenic inhibitors and thus may contribute to the vascular activity of K5. Later, kallistatin and angiostatin were found to block the overexpression of VEGF in the retina under ischemia and diabetic conditions, but do not affect VEGF levels in normal retinas. These angiogenic inhibitor-induced downregulations of VEGF correlate with their antiangiogenic activities *(23,128)*. Although it is not certain how these angiogenic inhibitors regulate VEGF expression, K5 has been shown to block the nuclear translocation of HIF-1α and thus inhibit the activation of HIF-1. Angiostatin has also been shown to diminish the activation of MAP kinase ERK1 and ERK2 in endothelial cells *(155)*. As HIF-1 and MAP kinase are both known to play roles in the regulation of VEGF, the blockade of the HIF-1 and MAP kinase activation may contribute to the K5-induced downregulation of VEGF expression. Recently, K5 was found to bind with voltage-dependent anion channel (VDAC1) on the membrane of endothelial cells and thus, VDAC1 was proposed to serve as the K5 receptor on endothelial cells *(160)*. It is unknown, however, how this receptor mediates the K5-induced regulation of VEGF expression.

In addition, endostatin has been shown to downregulate many other proangiogenic genes and pathways but upregulate many antiangiogenic genes *(161)*. Unlike K5, however, the antiangiogenic activity of endostatin has been shown to be HIF-1-independent. Therefore, it is likely that different angiogenic inhibitors may interact with VEGF via distinct mechanisms.

The interactions between angiogenic inhibitors with angiogenic factors are not limited at the regulation of gene expression. Recent studies have shown that some angiogenic inhibitors also block VEGF signaling. Kim et al. *(162)* showed that endostatin blocks VEGF signaling via direct interactions with VEGF receptor KDR on HUVEC. Binding of endostatin with KDR can block VEGF binding to its receptor and thus block the function of VEGF in endothelial cells. Recently, kallistatin has also been shown to compete with VEGF for binding to its receptors on endothelial cells *(23)*. Under the same conditions, however, K5 does not compete with VEGF for receptor binding. These findings further confirm that different angiogenic inhibitors may have distinct mechanisms of action or molecular targets. Combinations of two or more angiogenic inhibitors with different mechanisms or targets may achieve synergistic effects on vascular leakage and retinal NV.

In summary, our understanding about molecular mechanisms underlying the vascular activities of the angiogenic inhibitors and the regulation of their expression are very limited, compared with those of angiogenic factors such as VEGF signaling. Normal angiogenic regulation and the development of retinal NV are complicated processes and involve multiple, interacting factors.

FUTURE PERSPECTIVE

The disturbed balance between angiogenic stimulators and inhibitors represents a new pathogenic mechanism for DR. Identification of the involvement of angiogenic inhibitors in DR has not only opened a new field for investigation of the pathogenesis of diabetes, but also has revealed a new target for pharmacological interventions. However, there are many unknown features about the implication of angiogenic inhibitors in DR. First, it remains to be investigated how these inhibitors are decreased in DR. Second, their molecular targets and signaling pathways need to be identified. Third, as evidence has shown that there are interactions between different angiogenic inhibitors and between the inhibitors and angiogenic stimulators, it is important to examine these interactions and to study how these interactions are achieved.

The therapeutic approaches using peptide angiogenic inhibitors for the treatment of DR raise both hopes and challenges. Possible therapies using endogenous angiogenic inhibitors for the treatment of DME and retinal NV should offer some advantages over the current treatments. In general, the treatment of DME using angiogenic inhibitors is more promising than the treatment of retinal NV, as the doses required are substantially lower for the DME than that needed for antiangiogenic activity. These approaches may lead to the development of noninvasive, effective, economic, and safe treatments to prevent vision loss from DR.

Despite the encouraging results from animal models, the therapeutic application of these angiogenic inhibitors is still facing many challenges. First, diabetic retinopathy, unlike cancer, requires a local antiangiogenic treatment. The reason is that diabetic patients, although developing abnormal NV in the retina, have common wound-healing problems in peripheral tissues. This can result in foot ulcer, which represents a major challenge in diabetes care. Therefore, systemic administration of angiogenic inhibitors may exacerbate wound-healing problems in diabetic patients. Efficient local drug administration is desirable and needs to be developed. Second, diabetic retinopathy is a chronic disorder and requires a long-term administration of drugs. A sustained, long-term ocular drug delivery system needs to be developed. Third, most of the existing angiogenic inhibitors are large proteins or peptides. Efforts are needed to improve their delivery into the retina and prolong their bioavailability in the retina. Fourth, the costs of production of these large peptides are high. The minimal functional domains responsible for the vascular activities of these inhibitors need to be defined, as the production of small peptides is more economic and less problematic in general.

Taken together, more intensive, multidisciplinary research efforts are needed to reveal the pathogenesis of DR and to develop new, noninvasive therapies to prevent vision loss from this diabetic complication.

REFERENCES

1. Fong DS, Aiello L, Gardner TW, et al. and American Diabetes Association. Diabetic retinopathy. Diabetes Care 2003;26:226–229.
2. Anonymous. The effect of intensive treatment of diabetes on the development and progression of long-term complications in insulin-dependent diabetes mellitus. The Diabetes Control and Complications Trial Research Group [see comment]. N Engl J Med 1993; 329:977–986.
3. Anonymous. Effect of intensive diabetes treatment on nerve conduction in the Diabetes Control and Complications Trial. Ann Neurol 1995;38:869–880.
4. Anonymous. Effect of intensive therapy on the development and progression of diabetic nephropathy in the Diabetes Control and Complications Trial. The Diabetes Control and Complications (DCCT) Research Group. Kidney Int 1995;47:1703–1720.
5. Anonymous. Progression of retinopathy with intensive versus conventional treatment in the Diabetes Control and Complications Trial. Diabetes Control and Complications Trial Research Group. Ophthalmology 1995;102:647–661.
6. Anonymous. The effect of intensive diabetes treatment on the progression of diabetic retinopathy in insulin-dependent diabetes mellitus. The Diabetes Control and Complications Trial. Arch Ophthalmol 1995;113:36–51.
7. Anonymous. Influence of intensive diabetes treatment on quality-of-life outcomes in the diabetes control and complications trial [see comment]. Diabetes Care 1996;19:195–203.
8. Anonymous. Early photocoagulation for diabetic retinopathy. ETDRS report number 9. Early Treatment Diabetic Retinopathy Study Research Group. Ophthalmology 1991;98:766–785.
9. Anonymous. Preliminary report on effects of photocoagulation therapy. The Diabetic Retinopathy Study Research Group. Am J Ophthalmol 1976;81:383–396.
10. Anonymous. Photocoagulation treatment of proliferative diabetic retinopathy. Clinical application of Diabetic Retinopathy Study (DRS) findings, DRS Report Number 8. The Diabetic Retinopathy Study Research Group. Ophthalmology 1981;88:583–600.

11. Anonymous. Photocoagulation for diabetic macular edema. Early Treatment Diabetic Retinopathy Study report number 1. Early Treatment Diabetic Retinopathy Study research group. Arch Ophthalmol 1985;103:1796–1806.
12. Anonymous. Photocoagulation therapy for diabetic eye disease. Early Treatment Diabetic Retinopathy Study Research Group. JAMA 1985;254:3086–3086.
13. Funatsu H, Yamashita H, Ikeda T, Mimura T, Eguchi S, Hori S. Vitreous levels of interleukin-6 and vascular endothelial growth factor are related to diabetic macular edema. Ophthalmology 2003;110:1690–1696.
14. Gao G, Li Y, Zhang D, Gee S, Crosson C, Ma J. Unbalanced expression of VEGF and PEDF in ischemia-induced retinal neovascularization. FEBS Lett 2001;489:270–276.
15. Gao G, Li Y, Gee S, et al. Down-regulation of VEGF and up-regulation of PEDF: a possible mechanism for the anti-angiogenic activity of plasminogen kringle 5. J Biol Chem 2002;277:9492–9497.
16. Robinson GS, Aiello LP. Angiogenic factors in diabetic ocular disease: mechanisms of today, therapies for tomorrow. Int Ophthalmol Clin 1998;38:89–102.
17. Battegay EJ. Angiogenesis: mechanistic insights, neovascular diseases, and therapeutic prospects. J Mol Med 1995;73:333–346.
18. Lao YH. Endogenous angiogenesis inhibitors and their therapeutic implications [review]. Int J Biochem Cell Biol 2001;33:357–369.
19. Dawson DW, Volpert OV, Gillis P, et al. Pigment epithelium-derived factor: a potent inhibitor of angiogenesis. Science 1999;285:245–258.
20. Cao Y. Endogenous angiogenesis inhibitors and their therapeutic implications. Int J Biochem Cell Biol 2001;33:357–369.
21. Cao Y. Endogenous angiogenesis inhibitors: angiostatin, endostatin, and other proteolytic fragments. Prog Mol Subcell Biol 1998;20:161–176.
22. Duh EJ, Yang HS, Suzuma I, et al. Pigment epithelium-derived factor suppresses ischemia-induced retinal neovascularization and VEGF-induced migration and growth. Invest Ophthalmol Vis Sci 2002;43:821–829.
23. Gao G, Shao C, Zhang SX, Dudley A, Fant J, Ma J-X. Kallikrein-binding protein: a novel angiogenic inhibitor of the serpin family. Diabetologia 2003;46:689–698.
24. Zhang D, Kaufman PL, Gao G, Saunders RA, Ma J-X. Intravitreal injection of plasminogen kringle 5, an endogenous angiogenic inhibitor, arrests retinal neovascularization in rats. Diabetologia 2001;44:757–765.
25. O'Reilly MS, Holmgren L, Shing Y, et al. Angiostatin: a novel angiogenesis inhibitor that mediates the suppression of metastases by a Lewis lung carcinoma. Cell 1994;79:315–328.
26. O'Reilly MS, Boehm T, Shing Y, et al. Endostatin: an endogenous inhibitor of angiogenesis and tumor growth. Cell 1997;88:277–285.
27. O'Reilly MS, Pirie-Shepherd S, Lane WS, Folkman J. Antiangiogenic activity of the cleaved conformation of the serpin antithrombin. Science 1999;285:1926–1928.
28. Ogata N, Tombran-Tink J, Nishikawa M, et al. Pigment epithelium-derived factor in the vitreous is low in diabetic retinopathy and high in rhegmatogenous retinal detachment. Am J Ophthalmol 2001;132:378–382.
29. Spranger J, Hammes HP, Preissner KT, Schatz H, Pfeiffer AF. Release of the angiogenesis inhibitor angiostatin in patients with proliferative diabetic retinopathy: association with retinal photocoagulation. Diabetologia 2000;43:1404–1407.
30. Wild S, Roglic G, Sicree R, Green A, King H. Global burden of diabetes mellitus in the year 2000. In: Global Burden of Disaese, WHO, Geneva.
31. American Diabetes Association. Diabetic retinopathy [see comment]. Diabetes Care 2000;23:S73–S76.
32. The Eye Diseases Prevalence Research Group. Causes and prevalence of visual impairment among adults in the United States. Arch Ophthalmol 2004;122:477–485.

33. The Eye Diseases Prevalence Research Group. The prevalence of diabetic retinopathy among adults in the United States. Arch Ophthalmol 2004;122:552–563.
34. Ferris FL 3rd. Results of 20 years of research on the treatment of diabetic retinopathy. Prev Med 1994;23:740–742.
35. Cunha-Vaz JG. Diabetic retinopathy: surrogate outcomes for drug development for diabetic retinopathy. Ophthalmologica 2000;214:377–380.
36. Harris EL, Feldman S, Robinson CR, Sherman S, Georgopoulos A. Racial differences in the relationship between blood pressure and risk of retinopathy among individuals with NIDDM. Diabetes Care 1993;16:748–754.
37. Harris EL, Sherman SH, Georgopoulos A. Black–white differences in risk of developing retinopathy among individuals with type 2 diabetes. Diabetes Care 1999;22:779–783.
38. Harris MI. Diabetes in America: epidemiology and scope of the problem [see comment]. Diabetes Care 1998;21:C11–C14.
39. Harris MI, Klein R, Cowie CC, Rowland M, Byrd-Holt DD. Is the risk of diabetic retinopathy greater in non-Hispanic blacks and Mexican Americans than in non-Hispanic whites with type 2 diabetes? A US population study. Diabetes Care 1998;21:1230–1235.
40. Arfken CL, Reno PL, Santiago JV, Klein R. Development of proliferative diabetic retinopathy in African-Americans and whites with type 1 diabetes. Diabetes Care 1998;21:792–795.
41. Anonymous. Clustering of long-term complications in families with diabetes in the diabetes control and complications trial. The Diabetes Control and Complications Trial Research Group. Diabetes 1997;46:1829–1839.
42. Gao G, Li Y, Fant J, Crosson CE, Becerra SP, Ma J-X. Difference in ischemic regulation of vascular endothelial growth factor and pigment epithelium-derived factor in brown Norway and Sprague Dawley rats contributing to different susceptibilities to retinal neovascularization. Diabetes 2002;51:1218–1225.
43. Kao YL, Donaghue K, Chan A, Knight J, Silink M. A novel polymorphism in the aldose reductase gene promoter region is strongly associated with diabetic retinopathy in adolescents with type 1 diabetes. Diabetes 1999;48:1338–1340.
44. Kao YL, Donaghue K, Chan A, Knight J, Silink M. An aldose reductase intragenic polymorphism associated with diabetic retinopathy. Diabetes Res Clin Prac 1999;46:155–160.
45. Cisse A, Chevenne D, Chauffert M, Ndiaye MR, Wade A, Trivin F. HLA-markers and diabetic retinopathy in the Senegalese population. Dakar Medical 1998;43:29–33.
46. Stewart LL, Field LL, Ross S, McArthur RG. Genetic risk factors in diabetic retinopathy. Diabetologia 1993;36:1293–1298.
47. Cruickshanks KJ, Vadheim CM, Moss SE, et al. Genetic marker associations with proliferative retinopathy in persons diagnosed with diabetes before 30 yr of age. Diabetes 1992;41:879–885.
48. Dharma SK, D'Amico DJ. HLA antigens and the development of diabetic retinopathy. Int Ophthalmol Clin 1993;33:93–99.
49. Quiroz-Mercado H, Suarez-Licona A, Fromow-Guerra J, et al. Human lymphocyte antigen DR7 protects against proliferative retinopathy with type II diabetes mellitus. Arch Med Res 2002;33;123–127.
50. Birinci A, Birinci H, Abidinoglu R, Durupinar B, Oge I. Diabetic retinopathy and HLA antigens in type 2 diabetes mellitus. Eur J Ophthalmol 2002;12:89–93.
51. Warpeha KM, Chakravarthy U. Molecular genetics of microvascular disease in diabetic retinopathy. Eye 2003;17:305–311.
52. Jain SK, Kannan K, Lim G, Matthews-Greer J, McVie R, Bocchini JA Jr. Elevated blood interleukin-6 levels in hyperketonemic type 1 diabetic patients and secretion by acetoacetate-treated cultured U937 monocytes. Diabetes Care 2003;26:2139–2143.

53. Kamiuchi K, Hasegawa G, Obayashi H, et al. Intercellular adhesion molecule-1 (ICAM-1) polymorphism is associated with diabetic retinopathy in Type 2 diabetes mellitus. Diabetic Med 2002;19:371–376.
54. Beranek M, Kankova K, Benes P, et al. Polymorphism R25P in the gene encoding transforming growth factor-beta (TGF-beta1) is a newly identified risk factor for proliferative diabetic retinopathy. Am J Med Genet 2002;109:278–283.
55. De La Cruz JP, Gonzalez-Correa JA, Guerrero A, De La Cuesta FS. Pharmacological approach to diabetic retinopathy. Diabetes Metab Res Rev 2004;20:91–113.
56. Moss SE, Klein R, Klein BE. The 14-year incidence of visual loss in a diabetic population. Ophthalmology 1998;105:998–1003.
57. Klein R, Klein BE, Moss SE. Visual impairment in diabetes. Ophthalmology 1984;91:1–9.
58. Klein R, Klein BE, Moss SE, Davis MD, DeMets DL. The Wisconsin epidemiologic study of diabetic retinopathy. IV. Diabetic macular edema. Ophthalmology 1984;91:1464–1474.
59. Klein R, Klein BE, Moss SE, Cruickshanks KJ. The Wisconsin Epidemiologic Study of Diabetic Retinopathy. XV. The long-term incidence of macular edema. Ophthalmology 1995;102:7–16.
60. Gupta A, Gupta V. Diabetic maculopathy and cataract surgery. Ophthalmol Clin N Am 2001;14:625–637.
61. Klein R. Prevention of visual loss from diabetic retinopathy [review]. Surv Ophthalmol 2002;47:S246–S252.
62. Fong DS. Changing times for the management of diabetic retinopathy. Surv Ophthalmol 2002;47:S238–S245.
63. Ferris FL 3rd. Photocoagulation for diabetic retinopathy. Early Treatment Diabetic Retinopathy Study Research Group. JAMA 1991;266:1263–1265.
64. Anonymous. Photocoagulation for diabetic macular edema. Early Treatment Diabetic Retinopathy Study Report no. 4. The Early Treatment Diabetic Retinopathy Study Research Group. Int Ophthalmol Clin 1987;27:265–272.
65. Ciulla TA, Danis RP, Harris A. Age-related macular degeneration: a review of experimental treatments. Surv Ophthalmol 1998;43:134–146.
66. Antonetti DA, Lieth E, Barber AJ, Gardner TW. Molecular mechanisms of vascular permeability in diabetic retinopathy. Semin Ophthalmol 1999;14:240–248.
67. Klein R. Diabetic retinopathy. Annu Rev Public Health 1996;17:137–158.
68. Cunha-Vaz JG, Gray JR, Zeimer RC, Mota MC, Ishimoto BM, Leite E. Characterization of the early stages of diabetic retinopathy by vitreous fluorophotometry. Diabetes 1985;34:53–59.
69. Yoshida A, Ishiko S, Kojima M, Ogasawara H. Permeability of the blood-ocular barrier in adolescent and adult diabetic patients. Br J Ophthalmol 1993;77:158–161.
70. Gardner TW, Antonetti DA, Barber AJ, LaNoue KF, Levison SW. Diabetic retinopathy: more than meets the eye [review]. Surv Ophthalmol 2002;47:S253–S262.
71. Murata T, Nakagawa K, Khalil A, Ishibashi T, Inomata H, Sueishi K. The relation between expression of vascular endothelial growth factor and breakdown of the blood-retinal barrier in diabetic rat retinas. Lab Invest 1996;74:819–825.
72. Lund-Andersen H. Mechanisms for monitoring changes in retinal status following therapeutic intervention in diabetic retinopathy [review]. Surv Ophthalmol 2002;47:S270–S277.
73. Qaum T, Xu Q, Joussen AM, et al. VEGF-initiated blood-retinal barrier breakdown in early diabetes. Invest Ophthalmol Vis Sci 2001;42:2408–2413.
74. Barber AJ, Antonetti DA. Mapping the blood vessels with paracellular permeability in the retinas of diabetic rats. Invest Ophthalmol Vis Sci 2003;44:5410–5416.
75. Antonetti DA, Barber AJ, Khin S, Lieth E, Tarbell JM, Gardner TW. Vascular permeability in experimental diabetes is associated with reduced endothelial occludin content: vascular

endothelial growth factor decreases occludin in retinal endothelial cells. Penn State Retina Research Group. Diabetes 1998;47:1953–1959.
76. Barber AJ, Antonetti DA, Gardner TW. Altered expression of retinal occludin and glial fibrillary acidic protein in experimental diabetes. The Penn State Retina Research Group. Invest Ophthal Vis Sci 2000;41:3561–3568.
77. Kent D, Vinores SA, Campochiaro PA. Macular oedema: the role of soluble mediators. Br J Ophthalmol 2000;84:542–545.
78. Cooper ME, Vranes D, Youssef S, et al. Increased renal expression of vascular endothelial growth factor (VEGF) and its receptor VEGFR-2 in experimental diabetes. Diabetes 1999;48:2229–2239.
79. Engerman RL, Kern TS. Retinopathy in animal models of diabetes. Diabetes-Metab Rev 1995;11:109–120.
80. Yu DY, Cringle SJ, Su EN, Yu PK, Jerums G, Cooper ME. Pathogenesis and intervention strategies in diabetic retinopathy. Clin Exp Ophthalmol 2001;29:164–166.
81. Vinores SA, Seo MS, Okamoto N, et al. Experimental models of growth factor-mediated angiogenesis and blood-retinal barrier breakdown. Gen Pharmacol 2000;35: 233–239.
82. Vinores SA, Derevjanik NL, Vinores MA, Okamoto N, Campochiaro PA. Sensitivity of different vascular beds in the eye to neovascularization and blood-retinal barrier breakdown in VEGF transgenic mice. Adv Exp Med Biol 2000;476:129–138.
83. Kern TS, Engerman RL. Galactose-induced retinal microangiopathy in rats [see comment]. Invest Ophthalmol Vis Sci 1995;36:490–496.
84. Kador PF, Takahashi Y, Wyman M, Ferris F 3rd. Diabeteslike proliferative retinal changes in galactose-fed dogs [see comment]. Arch Ophthalmol 1995;113:352–354
85. Neuenschwander H, Julia C, Wyman M, Kador PF. Endothelial changes in galactose-fed dogs. Curr Eye Res 1995;14:319–322.
86. McLeod DS, D'Anna SA, Lutty GA. Clinical and histopathologic features of canine oxygen-induced proliferative retinopathy. Invest Ophthalmol Vis Sci 1998;39:1918–1932.
87. Phelps DL. Oxygen and developmental retinal capillary remodeling in the kitten. Invest Ophthalmol Vis Sci 1990;31:2194–2200.
88. Aiello LP, Wong JS. Role of vascular endothelial growth factor in diabetic vascular complications. Kidney Int Suppl 2000;77:S113–S119.
89. Nicaeus TE, Tolentino MJ, Adamis AP, Rubin PA. Sucralfate and basic fibroblast growth factor promote endothelial cell proliferation around porous alloplastic implants in vitro. Ophthalmic Plast Reconstruct Surg 1996;12:235–239.
90. Smith LE, Shen W, Perruzzi C, et al. Regulation of vascular endothelial growth factor-dependent retinal neovascularization by insulin-like growth factor-1 receptor. Nat Med 1999;5:1390–1395.
91. Chakrabarti S, Cukiernik M, Hileeto D, Evans T, Chen S. Role of vasoactive factors in the pathogenesis of early changes in diabetic retinopathy. Diabetes Metab Res Rev 2000;16:393–407.
92. Hammes HP, Lin J, Bretzel RG, Brownlee M, Breier G. Upregulation of the vascular endothelial growth factor/vascular endothelial growth factor receptor system in experimental background diabetic retinopathy of the rat. Diabetes 1998;47:401–406.
93. Ferrara N, Houck KA, Jakeman LB, Winer J, Leung DW. The vascular endothelial growth factor family of polypeptides. J Cell Biochem 1991;47:211–218.
94. Dvorak HF, Brown LF, Detmar M, Dvorak AM. Vascular permeability factor/vascular endothelial growth factor, microvascular hyperpermeability, and angiogenesis. Am J Pathol 1995;146:1029–1039.
95. Senger DR, Galli SJ, Dvorak AM, et al. Tumor cells secrete a vascular permeability factor that promotes accumulation of ascites fluid. Science 1983;219:983–985.

96. Aiello LP, Bursell SE, Clermont A, et al. Vascular endothelial growth factor-induced retinal permeability is mediated by protein kinase C in vivo and suppressed by an orally effective beta-isoform-selective inhibitor. Diabetes 1997;46:1473–1480.
97. Senger DR, Ledbetter SR, Claffey KP, Papadopoulos-Sergiou A, Peruzzi CA, Detmar M. Stimulation of endothelial cell migration by vascular permeability factor/vascular endothelial growth factor through cooperative mechanisms involving the alphavbeta3 integrin, osteopontin, and thrombin. Am J Pathol 1996;149:293–305.
98. Pe'er J, Shweiki D, Itin A, Hemo I, Gnessin H, Keshet E. Hypoxia-induced expression of vascular endothelial growth factor by retinal cells is a common factor in neovascularizing ocular diseases. Lab Invest 1995;72:638–645.
99. Dorey CK, Aouididi S, Reynaud X, Dvorak HF, Brown LF. Correlation of vascular permeability factor/vascular endothelial growth factor with extraretinal neovascularization in the rat. Arch Ophthalmol 1996;114:1210–1217.
100. Lu M, Amano S, Miyamoto K, et al. Insulin-induced vascular endothelial growth factor expression in retina. Invest Ophthalmol Vis Sci 1999;40:3281–3286.
101. Pierce EA, Avery RL, Foley ED, Aiello LP, Smith LE. Vascular endothelial growth factor/vascular permeability factor expression in a mouse model of retinal neovascularization. Proc Natl Acad Sci USA 1995;92:905–909.
102. de Vries C, Escobedo JA, Ueno H, Houck K, Ferrara N, Williams LT. The fms-like tyrosine kinase, a receptor for vascular endothelial growth factor. Science 1992;255: 989–991.
103. Terman BI, Dougher-Vermazen M, Carrion ME, et al. Identification of the KDR tyrosine kinase as a receptor for vascular endothelial cell growth factor. Biochem Biophys Res Comm 1992;187:1579–1586.
104. Adamis AP, Miller JW, Bernal MT, et al. Increased vascular endothelial growth factor levels in the vitreous of eyes with proliferative diabetic retinopathy. Am J Ophthalmol 1994;118:445–450.
105. Malecaze F, Clamens S, Simorre-Pinatel V, et al. Detection of vascular endothelial growth factor messenger RNA and vascular endothelial growth factor-like activity in proliferative diabetic retinopathy. Arch Ophthalmol 1994;112:1476–1482.
106. Ozaki H, Yu AY, Della N, et al. Hypoxia inducible factor-1alpha is increased in ischemic retina: temporal and spatial correlation with VEGF expression. Invest Ophthalmol Vis Sci 1999;40:182–189.
107. Ambati J, Chalam KV, Chawla DK, et al. Elevated gamma-aminobutyric acid, glutamate, and vascular endothelial growth factor levels in the vitreous of patients with proliferative diabetic retinopathy. Arch Ophthalmol 1997;115:1161–1166.
108. Funatsu H, Yamashita H, Noma H, Mimura T, Yamashita T, Hori S. Increased levels of vascular endothelial growth factor and interleukin-6 in the aqueous humor of diabetics with macular edema. Am J Ophthalmol 2002;133:70–77.
109. Aiello LP, Avery RL, Arrigg PG, et al. Vascular endothelial growth factor in ocular fluid of patients with diabetic retinopathy and other retinal disorders. N Engl J Med 1994;331:1480–1487.
110. Braun L, Kardon T, Reisz-Porszasz ZS, Banhegyi G, Mandl J. The regulation of the induction of vascular endothelial growth factor at the onset of diabetes in spontaneously diabetic rats. Life Sci 2001;69:2533–2542.
111. Tolentino MJ, Miller JW, Gragoudas ES, et al. Intravitreous injections of vascular endothelial growth factor produce retinal ischemia and microangiopathy in an adult primate. Ophthalmology 1996;103:1820–1828.
112. Tolentino MJ, Miller JW, Gragoudas ES, Chatzistefanou K, Ferrara N, Adamis AP. Vascular endothelial growth factor is sufficient to produce iris neovascularization and neovascular glaucoma in a nonhuman primate. Arch Ophthalmol 1996;114:964–970.

113. Tolentino MJ, Adamis AP. Angiogenic factors in the development of diabetic iris neovascularization and retinopathy. Int Ophthalmol Clin 1998;38:77–94.
114. Aiello LP. Keeping in touch with angiogenesis [comment]. Nat Med 2000;6:379–381.
115. Folkman J, Ingber D. Inhibition of angiogenesis. Semin Cancer Biol 1992;3:89–96.
116. Ferrara N. The role of vascular endothelial growth factor in pathological angiogenesis. Breast Cancer Res Treat 1995;36:127–137.
117. Gao G, Ma J. Tipping the balance for angiogenic disorders. Drug Discov Today 2002;7: 171,172.
118. Wahl ML, Moser TL, Pizzo SV. Angiostatin and anti-angiogenic therapy in human disease. Recent Prog Horm Res 2004;59:73–104.
119. Preis I, Langer R, Brem H, Folkman J. Inhibition of neovascularization by an extract derived from vitreous. Am J Ophthalmol 1977;84:323–328.
120. Lutty GA, Thompson DC, Gallup JY, Mello RJ, Patz A, Fenselau A. Vitreous: an inhibitor of retinal extract-induced neovascularization. Invest Ophthalmol Vis Sci 1983;24:52–56.
121. Lutty GA, Mello RJ, Chandler C, Fait C, Bennett A, Patz A. Regulation of cell growth by vitreous humour. J Cell Sci 1985;24:53–65.
122. Noma H, Funatsu H, Yamashita H, Kitano S, Mishima HK, Hori S. Regulation of angiogenesis in diabetic retinopathy: possible balance between vascular endothelial growth factor and endostatin. Arch Ophthalmol 2002;120:1075–1080.
123. Fukai N, Eklund L, Marneros AG, et al. Lack of collagen XVIII/endostatin results in eye abnormalities. EMBO J 2002;21:1535–1544.
124. Claesson-Welsh L, Welsh M, Ito N, et al. Angiostatin induces endothelial cell apoptosis and activation of focal adhesion kinase independently of the integrin-binding motif RGD. Proc Natl Acad Sci USA 1998;95:5579–5583.
125. Meneses PI, Hajjar KA, Berns KI, Duvoisin RM. Recombinant angiostatin prevents retinal neovascularization in a murine proliferative retinopathy model. Gene Ther 2001;8: 646–648.
126. Lai CC, Wu WC, Chen SL, et al. Suppression of choroidal neovascularization by adeno-associated virus vector expressing angiostatin. Invest Ophthalmol Vis Sci 2001;42:2401–2407.
127. Drixler TA, Rinkes IH, Ritchie ED, et al. Angiostatin inhibits pathological but not physiological retinal angiogenesis. Invest Ophthalmol Vis Sci 2001;42:3325–3330.
128. Sima J, Zhang SX, Shao C, Fant J, Ma J-X. The effect of angiostatin on vascular leakage and VEGF expression in rat retina. FEBS Lett 2004;564:19–23.
129. Tombran-Tink J, Johnson LV. Neuronal differentiation of retinoblastoma cells induced by medium conditioned by human RPE cells. Invest Ophthalmol Vis Sci 1989;30:1700–1707.
130. Ogata N, Tombran-Tink J, Jo N, Mrazek D, Matsumura M. Upregulation of pigment epithelium-derived factor after laser photocoagulation. Am J Ophthalmol 2001;132: 427–429.
131. Doll JA, Stellmach VM, Bouck NP, et al. Pigment epithelium-derived factor regulates the vasculature and mass of the prostate and pancreas. Nat Med 2003;9:774–780.
132. Spranger J, Osterhoff M, Reimann M, et al. Loss of the antiangiogenic pigment epithelium-derived factor in patients with angiogenic eye disease. Diabetes 2001;50:2641–2645.
133. Duh EJ, Yang HS, Haller JA, et al. Vitreous levels of pigment epithelium-derived factor and vascular endothelial growth factor: implications for ocular angiogenesis. Am J Ophthalmol 2004;137:668–674.
134. Boehm BO, Lang G, Volpert O, et al. Low content of the natural ocular anti-angiogenic agent pigment epithelium-derived factor (PEDF) in aqueous humor predicts progression of diabetic retinopathy. Diabetologia 2003;46:394–400.
135. Stellmach V, Crawford SE, Zhou W, Bouck N. Prevention of ischemia-induced retinopathy by the natural ocular antiangiogenic agent pigment epithelium-derived factor. Proc Natl Acad Sci USA 2001;98:2593–2597.

136. Raisler BJ, Berns KI, Grant MB, Beliaev D, Hauswirth WW. Adeno-associated virus type-2 expression of pigmented epithelium-derived factor or kringles 1–3 of angiostatin reduce retinal neovascularization. Proc Natl Acad Sci USA 2002;99:8909–8914.
137. Mori K, Gehlbach P, Yamamoto S, et al. AAV-mediated gene transfer of pigment epithelium-derived factor inhibits choroidal neovascularization. Invest Ophthalmol Vis Sci 2002;43: 1994–2000.
138. Liu H, Ren JG, Cooper WL, Hawkins CE, Cowan MR, Tong PY. Identification of the anti-vasopermeability effect of pigment epithelium-derived factor and its active site. Proc Natl Acad Sci USA 2004;101:6605–6610.
139. Funatsu H, Yamashita H, Noma H, Shimizu E, Yamashita T, Hori S. Stimulation and inhibition of angiogenesis in diabetic retinopathy. Jpn J Ophthalmol 2001;45:577–584.
140. Mori K, Duh E, Gehlbach P, et al. Pigment epithelium-derived factor inhibits retinal and choroidal neovascularization. J Cell Physiol 2001;188:253–263.
141. Auricchio A, Behling KC, Maguire AM, et al. Inhibition of retinal neovascularization by intraocular viral-mediated delivery of anti-angiogenic agents. Molecular Therapy: J Am Soc Gene Ther 2002;6:490–494.
142. Takahashi K, Saishin Y, Silva RL, et al. Intraocular expression of endostatin reduces VEGF-induced retinal vascular permeability, neovascularization, and retinal detachment. FASEB J 2003;6:896–898.
143. Castellino FJ, McCance SG. The kringle domains of human plasminogen. Ciba Found Symp 1997;212:46–60.
144. Cao Y, Ji RW, Davidson D, et al. Kringle domains of human angiostatin. Characterization of the anti-proliferative activity on endothelial cells. J Biol Chem 1996:271:29,461–29,467.
145. Cao Y, Chen A, An SS, Ji RW, Davidson D, Llinas M. Kringle 5 of plasminogen is a novel inhibitor of endothelial cell growth. J Biol Chem 1997;272:22,924–22,928.
146. Zhang SX, Sima J, Shao C, et al. Plasminogen kringle 5 reduces vascular leakage in the retina of rat model of the oxygen-induced retinopathy and diabetes. Diabitologia 2004;47:124–131.
147. Zhou GX, Chao L, Chao J. Kallistatin: a novel human tissue kallikrein inhibitor. Purification, characterization, and reactive center sequence. J Biol Chem 1992:267:25,873–25,880.
148. Chai KX, Ma J-X, Murray SR, Chao J, Chao L. Molecular cloning and analysis of the rat kallikrein-binding protein gene. J Biol Chem 1991;266:16,029–16,036.
149. Chao J, Tillman DM, Wang MY, Margolius HS, Chao L. Identification of a new tissue-kallikrein-binding protein. Biochem J 1986;239:325–331.
150. Chao J, Chai KX, Chen LM, et al. Tissue kallikrein-binding protein is a serpin. I. Purification, characterization, and distribution in normotensive and spontaneously hypertensive rats. J Biol Chem 1990;265:16,394–16,401.
151. Ma J-X, Yang Z, Chao J, Chao L. Intramuscular delivery of rat kallikrein-binding protein gene reverses hypotension in transgenic mice expressing human tissue kallikrein. J Biol Chem 1995;270:451–455.
152. Hatcher HC, Ma J-X, Chao J, Chao L, Ottlecz A. Kallikrein-binding protein levels are reduced in the retinas of streptozotocin-induced diabetic rats. Invest Ophthalmol Vis Sci 1997;38:658–664.
153. Ma J-X, King L, Yang Z, Crouch RK, Chao L, Chao J. Quantitative comparison of kallistatin in non-diabetic and diabetic vitreous fluids. Curr Eye Res 1996;15:1117–1123.
154. Moser TL, Stack MS, Asplin I, et al. Angiostatin binds ATP synthase on the surface of human endothelial cells. Proc Natl Acad Sci USA 1999;96:2811–2816.
155. Redlitz A, Daum G, Sage EH. Angiostatin diminishes activation of the mitogen-activated protein kinases ERK-1 and ERK-2 in human dermal microvascular endothelial cells. J Vasc Res 1999;36:28–34.
156. Eliceiri BP, Cheresh DA. The role of alpha v integrins during angiogenesis: insights into potential mechanisms of action and clinical development. J Clin Invest 1999;103:1227–1230.

157. Eliceiri BP, Klemke R, Stromblad S, Cheresh DA. Integrin alphavbeta3 requirement for sustained mitogen-activated protein kinase activity during angiogenesis. J Cell Biol 1998;140:1255–1263.
158. Tarui T, Miles LA, Takada Y. Specific interaction of angiostatin with integrin alpha(v)beta(3) in endothelial cells. J Biol Chem 2001;276:39,562–39,568.
159. Sudhakar A, Sugimoto H, Yang C, Lively J, Zeisberg M, Kalluri R. Human tumstatin and human endostatin exhibit distinct antiangiogenic activities mediated by alpha v beta 3 and alpha 5 beta 1 integrins. Proc Natl Acad Sci USA 2003;100:4766–4771.
160. Gonzalez-Gronow M, Kalfa T, Johnson CE, Gawdi G, Pizzo SV. The voltage-dependent anion channel is a receptor for plasminogen kringle 5 on human endothelial cells. J Biol Chem 2003;278:27,312–27,318.
161. Abdollahi A, Hahnfeldt P, Maercker C, et al. Endostatin's antiangiogenic signaling network. Mol Cell 2004;13:649–663.
162. Kim YM, Hwang S, Pyun BJ, et al. Endostatin blocks vascular endothelial growth factor-mediated signaling via direct interaction with KDR/Flk-1. J Biol Chem 2002;277: 27,872–27,879.

3
Corneal Angiogenesis

Trevor R. Carmichael, MBBCh, FCS, PhD (Med)

CONTENTS

INTRODUCTION

Corneal neovascularization (angiogenesis) results from the formation of new vascular structures from the limbal vasculature at the corneal edge. These new blood vessels may invade the normally avascular corneal stroma at different levels within the cornea (*see* Fig. 1).

The structure of the cornea may be viewed as a lipid–water–lipid sandwich in which the thick hydrophilic stroma is wedged between the epithelial layer of cells anteriorly and the single layer of endothelial cells posteriorly. The surface epithelium rests on Bowman's layer of compressed superficial stromal tissue, whereas the endothelial layer is separated from the stroma by the elastic Descemet's membrane.

In most cases a neovascularization network within the cornea is supplied by arteries entering the cornea into the stroma; it has been shown that in fewer than 10% of corneal graft buttons were the vessels only between the surface epithelium and Bowman's layer *(1)*. The course followed by the vessels in the cornea is determined somewhat by the anatomy of the corneal layers *(2)*. Clinically it can be observed that in stromal neovascularization, many of the visible large blood vessels are veins and the blood can be seen streaming toward the periphery. Arteries tend to be smaller and less obvious (*see* Fig. 2A).

New vessels in the cornea might be helpful in combating infections and assisting corneal healing, but they are usually undesirable because of their association with reduced corneal clarity and consequent reduction in vision. Vascularization of the cornea removes the privilege that the cornea enjoys in terms of corneal transplantation

From: *Ophthalmology: Ocular Angiogenesis: Diseases, Mechanisms, and Therapeutics*
Edited by: J. Tombran-Tink and C. J. Barnstable © Humana Press Inc., Totowa, NJ

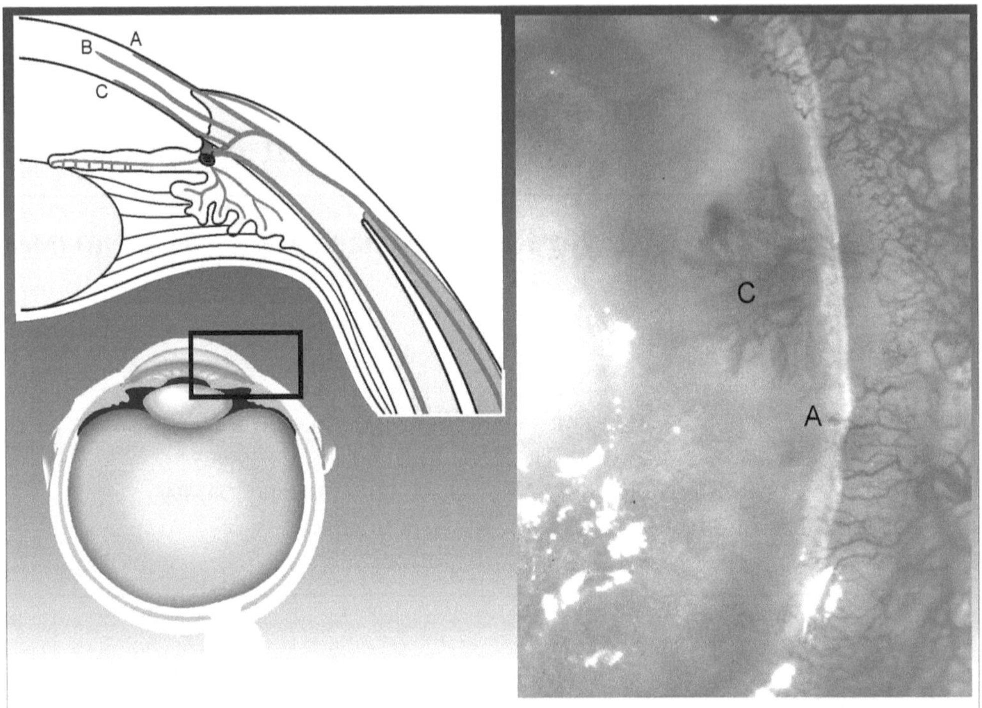

Fig. 1. Cross-sectional illustration showing levels of vessels entering the cornea. A slit-lamp section in the photograph shows superficial **(A)** and deep **(C)** vessels invading the peripheral cornea in response to a deep stromal abscess caused by herpetic infection. *See* color version on companion CD.

(grafting), and the chances of subsequent graft rejection increase according to the number of quadrants of cornea vascularized *(3)*.

Neovascularization of the cornea is observed, and has been reported, in disparate corneal pathologies, with the vessels sometimes seeming to play different roles in the pathology. From corneal graft failure and pterygium to lipid keratopathy in herpetic keratitis, the common endpoint is a threat to vision, either directly or by a reduced chance of successful surgery and maintaining a clear corneal graft. Trachoma and oncocerciasis (river blindness) are significant public health problems in some developing countries and corneal neovascularization plays a role in these diseases, although the cure will more likely result from control of the causative organisms and changes in socioeconomic conditions rather than from an antiangiogenic factor.

The relationship between inflammation and neovascularization in the cornea is complex. In the eye, inflammation usually manifests clinically as a red eye due to dilation of conjunctival and episcleral blood vessels (mostly veins) and involves inflammatory cells and cytokines mediating the inflammation. Inflammation in the cornea is often associated with edema of the corneal stroma, which facilitates stromal neovascularization; and all three play a role in reducing corneal clarity and vision. The fourth element is leakage from new vessels within the cornea, allowing lipid deposition in the stroma, which might further affect vision.

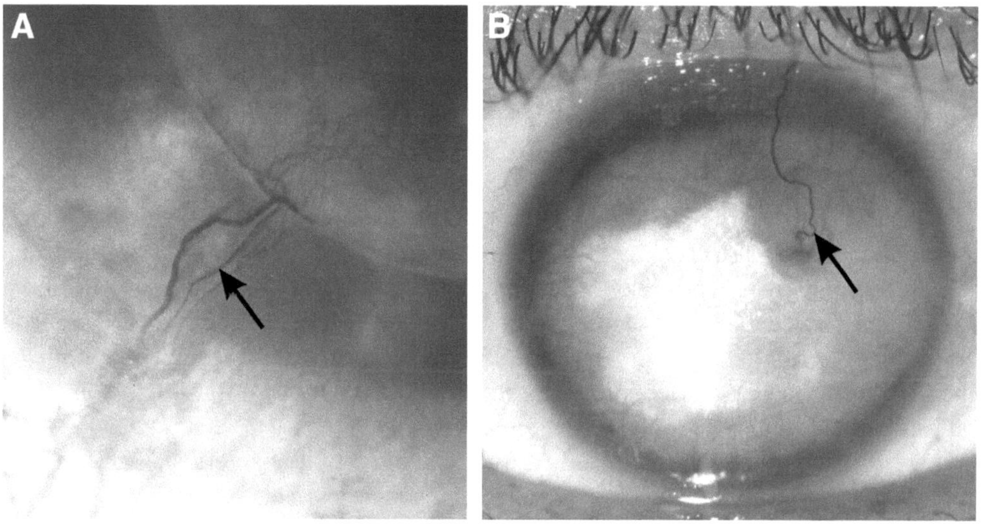

Fig. 2. (**A**) Superficial new vessels induce corneal graft rejection. A small artery (arrow) is flanked by a thick and a thin vein. (**B**) White deposit of lipid in the stroma indicates a lipid keratopathy following long-standing stromal herpes simplex infection of the cornea. Neovascularization in all four quadrants occurs in the middle and deep stroma and a prominent vein is seen arising deep in the center and draining superficially toward 12 o'clock (arrow). *See* color version on companion CD.

In treating the many unrelated corneal diseases, these different elements need to be addressed; this sometimes requires more than one therapeutic approach.

In this chapter the mechanisms for neovascularization of the cornea will be examined; this will include the clinical importance of the associated conditions and the molecular mechanisms, as well as possible therapeutic options that are currently becoming reality.

FACTORS IN CORNEAL AVASCULARITY AND FORMATION OF NEW VESSELS

Excellent vision requires a crystal-clear cornea. The cornea is uniquely constructed to achieve and maintain almost perfect clarity. There are few clear tissues in the body; the cornea, however, has anatomical features that allow light to pass through with minimal scattering. Corneal structure is evenly arranged with few cells blocking the transmission of light. Most of the corneal thickness (about 90%) consists of regular layers of collagen set apart in a gel matrix of mucopolysaccharides. The collagen fibrils are remarkable for their uniform diameter and spacing from surrounding fibers and include various types of collagen, mostly type I, but also types V and VI *(4)*. A total of 10 types of collagen are expressed in the human cornea *(5)*. The corneal stroma contains relatively few cells; these consist mostly of collagen-producing keratocytes. The ground substance between the collagen fibrils consists of proteoglycans, also produced by the keratocytes.

It has been estimated that less than 1% of incident light is scattered by the cornea; part of the reason is that the collagen fibers are held in a grid or "lattice" structure, improving the clarity of the cornea by eliminating scattered light by destructive interference *(6)*. The cornea is maintained in a compact state of dehydration, which not only allows light to pass through efficiently and prevents distortion of the grid structure, but also inhibits vascularization *(7)*. With stromal edema the collagen structure assumes a less compact arrangement, scatters incoming light, and also allows blood vessels to penetrate. This causes additional light scatter, which may reduce vision.

Origin of New Corneal Vessels

Corneal neovascularization arises from the existing vascular network of arteries and their corresponding veins, as well as capillaries at the limbus, by a process referred to as angiogenesis. The anterior segment blood supply may be thought of as arising from several circular ringlike systems that surround the cornea and communicate with each other. In reality these are theoretical ring-like communications, rather than something that can be identified as a complete ring anatomically.

There is a superficial episcleral ring system supplied by the anterior ciliary arteries, brought in from the ophthalmic artery by the rectus muscles. This superficial ring lies on and below the scleral surface 1 to 5 mm behind the limbus *(8)*. From this superficial episcleral ring arise the vascular arcades normally seen at the edge of the cornea, as well as the conjunctival vessels. The episcleral region immediately posterior to the limbus is particularly well vascularized, although many of the vessels are not normally visible. There are two deep ring systems lying in the ciliary muscle. The major arterial circle of the iris is supplied from the long posterior ciliary arteries, which themselves originate as two branches, medial and lateral, from the ophthalmic artery. The intramuscular ring lies posterior to the major circle and is supplied by deep perforating branches of the anterior ciliary arteries *(9)*. These ringlike systems surround the deep part of the cornea and anastomose with the more superficial episcleral ring created by the anterior ciliary arteries. The blood flow in the deep and superficial ring systems connect but flow is considered to occur mostly (60%) from the deep to superficial ring systems *(10)*. Although such an interconnected system may appear infallible in supplying blood to the anterior segment, the nature of the anastomoses between posterior and anterior ciliary vessels is somewhat doubtful because the blood supply to the posterior segment of the eye can be interrupted in a segmental way, leaving watershed areas *(11)*.

Clinically, in neovascularized corneas, many of the visible corneal vessels are veins that tend to have a thicker, more tortuous appearance than arteries and on slit-lamp examination, blood can be seen streaming out centrifugally, from the center of the cornea toward the corneal periphery. It can be difficult at the slit-lamp to identify the thinner, straighter, feeder arteries in the system of vessels. Sometimes the arteries arise deep in the cornea, with the venous outflow prominently visible and more superficial (*see* Fig. 2B).

When viewed by slit-lamp examination in the clinic, blood vessels can be seen to invade the cornea superficially, as a pannus extending a variable distance onto the cornea and associated with subepithelial or stromal scarring that may affect vision *(12)*, or as stromal vascularization, which may occur at any level in the stroma, depending on the cause (stimulus for neovascularization) *(1,12)*. The attractive patterns created by new vessels in the cornea were classified by the early ophthalmologists and given names, such as the umbel, or flower-cluster type (*see* Fig. 3A) *(12)*.

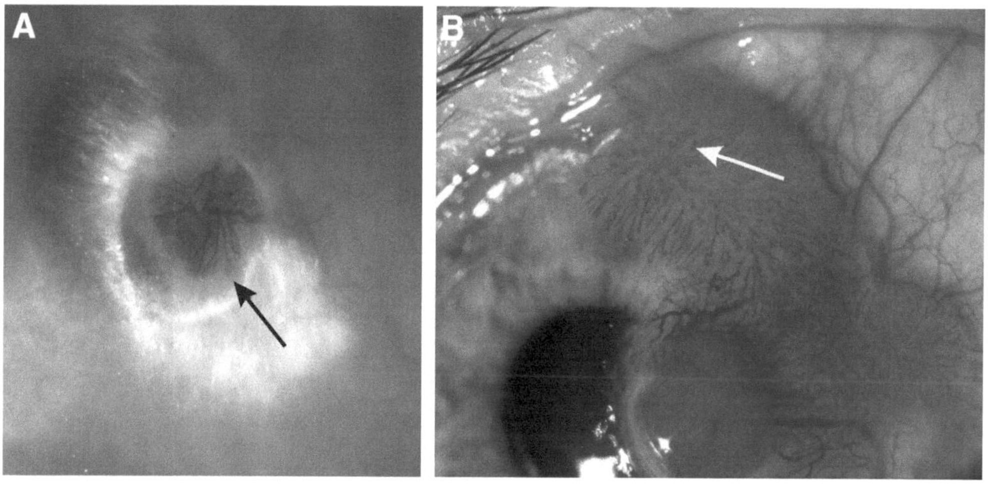

Fig. 3. (A) Stromal lipid (white feathery deposit) surrounds an "umbel" configuration of corneal neovascularization appearing as a flower-cluster (arrow). **(B)** A recurrent carcinoma *in situ* (noninfiltrative) spreading onto the cornea. Budding new vessels can be seen that arise deep and supply the tumor (arrow). Vessel loops are seen in the clear cornea. Fig. 8b shows the whole eye. *See* color version on companion CD.

Pannus occurs commonly in diseases like trachoma, atopic keratoconjunctivitis, and staphylococcal blepharitis, as well as vernal conjunctivitis and with contact lens wear, but there are many other causes *(13)*. When pannus develops, the new blood vessels originate from the vascular arcades derived from the superficial ring of episcleral blood vessels and may sometimes be seen extending from conjunctival branches of the ring. Superficial stromal vascularization occurring in the periphery of the cornea is quite commonly seen in soft contact lens wearers and is regarded as fairly benign, although undesirable *(14)*. With tumor growth at the limbus, the budding new vessels can be seen growing into the superficial spreading tumor (Fig. 3B).

Deeper vascularization occurring in the corneal stroma with interstitial keratitis originates from the anterior ciliary arteries *(8)* (and their deep anastomoses with the ciliary muscle intramuscular ring and major circle of the iris). Presumably the extensive connections between these two systems, the deeper rings fed by the long posterior ciliary arteries and the superficial episcleral ring fed by the anterior ciliary arteries, allow new blood vessels to enter the stroma at any level, although clinicians may place diagnostic significance on the exact level of corneal vascularization. Deep stromal vascularization has been considered virtually pathognomonic of syphilis *(13)*, but has also been reported in association with extended contact lens use in monkeys *(15)* and with soft contact lens use by patients *(16)*. It has been reported that an angiogenic factor related to basic fibroblast growth factor might occur naturally in Descemet's membrane *(17)*. The release of sequestered angiogenic factors by inflammation or other means might explain some of the clinical findings. There are many listed causes of corneal neovascularization *(12,13,18–20)*.

The actual new vessels seen in the cornea are derived from capillaries and veins *(2,21,22)*. The arteries show some proliferative activity, but this occurs later than the endothelial proliferation in veins and capillaries *(23)*.

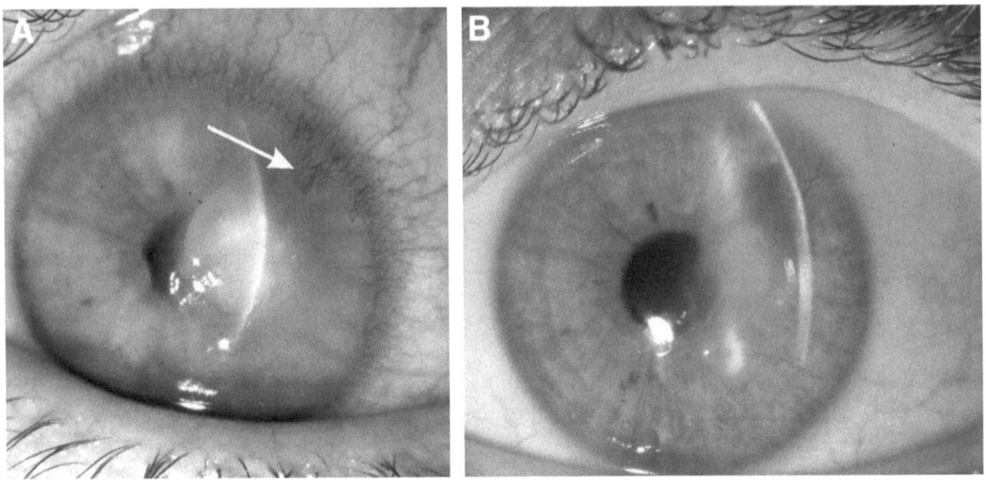

Fig. 4. **(A)** Superficial neovascularization (pannus) in a triangular shape (arrow) in response to a superficial stromal herpes infection. Ulceration is seen in the slit-lamp beam as a greenish opacity (due to fluorescein dye). **(B)** After 4 d of treatment with topical 1% dexamethasone eyedrops and acyclovir ointment, the dilated conjunctival vessels have constricted and regression of the corneal neovascularization has begun. The corneal ulcer is shown as green due to fluorescein dye enhancement. *See* color version on companion CD.

Conditions and Timing for New Vessel Formation in the Cornea

Michaelson *(24)* proposed a retinal factor with certain properties that appeared to stimulate the formation of retinal capillaries from veins in the developing retina. He showed that the capillary nets avoid arteries and arteries send only a few feeder vessels to connect with the net. He showed that the development of the vessel nets was in a triangular shape with the base toward the retinal periphery. Later work by Ashton suggested that the capillary net was developed first, and this was followed by differentiation into arteries and veins related to their role in carrying blood and also the oxygen concentration *(25)*.

Corneal neovascularization appears to have some parallels with the retinal vasculature, with many visible veins and few feeder arteries. The development of vascular structures in the cornea can have a triangular pattern, but with the base toward the limbus. This occurs in response to an angiogenic stimulus at the apex of the triangle and has been observed in animal experiments *(26)* and also clinically (*see* Fig. 4A,B). Careful study of the development of corneal vascularization in rabbits showed that stromal edema, usually near the limbus, preceded new vessel formation and that the first change seen was engorgement of capillaries and venules *(7)*. A clinical analogy to this was noted in acute corneal hydrops, where neovascularization was seen if corneal edema occurred close to the limbus *(27)*. Neovascularization in the more usual central corneal hydrops is considered uncommon. Scanning electron microscopy of casts made of new vessels in rat corneas showed that, in response to chemical cautery, new vessels bud from venules and, to a lesser extent, capillaries *(28)*. In this model, the first buds appeared at 27 h following the injury and differentiation into identifiable arteries and veins took 9 to 21 d. It was considered that this differentiation might be dependant on flow-through or pressure within the vessels.

Direct observation of the blood vessels in rabbit corneas that develop following suture placement in the cornea shows similar developments *(22)*. The initial budding from capillaries began by 18 h, with blood flow through the new vessels about 72 h later. Researchers found that the new vessel sprouts were located along corneal nerves. They felt that corneal edema was not a necessary component for corneal neovascularization. It has also been shown that when basic fibroblast factor with sucralfate was placed in the corneal stroma it induced angiogenesis in the mouse model without inflammation or edema *(29)*. Clinically there are conditions, such as congenital hereditary endothelial dystrophy and Fuchs' dystrophy *(22)*, in which quite severe corneal edema is seen without neovascularization, although neovascularization may occur with long-standing disease.

Role of Corneal Inflammation and Repair

A multitude of cytokines, extracellular matrix proteins, and growth factors have been found in the cornea *(5,30,31)*; their complex interactions might provide further opportunity for intervention in preventing opacification of the cornea, as well as blocking angiogenesis. This system of normal corneal maintenance and repair is invoked in response to various injuries and insults, including the most recent insult, refractive surgery. Corneal repair is usually described as it occurs by corneal layer *(31,32)* and although complex, is somewhat simplified by the relatively straightforward organization of the cornea. Much of the current interest focuses on what happens in the corneal stroma, epithelial regeneration and healing, and how the stroma and epithelium interact. Several of the layers heal with less effect on vision than the more critical healing of corneal stroma and epithelium.

The corneal endothelium, a single layer of cells coating the posterior surface of the cornea, does not replicate; repair is by the sliding of cells to cover areas of damage. Corneal endothelial cell density decreases with aging but is normally 3000 to 3500 cells/mm^2 in young adults. The corneal endothelial cells secrete Descemet's membrane, which has elastic properties and lies between the endothelium and the stroma, like a basement membrane. If Descemet's membrane is damaged it will slowly be replaced by the endothelium. Bowman's membrane, on the other hand, is not replaced once it is damaged or removed by excimer laser ablation.

Corneal epithelium is regenerated centripetally from the limbal stem cells, and the surface squamous cells are replaced from the underlying basal cells, which are attached to a basement membrane. The basement membrane of the corneal epithelium rests on Bowman's layer, a compressed zone of corneal stroma. Damage to the limbal stem cell area, the source of new corneal epithelial cells, may result in a change to a conjunctival type of epithelium covering the corneal surface. The reduced optical quality of this conjunctivalized surface may result in light scatter and reduced vision, as well as sometimes being the source of chronic inflammation and associated superficial corneal vascularization *(33)*.

In the stroma repair involves regeneration of both the collagen fibrils and regeneration of proteoglycans. Necrosis of stromal tissue due to trauma or an inflammatory disease process can cause corneal thinning, the clinical manifestation of tissue loss, seen by slit-lamp examination. Replacement collagen fibers may appear as permanent white stromal scarring, scattering incoming light and degrading vision. Control of inflammatory damage and scarring is a key factor in reducing morbidity due to eye disease or following refractive surgery.

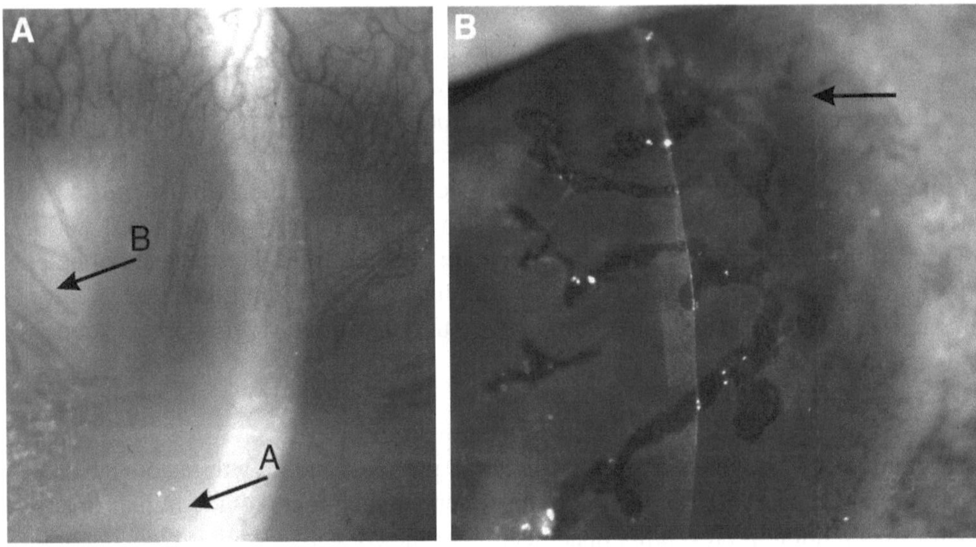

Fig. 5. (A) A neurotrophic ulcer (arrow **a**) has induced midstromal neovascularization of the cornea with vessel loops (arrow **b**) growing in from the corneal limbus. **(B)** A dendritic ulcer is shown as a reddish-purple branching pattern in the corneal epithelium by the slit-lamp beam. Early neovascularization from the limbus is beginning to encroach superficially into the cornea (arrow). *See* color version on companion CD.

Various factors are released by corneal epithelial cells or stromal keratocytes, or both; these factors may affect their own function (autocrine) or functioning of another cell (paracrine). Cytokines may be brought in via inflammatory cells from limbal vessels or new vessels invading the area, from the tear film, or even from the aqueous. The cytokines have been classified according to their site of production and where they exert their effect. The signaling system between corneal epithelium and stroma was reviewed by Nishada and Tanaka *(30)*. Keratocyte apoptosis follows epithelial damage; the results on the stroma of what happens to the epithelium are beginning to be understood *(5)*. This interactive relationship has been observed by clinicians who have frustratingly watched dramatically deteriorating situations that may have started out appearing fairly innocuous. A chronic corneal epithelial defect may trigger an inflammatory reaction in the stroma, stromal melting, stromal vascularization, or a combination of these (*see* Fig. 5A). In the 26-yr-old male depicted in Fig. 5A, the cornea was neurotrophic (absent corneal sensation) following head trauma, which also restricted eye movement. An epithelial defect was followed some weeks later by rapid stromal vascularization, which regressed following amniotic membrane graft to achieve healing of the epithelial defect. This was the patient's only eye.

There appears to be a regulatory mechanism involving interleukin-1 and matrix metalloproteinase-9 for remodeling of the corneal stroma, and interaction between stromal keratocytes and corneal epithelial cells seems part of the control mechanism *(30)*. Corneal stromal repair by keratocytes involves collagen and proteoglycan production; this process is at least partially controlled by cytokines *(31)*.

This interactive triad of edema, inflammation, and neovascularization of the cornea appears commonly in many conditions.

The current evidence suggests, in broad terms, that there are substances released within the cornea that initiate the process of new vessel formation and other substances that oppose the formation of blood vessels. The balance of these two opposing influences, as well as other elements such as edema of the corneal stroma and inflammation, would determine the extent and pace of vascularization. Conceptually, it may be useful to consider a switch *(34)* to the angiogenic phenotype under certain conditions, with interplay of many possible factors providing for a complex scenario. Some of the better known proangiogenic and antiangiogenic factors were recently listed, showing 21 pro- and 17 antiangiogenic factors *(35)*.

It is probably reasonable to differentiate between superficial vascularization and deeper vascularization of the corneal stroma. Superficial new vessels include situations in which there is conjunctivalization of the surface of the cornea and also the superficial vessel ingrowth that clinicians refer to as pannus. This separation is advisable because surface disorders have quite a different significance to clinicians. Both are problematic and surfacc disorders may be even more difficult to treat than the ominous stromal vessels that make corneal grafting difficult. The causes of these two groups of conditions are also generally different.

CORNEAL NEOVASCULARIZATION: ITS ROLE IN BLINDING DISEASES

Corneal Blindness

There are at least three direct mechanisms for vision loss: conjunctivalization of the corneal epithelium, causing a poor optical surface; leakage of lipids into the cornea; and direct growth of vessels with fibrous tissue obstructing vision *(36)*.

The extent of the worldwide problem of corneal neovascularization cannot easily be determined *(20)*. Corneal disease is responsible for unilateral or bilateral blindness in about 10 million people, many of whom live in developing countries *(37)*. It is second only to cataracts as a worldwide cause of blindness, and trachoma is responsible for half the cases of corneal blindness.

In developed countries, some degree of peripheral superficial vascularization associated with contact lens wear *(14,20)* or blepharitis might be accepted as fairly harmless, whereas stromal vascularization following herpes simplex, or other infections, may be associated with visual morbidity and poorer outcomes for corneal grafting *(20)*. Bacterial corneal ulceration may be associated with contact lens wear in developed countries *(38)* and may result in vascularized corneal scarring *(1)*.

In developing countries, corneal disease, with its associated corneal scarring and vascularization, is a major factor in blindness in both children and adults *(37)*. Surveys of schools for the blind in east Africa have shown that corneal blindness resulting from vitamin A deficiency and measles infection accounted for 35% of severe vision loss or blindness in 244 children under age 16 yr *(39)*. In Zimbabwe a survey of 430 students at schools for the blind showed 75% of blindness to be caused by bilateral corneal opacities *(40)*. The corneal disease was considered to have been a sequel of previous measles infection. The problem of corneal ulceration in children and the complex relationships among malnutrition, measles, and herpes simplex infection have received considerable attention *(41–43)*. The end result is often vascularized corneal scarring, which is difficult to treat with corneal grafting and is largely preventable. Corneal ulceration due to bacterial and fungal infections in adults, often associated with corneal trauma and degenerations, is an important cause of corneal blindness in adults in developing countries *(44,45)*.

Population surveys for corneal blindness are less common. A cluster survey of 18,962 inhabitants in the northern areas of South Africa found a blindness prevalence rate of 0.57%, with corneal scarring due to trachoma causing 10% of blindness *(46)*. This was a survey of bilateral blindness with vision less than 3/60; the corneal vascularization associated with trachoma makes corneal grafting difficult in these patients.

Corneal Neovascularization in Corneal Grafts

In addition to the direct problem that corneal vascularization causes for vision, it may jeopardize subsequent rehabilitation by corneal grafting. The importance of corneal vascularization as a risk factor for corneal grafts was demonstrated by the significant relationship between the numbers of quadrants vascularized and the chance of rejection *(3)*. In this study of 702 corneal grafts, one or two quadrants (or 1 to 15 vessels) were considered "high risk" for graft failure, whereas three or four quadrants (16 or more vessels) were considered "very high risk" for graft failure. Another study has shown significantly more corneal neovascularization in patients having a repeat graft (23%) than a primary graft (13%) and poorer outcomes at 2 and 5 yr in the repeat graft patients *(47)*. Peripheral anterior synechiae were also blamed for the poorer outcome in this group of repeat graft patients. In this study, corneal neovascularization was associated with double the risk of a poor outcome in both primary and regraft patients on multivariate analysis. About half the grafts in both groups were for bullous keratopathy following cataract surgery. Recently, deep stromal vascularization was shown to be a risk factor for corneal graft failure in a large case series of 3992 consecutive grafts *(48)*.

In first-world countries a 5-yr graft survival rate of 70% has been reported *(49)* but in developing areas, where data collection and patient follow-up are not as precise, the results are generally not as good. In developing countries, the procedure is reasonable in the good-prognosis nonvascularized corneas with keratoconus but drops to 65% at 2 yr in eyes with conditions associated with vascularization *(50)*.

Herpetic Corneal Disease

Herpes simplex and zoster corneal disease are a cause of substantial morbidity in both developed and developing populations. Herpes simplex has been estimated to cause recurrent infections in more than one-third of the world's population and causes 300,000 cases of ocular infection per year in the United States *(51)*. Probably about 90% of persons with recurrent ocular infections will maintain good vision *(52)*, but corneal scarring might result from corneal epithelial infection in the form of dendritic ulceration. This tends to be superficial *(53)* but following episodes of the deeper stromal type of herpes simplex keratitis, there can be associated deep stromal scarring and vascularization. The marginal type of dendrite is usually associated with greater corneal edema and inflammatory infiltrate in the superficial stroma *(53)*, and this may be

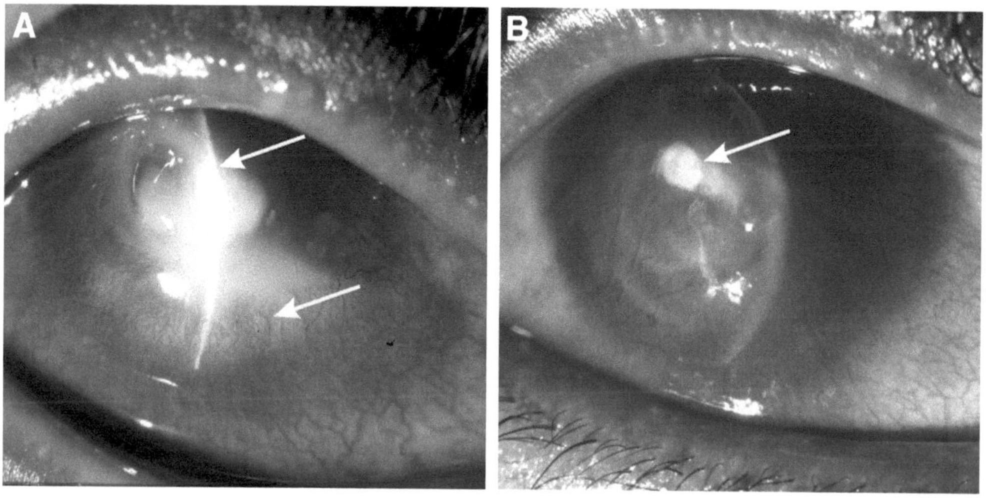

Fig. 6. (A) A necrotic stromal herpes simplex infection with corneal ulcer in an immunocompromised patient showing an abscess (upper arrow) and hypopyon. Florid superficial and deep corneal vascularization (lower arrow) is seen. **(B)** After 3 wk of a combination of dexamethasone drops and acyclovir ointment the ulcer is almost healed (arrow) and the neovascularization has partially regressed. *See* color version on companion CD.

associated with superficial corneal vascularization (*see* Fig. 5B). The deeper necrotic stromal disease may be associated with an intense inflammatory focus in the corneal stroma. There may be stromal edema and rapid mid- or deep-stromal vascularization, which can respond fairly dramatically to a combination of antiviral and topical steroid treatment (*see* Figs. 4A,B, 6A,B).

The strain of herpes simplex virus and its glycoprotein product has been shown to determine the intensity of the host inflammatory response and, thus, vascularization *(54)*. Experimentally, using a rabbit model, medroxyprogesterone was shown to decrease corneal neovascularization and this corresponded to a reduction in polymorphonuclear leukocyte (PMN) infiltration in the stroma *(55)*. There was a simultaneous reduction in "total collagenase" in the corneas. Later work using a mouse model to study the inflammatory infiltrate in stromal keratitis showed a peak of PMNs by day 7 after infection was induced *(56)*. After this, the response depended on the immune response of the mouse. If there was no cell-mediated immune response to herpes simplex virus type 1, the inflammation would subside. If there was a response, a mononuclear cell infiltrate (predominantly plasma cells) was seen, with associated neovascularization and necrosis in the stroma. There has been recent speculation on whether the prominent neovascularization seen in necrotic stromal herpes keratitis is a necessary part of the pathogenesis, or whether it is a secondary effect resulting from the intense inflammation induced in the stroma. In a mouse model, Zheng et al. *(57)* showed that vascular endothelial growth factor (VEGF) originated from either noninfected corneal epithelial cells or inflammatory cells, PMNs, or macrophage-like cells. VEGF antagonists partially blocked the angiogenesis and reduced the severity of the stromal lesions. It is of interest that VEGF-stimulated angiogenesis results in leaky vessels and lipid keratopathy is a fairly common sequel of chronic herpetic stromal keratitis.

The role of collagenases and gelatinases in the pathogenesis of stromal necrosis induced by herpes simplex infections is not fully understood. These enzymes, now grouped as the matrix metalloproteinases (MMPs) *(58)*, comprise at least 18 members in humans and are regulated by several mechanisms including tissue inhibitors of metalloproteinases (TIMPs). There are at least four TIMPs; TIMP-3 has been found to be antiangiogenic. MMP-9 and -8 are exceptional in that they are stored in the secretory granules of neutrophils and eosinophils *(58)*. MMP-9 is not found in normal corneas but has been shown to be a mediator of angiogenesis in herpes simplex keratitis *(59)*. In a mouse experiment, MMP-9, but not MMP-2, was expressed and was shown to originate from neutrophils that were part of the inflammatory infiltrate induced by the infection. Inhibition of MMP-9 by TIMP-1 resulted in a reduction in angiogenesis. The authors suggest the possible necessary role of angiogenesis in the pathogenesis of necrotic stromal herpetic keratitis and suggest that an "antiangiogenic cocktail" might be required to block angiogenesis at various points.

In contrast to the rapid vascularization seen in response to herpesvirus infections, chronic acanthamoeba *(60)* corneal infections have been observed to show little tendency to neovascularization in spite of a polymorphonuclear inflammatory response in the stroma. The reasons for this were not fully elucidated but were thought to be due to the nature of the immune response generated by the organism.

Mooren's Peripheral Corneal Ulceration

The Mooren's type of peripheral ulceration of the cornea is regarded as an autoimmune process, with the process directed toward an antigen in the corneal stroma *(61)*. The typical Mooren's ulcer of the cornea occurs more frequently in males, often affects the medial or lateral quadrants of the limbus, and affects the cornea and not the sclera (*see* Fig. 7A,B) *(62,63)*. The process involves intense inflammation adjacent to the ulcer with some neovascularization of the base of the ulcer. The blood vessels may be reactive, caused by the inflammatory reaction in the stroma, or they may be necessary and allow the antibody to get into the stroma, perpetuating the ulceration. Some forms are refractory to treatment but surgical removal of the vessels by conjunctival resection with or without corneal lamellar keratoplasty and immune suppression has been associated with cure in some of these patients *(62,64)*. The implication, as with herpetic infection, is that perhaps these blood vessels deliver factors or enzymes necessary in the pathogenesis of the ulceration. Studies of limbal vasculature in patients with peripheral corneal ulceration may show nonperfusion, neovascularization, or leakage from deep vessels, depending on the clinical type and associated systemic conditions *(63)*. In these studies using low-dose fluorescein angiography, it appeared that deep limbal vessels leak fluorescein in Mooren's ulcers. This group of conditions may be difficult to treat, but being able to medically interfere with the neovascularization might play a role in treatment of the condition.

Conjunctivalization of Corneal Surface

Alkali burn injury of the anterior segment of the eye, with limbal ischemia affecting more than four clock hours of limbus, was shown to be associated with worse outcomes than lesser ischemia, and requires intensive treatment *(65)*. Extensive corneal injury

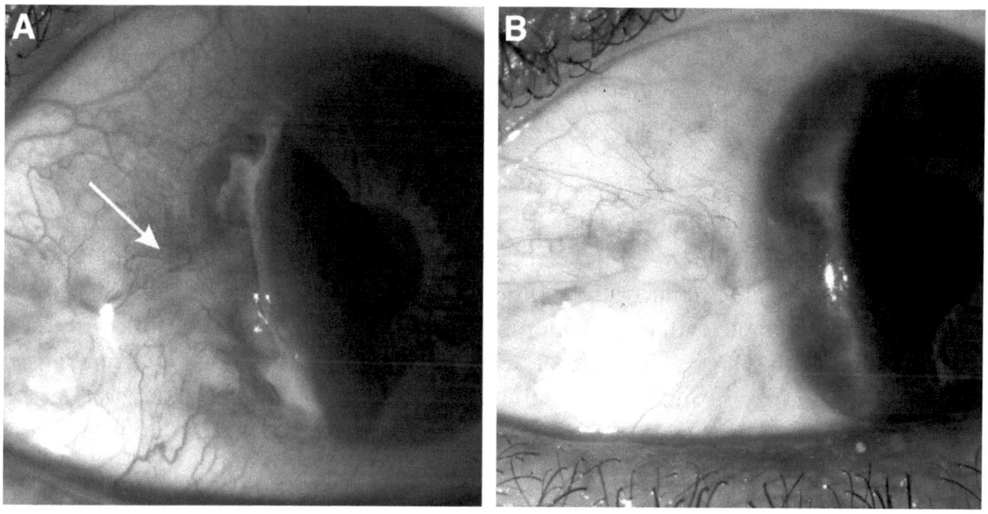

Fig. 7. (**A**) Mooren's peripheral corneal ulcer on presentation with superficial neovascularization in the ulcer bed and dilated episcleral vessels (arrow). (**B**) Following topical steroid treatment and conjunctival recession with thermal cautery to the episcleral vessels the ulcer healed over 2 mo, leaving some peripheral scarring but good vision (9 mo after presentation). *See* color version on companion CD.

associated with chemical burns may lead to conjunctivalization of the epithelial surface of the cornea, with reduced vision due to scarring *(20)*. This is also seen in aniridia *(66)* and Stevens-Johnson syndrome, in which limbal stem cell deficiency results in an altered corneal surface that contains goblet cells and often shows vascularization. The presence of goblet cells in the surface epithelium is an indication that a conjunctival phenotype is present and occlusion of corneal neovascularization has led to transdifferentiation to a corneal phenotype with improved corneal clarity *(67)*.

Conjunctivalization with neovascularization of the superficial cornea has been shown to be mediated by VEGF *(68)*. VEGF was also shown to play a key role in a rabbit model of corneal neovascularization, in which the vascularization (and inflammation) was induced by removal of corneal and limbal epithelium *(69)*. The vascularization in this model could be suppressed by anti-VEGF antibodies that were implanted in the cornea in a hydron pellet. The role of cytokines in this sequence of events was not clear. Subsequently, using a rabbit model in which the surface epithelium was removed by application of sodium hydroxide and surgical debridement, goblet cells appeared with reepithelialization and Flt-1 (VEGF-R1) receptors were found in goblet cells in the conjunctivalized epithelium. It was postulated that VEGF controlled the invasion of this conjunctiva-type epithelium as well as new vessels onto the corneal surface.

In alkali burns, inflammation may accompany conjunctivalization and new vessel formation and the inflammatory response may also be a target for intervention *(33)*. The introduction of substances such as the antiinflammatory cytokine, IL-1 RA, by intrastromal injection has been shown to reduce the inflammatory response to the alkali injury in this mouse model, and intrastromal injections would be feasible in the clinical environment.

Other possible ways to prevent angiogenesis in alkali burns might involve the integrins and matrix metalloproteinases. In the rat model, the angiogenesis associated with alkaline burns has been associated with the upregulation of VEGF and the integrin $\alpha_v\beta_5$, along with the matrix metalloproteinases MMP-2 and MTI-MMP *(70)*.

Lipid Keratopathy

Lipids may leak from abnormal blood vessels in the cornea, and the resulting opacification may affect vision (*see* Fig. 2B). This is usually associated with situations in which there is corneal vascularization, either following limbal inflammatory disease, as in vernal keratoconjunctivitis or trachoma, or stromal vascularization following herpetic infection, either herpes simplex or zoster. Primary lipid keratopathy occurring as a storage disease may result in the accumulation of lipid without corneal vascularization. Lipid deposition has been described with deep corneal vascularization in soft contact lens wearers, where the mechanisms involved are thought to be hypoxia, inflammation, and corneal edema *(16)*.

The accumulation of lipids in the cornea is equivalent to the circinate deposition of lipids in the retina, seen in diabetes and other conditions in which the retinal vasculature is abnormally permeable. The process in the cornea has also been referred to as circinate and described in two patterns: parallel to the limbus with an intervening clear zone, and as a ring of lipid around a sheath of vessels *(71)*. In tumors, angiogenesis gives rise to leaky vessels and focal hemorrhages and leakage is common within the tumors *(72)*. In neovascularization of the cornea, lipids may leak but focal hemorrhages are uncommon, probably because the fairly rigid corneal substance supports and protects the new vessels.

Lipid deposition associated with neovascularization in chronic herpetic infection is clinically the most problematic form, with the inherent threat of rejection or herpes recurrence should rehabilitation by corneal grafting be attempted. Peroxidized lipids themselves induce angiogenesis through a cytokine mechanism *(73)*; it is unknown if this is a factor resulting in a perpetuating cycle in chronic herpetic disease of the cornea. Further lipid leakage from corneal blood vessels may be suppressed by the ongoing use of topical steroid drops, with antiviral medication sometimes also being required. Direct treatment to the vessels has been attempted using argon laser *(74)* and, more recently, nonthermal laser light at 689 nm following the administration of verteporfin, a photosensitizing dye *(75)*. A technique of fine-needle cauterization of vessels may be helpful in allowing successful corneal grafting and stabilizing lipid keratopathy *(76)*. It has also been shown that using fluorescein dye as a sensitizer and applying argon laser treatment to vessels may be beneficial in terms of cosmesis and reduced topical steroid use *(77)*. These treatments, as with surgical cutdown and cautery, may fail due to recurrence of vessels, or repeat treatment may be required.

Pterygium

A pterygium is a degenerative process in which there is a triangular fibrovascular invasion into the cornea at the level of Bowman's membrane and that frequently recurs following excision. Zauberman *(78)* suggested that a "pterygium factor" was present that, once stimulated, caused the inevitable recurrence of the growth onto the cornea.

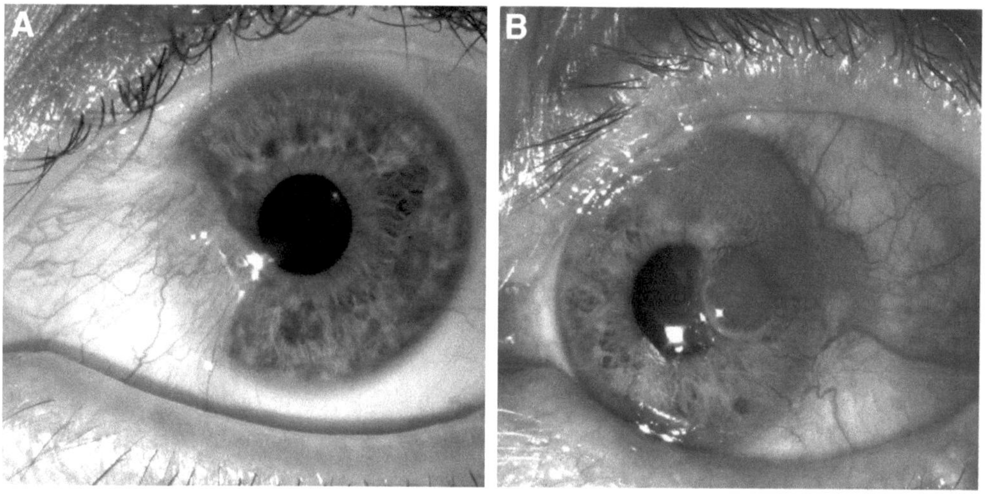

Fig. 8. **(A)** A large vascular pterygium that may show high recurrence rates in young adult patients following simple excision. **(B)** A carcinoma of the limbus extends onto the cornea (Fig. 3B shows close-up). *See* color version on companion CD.

Vascularization of the cornea has been considered to play a role in the pathogenesis of pterygium *(79)*, although other factors including ultraviolet (UV) light *(80,81)* and genetic predisposition *(82,83)* might also play a part. It has been hypothesized *(79)* that the ultraviolet radiation and other irritants might cause an inflammatory cell infiltrate leading to corneal angiogenesis, which results in the fibrovascular response seen clinically as pterygium (*see* Fig. 8A). The possibility of a "pterygium angiogenesis factor" has been proposed *(84)* and the possible absence of an inhibitor of vascularization of the cornea previously suggested *(85)*. More recently it has been shown that VEGF might be all or part of the pterygium angiogenesis factor and pigment epithelium-derived factor (PEDF) might play the role of the absent inhibitor of vascularization. In this study, Jin et al. showed increased VEGF levels in pterygium samples compared with normal individuals and a corresponding dramatic downregulation of PEDF *(86)*. It was not stated whether the control conjunctiva in this study was also harvested from the limbal area. The link between environmental and other factors in causing this disturbance in angiogenic factors is being explored. In a study of epithelial cells and fibroblasts from pterygia, it was shown that UV light upregulated heparin-binding epidermal growth factor-like growth factor *(87)*.

The full complexity and cellular mechanisms for pterygium development are being unraveled and as they are, the potential for intervention in both primary and recurrent pterygium may increase.

Trachoma

Limbal inflammatory disease may give rise to corneal neovascularization with or without lipid deposition. Trachoma, a chronic keratoconjunctivitis, was first described Egypt in 1900 BC, and remains a public health issue in developing countries *(37)*. In blinding trachoma, secondary bacterial infections of the cornea result in corneal scarring and subsequent blindness *(88)*.

Trachoma and other chlamydial diseases have been regarded as risk factors for corneal neovascularization. In trachoma it was found that superficial vascular pannus occurred superiorly in most children with the infection, with further extension onto the cornea as the child got older *(89)*. The neovascularization was thought to follow corneal infiltrates seen in the peripheral cornea, which were suspected of releasing angiogenic factors. The superior pannus preceded the development of conjunctival scarring in this group and was seen in children as young as 1 yr of age.

ANGIOGENESIS AND STIMULUS FOR NEOVASCULARIZATION IN CORNEA

Corneal neovascularization is presumed to be at least similar to angiogenesis in other areas of the eye and body, although exact mechanisms may differ depending on the vascular bed involved *(90)*. Our current understanding has been assisted by extensive experimental and clinical work done in other areas of medicine, including mechanisms of tumor growth *(34,72,91)*. Cells need to be within 200 μm of their blood supply, their source of oxygen, to grow *(72)*. The issue of angiogenesis and tumor blood supply might be critical to tumors occurring at the limbus and growing onto the avascular cornea (*see* Fig. 8B).

The stimulus for neovascularization seemingly differs according to the disease but some common factors are apparent. The association of stromal edema occurring near the limbus has long been proposed as necessary to allow blood vessels into the usually compact corneal stroma *(7)*. This might be of importance in chronic postoperative bullous keratopathy and advanced Fuchs' endothelial dystrophy. It has been suggested as being important in the pathogenesis of contact lens-induced neovascularization of the cornea *(14)*. Hypoxia, the trigger to retinal angiogenesis in diabetes mellitus and other conditions, has also been suggested for contact lens-induced vascularization *(15,16)*. Inflammation might be a requirement for angiogenesis or at least facilitate angiogenesis in pathological conditions and repair *(92)*. Inflammatory cells, in either sterile or infective inflammation, are often present and have been postulated as being a key factor *(19)*.

A substance such as basic fibroblast growth factor placed experimentally into a pocket in the corneal stroma *(29)* can effectively and efficiently stimulate new vessel formation, or the disease mechanism might involve a pathway that is more complex and indirect.

This may involve either the upregulation of angiogenic growth factors, such as VEGF in herpes simplex keratitis *(57)*, or an infective organism, such as Oncocerca volvulus, producing a protein that causes the downregulation of antiangiogenic factors *(93)*.

The current model for corneal angiogenesis has been suggested in various forms by several authors *(19,32,91,94–96)* but might contain the flowing elements:

1. The stimulus or initiating factor, e.g., herpes simplex infection or an alkali burn.
2. The latent period.
3. Dilation of limbal vessels.
4. Enzymatic digestion of the basement membrane of venules and capillaries.
5. Endothelial cell proliferation and migration toward the stimulus.
6. Elongation of endothelial cells to form a solid sprout, formation of a lumen followed by sprouts joining together to form vascular loops with blood flow.
7. Maturation of the afferent and efferent sides of the loop to form blood vessels that resemble mature arterioles and venules.

Initial Stimulus

The idea that there might be an angiogenic factor was conceptualized at the end of the 19th century and beginning of the 20th century *(19)* with Goldmann *(97)* mentioning the blood supply of tumors in tumor growth, although this appears to have been very much a vague idea. More specifically, the suggestion that tumor growth might be determined by its blood supply and the concept that this process might be interfered with medically to inhibit or cure cancers was suggested later by Folkman *(98)* and others *(72)*.

In 1948, Michaelson *(24)* suggested that a factor present in the retina was the link between ischemia of the retina in conditions such as diabetes mellitus and the new blood vessels that were sometimes observed on the retina and iris. The search for this substance or substances has been ongoing since that time. An exhaustive review of the subject in 1991 by Klintworth *(19)* identified possible corneal angiogenic growth factors and by 1994 there was still some indecision as to the most likely "Factor X." Three main possibilities were considered: basic fibroblast growth factor (bFGF), insulin-like growth factor (IGF)-I, and VEGF *(99)*.

VEGF, a cytokine, was described in 1989 *(100,101)* and appears to be the key angiogenic factor *(90,95,102)*. It has been shown to be upregulated in many clinical conditions involving the eye where angiogenesis is apparent. VEGF production may be upregulated during tumor growth by certain oncogenes such as K-ras, H-ras, and bcl-2 *(103)*. VEGF and its receptors, VEGFR-1 (Flt-1) and VEGFR-2 (Flk-1/KDR), have been shown to be expressed in vascularized human corneas obtained at the time of keratoplasty *(104)*. It was also suggested that VEGF was produced by epithelial cells adjacent to corneal ulcers in addition to corneal endothelium and the endothelium of limbal and corneal blood vessels.

Of the six known isoforms of VEGF, the one that seems most involved with ocular pathology is $VEGF_{164\,(165)}$ *(105)*. VEGF plays a central role surrounded by many other factors that might differ according to disease and tissue *(90)*. In a microarray analysis of corneal injury an excimer laser was used to create a wound, and the corneal responses of 588 genes examined *(106)*. On day 3 following the laser, the VEGF levels were maximally raised; this corresponded to the time at which the epithelium was absent. At day 7 the VEGF levels were lower; at this time epithelial healing had taken place, although stromal healing was continuing. Possibly this might indicate a tendency to neovascularization when the corneal epithelium is absent. VEGF does appear to be a necessary component of the neovascular response in the cornea. In an inflammatory model using rats, neutralization of VEGF with antibodies blocked the angiogenic response to corneal injury *(69)*.

In hypoxic conditions in the cornea, such as overuse of soft contact lenses, neovascularization may occur *(16)*. This might result from increased VEGF mediated by hypoxia-inducible factor (HIF)-1. This system of oxygen-regulated gene expression is similar to that seen in the development of the tracheal system in *Drosophila (92)*.

The actual initiation of corneal neovascularization is likely not a simple mechanism involving a single growth factor in all cases. It appears that the growth factor or factors inducing angiogenesis may be produced or released in the cornea by different mechanisms in different diseases.

Subsequent Events

The events following the initial stimulus have been described mainly for VEGF and the angiopoietins, although the family of ephrins has also been recently been implicated *(95)*. There might be other angiogenic factors or systems but VEGF seems to hold a key position. Following the stimulus to vascularization, there is a latent period of some 27 h during which VEGF levels rise. Current knowledge is incomplete and has been interpreted from knockout mice *(96)*. This suggests that VEGF via the VEGFR-2 receptor is involved in the migration and proliferation of endothelial cells while it acts via the –R1 receptor to promote tube formation from the solid sprouts. PEDF opposes this early stage, preventing proliferation of endothelial cells by inducing apoptosis in proliferating endothelial cells *(35)*.

The endothelial budding or sprouting is due to elongation of endothelial cells and is accompanied by focal areas of dissolution of the basement membrane of the vessel, allowing the endothelial cells to move into the corneal substance. The elongating solid sprouts become tubes by curving of endothelial cells *(94)* and these connect with other tubes to make a loop. This is followed by blood flow through the loop, and the afferent and efferent limbs take on the appearance of straighter thinner arterioles or thicker more prominent and numerous venules.

Subsequent vessel maturation is directed by VEGF and the angiopoietins via soluble tyrosine kinase TIE receptors *(72,92)*. The signaling between the angiopoietin Ang 1 and the TIE-2 receptor serves to promote maturation of blood vessels with thickening of the cell wall *(96)*. This would serve to lay down basement membrane, increase pericytes, and create a nonleaky blood vessel wall. Ang 2 also acts on the TIE-2 receptor but might promote the interaction of angiogenic stimulators like VEGF with endothelial cells, by loosening the walls of blood vessels. Ang 2 thus appears to act by preventing kinase activation in TIE-2 receptors on endothelial cells and hence blocks the effects of Ang 1. In spite of this blocking effect, it has been suggested that Ang 2 might actually promote new blood vessel growth by activation of the TIE-2 receptor depending on duration and strength of exposure *(91)*. Ang 2 might also be active in situations in which regression of established blood vessels occurs, and it might promote regression *(96)*. The role of other signaling pathways such as the ephrins in the development of corneal neovascularization awaits further investigation but might also provide opportunity for intervention *(107)*. Ephrin-B2 seems a requirement early and late in blood vessel formation and may also play a late role in the maturation of vessels *(72,95)*. Ephrin-B2 and -B4 seem to play a differentiating role in blood vessel formation and mark the endothelium of primordial arteries and veins, respectively *(72)*.

The latent period following the angiogenic trigger represents a window of opportunity for treatment if angiogenesis is to be blocked. Depending on the cause, and events in the cornea, this period would vary quite considerably, as it is mostly difficult to judge clinically how strong the tendency to neovascularization will be in an individual patient. Dilation of limbal blood vessels is an early feature during the process of corneal neovascularization, so clinically a red eye would precede corneal neovascularization, in most situations. The clinician would traditionally be addressing the primary cause of the corneal infection or inflammation and has thus far not been able to preempt the formation of new vessels but rather can record their presence and sometimes use their clinical appearance in a diagnostic way.

Endogenous inhibitors of angiogenesis, as well as a flood of new agents being developed, may allow the clinician to add antiangiogenic therapy in high-risk situations or be able to better induce regression of established blood vessels in the cornea.

Amid the complexities there seems one ray of hope: While it is seemingly a complex process to promote new vessel growth in ischemic diseases, it seems as if it is easier to block the process and that blockage of one key factor (VEGF) has the required result *(95)*.

REDUCING (OR INCREASING) CORNEAL NEOVASCULARIZATION

The usual therapeutic approach would be to prevent, eliminate, or at least reduce blood vessels in the cornea. In uncontrolled infections of the cornea an increase in blood supply might be required; this may be attained surgically by the use of a conjunctival flap to bring the body's antimicrobial factors into close proximity to the infective organisms to neutralize them.

The prevention of corneal neovascularization assumes that the event can be predicted, as is the situation in repeat corneal grafting in an already vascularized cornea. Otherwise, the initial stages of vascularization might be observed clinically and an antiangiogenic strategy employed. In such a clinical situation there might be other more urgent considerations such as nonhealing epithelial erosions and stromal melting that might take priority in management. In many instances it would be more useful to be able to induce regression of existing vascularization than to prevent it because patients often present with existing corneal vessels in many of the diseases that cause corneal blindness. The cornea is readily accessible for a wide range of therapeutic delivery methods, including drops, ointments and gels, and injections, either intracorneal, subconjunctival or under Tenon's capsule. More innovative methods have included collagen shields impregnated with medication *(108)*. Slow-release devices may also be placed in close proximity to the cornea.

Depending on the role of the corneal angiogenesis in the pathogenesis of the disease, different strategies might be appropriate and some have already been used successfully.

Surgical Methods

Removal of the conjunctiva from the limbus, called peritomy, with cauterization of limbal blood vessels has been the classical surgical approach to combat corneal neovascularization *(12)*. The technique of amniotic membrane grafting is a more recent approach and may act by reducing proinflammatory cytokines with a reduced tendency for neovascularization and also fibrosis *(109)*. The use of laser treatment *(74,75,77)* or other direct methods of blood vessel occlusion *(76)* might assist in certain cases, but these are plagued by recurrence of neovascularization where the angiogenic stimulus persists.

Steroid Medications as Antiangiogenic Intervention

The prototype antiangiogenic medication has been the corticosteroid group of drugs developed around 1950. The mechanisms and patterns of angiogenesis in the cornea have been investigated since the early part of the 20th century *(2)*. The cornea has been particularly useful for the investigation of angiogenesis and interventions, owing to its avascularity and the fact that it can be easily observed and photographed. Early reports suggested that cortisone could inhibit angiogenesis in diseased corneas *(110,111)*. It was assumed that the angiogenesis factor, suggested by Michaelson *(24)*, which caused retinal neovascularization, was also responsible for corneal neovascularization, and that appears to have been a correct surmise.

Corticosteroids have been shown to have an effect on inflammation and corneal edema and also to have a direct effect on angiogenesis. Using a model of alkali burns in rabbit corneas, it was shown that subconjunctival injections of cortisone suppressed the superficial neovascular response to the alkali injected superficially in the cornea *(110)*. The severity of the inflammation produced by a very concentrated alkali somewhat masked the cortisone effect, so a model using alloxan was tested *(111)*. The corneal vascularization was induced by injecting alloxan into the anterior chamber and the partially protective effect of sub-conjunctival cortisone injections was demonstrated. There was also reduced corneal swelling (edema) and opacification. It was subsequently shown that 1% prednisolone drops significantly reduced the neovascular response to thermal burns to the cornea *(112)*. This antiangiogenic effect was not seen with 1% medroxyprogesterone drops.

More recently, useful models have been developed for the study of angiogenesis in the cornea. These have included noninflammatory models in which angiogenesis can be studied without associated edema and inflammation *(29)*. The chick embryo chorioallantoic membrane (CAM) assay method has been shown to produce similar results to the rabbit corneal pocket model when testing angiostatic agents *(113)*.

Corticosteroids have been used clinically for ocular inflammation since their appearance in about 1950; their indications in infectious diseases have been controversial and benefits surprisingly difficult to demonstrate *(114,115)*. The significant side effects associated with their use make an alternative medication to prevent and reverse neovascularization of the cornea desirable.

Recent Development of Angiostatic Steroids

Angiostatic steroids are inhibitors of the angiogenic process but lack the glucocorticoid effects and side effects that make glucocorticoid use problematic. After extensive testing of more than 100 compounds the two most effective, AL-3789 and AL-4940, were selected for further study *(113)*. The two drugs appear to act as inhibitors of proteolytic enzymes, although their full mode of action is not clear. They specifically do not appear to work through cytokine and antiinflammatory mechanisms *(113)*. Both were tested in a rabbit corneal model, in which the cortisol acetate analog form (AL-3789) was found slightly more effective *(116)*. The delivery method used was very simple. An eyedrop containing AL-3789 in a 1% strength at two drops daily resulted in almost complete inhibition of the lipopolysaccharide-induced corneal neovascularization. The simplicity and effectiveness make this an attractive proposition, although the slow-release form might prove even more efficacious in situations such as high-risk corneal graft patients, in whom ongoing suppression of neovascularization is required.

Currently trials using anecortave acetate for the treatment of choroidal neovascularization are testing the efficacy of this delivery device and it is hoped that it can be tested in corneal neovascularization.

Other Approaches to Blocking Angiogenesis

Nonsteroidal agents have been shown to suppress angiogenesis in the eye. Nepafenac, a cyclooxygenase-1 and -2 inhibitor, was used in mice and shown to be effective as a drop to treat choroidal neovascularization because of its excellent corneal penetration *(117)*.

Cyclosporine given systemically to mice was shown to block corneal neovascularization induced by interleukin-2 *(118)*. Cyclosporine, given systemically, has been shown to prevent corneal graft rejection in patients who were at high risk. These patients had all four corneal quadrants vascularized with superficial and deep corneal vessels. No comment was made on the effect on neovascularization, but presumably the grafts did not vascularize because graft rejection usually follows vessel invasion of the graft tissue.

Several antibiotic medications have been shown to have antiangiogenic activity. Fumagillin, secreted by *Aspergillus fumigatus*, has shown inhibition of endothelial cell proliferation and its analog, TNP-470, was shown to have a similar effect in mice *(119)*. Reduced corneal VEGF levels were found in treated animals. The authors suggest that the medication might play a role in the treatment of corneal neovascularization, pterygium, and following filtering glaucoma surgery in humans.

Targeting VEGF by several novel approaches has been shown to block angiogenesis. This single-intervention strategy might be effective in ocular angiogenesis or we might find that other pathways open up and bypass our intervention. In particular, it might be naive to think that it would be this simple in cancer therapy where more angiogenic factors are expressed with time, and more than one intervention might be required *(72)*.

Inflammatory cells play a prominent role in corneal angiogenesis in many situations *(19)* and the chemokine control of leukocyte chemotaxis presents a possible target for intervention. Monocytes are attracted by the monocyte chemoattractant proteins (MCP, types 1–5) that bind to the C-C chemokine receptor 2 (CCR2). The receptor CCR2 is found on endothelial cells and monocytes and corneal neovascularization is inhibited in mice made deficient for CCR2 *(120)*. The inhibitory effect was possibly due to a decrease in endothelial migration. A similar partial inhibition of corneal neovascularization was also found in mice deficient in CCR5, the receptor for macrophage inflammatory protein 1α *(121)*.

Transfection of mouse cornea with cytokine interleukin-1 receptor antagonist produced a transient reduction in angiogenesis up to 21 d *(33)*. This was postulated to result from reduced leukocyte infiltration. The method used was a single intrastromal injection, a feasible approach in human eyes.

Interference with gene expression by double-stranded RNA *(122,123)* introduced into cells by transfection is a new approach that might be successfully employed to potently silence VEGF expression.

Natural Inhibitors of Angiogenesis

There are several well-described factors that oppose angiogenesis. It has been demonstrated that somatostatin, a neuropeptide, synthesized in the hypothalamus can block corneal angiogenesis induced by bFGF in a rat model *(124)*. This inhibition was dose-dependent and was seen at a dose of 200 ng somatostatin, but not 20 ng. The somatostatin was delivered in the pellet that contained the bFGF.

Transduction of donor corneal buttons with antiangiogenic factors might reduce the chances of graft rejection, although it is not known how long such an effect might last in the human eye. Using a lentivirus vector a combination of endostatin and kringle-5 were transfected by storing the donor corneas in Optisol GS corneal storage medium spiked with the combination gene and vector for 18 h *(125)*. The corneas were then grafted into rabbits and a reduction in graft vascularization was shown. This technique might have application in high-risk corneal grafting. Endostatin, a fragment of collagen XVIII that is found in vessel walls and basement membranes, exerts its antiangiogenic effect by inducing endothelial cell apoptosis *(72)*.

Combretastatin A-4, a tubulin-binding agent, can cause regression of established new vessels *(90)*.

The most important natural factor opposing angiogenesis currently known is PEDF *(126,127)*. PEDF also plays other roles in cell biology, including neuroprotective functions *(128)*. PEDF has been shown to be downregulated in pterygia *(86)*. The authors also showed that VEGF was upregulated, but less dramatically than the effect seen with PEDF. It was speculated that the disturbance in the usual balance of angiogenic control factors played a role in the pathogenesis of pterygium.

PEDF given by subretinal injection has been shown to reduce neovascularization in both new and established choroidal neovascularization *(129)*. The established blood vessels showed apoptosis of the endothelium caused by the PEDF gene therapy. It is not known whether this effect would still be seen on very mature blood vessels, because endothelial apoptosis was not seen in normal vessels in this model. If this strategy were to be used in vascularized corneas, the duration of neovascularization might be a limiting factor. It also seems likely that PEDF has antiangiogenic effects other than causing apoptosis in endothelial cells *(35)*. Campochiaro and Hackett *(90)* have suggested that PEDF given by gene transfer might be useful in both the prevention of neovascularization and in the treatment of established neovascularization.

Future therapeutic approaches might include Ang 1 to promote the stabilization of leaky vessels *(95)*. This might assist in patients with lipid keratopathy along with treatment aimed at inducing vessel regression.

REFERENCES

1. Cursiefen C, Kuchle M, Naumann GOH. Angiogenesis in corneal diseases: histopathologic evaluation of 254 human corneal buttons with neovascularization. Cornea 1998;17:611–613.
2. Ehlers H. Some experimental researches on corneal vessels. Acta Ophthalmol 1927; 5:99–112.
3. Hill JC. The relative importance of risk factors used to define high-risk keratoplasty. Ger J Ophthalmol 1996;5:36–41.
4. Edelhauser HF, Ubels JL. The cornea and the sclera. In: Adler's physiology of the Eye, Kaufman PL, Alm A, eds. Mosby, St. Louis, MO: 2003:47–114.
5. Zieske JD. Extracellular matrix and wound healing. Curr Opin Ophthalmol 2001; 12:237–241.
6. Maurice DM. The structure and transparency of the cornea. J Physiol 1957;136:263–286.
7. Cogan DG. Vascularization of the cornea. Its experimental induction by small lesions and a new theory of its pathogenesis. Arch Ophthalmol 1949;41:406–416.
8. Bron AJ, Tripathi RC, Tripathi BJ. Wolff's anatomy of the eye and orbit. Chapman & Hall, London, 1997.
9. Funk R, Rohen JW. Scanning electron microscopic study on the vasculature of the human anterior eye segment, especially with respect to the ciliary processes. Exp Eye Res 1990;51:651–661.
10. Meyer PAR. The circulation of the human limbus. Eye 1989;3:121–127.

11. Hayreh SS. Posterior ciliary artery circulation in health and disease. The Weisenfeld lecture. Invest Ophthalmol Vis Sci 2004;45:749–757.
12. Duke-Elder S, Leigh AG. System of Ophthalmology. Mosby, St. Louis, MO: 1965:676–691.
13. Arffa RC. Grayson's Diseases of the Cornea. Mosby-Year Book, St. Louis, MO: 1991.
14. Dixon JM, Lawaczeck E. Corneal vascularization due to contact lenses. Arch Ophthalmol 1963;69:72–75.
15. Madigan MC, Penfold PL, Holden BA, Billson FA. Ultrastructural features of contact lens-induced deep corneal neovascularization and associated stromal leukocytes. Cornea 1990;9:144–151.
16. Rozenman Y, Donnenfeld ED, Cohen EJ, Arentsen JJ, Bernardino VJ, Laibson PR. Contact lens-related deep stromal neovascularization. Am J Ophthalmol 1989;107:27–32.
17. Folkman J, Klagsbrun M, Sasse J, Wadzinski M, Ingber D, Vlodavsky I. Storage of a heparin-binding angiogenic factor in the cornea: a new mechanism for corneal neovascularisation. Invest Ophthalmol Vis Sci 1987;28 (Suppl): 230.
18. Chang J, Gabison EE, Kato T, Azar DT. Corneal neovascularization. Curr Opin Ophthalmol 2001;12:242–249.
19. Klintworth GK. Corneal Angiogenesis. A Comprehensive Review. Springer-Verlag, New York: 1991.
20. Lee P, Wang CC, Adamis AP. Ocular neovascularization: an epidemiologic review. Surv Ophthalmol 1998;43:245–269.
21. Burger PC, Chandler DB, Klintworth GK. Experimental corneal neovascularization: biomicroscopic, angiographic, and morphological correlation. Cornea 1985;4:35–41.
22. Yaylali V, Ohta T, Kaufman SC, Maitchouk DY, Beuerman RW. In vivo confocal imaging of corneal neovascularization. Cornea 1998;17:646–653.
23. Junghans BM, Collin HB. The limbal vascular response to corneal injury. An autoradiographic study. Cornea 1989;8:141–149.
24. Michaelson IC. The mode of development of the vascular system of the retina, with some observations on its significance for certain retinal diseases. Trans Ophthalmol Soc UK 1948;68:137–180.
25. Ashton N. Retinal angiogenesis in the human embryo. Br Med Bull 1970;26:103–106.
26. Campbell FW, Michaelson IC. Blood-vessel formation in the cornea. Br J Ophthalmol 1949;33:248–255.
27. Rowson NJ, Dart JKG, Buckley RJ. Corneal neovascularisation in acute hydrops. Eye 1992;6:404–406.
28. Burger PC, Chandler DB, Klintworth GK. Corneal neovascularization as studied by scanning electron microscopy of vascular casts. Lab Invest 1983;48:169–180.
29. Kenyon BM, Voest EE, Chen CC, Flynn E, Folkman J, D'Amato RJ. A model of angiogenesis in the mouse cornea. Invest Ophthalmol Vis Sci 1996;37:1625–1632.
30. Nishida T, Tanaka T. Extracellular matrix and growth factors in corneal wound healing. Curr Opin Ophthalmol 1996;7:2–11.
31. Ahmadi AJ, Jakobiec FA. Corneal wound healing: cytokines and extracellular matrix proteins. Int Ophthalmol Clin 2002;42:13–22.
32. Pepose JS, Ubels JL. The cornea. In: Adler's Physiology of the Eye, Hart WM Jr, ed. Mosby Year Book, St. Louis, MO:1992:29–70.
33. Moore JE, McMullen TCB, Campbell IL, et al. The inflammatory milieu associated with conjunctivalized cornea and its alteration with IL-1 RA gene therapy. Invest Ophthalmol Vis Sci 2002;43:2905–2915.
34. Folkman J. Angiogenesis in cancer, vascular, rheumatoid and other disease. Nat Med 1995;1:27–31.
35. Tombran-Tink J, Barnstable CJ. Therapeutic prospects for PEDF: more than a promising angiogenesis inhibitor. Trends Mol Med 2003;9:244–250.

36. Adamis AP, Aiello LP, D'Amato RA. Angiogenesis and ophthalmic disease. Angiogenesis 1999;3:9–14.
37. Whitcher JP, Srinivasan M, Upadhyay MP. Corneal blindness: a global perspective. Bull World Health Org 2001;79:214–221.
38. Bourcier T, Thomas F, Borderie V, Chaumeil C, Laroche L. Bacterial keratitis: predisposing factors, clinical and microbiological review of 300 cases. Br J Ophthalmol 2003;87:834–838.
39. Gilbert CE, Wood M, Waddel K, Foster A. Causes of childhood blindness in east Africa: results in 491 pupils attending 17 schools for the blind in Malawi, Kenya and Uganda. Ophthalmic Epidemiol 1995;2:77–84.
40. Schwab L, Kagame K. Blindness in Africa: Zimbabwe schools for the blind survey. Br J Ophthalmol 1993;77:410–412.
41. Foster A, Sommer A. Childhood blindness from corneal ulceration in Africa: causes, prevention, and treatment. Bull World Health Org 1986;64:619–623.
42. Foster A, Sommer A. Corneal ulceration, measles, and childhood blindness in Tanzania. Br J Ophthalmol 1987;71:331–343.
43. Sandford-Smith JH, Whittle HC. Corneal ulceration following measles in Nigerian children. Br J Ophthalmol 1979;63:720–724.
44. Carmichael TR, Wolpert M, Koornhof HJ. Corneal ulceration at an urban African hospital. Br J Ophthalmol 1985;69:920–926.
45. Upadhyay MP, Karmacharya PCD, Koirala S, et al. Epidemiologic characteristics, predisposing factors, and etiologic diagnosis of corneal ulceration in Nepal. Am J Ophthalmol 1991;111:92–99.
46. Bucher PJM, Ijsselmuiden CB. Prevalence and causes of blindness in the northern Transvaal. Br J Ophthalmol 1988;72:721–726.
47. Weisbrod DJ, Sit M, Naor J, Slomovic AR. Outcomes of repeat penetrating keratoplasty and risk factors for graft failure. Cornea 2003;22:429–434.
48. Price MO, Thompson RW Jr, Price FW Jr. Risk factors for various causes of failure in initial corneal grafts. Arch Ophthalmol 2003;121:1087–1092.
49. Williams KA, Muehlberg SM, Lewis RF, Coster DJ. How successful is corneal transplantation? A report from the Australian corneal graft register. Eye 1995;9:219–227.
50. Yorston D, Wood M, Foster A. Penetrating keratoplasty in Africa: graft survival and visual outcome. Br J Ophthalmol 1996;80:890–894.
51. Whitley RJ, Kimberlin DW, Roizman B. Herpes simplex viruses. Clin Infect Dis 1998; 26:541–553.
52. Liesegang TJ. Herpes simplex virus epidemiology and ocular importance. Cornea 2001; 20:1–13.
53. Dawson CR, Togni B. Herpes simplex eye infections: clinical manifestations, pathogenesis and management. Surv Ophthalmol 1976;21:121–135.
54. Centifanto-Fitzgerald YM, Fenger T, Kaufman HE. Virus proteins in herpetic keratitis. Exp Eye Res 1982;35:425–441.
55. Lass JH, Berman MB, Campbell RC, Pavan-Langston D, Gage J. Treatment of experimental herpetic interstitial keratitis with medroxyprogesterone. Arch Ophthalmol 1980;98:520–527.
56. Hendricks RL, Epstein RJ, Tumpey T. The effect of cellular immune tolerance to HSV-1 antigens on the immunopathology of HSV-1 keratitis. Invest Ophthalmol Vis Sci 1989;30:105–115.
57. Zheng M, Deshpande S, Lee S, Ferrara N, Rouse BT. Contribution of vascular endothelial growth factor in the neovascularization process during the pathogenesis of herpetic stromal keratitis. J Virol 2001;75:9828–9835.
58. Sethi CS, Bailey TA, Luthert PJ, Chong NHV. Matrix metalloproteinase biology applied to vitreoretinal disorders. Br J Ophthalmol 2000;84:654–666.

59. Lee S, Zheng M, Kim B, Rouse BT. Role of matrix metalloproteinase-9 in angiogenesis caused by ocular infection with herpes simplex virus. J Clin Invest 2002;110: 1105–1111.
60. Kremer I, Cohen EJ, Eagle RC, Udell I, Laibson PR. Histopathologic evaluation of stromal inflammation in Acanthamoeba keratitis. CLAO J 1994;20:45–48.
61. Gottsch JD, Liu SH, Minkovitz JB, Goodman DF, Srinivasan M, Stark WJ. Autoimmunity to a cornea-associated stromal antigen in patients with Mooren's ulcer. Invest Ophthalmol Vis Sci 1995;36:1541–1547.
62. Chen J, Xie H, Wang Z, et al. Mooren's ulcer in China: a study of clinical characteristics and treatment. Br J Ophthalmol 2000;84:1244–1249.
63. Watson PG. Management of Mooren's ulceration. Eye 1997;11:349–356.
64. Carmichael TR, Mervitz MD, Bezwoda W, Rush PS. Plasma exchange in the treatment of Mooren's ulcer. Ann Ophthalmol 1985;17:311–314.
65. Brodovsky SC, McCarty CA, Snibson G, et al. Management of alkali burns. Ophthalmology 2000;107:1829–1835.
66. Nishida K, Kinoshita S, Ohashi S, Kuwayama Y, Yamamoto S. Ocular surface abnormalities in aniridia. Am J Ophthalmol 1995;120:368–375.
67. Huang AJW, Watson BD, Hernandez E, Tseng SCG. Induction of conjunctival transdifferentiation on vascularized corneas by photothrombotic occlusion of corneal neovascularization. Ophthalmology 1988;95:228–235.
68. Joussen AM, Poulaki V, Mitsiades N, et al. VEGF-dependent conjunctivalization of the corneal surface. Invest Ophthalmol Vis Sci 2003;44:117–123.
69. Amano S, Rohan R, Kuroki M, Tolentino M, Adamis AP. Requirement for vascular endothelial growth factor in wound- and inflammation-related corneal neovascularisation. Invest Ophthalmol Vis Sci 1998;39:18–22.
70. Zhang H, Li C, Baciu PC. Expression of integrins and MMPs during alkaline-burn-induced corneal angiogenesis. Invest Ophthalmol Vis Sci 2002;43:955–962.
71. Braude LS, Sugar J. Circinate-pattern interstitial keratopathy in daily wear soft contact lens wearers. Arch Ophthalmol 1985;103:1662–1665.
72. Tonini T, Rossi F, Claudio PP. Molecular basis of angiogenesis and cancer. Oncogene 2003;22:6549–6556.
73. Spaide RF, Ho-Spaide WC, Browne RW, Armstrong D. Characterization of peroxidized lipids in Bruch's membrane. Retina 1999;19:141–147.
74. Marsh RJ, Marshal J. Treatment of lipid keratopathy with the argon laser. Br J Ophthalmol 1982;66:127–135.
75. Fossarello M, Peiretti E, Zucca I, Serra A. Photodynamic therapy of corneal neovascularization with verteporphin. Cornea 2003;22:485–488.
76. Pillai CT, Dua HS, Hossain P. Fine needle diathermy occlusion of corneal vessels. Invest Ophthalmol Vis Sci 2000;41:2148–2153.
77. Gordon YJ, Mann RK, Mah TS, Gorin MB. Fluorescein-potentiated argon laser therapy improves symptoms and appearance of corneal neovascularization. Cornea 2002;21: 770–773.
78. Zauberman H. Pterygium and its recurrence. Am J Ophthalmol 1967;63:1780–1786.
79. Hill JC, Maske R. Pathogenesis of pterygium. Eye 1989;3:218–226.
80. Coroneo MT. Pterygium as an early indicator of ultraviolet insolation: a hypothesis. Br J Ophthalmol 1993;77:734–739.
81. Mackenzie FD, Hirst LW, Battistutta D, Green A. Risk analysis in the development of pterygia. Ophthalmology 1992;99:1056–1061.
82. Booth F. Heredity in one hundred patients admitted for excision of pterygia. Aust N Z J Ophthalmol 1985;13:59–61.
83. Carmichael TR. Genetic factors in pterygium in South Africans. S Afr Med J 2001;91:22.

84. Wong WW. A hypothesis on the pathogenesis of pterygiums. Ann Ophthalmol 1978;10: 303–308.
85. Ashton N, Cook C. Mechanism of corneal vascularization. Br J Ophthalmol 1953;37: 193–209.
86. Jin J, Guan M, Sima J, et al. Decreased pigment epithelium-derived factor and increased vascular endothelial growth factor levels in pterygia. Cornea 2003;22:473–477.
87. Nolan TM, Di Girolamo N, Coroneo MT, Wakefield D. Proliferative effects of heparin-binding epidermal growth factor-like growth factor on pterygium epithelial cells and fibroblasts. Invest Ophthalmol Vis Sci 2004;45:110–113.
88. Carmichael TR, Gibson IHN, Küstner HGV. Blinding trachoma—a public health challenge. S Afr Med J 1982;61:5–8.
89. Dawson CR, Juster R, Marx R, Daghfous MT, Djerad AB. Limbal disease in trachoma and other ocular chlamydial infections: risk factors for corneal vasclarisation. Eye 1989;3:204–209.
90. Campochiaro PA, Hackett SF. Ocular neovascularization: a valuable model system. Oncogene 2003;22:6537–6548.
91. Fam NP, Verma S, Kutryk M, Stewart DJ. Clinician guide to angiogenesis. Circulation 2003;108:2613–2618.
92. Risau W. Mechanisms of angiogenesis. Nature 1997;386:671–674.
93. Higazi TB, Pearlman E, Whikehart DR, Unnasch TR. Angiogenic activity of an *Onchocerca volvulus* Ancylostoma secreted protein homologue. Biochem Parasitol 2003;129:61–68.
94. Folkman J, Klagsbrun M. Angiogenic factors. Science 1987;235:442–447.
95. Yancopoulos GD, Davis S, Gale NW, Rudge JS, Wiegand SJ, Holash J. Vascular-specific growth factors and blood vessel formation. Nature 2000;407:242–248.
96. Hanahan D. Signaling vascular morphogenesis and maintenance. Science 1997;277:48–50.
97. Goldmann E. The growth of malignant disease in man and the lower animals, with special reference to the vascular system. Proc R Soc Med 1 (Surgical section) 1907;1–13.
98. Folkman J. Tumor angiogenesis: therapeutic implications. N Engl J Med 1971;285: 1182–1186.
99. Frank RN. Vascular endothelial growth factor—Its role in retinal vascular proliferation. N Engl J Med 1994;331:1519–1520.
100. Connolly DT, Heuvelman DM, Nelson R, et al. Tumor vascular permeability factor stimulates endothelial cell growth and angiogenesis. J Clin Invest 1989;84:1470–1478.
101. Leung DW, Cachianes G, Kuang W, Goeddel DV, Ferrara N. Vascular endothelial growth factor is a secreted angiogenic mitogen. Science 1989;246:1306–1309.
102. Aiello LP, Avery RL, Arrigg PG, et al. Vascular endothelial growth factor in ocular fluid of patients with diabetic retinopathy and other retinal disorders. N Engl J Med 1994; 331:1480–1487.
103. Folkman J. Fundamental concepts of the angiogenic process. Curr Mol Med 2003; 3:643–651.
104. Philipp W, Speicher L, Humpel C. Expression of vascular endothelial growth factor and its receptors in inflamed and vascularized human corneas. Invest Ophthalmol Vis Sci 2000;41:2514–2522.
105. Usui T, Ishida S, Yamashiro K, et al. VEGF 164(165) as the pathological isoform: differential leukocyte and endothelial responses through VEGFR1 and VEGFR2. Invest Ophthalmol Vis Sci 2004;45:368–374.
106. Varela JC, Goldstein MH, Baker HV, Schultz GS. Microarray analysis of gene expression patterns during healing of rat corneas after excimer laser photorefractive keratectomy. Invest Ophthalmol Vis Sci 2002;43:1772–1782.
107. Sullivan DC, Bicknell R. New molecular pathways in angiogenesis. Br J Cancer 2003;89:228–231.

108. Friedberg ML, Pleyer U, Mondino BJ. Device drug delivery to the eye. Collagen shields, iontophoresis, and pumps. Ophthalmology 1991;98:725–732.
109. Sippel KC, Ma JJK, Foster CS. Amniotic membrane surgery. Curr Opin Ophthalmol 2001;12:269–281.
110. Jones IS, Meyer K. Inhibition of vascularization of the rabbit cornea by local application of cortisone. Proc Soc Exp Biol Med 1950;74:102–104.
111. Ashton N, Cook C, Langham M. Effect of cortisone on vascularization and opacification of the cornea induced by alloxan. Br J Ophthalmol 1951;35:718–724.
112. Phillips K, Arffa R, Cintron C, et al. Effects of prednisolone and medroxyprogesterone on corneal wound healing, ulceration and neovascularization. Arch Ophthalmol 1983;101: 640–643.
113. McNatt LG, Weimer L, Yanni J, Clark AF. Angiostatic activity of steroids in the chick embryo CAM and rabbit cornea models of neovascularization. J Ocul Pharmacol Ther 1999;15:413–423.
114. Carmichael TR, Gelfand Y, Welsh NH. Topical steroids in the treatment of central and paracentral corneal ulcers. Br J Ophthalmol 1990;74:528–531.
115. Stern GA, Buttross M. Use of corticosteroids in combination with antimicrobial drugs in the treatment of infectous corneal disease. Ophthalmology 1991;98:847–853.
116. BenEzra D, Griffin BW, Maftzir G, Sharif NA, Clark AF. Topical formulations of novel angiostatic steroids inhibit rabbit corneal neovascularization. Invest Ophthalmol Vis Sci 1997;38:1954–1962.
117. Takahashi K, Saishin Y, Saishin Y, et al. Topical nepafenac inhibits ocular neovascularization. Invest Ophthalmol Vis Sci 2003;44:409–415.
118. Lipman RM, Epstein RJ, Hendricks RL. Suppression of corneal neovascularization with cyclosporine. Arch Ophthalmol 1992;110:405–407.
119. Joussen AM, Beecken WD, Moromizato Y, Schwartz A, Kirchhof B, Poulaki V. Inhibition of inflammatory corneal angiogenesis by TNP-470. Invest Ophthalmol Vis Sci 2001;42:2510–2516.
120. Ambati BK, Joussen AM, Kuziel WA, Adamis AP, Ambati J. Inhibition of corneal neovascularization by genetic ablation of CCR2. Cornea 2003;22:465–467.
121. Ambati BK, Anand A, Joussen AM, Kuziel WA, Adamis AP, Ambati J. Sustained inhibition of corneal neovascularization by genetic ablation of CCR5. Invest Ophthalmol Vis Sci 2003;44:590–593.
122. Fire A, Xu S, Montgomery MK, Kostas SA, Driver SE, Mello CC. Potent and specific genetic interference by double-stranded RNA in *Caenorhabditis elegans*. Nature 1998;391:806–811.
123. Winston WM, Molodowitch C, Hunter CP. Systemic RNAi in C. elegans requires the putative transmembrane protein SID-1. Science 2004;295:2456–2459.
124. Wu P-C, Liu C-C, Chen C-H, et al. Inhibition of experimental angiogenesis of cornea by somatostatin. Graefe's Arch Clin Exp Ophthalmol 2003;241:63–69.
125. Murthy RC, McFarland TJ, Yoken J, et al. Corneal transduction to inhibit angiogenesis and graft failure. Invest Ophthalmol Vis Sci 2003;44:1837–1842.
126. King GL, Suzuma K. Pigment-epithelium-derived factor—a key coordinator of retinal neuronal and vascular functions. N Engl J Med 2000;342:349–351.
127. Dawson DW, Volpert OV, Gillis P, et al. Pigment epithelium-derived factor: a potent inhibitor of angiogenesis. Science 1999;285:245–248.
128. Tombran-Tink J, Barnstable CJ. PEDF: a multifacted neurotrophic factor. Nat Rev Neurosci 2003;4:628–636.
129. Mori K, Gehlbach P, Ando A, McVey D, Wei L, Campochiaro PA. Regression of ocular neovascularization in response to increased expression of pigment epithelium-derived factor. Invest Ophthalmol Vis Sci 2002;43:2428–2434.

4
Polypoidal Choroidal Vasculopathy

Nahoko Ogata, MD, PhD and Kanji Takahashi, MD, PhD

CONTENTS

INTRODUCTION

Polypoidal choroidal vasculopathy (PCV) is a relatively new clinical entity characterized by multiple recurrent serous or hemorrhagic detachments of the retinal pigment epithelium (RPE) and retina in the posterior pole of the eye. PCV was formerly reported as a peculiar hemorrhagic disorder of the macula, characterized by recurrent subretinal and subretinal pigment epithelial bleeding found in middle-aged black women *(1–4)*. Yanuzzi initially suggested the term "idiopathic polypoidal choroidal vasculopathy" *(5)* because the pathogenesis was unknown, but in recent years this condition has simply been called "polypoidal choroidal vasculopathy."

PCV is characterized by an abnormal vascular network of choroidal vessels with polyplike dilations at the terminals of the branches. These polypoidal outpouchings are seen ophthalmoscopically as reddish-orange, spheroidal, polyplike structures at the terminals of the abnormal choroidal vessels *(5,6)*. Indocyanine green (ICG) angiography reveals the characteristics of PCV very clearly, and optical coherence tomography (OCT) has provided additional important information on the structure of the polypoidal lesions. PCV is much more common than previously appreciated *(3,7–9)*, and in recent years, the spectrum of PCV has been expanded *(7)*.

ETIOLOGY

Although the pathogenesis of PCV has still not been determined conclusively, it is generally thought to be a primary abnormality of the choroid. The network of abnormal

From: *Ophthalmology: Ocular Angiogenesis: Diseases, Mechanisms, and Therapeutics*
Edited by: J. Tombran-Tink and C. J. Barnstable © Humana Press Inc., Totowa, NJ

choroidal vessels is made up of two distinct components: (1) a complex of branching vessels and (2) multiple reddish-orange terminal aneurysmal or polypoidal lesions *(6–8)*.

Uyama et al. suggested that PCV was a peculiar form of subretinal pigment epithelial neovascularization *(10)*, and Yannuzzi et al. also believed that PCV represented a subtype of choroidal neovascularization (CNV) in age-related macular degeneration (AMD) *(8,11)*. On the other hand, Okubo et al. recently suggested that PCV represents degenerative changes or abnormalities of the choroidal vessels rather than neovascularization *(12)*. Whether PCVs represent abnormal vessels from the choroidal circulation or neovascularization from choroidal vessels is still being debated.

CLINICAL FEATURES

Age

PCV is most commonly found in patients between the ages of 50 and 65 yr; however, the age at diagnosis can range from 20 to 80 yr, with a mean age of 60.1 yr *(11)*. Caucasian patients usually present at an older age *(8)*.

Race and Sex

PCV was originally reported to occur in highly pigmented women *(2)*, but more recent cases include women of Caucasian descent as well as men *(4,7,13)*. Although PCV was originally described as usually peripapillary *(1–4,6,7,14)*, currently PCV has been reported to be prevalent in the macula of elderly people of any race and gender *(9,10,15–17)*.

Fundus

The diagnosis of PCV is made by the presence of reddish-orange subretinal nodules in the posterior pole, exudative manifestations such as hemorrhagic or serous pigment epithelial and retinal detachments, retinal edema, and lipid depositions (hard exudates) *(6,14)*.

In patients with PCV limited to the macula, the vascular network often arises in the macula and follows an oval distribution pattern (Figs. 1A and 5A). In patients with peripapillary lesions, the vascular channels usually follow a radial, arching pattern and may be interconnected with small spanning branches that are more evident and numerous at the edges of the lesion (Fig. 2A). It has been suggested that there are two patterns of clinical manifestation of PCV: hemorrhagic and exudative *(18)*. The hemorrhagic pattern is characterized by hemorrhagic pigment epithelial detachments (PEDs) and subretinal hemorrhages in the macula that mimic exudative age-related macular degeneration (AMD) (Fig. 3A). The exudative pattern is characterized by serous PEDs and serous retinal detachments associated with intraretinal lipid deposits in the macula. The fundus then resembles chronic central serous chorioretinopathy in the elderly (Fig. 4A).

The retinal manifestations of PCV resemble those of neovascular AMD. Serous retinal detachment and PEDs are most common (52%), followed by retinal hemorrhages (30%), hemorrhagic PEDs (18%), subretinal hematomas (12%), and RPE degeneration and atrophy (10%) *(9)*. There is a lower percentage of eyes with subretinal fibrovascular proliferations (7%) in patients with PCV than with AMD, probably because of the low level of fibrovascular proliferation and hyperplasia of the RPE *(7,9)*. When present, the subretinal fibrosis proliferation in the macula severely damages the sensory retina and RPE and leads to marked visual loss.

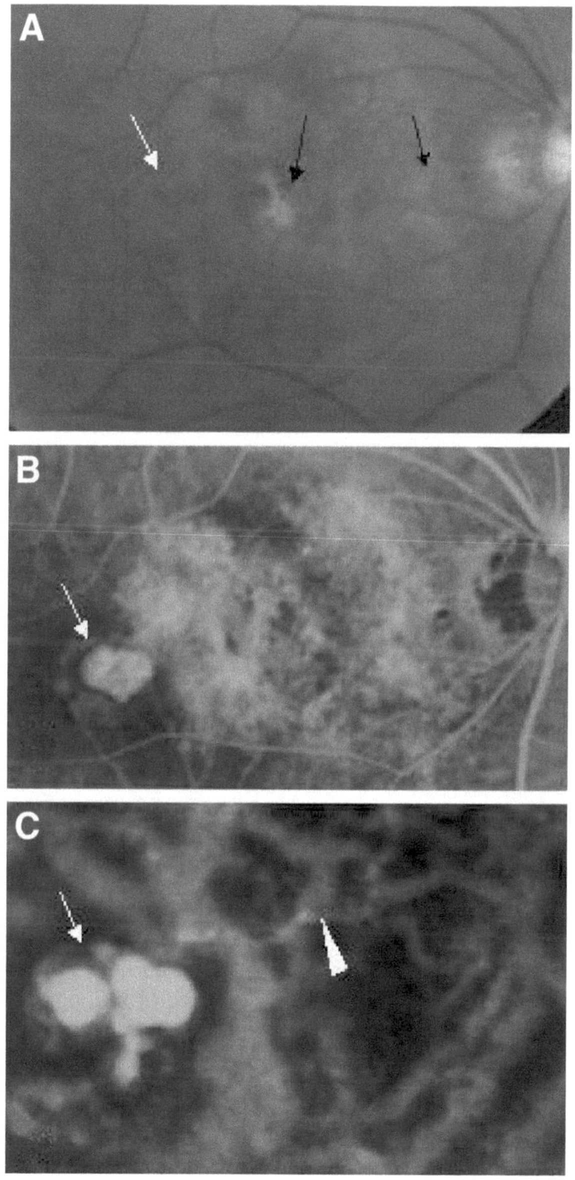

Fig. 1. Case 1, polypoidal choroidal vasculopathy in a macular lesion. **(A)** Fundus photograph. There are reddish-orange subretinal nodules (white arrow) associated with retinal pigment epithelium atrophy (black arrows). **(B)** Fluorescein angiography. The corresponding polypoidal dilations (white arrow) are seen as spotty hyperfluorescence. **(C)** Indocyanine green angiography. Shortly after the network (arrowhead) can be identified, hyperfluorescent "polyps" (white arrow) become easily identifiable within the choroid. *See* color version on companion CD.

Fluorescein Angiography

Most of the polypoidal dilations in PCV are detected as spotty hyperfluorescence, and some show slight leakages (Figs. 1B and 5B) *(19)*. The branching networks are not seen on fluorescein angiography because the network lies beneath the RPE. In a few eyes, the networks are visible as hyperfluorescence through the atrophic RPE.

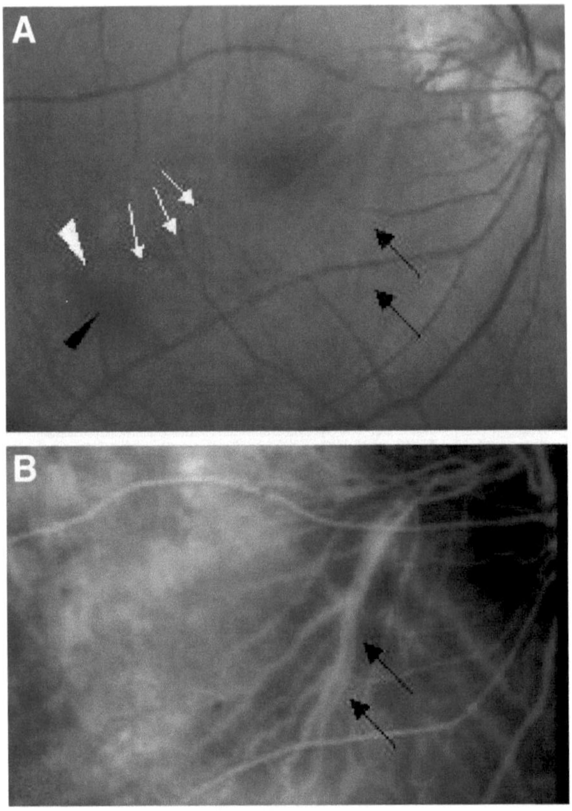

Fig. 2. Case 2, polypoidal choroidal vasculopathy in peripapillary lesion. **(A)** Fundus photography. Reddish-orange subretinal nodules (white arrows can be seen). The vascular channels follow a radial, arching pattern (black arrows). Pigment epithelial detachment (white arrow head) and subretinal pigment epithelium hemorrhage (black arrowhead) are seen. **(B)** Indocyanine green angiography. The structure of the radial, arching pattern of the network of vessels is clearly seen (black arrows). The vascular network has an umbrella-like appearance and spreads to beneath the retinal pigment epithelium layer. *See* color version on companion CD.

Indocyanine Green Angiography

Although the abnormal vascular choroidal changes in PCV can be detected by slit-lamp biomicroscopy with a contact lens, an exact diagnosis of PCV can be made only by ICG angiography. ICG angiography demonstrates the branching vascular network from the choroidal circulation and polypoidal or aneurysmal dilations at the terminal of the branching vessels *(7,10,14,15,17,20–22)*.

In the early stage of ICG angiography, the larger vessels of the PCV network are filled prior to the filling of the retinal vessels. Shortly after the network is identified, small hyperfluorescent "polyps" become easily identifiable within the choroid (Figs. 1C, 3B, 4B, 5B). The polypoidal structures seen on ICG angiography correspond to the reddish-orange lesions visible on biomicroscopy, although the network vessels may appear more extensive on ICG than on clinical examinations (Fig. 3B). The vascular network has an umbrellalike appearance and spreads beneath the RPE. The feeder artery to the PCV originates from the choroidal circulation and supplies the center of

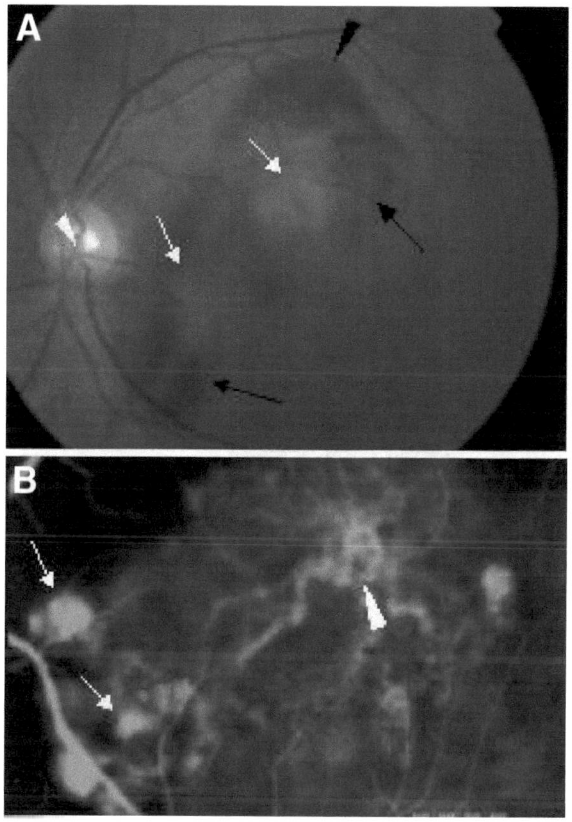

Fig. 3. Case 3, hemorrhagic polypoidal choroidal vasculopathy. **(A)** Fundus photograph. Reddish-orange subretinal nodules (white arrows can be seen). Hemorrhagic pigment epithelial detachments (black arrows) and subretinal hemorrhages (black arrowhead) are observed in the macula. **(B)** Indocyanine green (ICG) angiography. The branching vascular network (white arrowhead) from the choroidal circulation and polypoidal or aneurysmal dilations (white arrows) at the terminal of the branching vessels can be seen. The polypoidal structures seen on ICG angiography correspond to the reddish-orange lesions visible on biomicroscopy, although the network vessels appear more extensive on the ICG angiograms than on clinical examinations. *See* color version on companion CD.

the branching vascular network (Fig. 2B). The late phase of ICG angiography is associated with a reversal of the pattern of fluorescence previously observed.

Approximately half of the polypoidal vascular lesions found by ICG angiography are seen in the macula as reddish-orange nodular elevations of the RPE by ophthalmoscopy and slit-lamp biomicroscopy with a contact lens. However, the other half of the lesions are not seen by ophthalmoscopy because they are covered by subretinal hemorrhages, exudations, or PEDs.

Optical Coherence Tomography

OCT has also proven to be useful in the diagnosis of PCV *(23–25)*. The typical OCT image shows domelike elevations of the RPE and nodular structures beneath the RPE (Figs. 4C,5C). The walls of the orange nodules form a highly reflective band that has a tendency to bulge anteriorly beneath the detached retinal pigment epithelium.

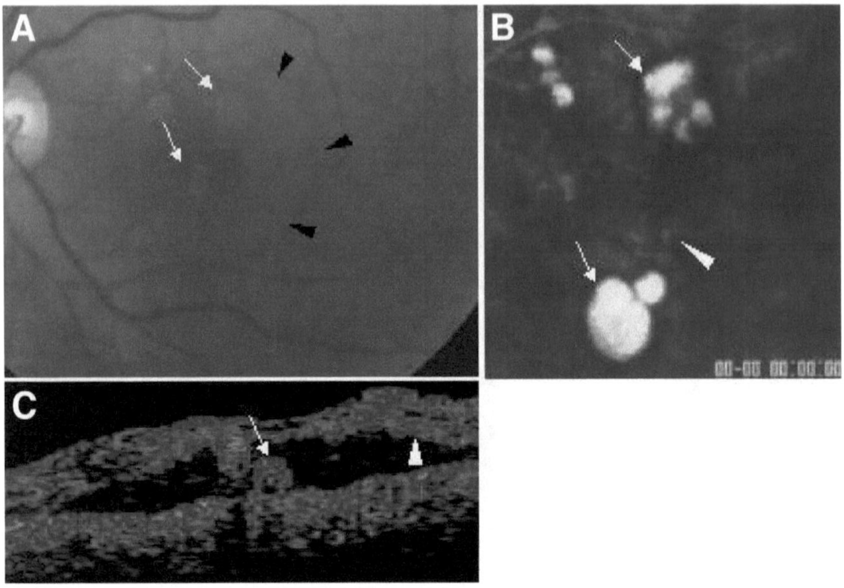

Fig. 4. Case 4, exudative polypoidal choroidal vasculopathy. **(A)** Fundus photograph. Reddish-orange subretinal nodules (white arrows) are associated with serous pigment epithelial detachments and serous retinal detachments (black arrowheads) in the macula. **(B)** Indocyanine green angiography. The vascular network arises in the macula (white arrowhead) and polypoidal dilations (white arrows) can be seen at the terminal of the branching vessels (white arrowhead). **(C)** Optical coherence tomography images show detached sensory retina (white arrowhead) and a nodular structure beneath the retinal pigment epithelium cell layer (white arrow). *See* color version on companion CD.

Natural Course

PCV often follows a remission-relapsing course, and is associated clinically with chronic multiple recurrent serosanguinous detachments of the RPE and neurosensory retina with long-term preservation of good vision. Uyama et al. followed 14 eyes with PCV without any treatment and found that 50% of the patients had a favorable course *(18)*. However, the other half had unfavorable outcomes because of repeated bleeding and leakage, resulting in macular degeneration and visual loss. Sho et al. also reported severe visual loss in 35% of the eyes *(9)*.

In cases of PCV, reactive fibrous proliferation resulting in a typical disciform degeneration, a characteristic of end-stage neovascular AMD, is rare *(6,9,18)*. PCVs progress more slowly than AMD. Thus, the visual outcome is markedly more favorable in PCV than in neovascular AMD.

Fig. 5. Case 5, surgically removed polypoidal choroidal vasculopathy. **(A)** Preoperative fundus photograph. Subretinal hemorrhage and pigment epithelial detachment (PED) can be seen (arrow). **(B)** Preoperative fluorescein angiography. Fluorescein angiography shows fluorescein leakage from the lesion and fluorescein pooling corresponding to the PED. **(C)** Optical coherence tomography. An elevation of the sensory retina by a highly reflective, domelike layer is displayed. **(D)** Preoperative indocyanine green (ICG) angiography. ICG angiography shows polyplike lesions (arrow) with an associated abnormal vascular network (white arrowhead). **(E)** Hematoxylin and eosin section.

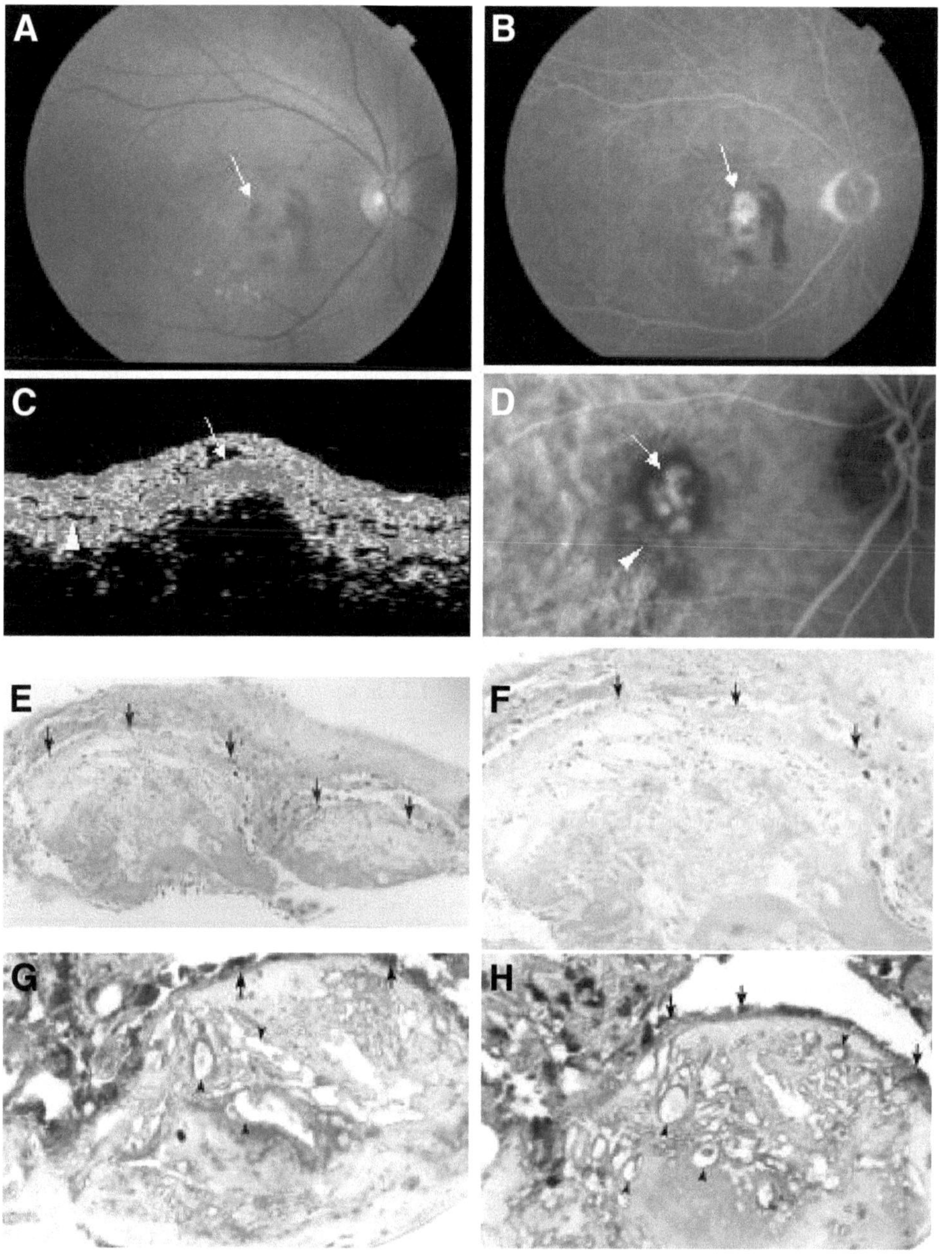

Fig. 5. *(Continued)* The fibrovascular tissue corresponds to the polypoidal lesion. Fibrovascular tissue is observed beneath the domelike elevation of the retinal pigment epithelium (RPE) layer (arrows). **(F)** A high-power photograph of E. The fibrovascular tissue contains numerous dilated thin-wall vessels and massive fibrin-like materials. **(G)** Pigment epithelium-derived factor (PEDF) expression. Strong immunoreactivity for PEDF is observed in the RPE (arrows) located above the fibrovascular membrane and also detected in the endothelial cells of the numerous abnormal vessels (arrowheads). **(H)** Vascular endothelial growth factor (VEGF) expression. Strong immunoreactivity for VEGF is observed in the RPE (arrows) located above the fibrovascular membrane and also in the endothelial cells of the numerous abnormal vessels (arrowheads). Scale bars, 100 μm. (Reproduced with permission from ref. *31*.) *See* color version on companion CD.

Differential Diagnosis

It is important to differentiate PCVs from AMDs. Some patients who were diagnosed with AMD and received ICG were found to actually have PCV rather than AMD on reviewing their ICG records. Vascular changes typical of PCV form a network of vessels ending with popypoidal lesions that are red to orange in color and are visible by slit-lamp biomicroscopy unless they are camouflaged by overlying exudates or blood. On the other hand, the vascular changes of the CNV associated with AMD tend to produce small-caliber vessels that have a grayish discoloration of the overlying retina. Flourescein angiography and ICG angiography can be used to distinguish the two entities. In both types of angiography, CNVs are characterized by diffuse late-staining plaques, whereas the choroidal network in PCVs is seen by ICG angiography as prominent vascular network in the early stages and a clearing of the dye in the late stage.

PCVs have been also reported to be associated with dry AMD *(26)*. However, characteristically, PCVs are rarely associated with conventional CNV (9%), suggesting that the pathogenesis of PCV differs from the CNV in AMD *(9)*.

In some patients, PCV presents as purely exudative changes and masquerades as a choronic decompensation of the RPE, a variant of central serous chorioretinopathy *(18,20)*. The polypoidal lesions resemble small PEDs both clinically and on flourescein angiography. The method of differentiating small serous PEDs from polypoidal lesions is by ICG angiography. The late staining of the PED is seen with flourescein angiography and hypofluorescence with ICG angiography. On the other hand, the polypoidal lesions are usually hyperfluorescent with ICG due to their vascular nature.

PATHOLOGY

The peculiar abnormality of PCV is believed to originate in the inner choroid. Whether PCVs represent abnormal vessels from the choroidal circulation or neovascularization from choroidal vessels is still being debated *(8,10,12)*.

Several clinicopathological studies of PCV have been reported *(12,15,27–31)*. MacCumber et al. showed extensive fibrovascular proliferation within Bruch's membrane and in the subretinal space *(27)*. Reynders et al. reported that the grossly dilated, thin-walled vessels in the specimen from one hemorrhagic AMD case were suggestive of PCV *(28)*. Lafaut et al. reported that the submacular tissue removed from an eye with PCV showed several dilated thin-walled vessels, and the aneurysmic vessels appeared to be of venular origin *(15)*. They suggested that PCVs represent a subtype of the CNV in AMD.

Okubo et al. on the other hand, found tortuous, unusually dilated venules in a surgically removed, submacular polypoidal vascular lesion *(15)*. The lesion consisted of degenerated RPE–Bruch's membrane–choriocapillaris complex and the inner choroids containing large dilated venules and arterioles. The diameters of the vessels (300 μm), and the structures and location of the tortuous venules associated with the arterioles, suggest that they were native, dilated choroidal venules rather than new vessels. Their findings suggested that PCV was a degenerative change or abnormality of the choroidal vessels. The authors hypothesized that the hyperpermeability and hemorrhages due to the stasis of blood in the vessel might cause edema and degeneration of the tissue.

Terasaki et al. reported clusters of dilated, thin-walled blood vessels surrounded by macrophages and fibrin material in two neovascular membranes obtained during macular translocation surgery for PCV *(30)*. They reported that the fibrovascular tissue was located under the basement membrane of the RPE and the elastic fiber layer of Bruch's membrane. The abnormal vessels were lined by a thin endothelium without pericytes. The vessels were surrounded by massive fibrin material. More recently, Matsuoka et al. examined a surgically removed PCV and found that the histological appearance of PCV differed from that of CNV membranes *(31)*. The fibrovascular tissues that appeared to correspond to the polypoidal lesions seen ophthalmoscopically and in ICG angiography were observed under the RPE and contained numerous dilated, thin-walled vessels and massive fibrin-like material (Fig. 3).

MOLECULAR MECHANISMS

Although the molecular mechanisms of PCV are still unknown, a recent investigation demonstrated that vascular endothelial growth factor (VEGF), a strong stimulus of angiogenesis, was expressed in the vascular endothelial cells and the RPE of eyes with PCV *(30)*.

More recently, we investigated the expression of VEGF and pigment epithelial-derived factor (PEDF), an endogenous inhibitor of angiogenesis, in surgically removed PCV tissues *(31)*. The specimens of PCV showed strong immunoreactivity for VEGF in the RPE located above the fibrovascular membrane and also in the endothelial cells of the numerous abnormal vessels (Fig. 5E,F). In addition, these VEGF-positive cells also showed strong immunoreactivity for PEDF (Fig. 5G,H). It has been reported that when subfoveal fibrovascular membranes are active, both VEGF and PEDF are strongly expressed in the endothelial cells *(32)*. Thus, this case of PCV has the characteristics of an active subfoveal fibrovascular membrane. These data strongly suggest that PEDF and VEGF play an important role in the development and/or maintenance of PCV.

THERAPEUTICS

Laser Photocoagulation

The treatment for PCV has not been well established. It is generally recommended that a conservative approach be taken unless the lesion is associated with persistent or progressive exudative changes threatening central vision. In these cases, conventional laser treatment of the leaking polypoidal vascular abnormalities may lead to the resolution of the serous-hemorrhagic manifestations *(10,33,34)*.

Yuzawa et al. reported that laser photocoagulation of the entire extrafoveal leasion showed improvement or no change in visual acuity *(34)*. This means that recurrent serosanguineous detachments are unlikely to occur after the entire lesion is coagulated. When only the polypoidal lesions were coagulated, the visual outcome was poor. However, definitive clinical trials to establish the efficacy of laser treatment are needed to confirm these observations.

Vitrectomy

In some cases, vitrectomy is required to clear the media to recover vision. Shiraga et al. reported anatomic success following vitrectomy to treat the submacular hemorrhage associated with PCV *(35)*. However, the value of submacular surgery has been questioned because of recurrence and poor visual outcomes *(36,37)*. In addition, the lesion of PCV is located beneath the RPE, and the removal of the PCV will result in a wide area of bare RPE. The visual outcome of the patients is poor.

Translocation

Macular translocation is another possible treatment for PCV *(30)*, but most patients with PCV have relatively large vascular lesions, and translocation is not valuable.

Transpupillary Thermotherapy

Transpupillary thermotherapy (TTT) shows some promise in treating occult choroidal neovasculatization with serous retinal detachment, but the value of TTT for PCV is unknown.

Photodynamic Therapy

Photodynamic therapy (PDT) with verteporfin has been reported to be effective and safe in patients with subfoveal PCVs *(38)*. However, definitive clinical trials to establish the efficacy and safety of PDT for PCV are needed to confirm these observations.

REFERENCES

1. Kleiner RC, Brucker AJ, Johnson RL. Posterior uveal bleeding syndrome. Ophthalmology 1984;91:110.
2. Stern RM, Zakow N, Zegarra H. Muptiple recurrent serous sanguineous retinal pigment epithelial detachments in black women. Am J Ophthalmol 1985;100:560–569.
3. Kleiner RC, Brucker AJ, Johnson RL. The posterior uveal bleeding syndrome. Retina 1990;10:9–17.
4. Perkovich BT, Zakov N, Berlin LA. An update on multiple recurrent serous sanguineous retinal pigment epithelial detachments in black women. Retina 1990;10:18–26.
5. Yannuzzi LA. Idiopathic popypoidal choroidal vasculopathy. Presented at the Macula Society meeting, Miami, Florida, 1982.
6. Yannuzzi LA, Sorenson J, Spaide RF, et al. Idiopathic popypoidal choroidal vasculopathy (IPCV). Retina 1990;10:1–8.
7. Yannuzzi LA, Ciardella A, Spaide RF, et al. The expanding clinical spectrum of idiopathic popypoidal choroidal vasculopathy. Arch Ophthalmol 1997;115:478–485.
8. Yannuzzi LA, Wong DW, Sforzolini BS, et al. Polypoidal choroidal vasculopathy and neovascularized age-related macular degenetration. Arch Ophthalmol 1999;117:1503–1510.
9. Sho K, Takahashi K, Yamada H, et al. Polypoidal choroidal vasculopathy. Incidence, demographic features, and clinical characteristics. Arch Ophthalmol 2003;121:1392–1396.
10. Uyama M, Matsubara T, Fukuchima I, et al. Idiopathic polypoidal choroidal vasculopathy in Japanese patients. Arch Ophthalmol 1999;117:1035–1042.
11. Ciardella AP, Donsoff IM, Hung SJ, Costa DL, Yannuzzi LA. Polypoidal choroidal vasculopathy. Surv Ophthalmol 2004;49:25–37.
12. Okubo A, Sameshima M, Uemura A, et al. Clinicopathological correlation of polypoidal choroidal vasculopathy revealed by ultrastructual study. Br J Ophthalmol 2002;86:1093–1098.
13. Lafaut BA, Ley AM, Snyers B, Rasquin F, Laey JJ. Popypoidal choroidal vasculopathy in Caucasians. Graefes Arch Clin Exp Ophthalmol 2002;238:752–759.
14. Spaide RF, Yannuzzi LA, Slakter JS, et al. Indocyanine angiography of idiopathic choroidal vasculopathy. Retina 1995;15:100–110.

15. Lafaut BA, Aisenbrey S, van den Broecke C. Polypoidal choroidal vasculopathy pattern in age-related macular degeneration. Retina 2000;20:650–654.
16. Yannuzzi LA, Nogueira FB, Spaide RF, et al. Idiopathic polypoidal choroidal vasculopathy: peripheral lesion. Arch Ophthalmol 1998;116:382,383.
17. Moorthy RS, Lyon AT, Tabb MF, et al. Idiopathic polypoidal choroidal vasculopathy of the macula. Ophthalmology 1998;105:1380–1385.
18. Uyama M, Wada M, Nagai Y, et al. Polypoidal choroidal vasculopathy: Natural history. Am J Ophthalmol 2002;133:639–648.
19. Iida T, Yannuzzi LA, Freund KB, Ciardella AP. Retinal angiography and popypoidal choroidal vasculopathy. Retina 2002;22:455–463.
20. Yannuzzi LA, Freud KB, Goldbaum M, et al. Popypoidal choroidal vasculopathy masquerading as central serous chorioretinopathy. Ophthalmology 2000;107:767–777.
21. Phillips WB II, Regillo CD, Mauire JI. Indocyanine angiography of idiopathic polypoidal choroidal vasculopathy. Ophthalmic Surg Lasers 1996;27:467–470.
22. Schneider U, Gelisken F, Kreissig I. Indocyanine angiography and idiopathic polypoidal choroidal vasculopathy. Br J Ophthalmol 1998;82:98,99.
23. Iijima H, Imai M, Gohodo T. Optical coherence tomography of idiopathic polypoidal choroidal vasculopathy. Am J Ophthalmol 1999;127:301–305.
24. Iijima H, Iida T, Imai M. Optical coherence tomography of orange-red subretinal lesions in eyes with idiopathic polypoidal choroidal vasculopathy. Am J Ophthalmol 2000;129: 21–26.
25. Otsuji T, Takahashi K, Fukushima I. Optical coherence tomography findings in idiopathic polypoidal choroidal vasculopathy. Ophthalmic Surg Lasers 2000;31:210–214.
26. Lois N. Idiopathic polypoidal choroidal vasculopathy in a patients with atrophic age-related macular degeneration. Br J Ophthalmol 2001;85:1011,1012.
27. MacCumber MW, Dastgheib K, Bressler NM. Clinicopathological correlation of the multiple recurrent serous anguineous retinal pigment epithelial detachments syndrome. Retina 1995;14:143–152.
28. Reynders S, Lafaut BA, Aisenbrey S, van den Broecke C. Clinicopathologic correlation in hemorrhagic age-related macular degeneration. Graefes Arch Clin Exp Ophthalmol 2002;240:279–285.
29. Rosa RH Jr, Davis JL, Eifrig CW. Clinicopathologic correlation of idiopathic polypoidal choroidal vasculopathy. Arch Ophthalmol 2002;120:502–508.
30. Terasaki H, Miyake Y, Nakamura M, et al. Polypoidal choroidal vasculopathy treated with macular translocation: clinical pathological correlation. Br J Ophthalmol 2002;86: 321–327.
31. Matsuoka M, Ogata N, Otsuji T, Nishimura T, Takahashi K, Matsumura M. Expression of pigment epithelium-derived factor and vascular endothelial growth factor in choroidal neovascular membranes and polypoidal choroidal vasculopathy. Br J Ophthalmol 2004;88: 809–815.
32. Ogata N, Wada M, Otsuji T, et al. Expression of pigment epithelium-derived factor in normal adult rat eye and experimental choroidal neovascularization. Invest Ophthalmol Vis Sci 2002;43:1168–1175.
33. Guyer DR, Yannuzzi LA, Ladas I. Indocyanine-green angiography guided laser photocoagulation of focal spots at the edge of plaques of choroidal neovascularization. Arch Ophthalmol 1996;114:693–697.
34. Yuzawa M, Mori R, Haruyama M. A study of laser photocoagulation for polypoidal choroidal vasculopathy. Jpn J Ophthalmol 2003;47:379–384.
35. Shiraga F, Matsuo T, Yokoe S. Surgical treatment of submacular hemorrhage associated idiopathic popypoidal choroidal vasculopathy. Am J Ophthalmol 1999;128:147–154.

36. Merill PT, LoRusso FJ, Lomeo MD. Surgically removed subfoveal choroidal neovascularization in age-related macular degeneration. Ophthalmology 1999;106:782–789.
37. Yuzawa M, Isomae T, Mori R. Surgical excision versus laser photocoagulation for subfoveal choroidal neovascular membranes with age-related macular degeneration. Jpn J Ophthalmol 2001;45:192–198.
38. Quaranta M, Maget-Faysse M, Coscas G. Exudative idiopathic popypoidal choroidal vasculopathy and photodynamic therapy with verteporfin. Am J Ophthalmol 2002;134:277–280.

5

Myopic Choroidal Neovascularization

Kyoko Ohno-Matsui, MD and Takashi Tokoro, MD, PhD

CONTENTS

INTRODUCTION

Pathological myopia is synonymous with high myopia and generally refers to a condition in which individuals have greater than 6 to 8 diopters of myopia or an axial length greater than 26 to 27 mm *(1,2)*. Pathological myopia is a major cause of legal blindness in many developed countries *(2–4)*, affecting 27 to 33% of all myopic eyes, which corresponds to a prevalence of 0.2 to 0.4% in the general population of the United States *(4)*. High myopia is especially common in Asia and the Middle East. In Japan, the number of cases of myopia is unknown, but pathological or high myopia affects 6 to 18% of the myopic population and approx 1% of the general population *(5)*.

Pathological myopia is associated with progressive and excessive elongation of the eyeball, which results in various funduscopic changes within the posterior staphyloma *(6,7)*. Among the various myopic fundus lesions, macular choroidal neovascularization (CNV) is the most common vision-threatening complication of high myopia *(8–10)*. Myopic CNV causes an abrupt decrease in central vision in highly myopic patients. After absorption of hemorrhage and transudate, a round or elliptical black lesion in the macula, the so-called "Fuchs' spot," is formed by hyperplasia of the retinal pigment epithelial cells over the subretinal neovascular membrane. Although the pathogenesis of CNV development in highly myopic eyes is unclear, much attention has recently focused on newly developed active treatments for myopic CNV, including photodynamic therapy and foveal translocation.

From: *Ophthalmology: Ocular Angiogenesis: Diseases, Mechanisms, and Therapeutics*
Edited by: J. Tombran-Tink and C. J. Barnstable © Humana Press Inc., Totowa, NJ

In this chapter, we describe the overview of myopic CNV, including its etiology, pathogenesis, fundus features, prognosis, and new treatments.

ETIOLOGY OF MYOPIC CNV

Pathological myopia is the most common cause of CNV in young patients. Cohen et al. *(11)* reported that high myopia accounts for 62% of CNV in patients younger than 50 yr of age. Therefore, there are social and economic consequences of CNV. Among the general population, Vongphanit et al. *(12)* reported the prevalence of myopic retinopathy among 3654 residents aged 49 yr or older who participated in the Blue Mountains Eye Study; myopic retinopathy was observed in 1.2% of the participants, and Fuchs' spot was observed in 0.1%. Curtin and Karlin *(13)* reported that CNV affects 5.2% of eyes whose axial length is greater than 26.5 mm, and Grossniklaus and Green *(14)* reported that CNV was histopathologically observed in 5.2% of 308 myopic eyes.

These lesions frequently affect both eyes. The length of the follow-up period, however, alters the reported frequency of bilaterality. The reported incidence of binocular Fuchs' spots varies with reports: 12% *(15)*, 18% *(13)*, and 41% *(9)*. Involvement of the fellow eye may occur within a matter of days or years. Fried and coworkers *(9)* reported an average interval of 2.4 yr between the formation of these lesions, with a maximum of 8 yr. Ohno-Matsui et al. *(16)* followed 46 eyes with preexisting unilateral myopic CNV for an average of 130.2 mo. During the follow-up period, CNV occurred in 16 of 46 fellow eyes (34.8%) within 91.7 ± 52.4 mo after the onset of myopic CNV in the first eye.

Most study populations of CNV indicate a predominance of females: 2:1 *(9,13)* and 3:2 *(8,15)*. Regarding the female predominance of myopic CNV, Kobayashi et al. *(17)*. reported the expression of estrogen receptors in surgically excised CNV in highly myopic eyes, and suggested that estrogen has important functions in the formation of myopic CNV. The influence of female sex on CNV in myopia remains uncertain, however, because myopic retinopathies other than myopic CNV are also predominant in women. Vongphanit et al. *(12)* determined the prevalence of myopic retinopathy in 3654 participants who were 49 yr or older in the Blue Mountains Eye Study. Myopic retinopathy was observed in 1.4% of women and 1.0% in men. All types of myopic retinopathy were more commonly observed in women than in men: posterior staphyloma 17:9, lacquer cracks 7:1, Fuchs' spot 2:1, and chorioretinal atrophy 4:3.

PATHOGENESIS

Although the condition is fairly common, the pathogenesis of CNV in high myopia is not well understood. Breaks in Bruch's membrane (lacquer cracks) are frequently observed in the vicinity of myopic CNV. Avila et al. *(8)* reported that 82% of the eyes with myopic CNV had lacquer cracks. Ohno-Matsui et al. *(16)* determined the predisposing findings of CNV in a large series of highly myopic patients. CNV developed in 29.4% of eyes with lacquer cracks during the follow-up period. These studies indicate that breaks in Bruch's membrane are strongly associated with the development of CNV in myopic patients, as in patients with angioid streaks or choroidal rupture *(18)*. Also, activation of retinal pigment epithelial cells by mechanical stretching might be involved in the pathogenesis of myopic CNV. Seko et al. *(19)* reported increased production of vascular endothelial growth factor induced by pulsatile stretching in retinal pigment epithelial cells. Increased production of angiogenic factors induced by mechanical stretching, in addition to mechanical breaks in Bruch's membrane, might lead to the development of CNV in myopic patients.

Data regarding the ocular abnormalities associated with the development of CNV are conflicting. Spitznas et al. *(20)* reported a proportional risk of CNV with increasing myopia both below and above –6 D. Hotchkiss and Fine *(15)*, however, reported no correlation between axial length or staphyloma and CNV. On the other hand, Steidl et al. *(7)* reported an increased risk of CNV in eyes with smaller staphyloma. Eyes with the shallowest staphyloma depth displayed the greatest frequency of CNV. Steidl et al. *(7)* hypothesized that the eyes with a shallow staphyloma might have a healthier and more metabolically active posterior pole with well-perfused chorioretinal tissue and good capacity to respond to injury by neovascular ingrowth. They suggest that the development of CNV might require preservation of the choriocapillaris, as in eyes with less advanced stages of posterior staphyloma formation.

Circulatory abnormalities occur in various ophthalmic neovascular conditions, including age-related maculopathy *(21)*. Dimitrova et al. *(22)* measured retrobulbar circulation in the affected and fellow eyes of patients with unilateral myopic CNV, and reported an increased resistivity index in the posterior ciliary artery of the affected eye, suggesting that increased peripheral vascular resistivity is associated with angiogenesis in pathological myopia. Indocyanine green (ICG) angiography reveals that choroidal vascular abnormalities are also observed in highly myopic eyes. Ohno-Matsui et al. *(23)* reported that in 25% of highly myopic eyes, the vortex vein near the macula or optic nervehead and choroidal veins draining to the posteriorly dislocated vortex vein were dilated and stagnated. These kinds of choroidal circulatory changes might influence the development of CNV in myopic eyes.

DIAGNOSIS (FUNDUS CHARACTERISTICS)

The onset of transudation or hemorrhage from myopic CNV is often associated with sudden metamorphopsia and central vision decrease. In ophthalmoscopic examination, subretinal hemorrhage, observed as a "rim" of subretinal blood around the neovascular membrane, is frequently observed with fresh lesions (Fig. 1). In myopic CNV, the neovascular membrane is usually not covered by blood. Ophthalmoscopic examination reveals a grayish fibrous membrane within the area of subretinal blood in most cases. Small areas of CNV, however, are sometimes missed by ophthalmoscopic examination alone (Fig. 2). In that case, fluorescein fundus angiography is a powerful tool to identify the small neovascular membrane. Almost all myopic CNV shows classic signs of CNV on fluorescein angiography. Fluorescein angiography demonstrates CNV as clear hyperfluorescence of the neovascular net in the early angiographic phase and staining or dye leakage in the late angiographic phase (Fig. 3). Sometimes a dark rim is observed around the CNV (Fig. 4). Fluorescein angiography is always recommended, however, when highly myopic patients complain of a sudden decrease in central vision or metamorphopsia. Although ICG angiography is also a powerful tool to demonstrate CNV, myopic CNV is not identified as hyperfluorescence by ICG angiography in many cases, partly owing to the low activity of the

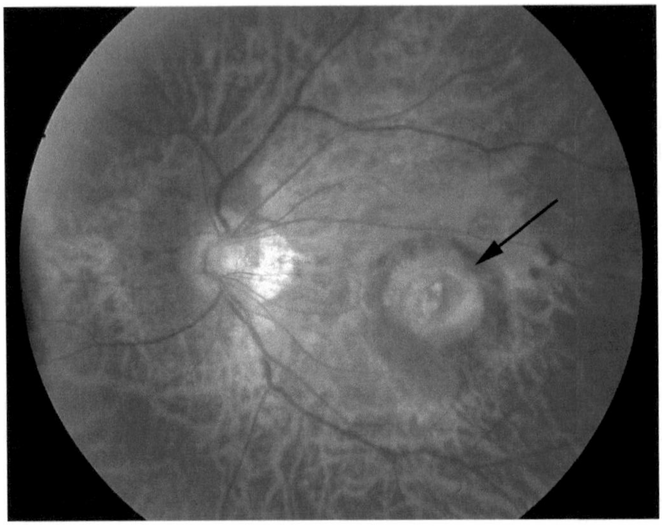

Fig. 1. Fundus photograph of typical myopic choroidal neovascular membrane at onset. Left fundus of a 70-yr-old woman. Refractive error is –15.0 D and the axial length is 30.5 mm in the right eye of the patient. Choroidal neovascular membrane (arrow) is recognized within the area of subretinal bleeding. *See* color version on companion CD.

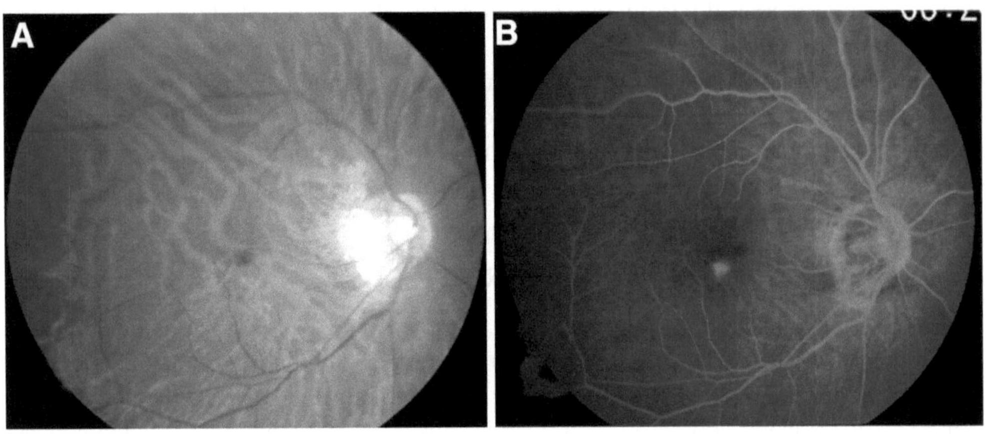

Fig. 2. Right fundus of a 52-yr-old woman. Refractive error is –16.0 D and axial length is 28.1 mm in the right eye of the patient. **(A)** Fundus photograph shows small subretinal bleeding below the fovea. Choroidal neovascular membrane is not obvious. **(B)** Fluorescein fundus angiogram shows clear hyperfluorescence due to choroidal neovascular membrane. *See* color version on companion CD.

neovascular membrane. Sometimes the intensity of myopic CNV in ICG angiography is similar to that of the choroidal background, and the CNV is detectable only because of the presence of the surrounding hypofluorescent rim (Fig. 5) *(24)*.

After absorption of the hemorrhage, round or elliptical black lesions occur in the macular area (Fuchs' spots) (Fig. 6). They are usually slightly elevated, sharply circumscribed, and vary in size. Fluorescein angiography findings in this phase include both blocked fluorescence due to pigmentation and hyperfluorescence due to staining of the neovascular membrane.

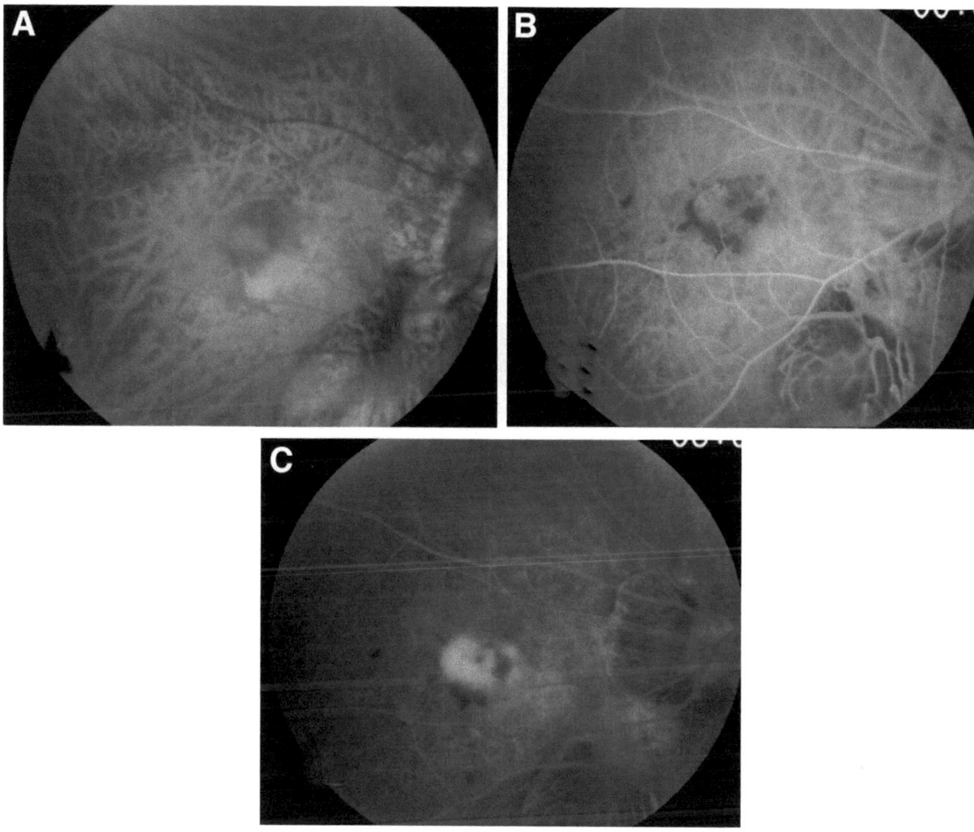

Fig. 3. Right fundus of a 59-yr-old woman. Refractive error is –11.5 D and the axial length is 25.5 mm in the right eye of the patient. (**A**) Fundus photograph shows a choroidal neovascular membrane surrounded by small area of subretinal bleeding. (**B**) The early phase of the fluorescein fundus angiogram shows a clear neovascular net within the choroidal neovascular membrane. (**C**) The late phase of fluorescein fundus angiogram shows tissue staining and slight dye leakage from the neovascular membrane. *See* color version on companion CD.

Optical coherence tomography (OCT) is a diagnostic imaging technique that produces cross-sectional images of the eye in a manner similar to ultrasound. OCT is a powerful tool for the identification of CNV and accompanying retinal edema. Baba et al. *(25)* reported OCT findings of myopic CNV, and demonstrated the effectiveness of OCT in evaluating the stage and activity of myopic CNV. OCT is also useful for detecting the effectiveness of therapy against CNV by examining the area decrease of CNV and the decrease in accompanying retinal edema.

DISEASE COURSE AND PROGNOSIS; NATURAL COURSE OF MYOPIC CNV

The natural history of CNV in high myopia is variable, and reports are somewhat conflicting. Some report a favorable prognosis for myopic CNV. Fried et al. *(9)* reported that in approx 63% of 55 eyes with myopic CNV, visual acuity was stabilized or improved without treatment within 36 to 180 mo after onset. Avila et al. *(8)* reported that in 96% of 70 eyes with myopic CNV, the CNV remained stable or regressed for an

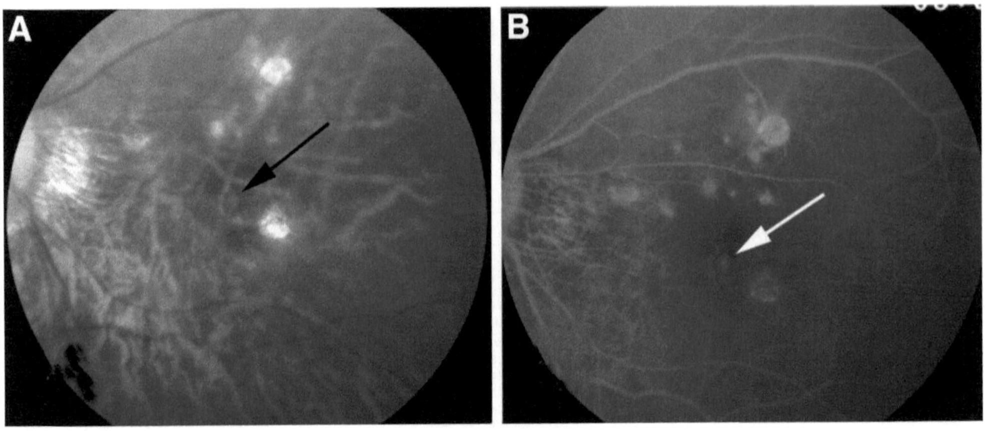

Fig. 4. Left fundus of a 43-yr-old woman. Refractive error is –11.0 D and the axial length is 27.3 mm in the left eye of the patient. (**A**) Fundus photograph shows a small pigmented fibrovascular membrane below the macula (arrow). Several whitish lesions of patchy chorioretinal atrophy are observed around the macula. (**B**) Fluorescein fundus angiogram shows hypofluorescent dark rim around the choroidal neovascular membrane (arrow). *See* color version on companion CD.

average of 40.9 mo, leaving an atrophic, nonexudative scar. Visual acuity remained stable or improved in 54% of the eyes. Others, however, report a poor prognosis. Hotchkiss and Fine *(15)* reported a series of 23 patients with myopic CNV observed for a mean of 26 mo and demonstrated that the final visual acuity was 20/200 or worse in 44%; however, 22% of the patients were treated with laser photocoagulation. Hampton et al. *(10)* observed 42 eyes with myopic CNV for 3 mo to 2 yr; the final visual acuity was 20/200 or worse in 60%.

Our clinical impression is that younger patients seem to maintain good vision compared with older patients. Tabandeh et al. *(26)* examined 22 patients older than 50 yr old with myopic CNV and reported that their visual prognosis was worse than that reported in previous studies that included patients of all ages. Yoshida et al. *(27)* examined 63 consecutive patients (73 eyes) with myopic CNV. They divided patients into two groups according to their ages (≤40 and >40 yr old) and followed them for more than 3 yr. Half the patients who were 40 yr old or less at onset retained a final visual acuity better than 20/40, and there was no significant change in the logarithm of the minimum angle of resolution (logMAR) during the follow-up period. On the other hand, logMAR worsened significantly during the follow-up in patients who were more than 40 yr old at onset of CNV, and more than half the patients in this group had a final visual acuity of less than 20/200. To further clarify the visual prognosis over a longer period, Yoshida et al. *(28)* next reviewed the medical records of 25 consecutive patients (27 eyes) with myopic CNV who were followed for at least 10 yr after the onset of CNV. The results indicated that at 3 yr after the onset of CNV, 55.5% retained a visual acuity of better than 20/200; however, at 5 and 10 yr after the onset, visual acuity dropped to 20/200 or less in 88.9 and 96.3% of the eyes, respectively (Fig. 7). Chorioretinal atrophy developed around the regressed CNV in 96.3% of eyes at 5 and 10 yr after the onset of CNV (Fig. 8). These studies indicated that if the patients are

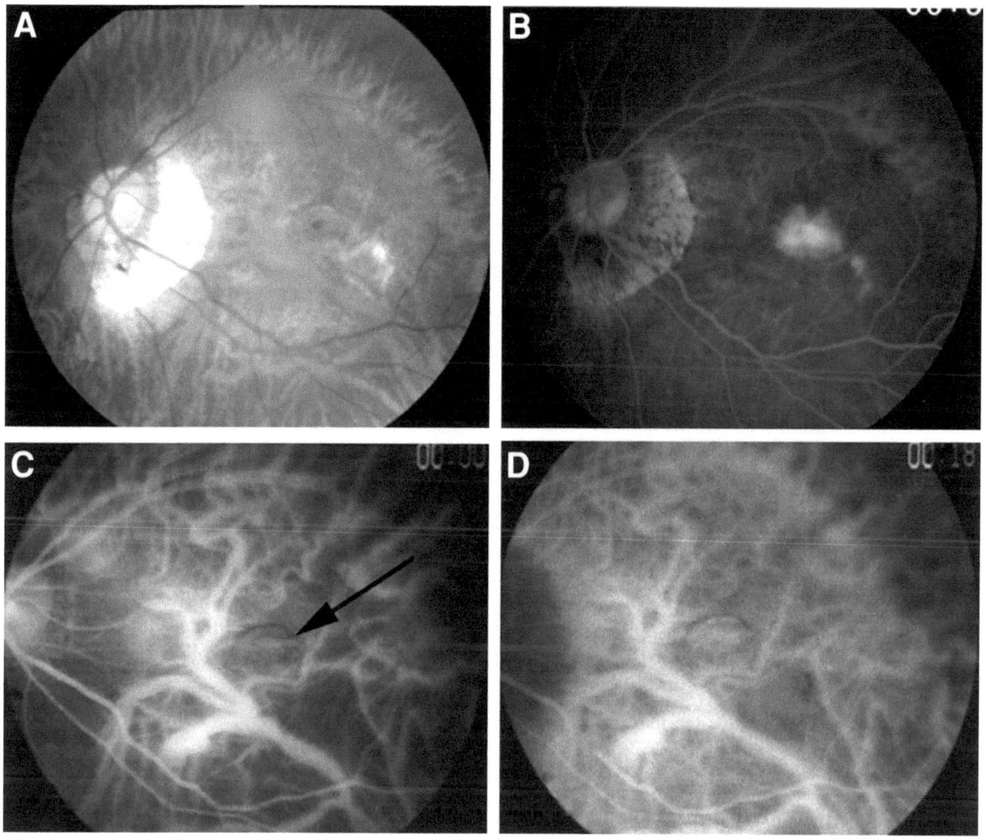

Fig. 5. Left fundus of a 63-yr-old woman. Refractive error is –9.0 D and the axial length is 28.7 mm in the left eye of the patient. **(A)** Left fundus shows a grayish fibrovascular membrane with small subretinal bleeding in the macula. **(B)** Fluorescein fundus angiogram shows hyperfluorescence at the corresponding site of choroidal neovascular membrane. **(C)** Early-phase indocyanine green (ICG) angiogram shows a hypofluorescent dark rim around the neovascular membrane (arrow). Dilated choroidal vein is observed in the vicinity of the neovascular membrane. **(D)** Late-phase ICG angiogram shows a choroidal neovascular membrane with similar intensity to surrounding choroidal tissue. A hyperfluorescent dark rim is observed around the neovascular membrane during the entire angiographic phase. *See* color version on companion CD.

young at the time of the onset of CNV, they might be able to retain good vision for a while. After a long period, however, most patients with myopic CNV eventually have a poor visual prognosis regardless of their age at onset, mainly due to an increased area of chorioretinal atrophy around the regressed CNV. To improve the long-term visual prognosis of myopic CNV, therefore, treatments that can also prevent the development of chorioretinal atrophy are necessary.

The mechanism underlying the later development of chorioretinal atrophy around myopic CNV is unclear, although this phenomenon seems characteristic of CNV caused by pathological myopia. Kojima et al. *(29)* examined factors affecting the development of chorioretinal atrophy in a large series of highly myopic patients using multivariate analysis. Multiple linear regression analysis revealed that patient age was the most

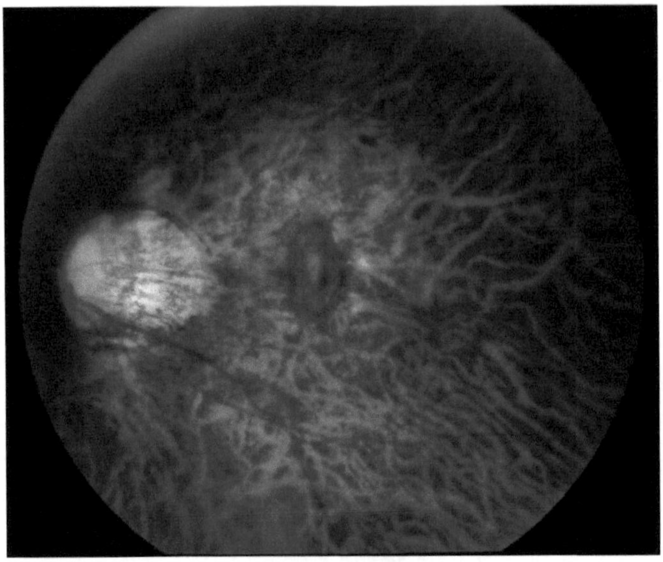

Fig. 6. Left fundus of a 46-yr-old woman. Refractive error is –12.5 D and the axial length is 30.0 mm in the left eye of the patient. Elliptical black lesion (so-called "Fuchs' spot") is observed in the macula. *See* color version on companion CD.

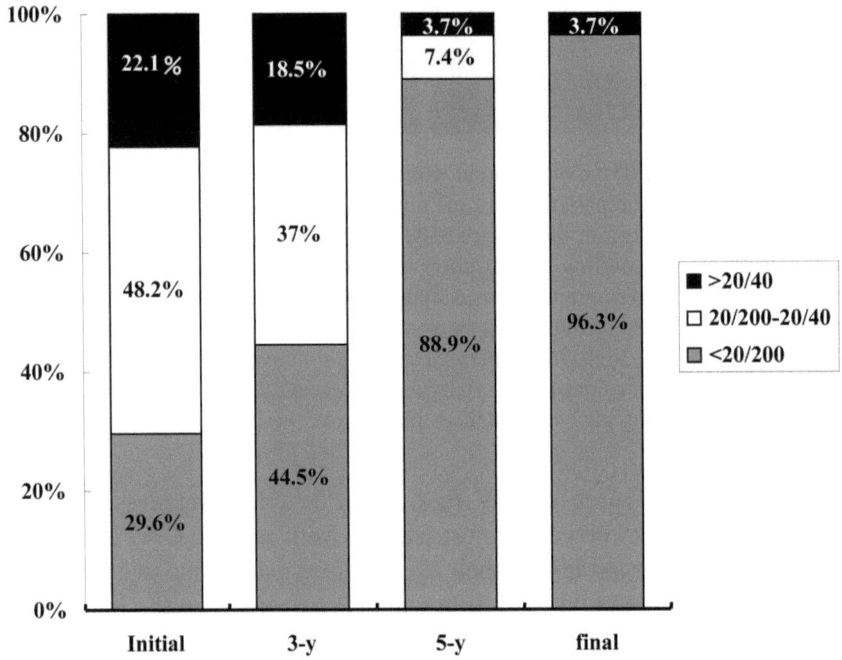

Fig. 7. Shift in the distribution of Snellen visual acuity in eyes with myopic choroidal neovascularization during the 10-yr follow-up period. (Reprinted with permission from ref. *28.*)

influential factor in the development of chorioretinal atrophy in all subjects. When the authors divided the subjects into two groups according to their age, however, CNV size was the only factor that influenced the development of chorioretinal atrophy in patients

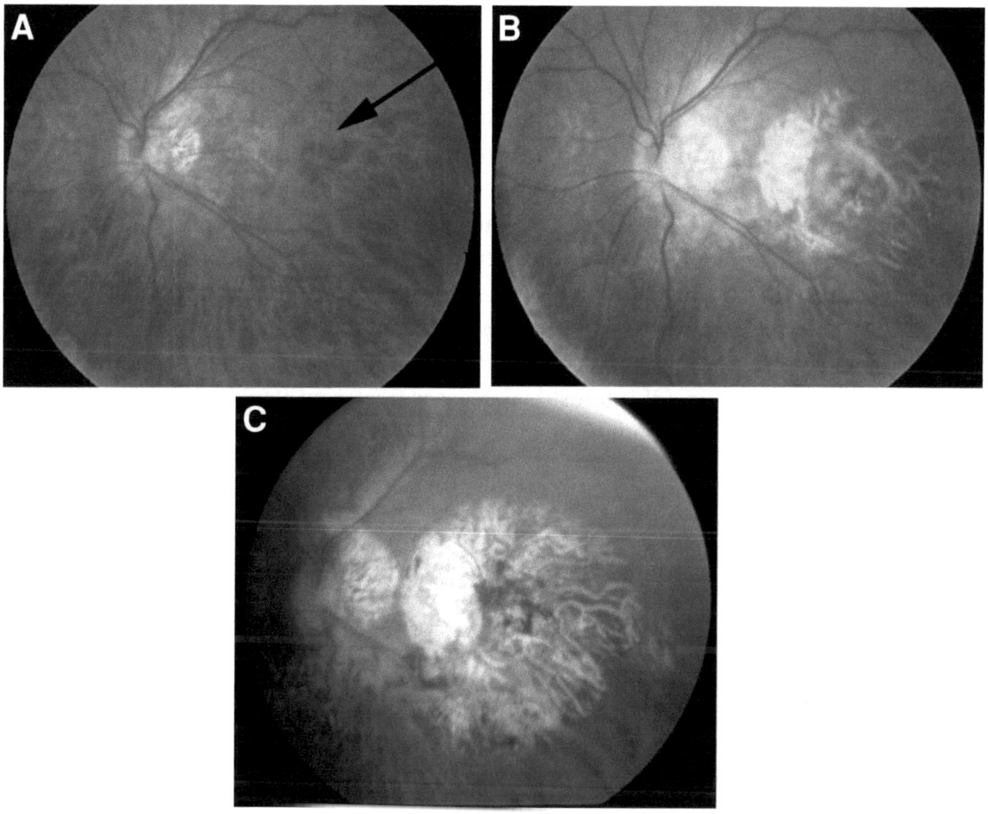

Fig. 8. Progression of chorioretinal atrophy in the left eye of a 56-yr-old woman with myopic choroidal neovascularization. Refractive error is –14.5 D and the axial length is 28.0 mm in the left eye of the patient. (**A**) Fundus photograph just after the onset of macular hemorrhage associated with choroidal neovascularization (arrow). Visual acuity was 20/60. (**B**) Fundus photograph of the same patient 4 yr after onset. Visual acuity decreased to 20/200. (**C**) Fundus photograph 10 yr after onset. Visual acuity was 20/200. *See* color version on companion CD.

younger than 40 yr, whereas age was still the only influencing factor in those older than 40 yr. This means that local factors, such as CNV size, determine the tendency to develop chorioretinal atrophy in young patients, whereas systemic factors, such as patient age, have a greater role in older subjects.

TREATMENT

Laser Photocoagulation

Patients with pathological myopia treated with laser photocoagulation can have a remarkable increase in the size of the area of chorioretinal atrophy over time *(30)*. This has led us to question the effectiveness of laser photocoagulation in patients with pathological myopia. In a retrospective study, Secretan et al. *(31)* examined eyes with pathological myopia and CNV. Of 50 eyes treated with laser photocoagulation and 50 untreated eyes, at 2 yr the treated eyes seemed to improve more than the untreated eyes. After 5 yr of follow-up, however, treatment improved only in eyes with an initial acuity of 20/40 or better. Ruiz-Moreno et al. *(32)* retrospectively analyzed 23 eyes with myopic CNV treated with laser photocoagulation. The results indicated that laser photocoagulation can improve visual acuity for between 2 and 24 mo. The improvement fades with time, and is no longer significant after the third year. Jalkh et al. *(33)* performed photocoagulation in 19 eyes with myopic CNV. All but two eyes had spontaneous progressive enlargement of the atrophic photocoagulation scar, which worsened visual acuity in 13 eyes (68%). Brancato et al. *(30)* performed a prospective study of 36 eyes affected by myopic CNV successfully treated by lasers. Scar expansion was noted in 97%. These studies indicate that although laser photocoagulation might cause occlusion of CNV and temporarily improve vision, it eventually causes prominent enlargement of the atrophic photocoagulation scar, which might result in worsening of the long-term visual prognosis. Of interest is that laser treatment itself might cause lacquer cracks in some patients with pathological myopia *(34)*.

Surgical Removal of Myopic CNV

Another therapeutic alternative is surgery to extract the area of CNV. Uemura et al. *(35)* retrospectively reviewed the medical records of 23 patients with high myopia who underwent vitrectomy with surgical removal of subfoveal CNV. The visual acuity improved by two or more Snellen lines in 39%, decreased in 35%, and remained unchanged in 26%, after a mean follow-up period of 24 mo. They suggest that surgical removal of CNV provides visual benefits in selected cases. Bottoni et al. *(36)* performed surgical removal of myopic CNV in 65 patients. Mean follow-up period was 16 mo. Mean postoperative visual acuity (0.18) was significantly better than mean preoperative visual acuity (0.09). On the other hand, Thomas et al. *(37)* reported that after a mean follow-up period of 7 mo, the final visual acuity in 10 patients with high myopia that was treated surgically was less than 20/70 in all cases and the mean change in visual acuity was a decrease by one ETDRS line.

Marked atrophic scar expansion is a major postoperative complication causing visual decrease in eyes treated with surgical removal of CNV *(36,37)*. Surgical extraction of CNV seems to cause mechanical damage to the retinal pigment epithelium (RPE) and choroid, and might induce atrophy of the RPE and choroid. Because of marked expansion of the atrophic scar after surgery, subretinal surgery is currently not an attractive option.

Foveal Translocation

Macular translocation is an innovative procedure first reported by Machemer and Steinhorst *(39)*. Unlike surgical removal, the new foveal location after macular translocation is in front of a healthier RPE at some distance from the choroidal atrophy or lacquer cracks. There are two translocation methods: limited macular translocation and translocation with a peripheral 360° retinotomy. Ichibe et al. *(40)* reviewed 10 eyes with myopic CNV treated with limited macular translocation (follow-up period ≥ 6 mo). Postoperatively, visual acuity improved more than three lines in logMAR measurement in all eyes. Fujii et al. *(41)* conducted a retrospective study of 11 eyes with myopic CNV treated by limited macular translocation. Visual acuity improvement of two lines or more was obtained in 36.4% during the 6- to 10-mo follow-up period. Glacet-Bernard et al. *(42)* reported the results of limited macular translocation in nine eyes with myopic

CNV. In six eyes (67%), there was an improvement of six lines or more during a mean follow-up period of 10 mo.

These two surgical approaches for foveal translocation have both advantages and disadvantages. A scleral imbrication has the advantage of being less invasive, because it does not require a large retinotomy. There are several problems, however. One problem is that the amount of foveal movement is difficult to control and is usually less than that obtained by translocation with peripheral retinotomy. If the translocated distance is too short, even if the myopic CNV itself is distant from the macula, the later expansion of an atrophic scar around the area of CNV or the recurrence of CNV might again involve the fovea.

Fujikado et al. *(43)* compared the visual outcome after foveal translocation by scleral shortening and that after 360° retinotomy in a patient with bilateral myopic neovascular maculopathy. Although postoperative visual acuity in both eyes was not different, there was improved reading ability in the eye that received peripheral retinotomy, because a larger retinal sensitive area was produced. Tano *(44)* performed macular translocation with a 360° retinotomy in 28 eyes with myopic CNV. The final visual acuity improved two lines or more in 64% of eyes, was unchanged in 14%, and decreased in 21% during the follow-up period of at least 6 mo.

In foveal translocation with peripheral retinotomy, the shift of the fovea is much greater, with vision ultimately being less affected in cases of CNV recurrence or later expansion of chorioretinal atrophy around the CNV. Tano *(44)* reported that postoperative retinal detachment, including proliferative vitreoretinopathy, developed in 29% of eyes following translocation with peripheral retinotomy. Therefore, the long-term results of these new surgical treatments regarding visual outcome as well as postoperative complications must be assessed before the true effectiveness of this treatment can be determined.

Photodynamic Therapy

Photodynamic therapy (PDT) is a relatively new treatment modality based on the use of light-sensitive drugs called photosensitizers; activation of photosensitizers by an appropriate-wavelength laser initiates multiple photochemical reactions culminating in vessel occlusion of the target tissue. Preliminary results of PDT on myopic CNV were first reported by Sickenberg et al. *(45)*. Ten myopic eyes with subfoveal CNV were enrolled. The follow-up period ranged from 12 to 43 wk. PDT with verteporfin caused short-term (1–4 wk) cessation of fluorescein leakage from myopic CNV without damage to retinal blood vessels. Improvement of best-corrected visual acuity of two lines or more was obtained in 50% of eyes. Based on their investigation, a randomized clinical trial, called the Verteporfin in Photodynamic Therapy (VIP) Trial, was initiated in Europe and North America. Patients with myopic CNV with a greatest linear dimension of no more than 5400 μm and best-corrected visual acuity of approx 20/100 or better were enrolled in the study ($N = 120$). The first report from the VIP Trial *(46)* describes the effects of verteporfin therapy compared with placebo therapy on all study visits through the 12-mo examination. At the 12-mo examination, 72% of the verteporfin-treated patients, compared with 44% of the placebo-treated patients, lost fewer than 8 letters ($p < 0.01$), including 32% (verteporfin-treated) vs 15% (placebo-treated) improving at least 5 letters. Recently, 2-yr results of PDT on myopic CNV were also reported from the same group *(45)*. At the 24-mo examination, 36% of verteporfin-treated patients, compared with 51% of the placebo-treated patients, lost at least 8 letters ($p = 0.11$). Improvement of visual acuity by at least 5 letters was obtained in 40% of the verteporfin-treated cases vs 13% of the placebo-treated cases and by at least 15 letters in 12% of verteporfin-treated cases vs 0% placebo-treated cases. They suggested that PDT with verteporfin can safely increase the chance of stabilizing or improving vision in patients with myopic CNV compared with placebo, although the primary outcome (visual acuity) was not significantly improved by verteporfin therapy at 2 yr as it had been at 1 yr following treatment.

The selection of eligible patients for PDT treatments might improve the effectiveness of this treatment. Montero and Ruiz-Moreno *(48)* performed PDT with verteporfin on 32 consecutive patients (33 eyes) with myopic CNV. The follow-up period was 1 yr. Patients who completed the follow-up study were divided into two groups according to their age: 55 yr old or less and more than 55 yr old. PDT was more effective for patients under 56 yr of age.

Histological studies, however, suggest that the PDT-induced occlusion might be temporary. Scupola et al. *(49)* reported histological findings of surgically excised myopic CNV after PDT. They did not find thrombus formation inside the vascular lumina in CNV, and suggested that PDT-induced occlusion might be temporary, and blood vessel regrowth or recanalization is possible. Therefore, whether PDT can lead to permanent occlusion of myopic CNV and maintain vision in treated eyes over the long term remains to be assessed. Also, it is necessary to determine whether PDT can prevent the later development of chorioretinal atrophy around the area of CNV, which is a major cause of long-term visual decrease in eyes with myopic CNV. Recently, favorable results of combination therapy of PDT and pharmaceutical treatments were reported for CNV caused by age-related macular degeneration *(50,51)*. These kinds of combination therapies are also expected to be useful for myopic CNV.

Pharmacological Approaches

Recently, various investigators have aggressively sought a pharmacological antiangiogenic treatment for CNV. Angiogenic factors, such as vascular endothelial growth factor (VEGF), are the major targets. Several approaches to neutralize VEGF are being explored, such as antisense oligonucleotides or anti-VEGF aptamers, which are now in phase 2 trials *(51)*. A newly described potent antiangiogenic factor, pigment-epithelium-derived factor (PEDF), might be another target to treat myopic CNV. Subretinal or intravitreous injection, or even periocular injection of a viral vector encoding PEDF, effectively inhibits CNV in animal models *(52,53)*.

Corticosteroid therapy is an effective treatment for CNV. Intravitreous triamcinolone acetonide injection is effective for the treatment of CNV *(54)*. Recently, subtenon injection was also tried. Our clinical impression is that subtenon injection of triamcinolone acetate is effective, especially for myopic CNV with prominent retinal edema. Nonsteroidal antiinflammatory drugs might be used to avoid the possible side effects of steroids. Takahashi et al. *(55)* reported that topical nepafenac (a potent cyclooxygenase inhibitor) significantly inhibited CNV in a mouse model. The effectiveness of anecortave acetate, which suppresses blood vessel growth by inhibiting the proteases required for vascular endothelial cell migration, has also been reported for CNV in age-related macular degeneration *(56)*. Most of these pharmacological approaches are ongoing; however, these might be useful approaches for myopic CNV in the future.

CONCLUSIONS

Myopic CNV is a major cause of CNV in young patients and is therefore an important problem socioeconomically. Myopic CNV has a characteristic natural course: chorioretinal atrophy develops and spreads after regression of CNV. Because of the spread of chorioretinal atrophy, vision decreases gradually and progressively over the long term. Various new active treatments have been tried for myopic CNV to improve its poor prognosis. Whether these new treatments can prevent secondary enlargement of chorioretinal atrophy as well and improve or maintain vision over the long term must be assessed before judging the true effectiveness of these treatments. It is expected that the pathogenic mechanism of myopic CNV will be clarified and effective treatments will be established in the near future.

REFERENCES

1. Pruett RC. Pathologic myopia. In: Principles and Practice of Ophthalmology, Albert DM, Jakobiec FA, eds. W.B. Saunders, Philadelphia: 1994.
2. Tokoro T. Criteria for diagnosis of pathologic myopia. In: Atlas of Posterior Fundus Changes in Pathologic Myopia, Tokoro T, ed. Springer, New York: 1981:p. 1.
3. Ghafour IM, Allan D, Foulds WS. Common causes of blindness and visual handicap in the west of Scotland. Br J Ophthalmol 1986;67:209–213.
4. Sperduto RD, Seigel D, Roberts J, et al. Prevalence of myopia in the United States. Arch Ophthalmol 1983;101:405–407.
5. Tokoro T. On the definition of pathologic myopia in group studies. Acta Ophthalmol Suppl 1988;185:107, 108.
6. Curtin BJ. Ocular findings and complications. In: Myopias, Curtin BJ, ed. Harper & Row, Philadelphia: 1985:277–347.
7. Steidl SM, Pruett RC. Macular complications associated with posterior staphyloma. Am J Ophthalmol 1997;123:181–187.
8. Avila MP, Weiter JJ, Jalkh AE, et al. Natural history of choroidal neovascularization in degenerative myopia. Ophthalmology 1984;91:1573–1581.
9. Fried M, Siebert A, Meyer-Schwickerath G, et al. Natural history of Fuchs' spot: a long-term follow-up study. Doc Ophthalmol 1981;28:215–221.
10. Hampton GR, Kohen D, Bird AC. Visual prognosis of disciform degeneration in myopia. Ophthalmology 1983;90:923–926.
11. Cohen SY, Laroche A, Leguen Y, et al. Etiology of choroidal neovascularization in young patients. Ophthalmology 1996;103:1241–1245.
12. Vongphanit J, Mitchell P, Wang JJ. Prevalence and progression of myopic retinopathy in an older population. Ophthalmology 2002;109:704–711.
13. Curtin BJ, Karlin DB. Axial length measurements and fundus changes of the myopic eye. Am J Ophthalmol 1971;71:42–53.
14. Grossniklaus HE, Green WR. Pathologic findings in pathologic myopia. Retina 1992;12:127–133.
15. Hotchkiss ML, Fine SL. Pathologic myopia and choroidal neovascularization. Am J Ophthalmol 1981;91:177–183.
16. Ohno-Matsui K, Yoshida T, Futagami S, et al. Patchy atrophy and lacquer cracks predispose to the development of choroidal neovascularization in pathologic myopia. Br J Ophthalmol 2003;87:570–573.
17. Kobayashi K, Mandai M, Suzuma I, et al. Expression of estrogen receptor in the choroidal neovascular membranes in highly myopic eyes. Retina 2002;22:418–422.

18. Pruett RC, Weiter JJ, Goldstein RB. Myopic cracks, angioid streaks, and traumatic tears in Bruch's membrane. Am J Ophthalmol 1987;103:537–543.
19. Seko Y, Seko Y, Fujikura H, et al. Induction of vascular endothelial growth factor after application of mechanical stress to retinal pigment epithelium of the rat in vitro. Invest Ophthalmol Vis Sci 1999;40:3287–3291.
20. Spitznas M, Boker T. Idiopathic posterior subretinal neovascularization is related to myopia. Graefes Arch Clin Exp Ophthalmol 1991;229:536–538.
21. Remulla JFC, Gaudio AR, Miller S, et al. Foveal electroretinograms and choroidal perfusion characteristics in fellow eyes of patients with unilateral neovascular age-related macular degeneration. Br J Ophthalmol 1995;79:558–561.
22. Dimitrova G, Tamaki Y, Kato S, et al. Retrobulbar circulation in myopic patients with or without myopic choroidal neovascularization. Br J Ophthalmol 2002;86:771–773.
23. Ohno-Matsui K, Morishima N, Ito M, et al. Posterior routes of choroidal blood outflow in high myopia. Retina 1996;16:419–425.
24. Quaranta M, Arnold J, Coscas G, et al. Indocyanine green angiographic features of pathologic myopia. Am J Ophthalmol 1996;122:663–671.
25. Baba T, Ohno-Matsui K, Yoshida T, et al. Optical coherence tomography of choroidal neovascularization in high myopia. Acta Ophthalmol Scand 2002;80:82–87.
26. Tabandeh H, Flynn HW, Scott IU, et al. Visual acuity outcome of patients 50 years of age and older with high myopia and untreated choroidal neovascularization. Ophthalmology 1999;106:2063–2067.
27. Yoshida T, Ohno-Matsui K, Ohtake Y, et al. Long-term visual prognosis of choroidal neovascularization in high myopia. A comparison between age groups. Ophthalmology 2002;109:712–719.
28. Yoshida T, Ohno-Matsui K, Yasuzumi K, et al. Myopic choroidal neovascularization. A 10-year follow-up. Ophthalmology 2003;110:1297–1305.
29. Kojima A, Ohno-Matsui K, Teramukai S, et al. Factors associated with the development of chorioretinal atrophy around choroidal neovascularization in pathologic myopia. Graefes Arch Clin Exp Ophthalmol 2004;242:114–119.
30. Brancato R, Pece A, Avanza P, et al. Photocoagulation scar expansion after laser therapy for choroidal neovascularization in degenerative myopia. Retina 1990;10:239–243.
31. Secretan M, Kuhn D, Soubrane G, et al. Long-term visual outcome of choroidal neovascularization in pathologic myopia: natural history and laser treatment. Eur J Ophthalmol 1997;7:307–316.
32. Ruiz-Moreno JM, Montero JA. Long-term visual acuity after argon green laser photocoagulation of juxtafoveal choroidal neovascularization in highly myopic eyes. Eur J Ophthalmol 2002;12:117–122.
33. Jalkh AE, Weiter JJ, Trempe CL, et al. Choroidal neovascularization in degenerative myopia: role of laser photocoagulation. Ophthalm Surg 1987;18:721–725.
34. Johnson DA, Yannuzzi LA, Shakin JL, et al. Lacquer cracks following laser treatment of choroidal neovascularization in pathologic myopia. Retina 1998;18:118–124.
35. Uemura A, Thomas MA. Subretinal surgery for choroidal neovascularization in patients with high myopia. Arch Ophthalmol 2000;118:344–350.
36. Bottoni F, Perego E, Airaghi P, et al. Surgical removal of subfoveal choroidal neovascular membranes in high myopia. Graefes Arch Clin Exp Ophthalmol 1999;237:573–582.
37. Thomas MA, Dickinson JD, Melberg NS, et al. Visual results after surgical removal of subfoveal choroidal neovascular membranes. Ophthalmology 1994;101:1384–1396.
38. Ruiz-Moreno JM, de la Vega C. Surgical removal of subfoveal choroidal neovascularization in highly myopic patients. Br J Ophthalmol 2001;85:1041–1043.
39. Machemer R, Steinhorst UH. Retinal separation, retinotomy, and macular relocation: 2. A surgical approach for age-related macular degeneration? Graefes Arch Clin Exp Ophthalmol 1993;231:635–641.

40. Ichibe M, Imai K, Ohta M, et al. Foveal translocation with scleral imbrication in patients with myopic neovascular maculopathy. Am J Ophthalmol 2001;132:164–171.
41. Fujii GY, Humayun MS, Pieramici DJ, et al. Initial experience of inferior limited macular translocation for subfoveal choroidal neovascularization resulting from causes other than age-related macular degeneration. Am J Ophthalmol 2001;131:90–100.
42. Glacet-Bernard A, Simon P, Hamelin N, et al. Translocation of the macula for management of subfoveal choroidal neovascularization: comparison of results in age-related macular degeneration and degenerative myopia. Am J Ophthalmol 2001;131:78–89.
43. Fujikado T, Ohji M, Hosohata J, et al. Comparison of visual function after foveal translocation with 360 degrees retinotomy and with scleral shortening in a patient with bilateral myopic neovascular maculopathy. Am J Ophthalmol 2000;130:525–527.
44. Tano Y. Pathologic myopia: where are we now? Am J Ophthalmol 2002;134:645–660.
45. Sickenberg M, Schmidt-Erfurth U, Miller JW, et al. A preliminary study of photodynamic therapy using verteporfin for choroidal neovascularization in pathologic myopia, ocular histoplasmosis syndrome, angioid streaks, and idiopathic causes. Arch Ophthalmol 2000;117:327–336.
46. Verteporfin in Photodynamic Therapy (VIP) Study Group. Photodynamic therapy of subfoveal choroidal neovascularization in pathologic myopia. 1-year results of a randomized clinical trial-VIP report no. 1. Ophthalmology 2001;108:841–852.
47. Verteporfin in Photodynamic Therapy (VIP) Study Group. Photodynamic therapy of subfoveal choroidal neovascularization in pathologic myopia. 2-year results of a randomized clinical trial-VIP report no. 3. Ophthalmology 2003;110:667–673.
48. Montero JA, Ruiz-Moreno JM. Verteporfin photodynamic therapy in highly myopic subfoveal choroidal neovascularization. Br J Ophthalmol 2003;87:173–176.
49. Scupola A, Ventura L, Tiberti AC, et al. Histological findings of a surgically excised myopic choroidal neovascular membrane after photodynamic therapy. A case report. Graefes Arch Clin Exp Ophthalmol 2004;242:605–610.
50. Spaide RF, Sorenson J, Maranan L. Combined photodynamic therapy with verteporfin and intravitreal triamcinolone acetonide for choroidal neovascularization. Ophthalmology 2003;110:1517–1525.
51. Eyetech Study Group. Anti-vascular endothelial growth factor therapy for subfoveal choroidal neovascularization secondary to age-related macular degeneration: phase 2 study results. Ophthalmology 2003;110:879–881.
52. Mori K, Gehlbach P, Yamamoto S, et al. AAV-mediated gene transfer of pigment epithelium-derived factor inhibits choroidal neovascularization. Invest Ophthalmol Vis Sci 2002; 43:1994–2000.
53. Gehlbach P, Demetriades AM, Yamamoto S, et al. Periocular injection of adenoviral vector encoding pigment epithelium-derived factor inhibits choroidal neovascularization. Gene Ther 2003;10:637–646.
54. Rechtman E, Danis RP, Pratt LM, et al. Intravitreal triamcinolone with photodynamic therapy for subfoveal choroidal neovascularization in age-related macular degeneration. Br J Ophthalmol 2004;88:344–347.
55. Takahashi K, Saishin Y, Saishin Y, et al. Topical nepafenac inhibits ocular neovascularization. Invest Ophthalmol Vis Sci 2003;44:409–415.
56. The Anecortave Acetate Clinical Study Group. Anecortave acetate as monotherapy for treatment of subfoveal neovascularization in age-related macular degeneration. Twelve-month clinical outcomes. Ophthalmology 2003;110:2372–2385.

6

Mechanisms of the Formation and Stability of Retinal Blood Vessels

Jonathan Stone, DSc, FAA, **Trent Sandercoe,** MBBS, PhD, **and Jan Provis,** PhD

CONTENTS

UNDERSTANDING RETINAL VESSEL FORMATION

As an introduction, we restate briefly several major themes of retinal vascularization. All have been reviewed previously. Some are common to the formation of vessels in any tissue; others are unique to the eye.

The Choroid Rules

From a survey of adult vertebrate eyes, Michaelson concluded that:

> the vascularisation of the inner eye may be affected by two influences: the choroid's capacity to nourish the retina and the activity in the retina of a factor which affects retinal growth. The former influence is presumably the primary, prepotent one *(1)*.

Michaelson noted that the choroidal circulation is a constant feature in the nutrition of the vertebrate eye, whereas the retinal circulation is more variable, being found in only of a subset of the mammals, in which it develops much later in ontogeny *(1)*. His suggestion that the development of the retinal circulation depends on the ability of the choroidal circulation to supply the nutritional requirements of the retina gained support from Chase's *(2)* survey of the thickness of mammalian retinas. In species lacking a retinal circulation (rabbit, guinea pig, horse), the retina was thin (<150 μm); in those in which a retinal circulation formed (humans, rats, cats, dogs), the retina was thicker (up to threefold) *(2)*.

From: *Ophthalmology: Ocular Angiogenesis: Diseases, Mechanisms, and Therapeutics*
Edited by: J. Tombran-Tink and C. J. Barnstable © Humana Press Inc., Totowa, NJ

These observations suggested that retinal circulation evolved to allow the retina to be thicker than the choroid could supply. The advantage of thickness was presumably an increase in the number of inner retinal neurons available to code the light-induced signals generated by the photoreceptors. Certainly, the mammalian species with the highest spatial and color resolution (the primates) all have vascularized, thick retinas. In foveate birds, in which retinal performance may be even greater than in the primates, the retina is also thick and the inner retina is nourished by the pecten specialization, via the choroid.

It is argued below that the powerful influence of the choroid on the development and adult structure of the retinal vasculature also drives several retinal diseases, including retinopathy of prematurity, retinopathy of detachment, and retinitis pigmentosa.

Regulation of Retinal Vessel Formation Is Local, Controlled by a "Factor"

This principle of vessel formation was first formulated for the retinal circulation by Michaelson *(1,3)*, and is still most clearly defined for this circulation. Influenced by the micro architecture of retinal vessels, particularly the capillary-free zones along arteries, Michaelson suggested that

> the … development of retinal vessels … indicates the probable presence of a factor or factors in the retina which affect the growth of vessels … (and) … is present in a gradient … such that it differs in arterial and venous neighbourhoods … (and) determines the ultimate extent as well as the initiation of capillary growth.

The most specific identification of a factor that controls the growth of retinal capillaries came from a series of studies, reviewed by Stone and Maslim *(4)*, which showed that vascular endothelial growth factor (VEGF) is expressed by a variety of retinal cells, especially the macroglia (astrocytes and Müller cells), in temporal and spatial patterns that indicate that it is important for the induction of vessel formation in the retina (Fig. 1). Further, the vasoformative action of VEGF in the retina is regulated by tissue oxygen levels, providing an understanding of how retinal metabolism, and more specifically the ability or inability of the choroidal circulation to support that metabolism, controls the retinal circulation.

Photoreceptor Metabolism Controls Vascularization of Inner Retina

Evidence of the importance of retinal metabolism in the formation of retinal vessels came from several sources. In a still-unique series of experiments, Graymore *(5)* showed that glycolysis in the rat retina (both aerobic and anaerobic) accelerates sharply from low postnatal to high adult levels, over a few days (postnatal days 12–13). This is the period in which, in this species, the eyes open, the electroretinogram (ERG) becomes detectable, and photoreceptors begin to differentiate their inner and outer segments. Graymore went on to show that the acceleration does not occur if the photoreceptor population is depleted by a toxin (iodoacetate) or by a genetically driven degeneration (in the RCS rat), showing that the metabolic acceleration occurs in the photoreceptors *(5,6)*.

The mechanisms linking the onset of photoreceptor metabolism to the formation of the retinal circulation were elucidated much more slowly and painfully. One major line of evidence emerged from the analysis of the blinding disease retrolental fibroplasia, which emerged in the 1940s in neonatal clinics and was eventually traced to the use of

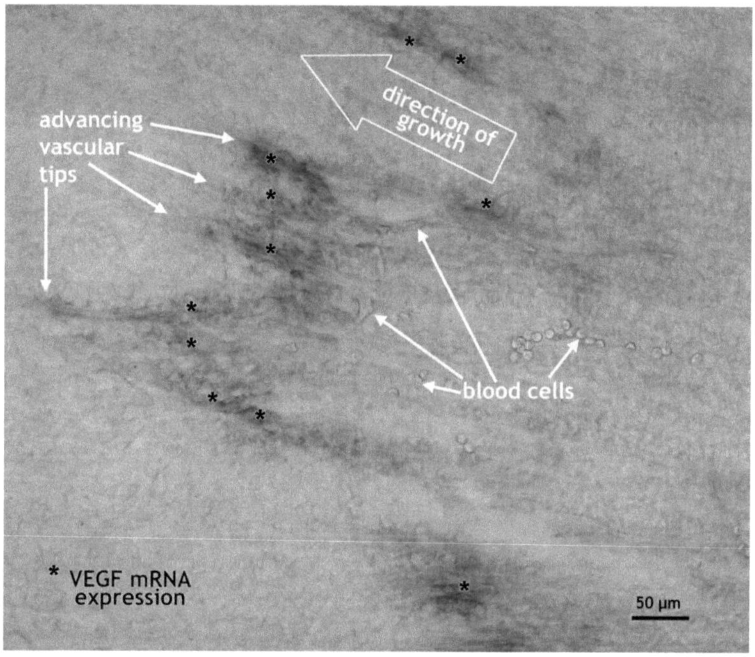

Fig. 1. Montage of a wholemount of a human fetal retina at 18 wk gestation, showing vascular endothelial growth factor (VEGF) mRNA expression associated with the formation of retinal vessels. The large arrow indicates the direction of growth; vascularized retina is to the right (showing the outlines of some blood cells, indicated), avascular retina to the left. The dark patches show the sites of expression of VEGF mRNA (asterisks). Note that VEGF mRNA is expressed at the tips of the vessels as they form, as well as in the retina immediately ahead of the vessels, consistent with the distribution of astrocytes. *See* color version on companion CD.

oxygen to relieve respiratory distress in neonates. This analysis, in which Ashton and colleagues in the United Kingdom and Patz and colleagues in the United States played major roles, has been reviewed many times *(4,7–9)*. Four "principles" of retinal angiogenesis emerge from the analysis.

1. **Dominance of the choroid:** Formation of the retinal circulation is regulated by the ability/inability of oxygen flowing from the choroid. Increases in the availability of choroidal oxygen inhibit, and decreases stimulate, vessel formation.
2. **Photoreceptor metabolism triggers retinal angiogenesis:** Photoreceptor metabolism is a major sink for choroidal oxygen. When that metabolism begins (quite suddenly, as Graymore showed), the inner retina becomes hypoxic, and that hypoxia (dubbed "physiological hypoxia" *[10]*) is the major stimulus for the genesis of the vessels of the retinal circulation.
3. **Early plasticity:** As they form, retinal vessels are highly plastic. The formation of these vessels can be completely prevented if, for example, higher than normal levels of oxygen flow from the choroid into the retina, and eliminate the episode of physiological hypoxia normally induced by the onset of retinal metabolism. Further, for some period, the vessels remain plastic and can be totally obliterated by an episode of hyperoxia.
4. **Late stability:** In adults, by contrast, capillary beds are much more stable in the face of hyperoxia. They constrict in high oxygen but are much slower to retract.

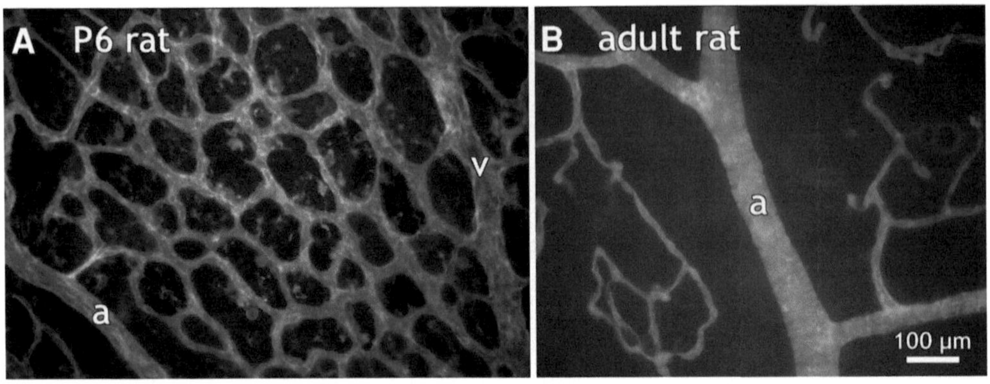

Fig. 2. Wholemounts of rat retina at P6 **(A)** and in adult **(B)** labeled with *Griffonia simplicifolia* lectin. **(A)** a dense capillary network is shown, flanked by an artery (a) and a vein (v). There are more capillary bed connections to the vein than the artery, although the capillary bed adjacent to the artery is quite dense. **(B)** An artery (a) in adult retina showing substantial remodeling of the vascular bed. *See* color version on companion CD.

Mechanisms of Oxygen Supply to Retina Are Also Mechanisms of Disease

Retinopathy of Prematurity

Ashton *(7)*, reviewing the role of oxygen in the development of retinal vessels, commented that "many of the pathological responses of the retinal vessels are not separate morbid processes, but exaggerations of normal behaviour." Essentially, he was suggesting that retinopathy of prematurity (at least in the "first epidemic" that he analyzed) results from the operation of the normal mechanisms of retinal vessel formation, after they are perturbed by an episode of hyperoxia. We now know *(10–12)* that the normal formation of retinal vessels is regulated by oxygen levels in the developing retina. The onset of a photoreceptor metabolism reduces oxygen entering the retina from the choroid (because a strong oxygen sink develops at the inner segments). The retina experiences a period of "physiological hypoxia" that induces the formation of retinal vessels *(10)*. The oxygen brought by these vessels limits the period of physiological hypoxia, and downregulates the activity or expression of oxygen-inducible factors (hypoxia-inducible factor [HIF]-1, VEGF) that mediate vessel formation. Enriching the oxygen breathed by neonates can save them from death and brain damage from respiratory distress; but it can also eliminate the episode of physiological hypoxia in the retina, without which retinal vessels will not form.

The analysis of retinopathy of prematurity highlighted two additional features of normal vessel formation. First, retinal vessels normally form in excess, and are somehow pruned back to a more sparse, adult pattern (Fig. 2). Key to this process is the ability of vessels to completely regress under the impact of high oxygen levels *(7)*. This oxygen-induced obliteration generates the capillary-free zones that form along arteries (above) and expand or contract with the level of oxygen available.

Second, this early plasticity of retinal vessels is transient. The end of the plasticity occurs in rats at about P30 (below), and is mediated by factors (platelet-derived growth factor [PDGF]-β, VEGF) released by pericytes, which extend over the retinal vessels at this age *(13)*. Thereafter, retinal vessels are more stable, constricting but resisting obliteration when exposed to high tissue oxygen levels. Retinal vessels in other species, such as the human, are known to be plastic in the young and more stable in the adult, but studies defining the age of transition, and giving evidence of the mechanism involved, have been reported only for the rat.

Retinopathy of prematurity highlights one rigidity of the retinal circulation. The choroidal circulation does not appear able to sense or respond to hypoxia of the retina, presumably because its capillaries do not lie in the retina, but supply oxygen to the retina by diffusion from a distance (across Bruch's membrane and the retinal pigment epithelium [RPE]) *(9)*.

Finally, two mechanisms come into play in the pathogenesis of retinopathy of prematurity that are not physiological, although they do highlight physiological mechanisms. One such mechanism is that retinal hypoxia (which occurs when the oxygen-exposed infant is returned to room air with the retina depleted of vessels) causes the death of retinal astrocytes *(14)*. Astrocytes express the principal factor regulating retinal angiogenesis (VEGF), are the normal template for vessel formation (below), induce barrier properties in vessels as they form *(15,16)*, and are an important element of the glia limitans of the retina (the inner limiting membrane) and its vessels *(17)*, which constrains vessel growth *(18)*. In the absence of astrocytes, VEGF expression is upregulated in neurons, particularly retinal ganglion cells *(12,19,20)*. The vessels induced to form are leaky, abnormal in morphology, and lacking the constraint of the inner limiting membrane, grow into the vitreous humor *(12)*.

Retinopathy of Detachment

Detachment of the retina typically occurs between the neural retina and the RPE. This separates the photoreceptors from the source of their nutrition (the choriocapillaris). A retinopathy results, which has been termed retinopathy of detachment *(21,22)*. This retinopathy comprises two major pathologies: the death of photoreceptors and gliosis of the retina, caused by the hypertrophy and proliferation of retinal neuroglia. Both contribute to a loss of retinal function, which can vary from minor to complete.

The death of photoreceptors and the gliosis caused by detachment are both mitigated by increasing the partial pressure of oxygen in the blood, by the inhalation of oxygen-enriched air *(21,22)*. Clinically, hyperoxia should be useful in reducing retinal damage until the retina is reattached. Analytically, the effectiveness of oxygen in mitigating both pathologies suggests that the detached retina becomes hypoxic, as predicted by models of oxygen supply to and consumption by the retina *(23)*. These models assume that the choroidal circulation cannot respond to the hypoxia that results from retinal detachment, the hypoxia resulting from the longer diffusion path to the detached retina. Conversely, if arterial pO_2 is increased by hyperoxia, the unresponsiveness of the choroid to oxygen conditions means that oxygen diffusion from the choroid should increase and mitigate the pathology, as observed empirically. Thus the lack of autoregulation in the choroid, which shapes the pattern of formation of the retinal circulation, drives the pathology and allows the treatment of retinopathy of detachment.

Retinitis Pigmentosa

The central pathology of retinitis pigmentosa (RP) is photoreceptor death, often consequent to a mutation in a gene important for photoreceptors. Nevertheless, the late stages of the disease are thought to result from the failure of the choroidal circulation to autoregulate, as the photoreceptor population is depleted (the oxygen toxicity hypothesis of ref. *24*). As the oxygen consumption by photoreceptors falls, oxygen levels build up in the outer nuclear layer *(25,26)*, and become toxic to photoreceptors *(27,28)*. Further, the accumulation of oxygen in the retina following photoreceptor degeneration causes thinning of retinal vessels in human RP *(29)*, and in animal models *(30)*. Again, the failure of the choroidal circulation to autoregulate has a major effect on a disease phenotype.

ROLES OF MACROGLIA

Both major classes of macroglial cells of the retina (astrocytes and Müller cells) are of importance in the formation of the retinal vasculature.

Astrocytes

Astrocytes Are Immigrants to the Retina

It is significant that astrocytes are not generated by the neuroepithelium of the retina. Early surveys showed that astrocytes are found only in a subset of mammals, those in which the retina becomes vascularized. They are present in the cat, dog, rat, mouse, ferret, monkey, and human, for example *(31–33)*. This selective entry of astrocytes suggests a mechanism evolved to allow a thicker retina, with more complex circuitry (*see* "The Choroid Rules"). Astrocytes are now thought to originate from glial lineage-restricted precursors cells derived from the neural tube *(34)* that migrate into the retina during development *(35–37)*.

In all species investigated, in which astrocytes are found in the retina—cat *(33,38)*, ferret *(39)*, rat *(40)*, mouse *(41,42)*, monkey *(43,44)*, and human *(45)*—astrocytes (identified by their expression of glial fibrillary acidic protein [GFAP]) spread from the optic disk to the edge of the retina. The presence in the retina of astrocyte precursor cells (APCs), cells committed to becoming astrocytes but not yet GFAP-immunoreactive, has also been suggested. APCs have been isolated by several groups *(34)*, including E17 rat optic nerve *(46)*. These optic nerve-derived APCs are express vimentin and the glial lineage epitope A2B5, as well as the paired homeobox gene Pax2, important for normal development of the urogenital tract, inner ear, CNS, optic nerve, and retina *(47)*. In vitro, optic nerve-derived APCs respond to serum and to platelet-derived growth factor (PDGF), which is also thought to play a role in astrocyte migration into the retina *(48,49)*. Both leukemia inhibitory factor (LIF) and ciliary neurotrophic factor (CNTF) are important in promoting differentiation of optic nerve-derived APCs into mature astrocytes *(46)*. Furthermore, endothelial cells have been shown to promote maturation of APC into GFAP+ve astrocytes via a LIF-dependent mechanism *(50)*. In vivo, Pax2+ve APC have been described in the human fetal retina, radiating from the optic nerve toward the periphery at 14 wk gestation (when GFAP immunoreactivity in the retina is low), and ahead of GFAP-positive astrocytes and the developing vessels in older retinas *(51)*. The findings suggest that the association of differentiated endothelial cells (ECs) with APCs promotes their maturation into mature, GFAP+ve astrocytes. In addition, it appears that both APCs and mature astrocytes continue to proliferate in the retina, as they spread toward the retinal edge *(52)*.

Timing of Astrocyte Migration

The timing of astrocyte migration is also critical for the formation of retinal vessels. In the cat *(53)* and rat *(36)* they enter the retina as the genesis of retinal neurons is in its final stages and retinal function is about to begin. The increase in metabolism associated with function then induces vessel formation (*see* Photoreceptor Metabolism Controls Vascularization of Inner Retina). In the rat, for example, astrocytes enter the retina from approximately P2, and approach the retinal edge 12 d later. By the time vessels start to form (P5), astrocytes have spread 1 to 2 mm into the retina and are in place to detect the hypoxia induced by the acceleration of retinal metabolism, to express the hypoxia-inducible factor VEGF *(40)*, and to form a template for the new vessels.

Template for Vessel Formation

As they spread, astrocytes create a physical template, on which vessels form. There are two steps in the formation of the template. Astrocytes enter the retina, and spread over its surface in a bipolar form, suitable for migration. If they do not encounter hypoxic conditions (for example, in experimental animals in hyperoxic conditions) they remain bipolar. When they encounter hypoxia, they become stellate and cease migration *(54)*. Second, stellate astrocytes interact with each other like epithelial cells. They space out their somas with considerable regularity, and also maintain contact with neighboring astrocytes, by intertwining of the tips of their processes ("contact-spacing") *(16,38)*. These properties are evident in vivo, and have been demonstrated in purified primary cultures *(16)*. With classical epithelial cells, flattened and processless, the result of contact-spacing behavior is an epithelium, a continuous sheet of cells. With stellate astrocytes, the result is a latticework of cells (Fig. 3). The molecular pathways controlling stellation of astrocytes and their contact-spacing behavior are not fully known, although roles have been proposed (*see* Timing of Astrocyte Migration) for hypoxia and contact with EC in the stellation process.

Formation of Innermost Layer of Retinal Vessels

The first retinal vessels to form extend from the hyaloid artery at the optic nerve head and grow along the inner surface of the retina. They become they innermost layer of retinal vessels (deeper layers form subsequently in the middle layers of the retina). The innermost vessels form the extension of filopodia of ECs along the outer surface of the astrocyte template *(40,42)*. This close apposition of growing endothelial cells allows astrocytes to control the proliferation of EC and the formation of vessels, by their expression of the vasoformative factor VEGF, and to induce the formation of the barrier properties in the ECs of newly formed vessels, by their expression of a still-unidentified barrier signal *(15,55,56)*. As a consequence of this close relationship, the initial capillary plexus formed in the retina is shaped by the astrocyte template; all vessels are initially capillaries, with larger vessels (arteries, veins) forming subsequently, by aggregation or growth of capillaries. Also as a result of this relationship, retinal vessels have barrier properties as soon as they are formed.

Astrocytes remain important for the blood-retinal barrier throughout life. Hypoxia in the retina causes astrocyte degeneration, at least in the cat *(14)*, and the retinal vessels that lose astrocyte cover become leaky. It is not known whether retinal hypoxia causes astrocyte degeneration in humans. If it does, then this degeneration is a much-neglected feature of hypoxic retinal diseases, such as diabetic retinopthy and venous occlusion.

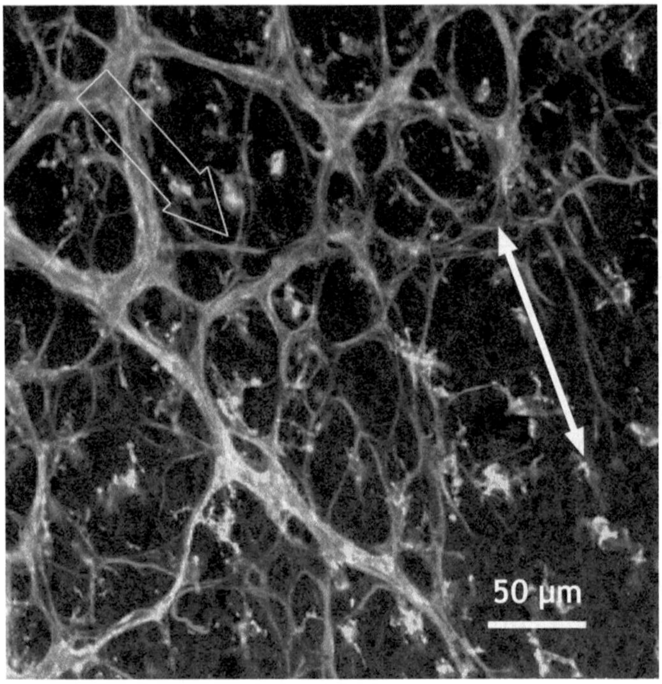

Fig. 3. A retinal wholemount showing the developing retinal vasculature (green) associated with the underlying astrocyte template (red). The open arrow indicates the direction of growth; the double-headed arrow, the GFAP+ve astrocyte template that lies ahead of the developing vessels (labeled with *Griffonia simplicifolia*). The branched cells (green) distributed throughout the field are the *Griffonia simplicifolia*+ve microglia. *See* color version on companion CD.

Astrocyte Participation in Inner Limiting Membrane

One final property of astrocytes essential for normal formation of retinal vessels is their participation in the inner glia limitans of the retina, the inner limiting membrane (ILM). This "membrane" is formed by the inner end feet of Müller cells, interspersed with astrocytes, all linked by adherent junctions *(57)*. The importance of the ILM for the retinal vasculature is seen in the severely hypoxic retina. In severe hypoxia, astrocytes die *(14,18)*, VEGF is strongly expressed by nearby neurons *(12)*, and vessels form rapidly without an astrocyte template. The inner limiting membrane is breached by the death of astrocytes and these rapidly growing vessels invade the vitreous humor *(18)* where, lacking astrocyte cover, they do not form the blood–retinal barrier.

Müller Cells as Template for Formation of Deep Vasculature

Astrocytes are confined to the innermost layer of the retina, and are related only to the innermost retinal vessels. The retinal vasculature extends deep into the retina (typically to the outer aspect of the inner nuclear layer [INL]), and the glia limitans of the deeper vessels is formed by Müller cells *(57)*. Developmentally, Müller cells are the end-stage differentiation of neural progenitor cells in the retina *(58,59)* and are thus intrinsic retinal cells. They also differ from astrocytes morphologically: Müller cells stretch radially across the thickness of the retina, whereas astrocytes are flattened cells restricted to the inner service of the retina. Nevertheless, in their relations to neurons, vessels and other Müller cells and astrocytes show many similarities *(57)*. One of those similarities is that during development, Müller cells also form a template for the growth of retinal vessels. The deeper vessels of the retinal circulation form as buds from the innermost (astrocyte-related) vessels. In the cat and rat the buds grow radially, following the radially oriented processes of Müller cells *(40,60)* before spreading in plexuses at the inner and outer aspects of the ILM.

Like astrocytes, Müller cells express VEGF in a spatiotemporal pattern just prior to the growth of capillaries through the inner plexiform layer, into the inner nuclear layer (rat, *40*; human, Sandercoe and Provis [unpublished], Fig. 4). Studies of monkey retina suggest that most of the EC proliferation associated with formation of the deeper retinal vessels occurs in the inner retina, in association with major vessels, rather than at the growing tips of the newly forming capillaries (Sandercoe and Provis [unpublished], Fig. 5B). From the site of their generation, ECs presumably migrate outward, and are assembled into vessels.

Why Both?

Astrocytes and Müller cells share the ability to form the glia limitans of vessels and of the retina *(57)*, and to detect hypoxia and express VEGF *(40)*. Why are both needed for the formation of the retinal vasculature, so that the evolution of the retinal vasculature required the preliminary step of a migration of astrocytes into the retina? Stone et al. *(40)* suggested that the answer to this questions lies in the distinct morphologies of the two classes of macroglia. Retinal astrocytes are flattened in morphology, and are confined to the innermost layers of the retina. They are well placed to detect hypoxia at the inner surface of the retina and to induce and guide the spread of vessels from the optic disk across the surface. Müller cells, in contrast, stretch across all cellular layers of the retina and cannot respond in a layer-specific way. They can, however, detect hypoxia in deeper layers, even after the vascularization of the inner surface, and their radial orientation is ideal to guide the outward growth of vessels, to form the deeper layers of the retinal circulation.

In the brain, in comparison, a comparable radial growth of vessels occurs, from the pial surface, where vessel first appear, toward the ventricular surface. This radial growth is guided by GFAP+ve astrocytes, which, at this stage of development, are in a radial form (*see* Fig. 3, ref. *4*). Cerebral astrocytes subsequently divide and change their morphology to the stellate form most common in the adult. In the retina, this early radial form of macroglia are called Müller cells, and they retain their radial morphology into adulthood.

THE MOLECULAR BASIS OF HYPOXIA-INDUCED BLOOD VESSEL FORMATION

Michaelson's *(1)* suggestion that retinal blood vessels form in response to the needs of retinal metabolism has been extensively confirmed (*see* The Choroid Rules), and has been expanded to show that the formation of blood vessels is part of a coordinated tissue response to hypoxia, which includes an upregulation of glycolysis and erythropoiesis. Much of this broader response to hypoxia is mediated by the transcription factor HIF-1 *(62–64)*.

Erythropoiesis

The recognition that hypoxia induces an increase in density of red (oxygen-carrying) cells in the blood goes back to Bert's report "*Sur la richesse en hémoglobine du sang*

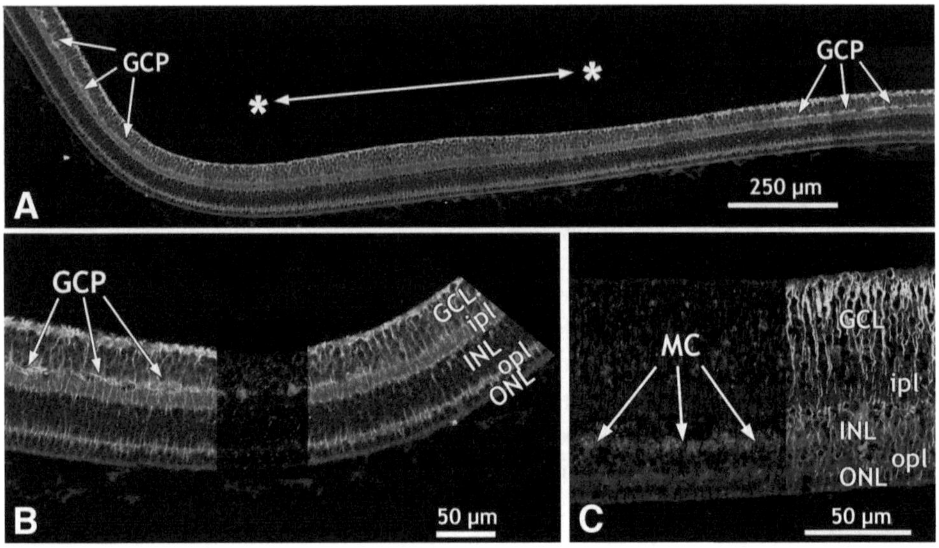

Fig. 4. Vascular endothelial growth factor (VEGF) mRNA expression associated with vascular development in primate retina. **(A)** Section through the incipient fovea of a Fd100 macaque retina. The asterisks and double-headed arrow indicate the thickened part of the retina associated with the pure cone area, where the fovea will form. Vessels expressing VEGF mRNA (red) are shown growing toward this area at the ganglion cell/inner plexiform layer interface (the ganglion cell layer plexus [GCP]) from both sides. **(B)** High-magnification view showing the GCP (from the left in **A**) in relation to the retinal layers. VEGF mRNA (red) is expressed in astrocytes with vimentin +ve processes (yellow). **(C)** Human fetal retina at 18 wk gestation showing VEGF mRNA expression in Müller cell bodies (MC), within the inner nuclear layer (INL). All sections are counter-immunolabeled with antibody to vimentin, to label Müller cell and astrocyte processes (green). GCL, ganglion cell layer; ipl, inner plexiform layer; ONL, outer nuclear layer; opl, outer plexiform layer. *See* color version on companion CD.

des animaux vivant sur les haux lieux" ("On the high haemoglobin content in the blood of animals living at high altitude") *(65)*. Evidence that the increase is mediated by a hormone, now called erythropoietin (EPO), goes back 100 yr *(63)*. Hemorrhage, hemolysis, failure of the bone marrow to produce sufficient red cells, and any factor (such as high altitude) that reduces arterial pO_2 all lead to an increase of EPO levels in the blood. It was analysis of the regulation of EPO that led to the isolation and characterization of HIF-1 as its major regulator *(62,63)*. Analysis of regulatory elements in the EPO gene showed an HIF-1 binding site at the 3′ end of the gene, which is essential for hypoxia-induced upregulation of EPO.

Glycolysis

A second hallmark response of mammalian tissue to hypoxia is the upregulation of glycolysis. Recently, evidence has been reported that HIF-1 controls glycolytic activity by regulation of the enzyme fructose-2,6-biphosphatase (PFK-2), which in turn regulates the key metabolite fructose-2,6-biphosphatase *(66)*. Obach et al. *(66)* described a hypoxia response element (HRE) in the 5′ flanking region of *pfkfb3*, one of four genes (*pfkfb1–4*) coding for different isoforms of the PKF-2. Further, they showed that this HRE binds HIF-1 and is essential for hypoxic induction of glycolysis.

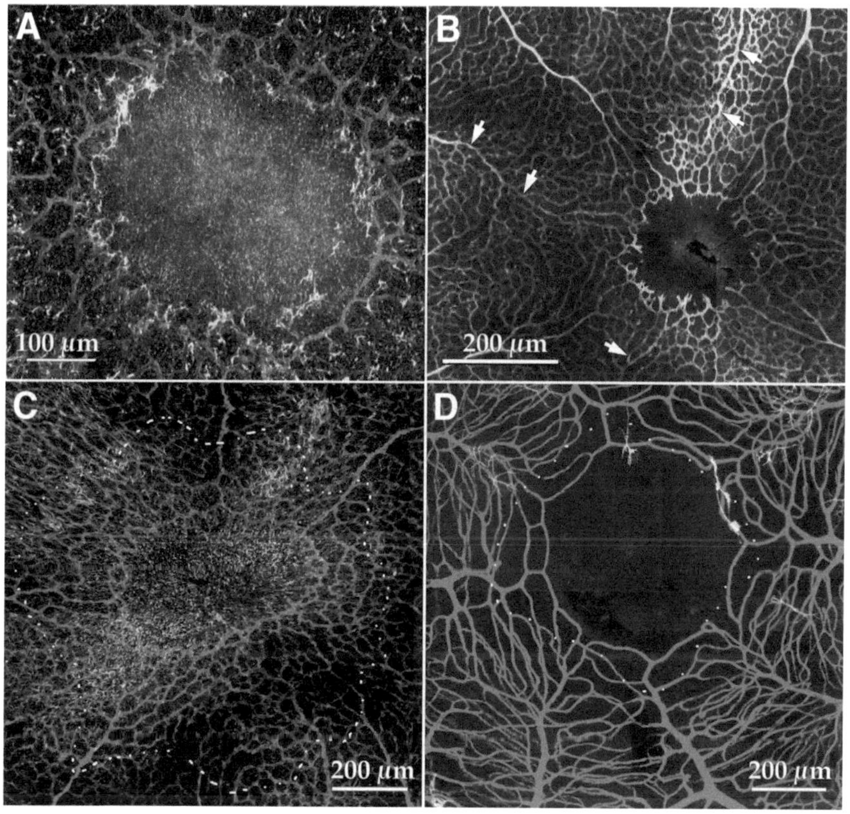

Fig. 5. Confocal microscope images of macaque retina showing different stages in formation of the perifoveal capillary plexus. **(A)** The foveal avascular zone at Fd105 showing the vascular endothelium labeled with antibody to CD31 (red) and GFAP-immunoreactive astrocytes (green). Neither endothelial cells nor astrocytes enter the foveal avascular zone at any stage of development. **(B)** The foveal region at Fd 142, showing CD31 immunorective vessels (green) and Ki67-immunoreactive, proliferating cells (red) in the inner layer of vessels (the ganglion cell layer plexus [GCP]). The majority of proliferating epithelial cells (ECs) (yellow) are distributed along the main vessels (arrows). Because vessels do not form in the GCP at this time it is concluded that the majority of daughter cells move outwards to contribute to the outer plexus, which is forming at this time (see **C**). **(C)** The CD31-immunoreactive inner vascular endothelium (red) at Fd145, also showing GFAP immunoreactivity in clusters of astrocytes, and in Müller cells within the foveal avascular zone. Note the absence of astrocytes associated with the free-endings of EC complexes (compared with **A**). There is no deep plexus within the region defined by the dotted line at this stage of development. **(D)** The perifoveal capillaries (red) in the retina of a 2-yr-old macaque. The full depth of the vasculature is shown. Only one layer of vessels is within the region defined by the dotted line. Note the scarcity of astrocytes (green) in the field. *See* color version on companion CD.

Vessel Formation

Successive investigators of the detail of the formation of retinal vessels *(1,9,68)* have noted the importance of oxygen in the normal development of retinal vessels, suggesting that hypoxia is a normal stimulus ("physiological" hypoxia) for vessel formation *(10)*. After the potent vasoformative factor VEGF was shown to be hypoxia-inducible, the role of VEGF as a hypoxia-inducible angiogenic factor, expressed by a template of astrocytes and Müller cells strategically located in the developing retina, was elucidated *(10,40)*. The demonstration that hypoxia-inducibility of VEGF results from the regulation of its expression by HIF-1 came with the definition of hypoxia response elements in the promoter region of the VEGF gene *(69,70)*, containing one or more binding sites for HIF-1.

HIF-1 Regulation and Tissue Oxygen Sensor

The analysis of HIF-1 regulation has given insight into the nature of the cellular "oxygen sensor." HIF-1 is a dimeric protein, composed of a HIF-1α subunit and a protein known as aryl hydrocarbon receptor nuclear translocator (ARNT). ARNT appears to be insensitive to changes in tissue oxygen, and the mRNAs for HIF-1α and ARNT appear to be expressed constitutively. Tissue oxygen regulates HIF-1 activity partly by regulating the ubiquitination and proteosomal breakdown of HIF-1α. This regulation is effected by the hydroxylation of two conserved proline residues in a region of HIF-1α called the oxygen-dependent domain *(62,63)*. Hydroxylation and subsequent ubiquitination of HIF-1α are inhibited by hypoxia, resulting in accumulation of HIF-1α and upregulation of its activity as a transcription factor. The inhibition occurs because oxygen is the rate-limiting factor for the activity of a family of enzymes, prolyl hydroxylases, which mediate the hydroxylation of the key proline residues in HIF-1α. It has been suggested *(62)* that these enzymes are the cellular oxygen sensors, with one of the family (prolyl hydroxylase 2) of particular importance. A second site of oxygen regulation of HIF-1α lies in C-terminal transactivation domain (CTAD). Hypoxia facilitates interaction of the HIF-1α CTAD with transcriptional activator proteins, thus upregulating the activity of HIF-1. This regulation results because tissue oxygen inhibits, and hypoxia disinhibits, the hydroxylation of a key asparigine residue in the CTAD *(62)*.

MECHANISMS OF FORMATION OF BLOOD VESSELS

Two alternative mechanisms of vascular development have been described: vasculogenesis, the formation of vessels in previously avascular tissue by endothelial precursor cells (EPCs) of mesodermal origin, and angiogenesis, the formation of new vessels by budding or extension from preexisting vasculature *(71,72)*. The distinction has proved a useful one. Michaelson's description of the growth of retinal vessels, for example, suggested an angiogenic mechanism *(1,3)*, whereas later authors *(11,60,67,68,73)* have argued that retinal vessels form from a preexisting population of "spindle" or endothelial precursor cells, which were believed to align and aggregate, forming solid endothelial cords, which subsequently develop lumens and differentiate into mature vasculature. Recent analysis of the bone marrow origins of endothelial cells, and of their incorporation into retinal vessels, however, draws attention away from this distinction.

Origin of Endothelial Cells

Because retinal vessels grow from the hyaloid artery, it was initially thought that retinal endothelial cells differentiate from primary mesoderm surrounding the hyaloid artery *(74)*. More recent work suggests, however, that endothelial cells found in the retina originate more directly from the bone marrow. The marrow is a rich source of multipotential cells of overlapping lineages *(75,76)*, with subpopulations shown to form blood vessels in vivo and in vitro *(77)*. Lineage negative (Lin-ve) hematopoietic, bone-marrow-derived stem cells (HSCs) give rise to EPCs capable of targeting and integrating into normal and pathological vasculature *(77–80)*. Lin-ve HSCs, injected intravitreally, selectively seek out astrocytes and are incorporated into developing retinal vessels, as well as into adult vasculature damaged experimentally or by pathological degeneration *(81,82)*. Although in other organ systems the mechanisms that facilitate targeting of EPCs to areas of neo- or revascularization are not known, R-cadherin (but not other members of the cadherin family) has been shown to have a role in targeting Lin-ve cells to the astrocyte template of the retinal vasculature. Dorrell and colleagues *(83)* have shown that approx 80% of Lin ve cells express R-cadherin, and that blocking R-cadherin by preincubation of Lin-ve cells with R-cadherin antibodies inhibits the targeting, but not the survival, of transplanted cells. Involvement of HSCs in experimental models of subretinal choroidal neovascularization (CNV) has also been demonstrated *(85)*. In these studies bone marrow was obtained from GFP transgenic mice and transplanted into wild-type mice, followed some time later by induction of CNV by laser treatment. The data show that GFP-labeled HSCs are incorporated into the newly formed vessels, comprise up to 50% of that vasculature *(85)*, and include desmin+ve and smooth muscle actin+ve cells, along with CD31+ve endothelial cells *(84)*.

There may, however, be diverse origins of EC. For example, bone marrow-derived stromal cells (BMSCs) are nonhematopoietic pluripotent cells that give rise to a variety of mesenchymal phenotypes *(86)*, including EC *(75)*. Unlike Lin-ve HSCs, BMSCs are regulated by fibroblast growth factor (FGF) 2 and less so by VEGF; grown in matrigel, BMSC form networks in response to FGF2, but not VEGF, and proliferate at double the rate in response to FGF2 compared with VEGF *(76)*. It has also been reported that although VEGF regulates cell behavior during vessel formation in the avian embryo, VEGF is not required for the initial differentiation of endothelial cells from mesoderm *(87)*.

Many Roles of VEGF

Formation of vasculature is now understood to involve a range of pro-angiogenic processes, including EPC differentiation, migration, proliferation, alignment, and tubulogenesis. VEGF has key roles in many of these processes. Mutations involving only a single VEGF allele have been shown to result in major vascular anomalies and lethality in mouse embryos at embryonic day 11 to 12 *(61,88,89)*. VEGFA, the predominant form in the developing retina, signals via two tyrosine kinase receptors, VEGFR-1 (*flt*) and VEGFR-2 (*flk*/KDR), as well as a coreceptor, neuropilin-1 *(90)*. VEGFR2 is thought to be the main receptor mediating VEGF signals in ECs, including proliferation, migration *(91)*, and survival *(92,93)*, whereas neuropilin-1 appears to have a specific role in retinal arteriolar development *(94)* and is upregulated in response to VEGF via VEGFR-2 *(95)*.

VEGF was initially identified as a vascular permeability factor *(96)*, but soon after was also cited as having key roles in endothelial cell proliferation, migration, and survival *(97–99)*, i.e., in facilitating *angiogenesis*. Other studies also indicated that VEGF was also required for endothelial cell differentiation *(61,88)*, thus suggesting a major role in *vasculogenesis (100)*. It is now understood that VEGF plays an important role in several aspects of vessel formation. Furthermore, formation of vascular endothelium from bone marrow-derived stem cells has, more recently, raised questions concerning the value of the distinction between angiogenesis and vasculogenesis, and the term "postnatal vasculogenesis" has been coined to refer to neovascular formations that incorporate HSC *(77,100)*. The pivotal role of VEGF in facilitating incorporation of HSCs into both developing vessels *(81,83)* and vessels growing pathologically or therapeutically in adult tissues *(82–85)* further blurs the distinction between angiogenic and vasculogenic mechanisms.

The effects of expression of low levels of VEGF in the developing central nervous system (CNS) have been investigated using double-transgenic mice in which one VEGF-A allele is deleted, specifically in the CNS *(101)*. In these animals, the initial stages of vascular migration into the retina and extension into the periphery take place, although the animals show abnormally high vascular plexus density (suggesting anomalies in vascular remodeling), aberrantly oriented EC filopodia, and lack of development of the outer retinal plexus. Thinning of the retina was correlated with degree of abnormality in the retinal vasculature *(101)*. The data suggest that although VEGF-A may not be required for recruitment of EPC into the retina or differentiation of EC in the optic stalk region, VEGF signaling to some degree mediates all other aspects of retinal vascular development, including remodeling *(101)*. This latter finding confirms the earlier suggestion that VEGF signaling via FGFR-2 enhances EC survival by inhibiting apoptosis *(92)* and more recently, that EPC survival is VEGF-mediated, via an autocrine mechanism *(102)*. As well as mediating survival, VEGF is has been shown in several studies to mobilize EPC from the bone marrow in mice *(100)* and in humans *(78,103)*, and to mediate EC extension and protrusion during vessel formation *(87)* and network formation in nonproliferating populations of EC *(104)*. Taken together, recent findings suggest that vascular development in the retina is highly, but probably not exclusively, VEGF-dependent.

A RETINAL SPECIALTY: DEFINING AVASCULAR AREAS

The vertebrate central nervous system is a richly vascularized tissue, reflecting its high metabolic activity. The retina is the only part of the CNS that lacks vessels, in whole or part. The exclusion of vessels from the vertebrate retina has the advantage that vessels do not form in the optical path; it was made possible by the evolution of the choroidal vascular bed to supply the retina by diffusion from behind. What mechanisms evolved to exclude vessels from growing into the retina? Conversely, what mechanisms evolved in later vertebrates (mammals) to allow vessels to grow into the inner layers of the retina, allowing greater thickness and complexity of the retina, yet still exclude them from the outer (photoreceptor) layers? Furthermore, what mechanisms evolved still later (in some primates) to exclude vessels from the highly specialized foveal region? Here we briefly review what is known of the mechanisms that define two, and in the case of anthropoid apes three, avascular regions of the retina.

Avascularity of Outer Retina

In all vascularized mammalian retina, the outer layers, formed by photoreceptors, are avascular. The rich vascular bed of the choroid lies just external to these deep layers, separated from them by the RPE; the deep plexus of retinal vessels lies immediately internal to them. Except in disease conditions, vessels do not invade the photoreceptors from either aspect. This exclusion of vessels from the photoreceptor layers facilitates visual acuity. Photoreceptors are aligned parallel to the light rays striking them, so photons pass directly along the photoreceptor to the outer segment. The photoreceptor array resembles, the array of pixels in the receptor plate of a digital camera, and determines the retina's ability to distinguish closely spaced visual stimuli (i.e., visual acuity). Inner and outer segments of the photoreceptors are 1 to 3 μm in cross-section. The smallest vessels are 7 μm in diameter, and would create significant gaps in the photoreceptor array. How is avascularity of the outer retina achieved and maintained? At least two factors appear to have roles in establishing the avascular zone in outer retina: R-cadherin and pigment-epithelium-derived factor (PEDF).

Further Role for R-Cadherin

R-cadherin has been shown to have a significant role in targeting EPCs to the astrocyte template *(83)*. In earlier studies from the same group, R-cadherin was shown to have a role in confining retinal vessels to the inner retinal layers *(42)*. R-cadherin is a member of the calcium-dependent family of adhesion molecules, is regulated by the homeobox gene, Pax-6 *(105)*, and expressed in the developing retina and brain *(105–109)*. In the retina, the expression of R-cadherin during development is dynamic *(109)*. In mouse development R-cadherin is upregulated between P0 and P4 during formation of the primary vasculature, and reaches a second peak expression at P12 during formation of the deep vascular layers *(42)*. R-cadherin is detected in the normally vascularized layers of the retina and is localized to astrocytes *(108)*, to ganglion cells *(42,109)*, to horizontal cells *(109)*, to the inner nuclear layer (INL) (amacrine cells), and to the inner plexiform layer (IPL). Only low levels of R-cadherin are present in the outer retina *(109)*. When antibodies to R-cadherin were injected into the eyes of mice at P2, normal development of the primary retinal vasculature (the inner layer) was disrupted and the area of vascularized retina reduced *(42)*. However, when anti-R-cadherin was injected *after* formation of the primary vasculature (at P7), vessels forming the deep layer of the retinal circulation grew past the INL/outer plexiform layer (OPL) boundary, where their outward growth normally stops, and entered the outer retina, extending throughout the OPL, the ONL and layer of inner and outer segments (bacillary layer) *(42)*. The astrocytic template, to which the primary retinal vasculature normally adheres, was not disrupted by injection of R-cadherin antibody, suggesting that cohesion between substrate and developing vasculature was affected, rather than the substrate itself.

Pigment-Epithelium-Derived Factor in Outer Retina

PEDF is a neurotrophic and antiangiogenic factor first isolated from the RPE *(110)* but expressed also in trabecular meshwork, sclera, and ciliary body and at low levels in orbital muscle, retina *(111)*, and vascular endothelial cells *(112)*. In the retina, PEDF protein is released predominantly from the apical aspect of the RPE and localized in the avascular, outer retina, within the interphotoreceptor matrix, and associated with cone sheaths *(111)*. Several studies have demonstrated the capacity of PEDF to inhibit vessel growth in a variety of models, including neovascularization of the cornea, vitreous and retina *(113–116)*, suggesting that its presence in outer retina may be directly inhibitory to vascular growth. It has also been suggested that under normal conditions VEGF and PEDF are in "critical balance" in the outer retina and RPE, and that this natural balance may be perturbed in some disease or unusual physiological states, contributing to the development of neovascular disease *(112,117,118)*. For example, it has been shown that retinoblastoma cells maintained in low oxygen show increased levels of VEGF but decreased levels of PEDF in conditioned media *(113)*.

Vascular Retraction From Edge of Retina

Even in well-vascularized retinas, such as those of the rat, cat, and human *(36,40,119)*, the edge of the retina is avascular. The width of the avascular region (i.e., the distance from the edge of the retina to the most peripheral vessel) varies from tens of microns to several millimeters. The occurrence and width of this avascular region are determined by two factors. First, the retina thins toward its edge, all three neuronal layers being reduced. Because the choroid can supply the oxygen needs of retinas up to 150 μm thick *(2)*, the retinal vessels are unnecessary, and do not form close to the edge. This idea is confirmed by the fact that the avascular zone is always wider for the deeper layers of the retinal circulation, which are closer to the choroid.

Second, the edge of the retina actively degenerates, beginning in early postnatal life, as soon as the retina starts to function *(119,120)* and continuing, in long-lived species such as the human, decade after decade. In the human this degeneration is well known clinically as cystoid degeneration. This degeneration "is of universal occurrence, having been found in virtually all eyes, including those of premature infants and octogenarians. The cysts increase in number with advancing age, rarely becoming numerous before the age of eight and becoming widespread only after the fourth decade" (*121*, p. 14). In the human the degeneration advances at approx 100 μm per year. As it advances, vessels retract from the edge, leaving the cystoid region, and the still-intact region of retina close to the cystoid region, avascular.

Detailed analysis of this edge degeneration *(119)* shows that it is slowly progressive, even while the retina remains recognizable and probably functional. At the earliest stages outer segments of photoreceptors shorten and are distorted, and vessels disappear. Then the ONL thins as photoreceptors die. Eventually, the few surviving photoreceptors lose their inner and outer segments completely, and cysts form within the retina. The last cells to remain recognizable are Müller cells. Eventually these too die, and pigmented cells, probably from the RPE, invade the residual skeleton of the retina.

Michaelson *(1)* had proposed that the onset of retinal metabolism was an important stimulus for the formation of retinal vessels. These observations show the converse, that the collapse of retinal metabolism is the stimulus for the deconstruction of retinal vessels.

Exclusion of Vessels From the Fovea Centralis

The *fovea centralis* ("fovea") is the part of the retina that allows us to discriminate detail in the visual field, particularly during close work. In primates, the fovea (latin for pit) is formed in early postnatal life by radial/centrifugal migration of the neurons of the two inner layers of retina (ganglion cells and inner nuclear layers) away from a central point in the foveal cone mosaic *(122,123)*, leaving a layer of cone photoreceptor nuclei lining the floor of the pit. The neurons displaced in this process retain their contacts with the central photoreceptors and pile up around the center of the specialization, on the foveal rim. Teleologically, it is believed that this arrangement allows optimal access of incident light to the foveal array of photoreceptors, thereby optimizing visual acuity. The mechanism of this adaptation has been much debated. One attractive recent idea is that the primary mechanism in foveal development is the definition of the foveal avascular zone *(44,124,125)*. The lack of vascularity, it is then argued, makes the foveal region more elastic than vascularized areas of retina, resulting in displacement of neurons of the inner layers away from the avascular zone *(125)*, toward the available vessels.

It needs to be stressed that the vascular specialization of the foveal region is not the absence of vessels from this region of the adult retina. In the adult, only the ONL is present in the central fovea, and this layer is avascular throughout the retina. The vascular specialization is evident in fetal life, when the foveal region has the full set of retinal layers (Fig. 4). It is striking that even with all layers present, the spreading retinal vessels approach the incipient fovea but never enter the region. The GFAP+ve astrocytes that spread ahead of retinal vessels mostly skirt the foveal region, and those that do approach the region where the fovea will develop also stop short of entering it (Fig. 5A).

The signals that guide astrocytes and retinal vessels around the fovea, and that exclude them from the foveal region, are not known. Detailed observations, however, suggest several of their properties. First, these signals guide the astrocytes and capillaries toward the fovea at a deeper level than in other parts of the retina. In other parts of the primate retina the inner layer of vessels is located at the nerve fiber layer/ganglion cell layer interface. The vessels growing toward the fovea, however, are positioned deep in the ganglion cell layer, at the ganglion cell/inner plexiform layer interface (Fig. 4). Second, the molecular barrier blocking entry to the foveal region may be primarily aimed at astrocytes. The astrocytes growing ahead of the vessels toward the foveal region are large and intensely GFAP+ve (Fig. 5; *44*) and strongly express VEGF mRNA (Fig. 4; *126*). They appear to pile up against an invisible barrier around the area where the fovea will form (Fig. 5A; *44*). Furthermore, over the following months, these astrocytes disappear or retreat from the macular region, leaving the perifoveal capillaries virtually devoid of GFAP+ve astrocytes postnatally *(44,127)*. It is possible that the primary block affects astrocytes, and that vessels cannot enter the foveal site because their template is not formed.

The second line of evidence comes from analysis of rates of cell proliferation in the vessels that grow along the horizontal meridian, from the optic disk toward the developing fovea, and in the vessels growing outward to form the deeper layers of the perifoveal capillary plexus. Both astrocytes and endothelial cells proliferate during formation of the primary vasculature in the human retina; pericytes and microglia appear to be nondividing populations in the retina *(52)*. When the density of proliferating cells (Ki67+ve cells/mm^2) is measured in retinal wholemounts, the highest levels of proliferation are found at the peripheral vascular front and along large vessels (peak value, 1296 cells/mm^2) (Figs. 5B,6). Even though vessels are actively growing toward the foveal region at Fd100, rates of cell proliferation surrounding the incipient fovea, and between the optic disk and incipient fovea, are the lowest in the retina (<590 cells/mm^2) (Fig. 6). When the proportion of proliferating cells also expressing the vascular marker CD31 is calculated, the levels of proliferation along the horizontal meridian are half the levels in peripheral retina (Table 1). Similar data were obtained from an animal at Fd142, but in this older animal, the difference in proportions

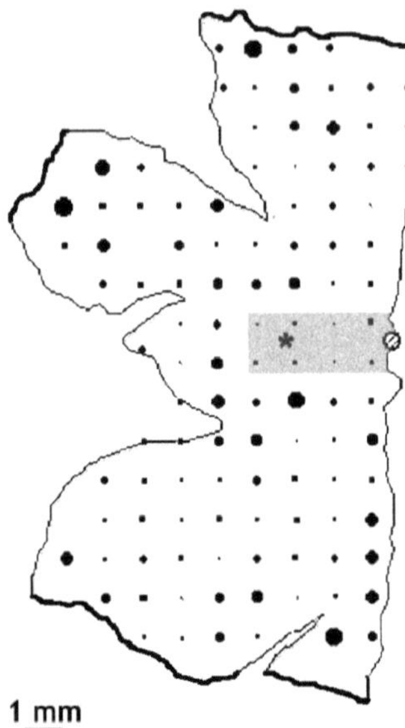

Fig. 6. A map showing the numbers of proliferating endothelial cells (ECs) (Ki67+ve/CD31+ve) cells in a macaque retina at Fd100 (*see* Fig. 5B). Dot size is proportional to the number of proliferating ECs/mm^2. The peak density of double-labeled cells is 1296/mm^2 (temporal superior periphery, i.e., upper left). The area from which "horizontal meridian" and "foveal region" counts were sampled is indicated in gray.

Table 1
Mean Density Labeled Cells (No./mm^2 ± SD) in Inner Retinal Vessels (Fd100)

Fd100	*Horizontal meridian* (N = *12)*	*Periphery* (N = *102)*	*p-value*
Total proliferating cells (Ki67-IR)	568.00 ± 289.65	814.74 ± 334.26	$p = 0.0146^a$
Proliferating endothelial cells (Ki67-IR/CD31-IR)	280.00 ± 156.84	473.72 ± 248.58	$p = 0.0032^a$
% Proliferating endothelial cells	49.88 ± 9.26	56.39 ± 12.73	$p = 0.0628$

Mann-Whitney U test.
[a]Significant, $p < 0.05$.

of proliferating endothelial cells in perifoveal compared with peripheral locations probably reflects the retreat of astrocytes from the central retina *(44,127)* rather than a specific antiangiogenic effect (Table 2). The data also show much lower levels of endothelial cell proliferation in the perifoveal deep plexus, which is just forming around this age, compared with the periphery (Table 2).

The data suggest that an *antiproliferative factor* is expressed along the horizontal meridian, and at peak concentration at the developing fovea, which slows the rate of proliferation in both the astrocyte and endothelial cell populations. This is also evident

Table 2
Mean Density Labeled Cells (No./mm² ± SD) in Inner Retinal Vessels (Fd142)

Fd142	*Perifoveal region & HM* (N = *19*)	*Periphery* (N = *36*)	p-*value*
Total proliferating cells (Ki67-IR)	346.11 ± 226.79	507.76 ± 277.16	$p = 0.0323^a$
Proliferating endothelial cells (Ki67-IR/CD31-IR)	265.26 ± 172.43	443.76 ± 33.97	$p = 0.0059^a$
% Proliferating endothelial cells	78.22 ± 8.7419	87.57 ± 10.91	$p - 0.0008^a$
Deep plexus (Ki67-IR/CD31-IR)	90.00 ± 75.98	188.6 ± 113.45	$p = 0.0096^a$

Mann-Whitney U test.
[a]Significant, $p < 0.05$.

during formation of the deep layers of the perifoveal capillary plexus; the rate of cell proliferation there (Fd142) is less than half that seen in sample areas at comparable stages of formation in the periphery (90.00 cells/mm² ± 75.98, vs 188.6 cells/mm² ± 113.45; Table 2). Although the identity of such a factor or factors remains to be determined, it is worth noting that the low levels of proliferation reflect the topographic distribution of cones, which concentrate at the developing fovea and along the horizontal meridian of the retina *(128)*. Whether a factor originating from cones, located in the outer nuclear layer, can influence events occurring in the inner retina remains speculative, however.

CONCLUSIONS

In evolutionary terms, the retinal circulation has developed late, and in only a subset of vertebrates (some mammalian species). Its evolution has allowed the retina in those species to be thicker and more complex, making possible the high spatial and chromatic acuity of primates. This evolution is fascinating in its detail, and the mechanisms that guide the formation and specialization of retinal vessels are importantly clinically, for much retinal disease is driven by those mechanisms. The nature of the interaction between the choroidal and retinal circulations, and the role of this interaction in retinopathy of prematurity, retinopathy of detachment, and retinitis pigmentosa have been understood for some time. The roles of retinal metabolism in precipitating the formation of retinal vessels, the developmental importance of physiological hypoxia and the damaging effects of hyperoxia, the diverse roles of macroglia, the operation of a local vasoformative factor, and the identification of that factor as VEGF, were all proposed more than a decade ago. In the last decade, (at least) three new concepts of retinal vasculature development have been established or proposed. One is that the formation of vessels is part of a broader response of the tissue (any tissue, not just retina) to hypoxia. The broader response involves erythropoiesis and glycolysis, as well as vessel growth, and is coordinated by transcription factors, in particular HIF-1, that are able to mobilize the range of genes involved. A second is that the endothelial cells that form new vessels, during development or in the adult, are derived from distant (bone marrow) as well as local sources. A third is that late-evolved specializations of retinal vasculature, such as those found at the foveal region, have required the development of new, and still only partially understood, mechanisms for the control of the migration of both macroglial cells (astrocytes) and endothelial cells in the inner layers of the retina. Identifying these mechanisms remains a scientific challenge. The understanding that will emerge as these mechanisms are revealed should also expand the opportunities for therapeutic intervention in still-intractable diseases of the retina.

REFERENCES

1. Michaelson IC. Retinal Circulation in Man and Animals. Charles C. Thomas, Springfield, IL, 1954.
2. Chase J. The evolution of retinal vascularization in mammals. Ophthalmology 1982;89: 1518–1525.
3. Michaelson IC. The mode of development of the vascular system of the retina, with some observations on its significance for certain retinal diseases. Transactions Ophthalmol Soc UK 1948;68:137–181.
4. Stone J, Maslim J. Mechanisms of Retinal Angiogenesis. Prog Retinal Eye Res 1997;16:157–181.
5. Graymore C. Metabolism of the developing retina. III. Respiration in the developing normal rat retina and the effect of an inherited degeneration of the retinal neuroepithelium. Br J Ophthalmol 1960;44:363–369.
6. Graymore C. Metabolism of the developing retina. Exp Eye Res 1963;3:5–8.
7. Ashton N. Oxygen and the growth and development of retinal vessels. Am J Ophthalmol 1966;62:412–435.
8. Patz A. The effect of oxygen on immature retinal vessels. In: Vascular Disorders of the Eye. Mosby, St. Louis:1966:16–27.
9. Chan-Ling T, Stone J. Retinopathy of prematurity: Its origins in the architecture of the retina. Prog Retinal Res 1993;12:155–178.
10. Chan-Ling T, Gock B, Stone J. The effect of oxygen on vasoformative cell division: Evidence that 'physiological hypoxia' is the stimulus for normal retinal vasculogenesis. Invest Ophthalmol Vis Sci 1995;36:1201–1214.
11. Ashton N. The mode of development of the retinal vessels in man. The William Mackenzie Centenary Symposium on Ocular Circulation in Health and Disease. Can JS. H. Kimpton, London:1969:7–17.
12. Stone J, Chan-Ling T, Pe'er J, Itin A, Gnessin H, Keshet E. Roles of vascular endothelial growth factor and astrocyte degeneration in the genesis of retinopathy of prematurity. Invest Ophthalmol Vis Sci 1996;37:290–299.
13. Benjamin LE, Hemo I, Kashet E. A plasticity window for blood vessel remodeling is defined by pericyte coverage of the preformed endothelial network and is regulated by PDGF-B and VEGF. Development 1998;125:1591–1598.
14. Chan-Ling T, Stone J. Degeneration of astrocytes in the feline model of retinopathy of prematurity causes failure of the blood-retinal barrier. Investi Ophthalmol Vis Sci 1992;33: 2148–2159.
15. Janzer RC, Raff MC. Astrocytes induce blood-brain barrier properties in endothelial cells. Nature 1987;325:253–257.
16. Tout S, Chan-Ling T, Hollander H, Stone J. The role of Muller cells in the formation of the blood-retinal barrier. Neuroscience 1993;55:291–301.
17. Greenwood J, Penfold PL, Provis JM. Evidence for the intrinsic innervation of retinal vessels: anatomical substrate of autoregulation in the retina? In: Nervous Control of the Eye. Burnstock GG, Sillito A, eds. 2001, Harwood Academic, Singapore: pp. 155–169.

18. Zhang Y, Stone J. Role of astrocytes in the control of developing retinal vessels. Investi Ophthalmol Vis Sci 1997;38:1653–1666.
19. Donahue ML, Phelps D, Watkins RH, LoMonaco MB, Horowitz S. Retinal vascular endothelial growth factor (VEGF) mRNA expression is altered in relation to neovasculatization in oxygen induced retinopathy. Curr Eye Res 1996;15:175–184.
20. Gerhardinger C, Brown LF, Roy S, Mizutani M, Zucker CL, Lorenzi M. Expression of vascular endothelial growth factor in the human retina and in nonproliferative diabetic retinopathy. Am J Pathol 1998;152:1453–1462.
21. Lewis G, Mervin K, Valter K, et al. Limiting the proliferation and reactivity of retinal müller cells during detachment: the value of oxygen supplementation. Am J Ophthalmol 1999;128:165–172.
22. Mervin K, Valter K, Maslim J, Lewis G, Fisher S, Stone J. Limiting photoreceptor death and deconstruction during experimental retinal detachment: the value of oxygen supplementation. Am J Ophthalmol 1999;128:155–164.
23. Linsenmeier RA, Padnick-Silver L. Metabolic dependence of photoreceptors on the choroid in the normal and detached retina. Invest Ophthalmol Vis Sci 2000;41:3117–3123.
24. Stone J, Maslim J, Valter-Kocsi K, et al. Mechanisms of photoreceptor death and survival in mammalian retina. Prog Retinal Eye Res 1999;18:689–735.
25. Yu DY, Cringle SJ, Su EN, Yu PK. Intraretinal oxygen levels before and after photoreceptor loss in the RCS Rat. Investi Ophthalmol Vis Sci, 2000;41:3999–4006.
26. Yu DY, Cringle S, Valter K, Walsh N, Lee D, Stone J. Photoreceptor death, trophic factor expression, retinal oxygen status, and photoreceptor function in the P23H rat. Invest Ophthalmol Vis Sci 2004;45:2013–2019.
27. Yamada H, Yamada E, Ando A, et al. Fibroblast growth factor-2 decreases hyperoxia-induced photoreceptor cell death in mice. Am J Pathol 2001;159:1113–1120.
28. Walsh N, Bravo-Nuevo A, Geller S, Stone J. Resistance of photoreceptors in the C57BL/6-C2J, C57BL/6J and BALB/CJ mouse strains to oxygen stress: evidence of an oxygen phenotype. Current Eye Research 2004;29:441–447.
29. Heckenlively J. Retinitis Pigmentosa. Lippincott, Philadelphia: 1988.
30. Penn JS, Li S, Naash MI. Ambient hypoxia reverses retinal vascular attenuation in a transgenic mouse model of autosomal dominant retinitis pigmentosa. Invest Ophthalmol Vis Sci 2000;41:4007–4013.
31. Schnitzer J. Retinal astrocytes: their restriction to vascularized parts of the mammalian retina. Neurosci Lett 1987;78:29–34.
32. Stone J, Dreher Z. Relationship between astrocytes, ganglion cells, and vasculature of the retina. J Comp Neurol 1987;255:35–49.
33. Schnitzer J. Astrocytes in the guinea pig, horse, and monkey retina: their occurence coincides with the presence of blood vessels. Glia 1988;1:74–89.
34. Liu Y, Rao MS. Glial progenitors in the CNS and possible lineage relationships among them. Biol Cell 2004;96:279–290.
35. Watanabe T, Raff MC. Retinal astrocytes are immigrants from the optic nerve. Nature 1988;332:834–837.
36. Ling T, Mitrofanis J, Stone J. The origin of astrocytes in the developing retina of the rat: evidence of a migration from the optic nerve. J Comp Neurol 1989;286:345–352.
37. Huxlin KR, Dreher Z, Schulz M, Dreher B. Glial reactivity in the retinal of adult rats. Glia 1995;15:105–118.
38. Chan-Ling T, Stone J. Factors determining the migration of astrocytes into the developing retina: migration does not depend on intact axons or patent vessels. J Comp Neurology 1991;303:375–386.
39. Kopatz K, Distler C. Astrocyte invasion and vasculogenesis in the developing ferret retina. J Neurocytol 2000;29:157–172.

40. Stone J, Itin A, Alon T, et al. Development of retinal vasculature is mediated by hypoxia-induced vascular endothelial growth factor (VEGF) expression by neuroglia. J Neurosci 1995;15:4738–4747.
41. Huxlin KR, Sefton AJ, Furby JH. The origin and development of retinal astrocytes in the mouse. J Neurocytol 1992;21:530–544.
42. Dorrell MI, Aguilar E, Friedlander M. Retinal vascular development is mediated by endothelial filopodia, a preexisting astrocytic template and specific R-cadherin adhesion. Invest Ophthalmol Vis Sci 2002;43:3500–3510.
43. Gariano RF, Sage EH, Kaplan HJ, Hendrickson AE. Development of astrocytes and their relation to blood vessels in fetal monkey retina. Invest Ophthalmol Vis Sci 1996;37: 2367–2375.
44. Provis JM, Sandercoe T, Hendrickson AE. Astrocytes and blood vessels define the foveal rim during primate retinal development. Invest Ophthalmol Vis Sci 2000;41:2827–2836.
45. Provis JM, Leech J, Diaz CM, Penfold PL, Stone J, Keshet E. Development of the human retinal vasculature: cellular relations and VEGF expression. Exp Eye Res 1997;65: 555–568.
46. Mi H, Barres BA. Purification and characterization of astrocyte precursor cells in the developing rat optic nerve. J Neurosci 1999;19:1049–1061.
47. Cunliffe HE, McNoe LA, Ward TA, Devriendt K, Brunner HG, Eccles MR. The prevalence of PAX2 mutations in patients with isolated colobomas or colobomas associated with urogenital anomalies. J Med Genet 1998;35:806–812.
48. Mudhar HS, Pollock RA, Wang C, Stiles CD, Richardson WD. PDGF and its receptors in the developing rodent retina and optic nerve. Development 1993;118:539–552.
49. Reneker WL, Overbeek PA. Lens-specific expression of PDGF-A in transgenic mice results in retinal astrocytic hamartomas. Invest Ophthalmol Vis Sci 1996;37: 2455–2466.
50. Mi H, Haeberle H, Barres BA. Induction of astrocyte differentiation by endothelial cells. J Neurosci 2001;21:1538–1547.
51. Chan-Ling T, McLeod DS, Hughes S, et al. Astrocyte-endothelial cell relationships during human retinal vascular development. Invest Ophthalmol Vis Sci 2004;45:2020–2032.
52. Sandercoe TM, Madigan MC, Billson FA, Penfold PL, Provis JM. Astrocyte proliferation during development of the human retinal vasculature. Exp Eye Res 1999;69:511–523.
53. Ling, T, Stone J. The development of astrocytes in the cat retina: Evidence of migration from the optic nerve. Dev Brain Res 1988;44:73–85.
54. Zhang Y, Porat RM, Alon T, Keshet E, Stone J. Tissue oxygen levels control astrocyte movement and differentiation in developing retina. Dev Brain Res 1999;118:135–145.
55. Risau W. Induction of blood-brain barrier endothelial cell differentiation. [review]. Ann NY Acad Sci 1991;633:405–419.
56. Gardner TW, Lieth E, Khin SA, et al. Astrocytes increase barrier properties and ZO-1 expression in retinal vascular endothelial cells. Invest Ophthalmol Vis Sci 1997;38:2423–2427.
57. Holländer H, Makarov F, Dreher Z, van Driel D, Chan-Ling T, Stone J. Structure of the macroglia of the retina: Sharing and division of labour between astrocytes and Müller cells. J Comp Neurol 1991;313:587–603.
58. Furukawa T, Mukherjee S, Bao Z, Morrow E, Cepko C. rax, Hes1, and notch1 promote the formation of Müller glia by postnatal retinal progenitor cells. Neuron 2000;26:383–394.
59. Walcott JC, Provis JM. Muller cells express the neuronal progenitor cell marker nestin in both differentiated and undifferentiated human foetal retina. Clin Exper Ophthalmol 2003;31:246–249.
60. Chan-Ling, T, Halasz P, Stone J. Development of retinal vasculature in the cat: processes and mechanisms. Curr Eye Res 1990;9:459–478.

61. Carmeliet P, Ferreira V, Breier G, et al. Abnormal blood vessel development and lethality in embryos lacking a single VEGF allele. Nature 1996;380:435–439.
62. Poellinger, L, Johnson RS. HIF-1 and hypoxic response: the plot thickens. Curr Opin Genet Dev 2004;14:81–85.
63. Fandrey J. Hypoxia-inducible gene expression. [review] [47 refs]. Respiration Physiol 1995;101:1–10.
64. Mazure NM, Brahimi-Horn MC, Berta MA, et al. HIF-1: master and commander of the hypoxic world. A pharmacological approach to its regulation by siRNAs. Biochem Pharmacol 2004;68:971–980.
65. Bert P. Sur la richesse en hémoglobine du sang des animaux vivant sur les haux lieux. CR. Acad Sci Paris 1882;94:805–807.
66. Obach M, Navarro-Sabate A, Caro J, et al. 6-Phosphofructo-2-kinase (pfkfb3) gene promoter contains hypoxia-inducible factor-1 binding sites necessary for transactivation in response to hypoxia. J Biol Chem 2004;279:53,562–53,570.
67. Ashton N. Retinal vascularization in health and disease. Am J Ophthalmol 1957;44(suppl): 7–17.
68. Ashton N. Retinal angiogenesis in the human embryo. Brit Med Bull 1970;26:103–106.
69. D'Angio CT, LoMonaco MB, Johnston CJ, Reed CK, Finkelstein JN. Differential roles for NF-kappa B in endotoxin and oxygen induction of interleukin-8 in the macrophage. Am J Physiol Lung Cell Mol Physiol 2004;286:L30–L36.
70. Josko J, Mazurek M. Transcription factors having impact on vascular endothelial growth factor (VEGF) gene expression in angiogenesis. Med Sci Monit 2004;10:RA89–RA98.
71. Ausprunk D, Folkman J. Migration and proliferation of endothelial cells in preformed and newly formed blood vessels during tumor angiogenesis. Microvasc Res 1977:14.
72. Risau W, Flamme I. Vasculogenesis. Ann Rev Cell Dev Biol 1995;11:73–91.
73. Hughes S, Yang H, Chan-Ling T. Vascularization of the human fetal retina: roles of vasculogenesis and angiogenesis. Invest Ophthalmol Vis Sci 2000;41:1217–1228.
74. Shakib M, De Oliveira LF, Henkind P. Development of retinal vessels. II Earliest stages of vessel formation. Invest Ophthalmol 1968;7:689–700.
75. Reyes M, Dudek A, Jahagirdar B, Koodie L, Marker PH, Verfaillie CM. Origin of endothelial progenitors in human postnatal bone marrow. J Clin Invest 2002;109:337–346.
76. Annabi B, Naud E, Lee Y, Eliopoulos N, Galipeau J. Vascular progenitors derived from murine bone marrow stromal cells are regulated by fibroblast growth factor and are avidly recruited by vascularizing tumors. J Cell Biochemis 2004;91:1146–1158.
77. Asahara T, Murohara T, Sullivan A, et al. Isolation of putative progenitor endothelial cells for angiogenesis. Science 1997;275:964–967.
78. Kalka C, Masuda H, Takahashi T, et al. Vascular endothelial growth factor(165) gene transfer augments circulating endothelial progenitor cells in human subjects. Circ Res 2000;86:1198–1202.
79. Isner JM, Kalka C, Kawamoto A, Asahara T. Bone marrow as a source of endothelial cells for natural and iatrogenic vascular repair. Ann NY Acad Sci 2001;953:75–84.
80. Csaky K, Baffi J, Byrnes G, et al. Recruitment of marrow-derived endothelial cells to experimental choroidal neovascularization by local expression of vascular endothelial growth factor. Exper Eye Res 2004;78:1107–1116.
81. Otani A, Kinder K, Ewalt K, Otero FJ, Schimmel P, Friedlander M. Bone marrow-derived stem cells target retinal astrocytes and can promote or inhibit retinal angiogenesis. [comment]. Nat Med 2002;8:1004–1010.
82. Otani A, Dorrell M, Kinder K, et al. Rescue of retinal degeneration by intravitreally injected adult bone marrow-derived lineage-negative hematopoietic stem cells. J Clin invest 2004;114:765–774.

83. Dorrell IM, Otani A, Aguilar E, Moreno SK, Friedlander M. Adult bone marrow-derived stem cells use R-cadherin to target sites of neovascularization in the developing retina. Blood 2004;103:3420–3427.
84. Espinosa-Heidmann GD, Caicedo A, Hernandez EP, Csaky KG, Cousins SW. Bone marrow-derived progenitor cells contribute to experimental choroidal neovascularization. Invest Ophthalmol Vis Sci 2003;44:4914–4919.
85. Sengupta N, Caballero S, Mames RN, Butler JM, Scott EW, Grant MB. The role of adult bone marrow-derived stem cells in choroidal neovascularization. Invest Ophthalmol Vis Sci 2003;44:4908–4913.
86. Prockop D. Marrow stromal cells as stem cells for nonhematopoietic tissues. Science 1997;27:71–74.
87. Drake JC, LaRue A, Ferrara N, Little CD. VEGF regulates cell behavior during vasculogenesis. Dev Biol 2000;224:178–188.
88. Ferrara N, Carver-Moore K, Chen H, et al. Heterozygous embryonic lethality induced by targeted inactivation of the VEGF gene. Nature 1996;380:439–442.
89. Gerber PH, Hillan KJ, Ryan AM, et al. VEGF is required for growth and survival in neonatal mice. Development 1999;126:1149–1159.
90. Witmer AN, Vrensen GF, Van Noorden CJ, Schlingemann RO. Vascular endothelial growth factors and angiogenesis in eye disease. Prog Retinal Eye Res 2003;22:1–29.
91. Thakker GD, Hajjar DP, Muller WA, Rosengart TK. The role of phosphatidylinositol 3-kinase in vascular endothelial growth factor signaling. J Biol Chem 1999;274:10,002–10,007.
92. Gerber HP, Dixit V, Ferrara N. Vascular endothelial growth factor induces expression of the antiapoptotic proteins Bcl-2 and A1 in vascular endothelial cells. J Biol Chem 1998;273: 13,313–13,316.
93. Gerber HP, McMurtrey A, Kowalski J, et al. Vascular endothelial growth factor regulates endothelial cell survival through the phosphatidylinositol 3'-kinase/Akt signal transduction pathway. Requirement for Flk-1/KDR activation. J Biol Chem 1998;273:30,336–30,343.
94. Stalmans I, Ng YS, Rohan R, et al. Arteriolar and venular patterning in retinas of mice selectively expressing VEGF isoforms. J Clin Invest 2002;109:327–336.
95. Oh H, Takagi H, Otani A, et al. Selective induction of neuropilin-1 by vascular endothelial growth factor (VEGF): a mechanism contributing to VEGF-induced angiogenesis. Proc Natl Acad Sci USA 2002;99:383–388.
96. Connolly DT, Heuvelman DM, Nelson R, et al. Tumor vascular permeability factor stimulates endothelial cell growth and angiogenesis. J Clin Invest 1989;84:1470–1478.
97. Ferrara N, Henzel W. Pituitary follicular cells secrete a novel heparin-binding growth factor specific for vascular endothelial cells. Biochem Biophys Res Commun 1989;161:851–858.
98. Plouet J, Schilling J, Gospodarowicz D. Isolation and characterization of a newly identified endothelial cell mitogen produced by AtT-20 cells. 3801–3806.
99. Alon T, Hemo I, Itin A, Pe'er J, Stone J, Keshet E. Vascular endothelial growth factor acts as a survival factor for newly formed retinal vessels and has implications for retinopathy of prematurity. Nat Med 1995;1:1024–1028.
100. Asahara T, Takahashi T, Masuda H, et al. VEGF contributes to postnatal neovascularization by mobilizing bone marrow-derived endothelial progenitor cells. EMBO J 1999;18:3964–3972.
101. Haigh JJ, Morelli PI, Gerhardt H, et al. Cortical and retinal defects caused by dosage-dependent reductions in VEGF-A paracrine signaling. Developmental Biology 2003;262: 225–241.
102. Gerber HP, Malik AK, Solar GP, et al. VEGF regulates haematopoietic stem cell survival by an internal autocrine loop mechanism. Nature 2002;417:954–958.
103. Kalka C, Tehrani H, Laudenberg B, et al. VEGF gene transfer mobilizes endothelial progenitor cells in patients with inoperable coronary disease. Ann Thorac Surg 2000;70:829–834.

104. Helmlinger G, Endo M, Ferrara N, Hlatky L, Jain RK. Formation of endothelial cell networks. Nature 2000;405:139–141.
105. Andrews GL, Mastick GS. R-cadherin is a Pax6-regulated, growth-promoting cue for pioneer axons. J Neurosci 2003;23:9873–9880.
106. Liu Q, Marrs JA, Raymond PA. Spatial correspondence between R-cadherin expression domains and retinal ganglion cell axons in developing zebrafish. J Comp Neurol 1999;410: 290–302.
107. Liu Q, Sanborn KL, Cobb N, Raymond PA, Marrs JA. R-cadherin expression in the developing and adult zebrafish visual system. J Comp Neurol 1999;410:303–319.
108. Gerhardt H, Rascher G, Schuck J, Weigold U, Redies C, Wolburg H. R- and B-cadherin expression defines subpopulations of glial cells involved in axonal guidance in the optic nerve head of the chicken. Glia 2000;31:131–143.
109. Honjo M, Tanihara H, Suzuki S, Tanaka T, Honda Y, Takeichi M. Differential expression of cadherin adhesion receptors in neural retina of the postnatal mouse. Invest Ophthalmol Vis Sci 2000;41:546–551.
110. Tombran-Tink, J, Chader GG, Johnson LV. PEDF: a pigment epithelium-derived factor with potent neuronal differentiative activity. Exper Eye Res 1991;53:411–414.
111. Becerra P, Fariss RN, Wu YQ, Montuenga LM, Wong P, Pfeffer BA. Pigment epithelium-derived factor in the monkey retinal pigment epithelium and interphotoreceptor matrix: apical secretion and distribution. Exper Eye Res 2004;78:223–234.
112. Tombran-Tink, J, Lara N, Apricio SE, et al. Retinoic acid and dexamethasone regulate the expression of PEDF in retinal and endothelial cells. Exper Eye Res 2004;78:945–955.
113. Dawson DW, Volpert OV, Gillis P, et al. Pigment epithelium-derived factor: a potent inhibitor of angiogenesis. Science 1999;285:245–248.
114. Mori K, Duh E, Gehlbach P, et al. Pigment epithelium-derived factor inhibits retinal and choroidal neovascularization. J Cell Physiol 2001;188:253–263.
115. Stellmach V, Crawford SE, Zhou W, Bouck N. Prevention of ischemia-induced retinopathy by the natural ocular antiangiogenic agent pigment epithelium-derived factor.[see comment]. Proc Nat Acad Sci USA 2001;98:2593–2597.
116. Mori K, Gehlbach P, Ando A, McVey D, Wei L, Campochiaro PA. Regression of ocular neovascularization in response to increased expression of pigment epithelium-derived factor. Invest Ophthalmol Vis Sci 2002;43:2428–2434.
117. Ohno-Matsui K, Morita I, Tombran-Tink J, et al. Novel mechanism for age-related macular degeneration: an equilibrium shift between the angiogenesis factors VEGF and PEDF. J Cell Physiol 2001;189:323–333.
118. Ohno-Matsui K, Yoshida T, Uetama T, Mochizuki M, Morita I. Vascular endothelial growth factor upregulates pigment epithelium-derived factor expression via VEGFR-1 in human retinal pigment epithelial cells. Biochem Biophys Res Comm 2003;303:962–967.
119. Stone J, Mervin K, Walsh N, Valter K, Provis J, Penfold P. Photoreceptor stability and degeneration in mammalian retina: lessons from the edge. In: Macular Degeneration. Penfold P, Provis J, eds. Springer, Berlin-Heidelberg-New York 2004;149–165.
120. Mervin K, Stone J. Developmental death of photoreceptors in the C57BL/6J mouse: association with retinal function and self-protection. Exp Eye Res 2002;75:703–713.
121. Bell FC, Stenstrom WJ. Atlas of the Peripheral Retina. WB Saunders Co., Philadelphia:1998.
122. Hendrickson AE, Yuodelis C. The morphological development of the human fovea. Ophthalmology 1984;91:603–612.
123. Hendrickson A. A morphological comparison of foveal development in man and monkey. Eye 1992;6:136–144.
124. Provis JM, Diaz CM, Dreher B. Ontogeny of the primate fovea: a central issue in retinal development. Prog Neurobiol 1998;54:549–580.

125. Springer A, Hendrickson A. Development of the primate area of high acuity.1. Use of finite element analysis models to idently mechanical variables affecting pit formation. Vis Neurosci 2004;21:53–62.
126. Sandercoe TM, Geller SF, Hendrickson AE, Stone J, Provis JM. VEGF expression by ganglion cells in central retina before formation of the foveal depression in monkey retina: evidence of developmental hypoxia. J Comp Neurol 2003;462:42–54.
127. Distler C, Kopatz K, Telkes I. Developmental changes in astrocyte density in the macaque perifoveal region. Eur J Neurosci 2000;12:1331–1341.
128. Curcio CE, Sloan KR, Kalina RE, Hendrickson A. Human photoreceptor topography. J Comp Neurol 1990;292:497–523.

7
Neovascular Glaucoma

James C. Tsai, MD and M. Bruce Shields, MD

CONTENTS

INTRODUCTION

Neovascular glaucoma (NVG) is a devastating ocular disease that results most often as an end-stage complication of retinal ischemia. The condition has been referred to by several other names, including rubeotic, hemorrhagic, congestive, or thrombotic glaucoma, although NVG is now the mostly commonly used term. Fibrovascular tissue proliferates in the anterior chamber, producing neovascularization of the iris (NVI), also known as rubeosis iridis, and/or neovascularization of the anterior chamber angle (NVA). The fibrovascular membrane eventually obstructs the trabecular meshwork and subsequently contracts to produce peripheral anterior synechiae (PAS) and progressive angle closure. The resulting increased intraocular pressure (IOP) is often difficult to control and frequently causes irreversible visual loss *(1)*.

Rubeosis iridis was initially described by Coats in 1906 *(1)*. Since his original description, NVI and NVA have been noted in a multitude of ocular diseases, the majority of which (up to 97%) are associated with an underlying process of retinal hypoxia and ischemia *(2)*. The remaining 3% of cases of NVG are associated with inflammatory diseases, such as chronic uveitis, and intraocular neoplasms. The most common conditions associated with NVG are proliferative diabetic retinopathy (PDR), central retinal vein occlusion (CRVO), and ocular ischemic syndrome. Patients with NVG often have advanced systemic vascular disease. In one series of 79 patients with NVG, 17 patients died within 3 yr of glaucoma surgery because of related systemic disorders *(3)*.

From: *Ophthalmology: Ocular Angiogenesis: Diseases, Mechanisms, and Therapeutics*
Edited by: J. Tombran-Tink and C. J. Barnstable © Humana Press Inc., Totowa, NJ

PREDISPOSING CONDITIONS/THEORIES OF MECHANISMS

The various ocular diseases in which NVI and NVG have been observed are listed in Table 1 *(1)*. Approximately one-third of patients with NVI have diabetic retinopathy *(2)*. The frequency with which rubeosis iridis occurs in association with diabetic retinopathy is influenced significantly by the status of the lens and vitreous. Following pars plana vitrectomy for diabetic retinopathy, the reported incidence of NVI and NVG has ranged from 25 to 42% and 10 to 23%, respectively *(4)*. Removal of the lens, especially if the posterior capsule is disrupted, has also been shown to be associated with a higher incidence of rubeosis and NVG *(5,6)*. In eyes with diabetic retinopathy, extracapsular cataract extraction with primary capsulotomy had a high incidence of postoperative NVI and NVG similar to that observed with intracapsular cataract surgery *(7)*. Leaving the posterior capsule intact appears to reduce this incidence, although subsequent neodymium-yttrium-aluminum-garnet (Nd-YAG) laser capsulotomy in diabetic patients may increase the risk of NVG *(8)*.

Neovascular glaucoma is also associated with retinal vascular occlusive diseases. It is for this reason that it was once called thrombotic glaucoma. In one large series, CRVO accounted for 28% of all cases of NVI *(9)*. Rubeosis iridis and NVG may also be associated with central retinal artery occlusion, although less commonly than with CRVO *(10)*. Other retinal diseases associated with an increased risk for the development of NVI and NVG include branch retinal artery occlusion, branch retinal artery occlusion, and rhegmatogenous retinal detachment *(4)*.

Because the majority (but certainly not all) of the ocular conditions associated with NVI and NVG involve diminished perfusion of the retina, hypoxia of the retina has been postulated to be a significant factor in the formation of new vessels on the iris and in the anterior chamber angle. Ischemia is known to trigger the release of factors that both inhibit and promote new vessel growth *(11)*. Moreover, for the neovascular process to occur, necessary conditions include viable retinal tissue, low oxygen tension, and venous drainage that allows for the accumulation of these angiogenic factors *(12)*. The retinal ischemia theory has been further supported by clinical observations that rubeosis iridis is more likely to occur in patients with PDR or CRVO, wherein there is significant capillary nonperfusion *(13,14)*. Altogether, these clinical observations have lent credibility to the concept that NVI and NVG result from the diffusion of neovascularization-inciting factor(s), which are most often stimulated by hypoxia in the posterior segment.

UNDERLYING MOLECULAR MECHANISMS

The concept of a diffusible factor that stimulates the budding of new vessels from preexisting vascular beds was proposed as early as 1948 *(15)*. Vascular endothelial cells play a crucial role in the process of angiogensis. In response to a specific stimulus (e.g., tissue hypoxia), proangiogenic factors, such as vascular endothelial growth factor (VEGF), basic fibroblast growth factor (bFGF), tumor necrosis factor (TNF)-α, insulin-like growth factor, and platelet-derived growth factor, are actively secreted by these endothelial cells (Fig. 1). This process in turn stimulates a cascade that results in the activation, proliferation, and migration of the endothelial cells, with the final result being formation of new, leaky, fragile blood vessels.

Table 1
Diseases in Which Rubeosis Iridis Has Been Reported *(1)*

Retinal ischemic diseases	
	Diabetes
	Central retinal vein occlusion
	Ocular ischemic syndrome/carotid occlusive disease
	Central retinal artery occlusion
	Retinal detachment
	Leber's congenital amaurosis
	Coats' disease
	Eales' disease
	Sickle-cell retinopathy
	Retinal hemangioma
	Persistent hyperplastic primary vitreous
	Norrie's disease
	Wyburn Mason
	Carotid-cavernous fistula
	Dural shunt
	Stickler's syndrome
	X-linked retinoschisis
	Takayasu's aortitis
	Justafoveal telangiectasis
Surgically induced	
	Carotid endarterectomy
	Cataract extraction
	Pars plana vitrectomy/lensectomy
	Silicone oil
	Scleral buckle
	Neodymium: yttrium–aluminium–garnet capsulotomy
	Laser coreoplasty
Tumors	
	Iris: melanoma, hemangioma, metastatic lesion
	Ciliary body: ring melanoma
	Retina: retinoblastoma, large cell lymphoma
	Choroid: melanoma
	Conjunctiva: squamous cell carcinoma
Radiation	
	External beam
	Charged particle: proton, helium
	Plaques
	Photoradiation
Inflammatory diseases	
	Uveitis: chronic iridocyclitis, Behçet's disease
	Vogt-Koyanagi-Harada syndrome
	Syphilitic retinitis
	Sympathetic ophthalmia
	Endophthalmitis
Miscellaneous	
	Vitreous wick syndrome
	Interferon-α

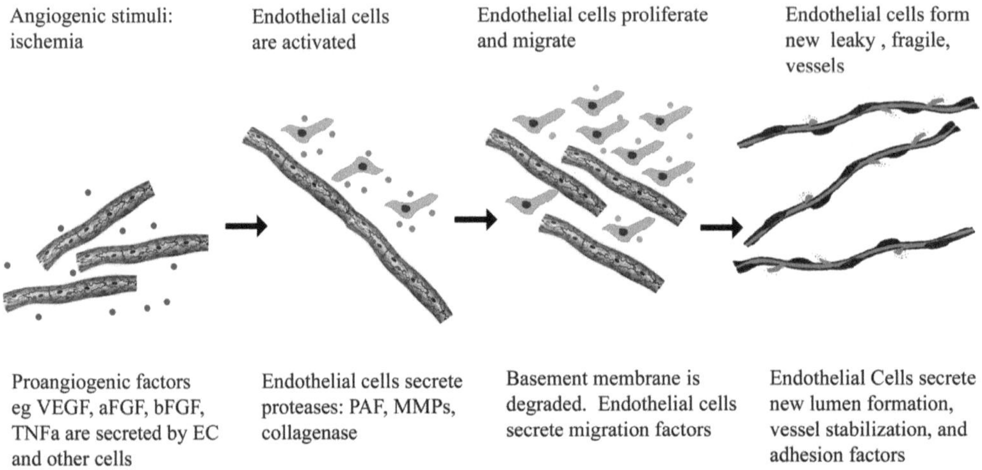

Fig. 1. Key events occurring during the process of angiogenesis. (Reprinted with permission from ref. *22.*) *See* color version on companion CD.

Vascular endothelial growth factor is the most extensively studied of the proangiogenic factors in the pathogenesis of NVG *(16–18)*. The factor is composed of four homodimeric polypeptides, produced through the alternative splicing of messenger RNA. Although VEGF is synthesized by various retinal cells, there is evidence that the Müller cells represent a significant source of the factor under conditions of retinal ischemia. The four VEGF isoforms (VEGF-A, -B, -C, and -D) contain consensus signal sequences for extracellular secretion, and each binds to specific receptor subtypes and stimulates tissue-specific angiogenesis (Fig. 2).

Elevated levels of VEGF have been identified in the aqueous humor of patients with NVG *(19)*. Higher levels of VEGF have also been observed in the aqueous humor of diabetic patients with NVG, compared with those with PDR only *(20)*. Experimental studies in nonhuman primates have shown that intravitreal injections of human recombinant VEGF (in amounts comparable to those measured in eyes with active neovascularization) are sufficient to produce noninflammatory NVI, ectropion uveae, and NVG *(21)*.

Although VEGF is intricately involved in the proangiogenic cascade, therapy targeted for VEGF alone would probably not be sufficient to fully counteract the process of angiogenesis. There are many reasons for this, including endothelial cell diversity, regional variation in tissue expression of the gene encoding VEGF, the complexity of the VEGF family isoforms and receptors, and the contribution of dozens of other factors in the angiogenesis cascade *(22)*. These other proangiogenic factors include insulin-like growth factors I and II *(23)* insulin-like growth factor binding proteins 2 and 3 *(23)*, basic fibroblast growth factor *(24)*, interleukin-6 *(25)*, and platelet-derived growth factor *(25)*.

In most tissues, the vasculature is maintained in a state of quiescence through a delicate balance between proangiogenic and antiangiogenic factors. In the eye, it appears that new vessel formation is affected to a great extent by the balance between VEGF and the antiangiogenic factor, pigment epithelium-derived factor (PEDF) *(22,26)*. PEDF is a naturally occurring and extremely potent angiogenesis inhibitor that not only targets

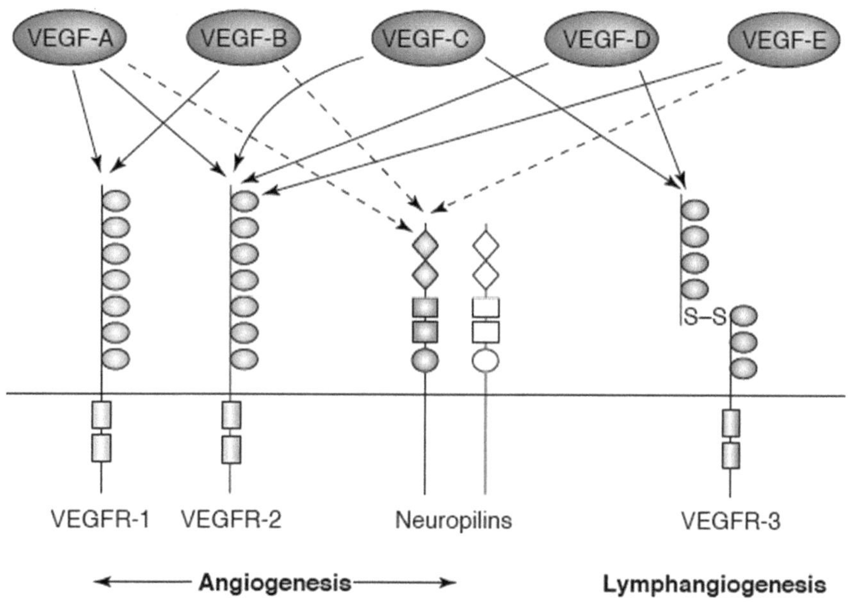

Fig. 2. Diversity of interactions of vascular endothelial growth factor (VEGF) with its receptors. (Reprinted with permission from ref. *22*.) *See* color version on companion CD.

new vessel growth but also has potent neuroprotective activities. The VEGF–PEDF homeostatic equilibrium theory is supported by studies that show increased VEGF and decreased PEDF levels in the vitreous of patients with PDR. Moreover, observations of reduced PEDF levels in the vitreous of patients with active diabetic retinopathy, compared with inactive retinopathy, further support this theory *(27–29)*. These observations suggest possible future therapeutic modalities for neovascular glaucoma that rely on modulation of this angiogenic balance (*see* "Future Therapeutic Options").

It has also been postulated that chronic dilation of ocular vessels is a stimulus for new vessel growth in response to hypoxia *(4,30)*. According to this theory, rubeosis iridis arises from localized hypoxia of iris tissue, which causes dilation of iris vessels and subsequent neovascularization.

CLINICOPATHOLOGICAL COURSE

The clinicopathological course of NVG can be conceptualized as proceeding from an initial preglaucoma stage (existing rubeosis iridis) through an intermediate open-angle stage to the advanced angle-closure stage (Fig. 3). In the preglaucoma stage, fine new vessel growth is observed on the iris, in the anterior chamber angle, or in both locations. Slit-lamp biomicroscopy usually reveals fine, randomly oriented vessels on the surface of the iris stroma near the pupillary margin *(4)*. The new vessels are also characterized by leakage of fluorescein *(31)*. Gonioscopy may reveal a normal anterior chamber angle or early neovascularization, characterized by single vascular trunks crossing the ciliary body band and scleral spur and arborizing on the trabecular meshwork *(4)*. The IOP is typically normal in this stage, unless preexisting open-angle glaucoma is present.

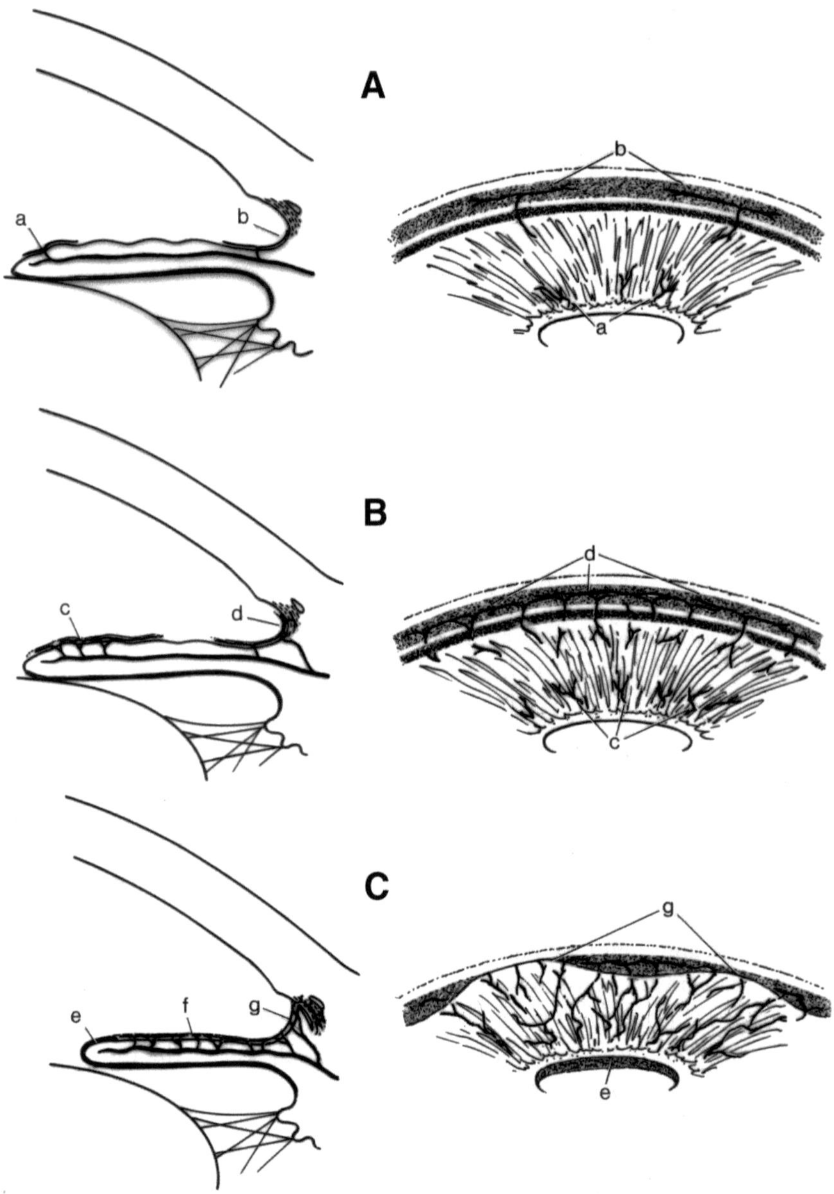

Fig. 3. Clinicopathological stages of neovascular glaucoma. **(A)** Preglaucoma stage (rubeosis iridis), characterized by new vessels on the surface of the iris (a) and in the anterior chamber angle (b). **(B)** Open-angle glaucoma stage, characterized by an increase in neovascularization and a fibrovascular membrane on the iris (c) and in the anterior chamber angle (d). **(C)** Angle-closure glaucoma stage, characterized by contracture of the fibrovascular membrane, causing corectopia, ectropion uvea (e), flattening of the iris (f), and peripheral anterior synechiae (g). (Reprinted with permission from ref. *4*.)

The rubeosis iridis process usually begins intrastromally and then develops on the anterior iris surface *(32)*. Experimental studies in monkey eyes with retinal vein occlusion have demonstrated that the rubeotic process begins with dilation of normal iris vessels, followed by a marked increase in the metabolism of vascular endothelial cells and subsequent new vessel growth *(33)*. Silicone injection studies suggest that the new vessels on the iris (NVI) arise from normal iris arteries and drain into iris and ciliary body veins, whereas new vessels in the angle (NVA) arise from arteries of the iris and ciliary body and drain via the peripheral neovascular network on the iris *(34)*. Histologically, the new vessels have thin fenestrated walls and are arranged in irregular patterns *(35–37)*. Light and electron microscopic studies of the ultrastructure of NVI associated with sickle-cell retinopathy, which is clinically similar to that observed in PDR and CRVO, showed open interendothelial cell junctions, attenuated intraendothelial cytoplasm, and pericyte formation *(38)*.

Rubeosis iridis does not invariably lead to the development of NVG. In rare cases, the rubeotic process may resolve spontaneously, especially in cases associated with PDR *(39)*. However, in eyes that do progress to the intermediate, open-angle glaucoma stage, the growth of fibrovascular tissue is typically florid, and the aqueous humor often reveals an inflammatory reaction *(4)*. It is this stage that once led to the term congestive glaucoma. Gonioscopy shows an open anterior chamber angle, but histological studies indicate that a fibrovascular membrane obstructs the trabecular meshwork, thereby decreasing aqueous outflow and leading to an open-angle form of glaucoma *(35,36)*. In this stage, the IOP may increase rapidly, presenting as an acute onset glaucoma. Hyphema may also be observed at this stage, which is why the disorder was once called hemorrhagic glaucoma.

In the advanced, angle-closure stage of NVG, the iris stroma becomes flattened, often with ectropion uveae, and the anterior chamber angle progressively closes. Myofibroblasts, transiently present in the fibrovascular tissue, proliferate and contract, thereby flattening the iris and pulling the angle closed *(40)*. Obstruction of the trabecular meshwork by progressive synechial closure of the angle leads to increasingly elevated IOP that is often recalcitrant to medical therapy and associated with a high proportion of vision loss *(4,41)*.

CLINICAL DIAGNOSIS

Early diagnosis of NVG offers the best chance of controlling the condition and preserving the patient's vision. This requires a high index of suspicion, especially if the patient has any of the predisposing disease processes (Table 1). Every patient who is at risk of NVG should undergo a comprehensive ocular evaluation with particular attention to the pupillary margin of the iris by undilated slit-lamp examination, gonioscopy, and dilated funduscopic examination. The IOP should be measured as accurately as possible, preferably by applanation tonometry.

In patients with CRVO, studies have shown that a relative afferent pupillary defect (RAPD) indicates an increased risk of developing rubeosis iridis *(42)*. Even patients with a greater degree of RAPD (mean score of 0.9 log units) were more likely to develop rubeosis, compared to those with a lesser pupillary defect (mean score of 0.3 log units) *(43)*. These findings may reflect the relative extent of retinal ischemia produced by the retinal vein occlusion.

A nondilated slit-lamp examination and gonioscopy are essential in the detection of NVI and NVA, respectively. Although NVI usually precedes NVA, new vessels may be found in the angle without slit-lamp evidence of iris neovascularization *(44)*. The Central Vein Occlusion Study (CVOS) revealed that approx 10% of eyes with non-ischemic CRVO and 6% of eyes with ischemic CRVO developed NVA without signs of iris neovasularization *(45)*. Other investigators reported that 4 of 34 eyes (12%) with CRVO developed NVA without signs of NVI *(46)*, hence the importance of careful gonioscopy in these patients.

Other diagnostic techniques for predicting the risk of developing rubeosis iridis in patients with CRVO include angiography and electroretinography (ERG). Retinal angiography may be useful in demonstrating capillary nonperfusion, but its value is limited because the peripheral retina is not included, and interpretation can be difficult owing to the presence of blood and media opacities. Iris angiography may be more useful by revealing early, subtle NVI. In a study of 200 randomly selected fluorescein angiograms of the iris, rubeosis iridis was detected in 97.2%, with a false-positive rate of 1% *(47)*. Moreover, in approximately one-third of the eyes, the angiography test allowed detection of rubeosis prior to its becoming clinically evident on slit-lamp biomicroscopy.

Another test for rubeosis iridis is goniofluorescein angiography. In 100 diabetic eyes studied with this technique, 56 eyes were shown to have angle rubeosis, even though it was evident in only approximately half of the patients by gonioscopy *(48)*.

Electroretinography has also proven to be useful in predicting the development of rubeosis iridis by providing a measure of the degree of retinal ischemia. Although data are conflicting as to the most predictive ERG parameter, a b-wave-implicit time delay and a reduced b-wave/a-wave amplitude ratio appear to be the most diagnostic findings *(49–52)*. The flicker ERG has also been reported to have diagnostic value in predicting the development of rubeosis *(53,54)*.

The differential diagnosis is dependent on the angle status of the NVG. In the open-angle stage, NVG must be distinguished from other glaucomas of acute onset (e.g., glaucoma associated with acute inflammation, angle-closure glaucoma). The diagnosis can usually be made based on the presence of the new vessels on the iris surface and/or angle (although in eyes with uveitic glaucoma, dilation of normal iris vessels may be confused for neovascularization). Moreover, eyes with Fuchs' heterochromic iridocyclitis also may have new vessels in the anterior chamber angle *(4)*. When NVG presents in the closed-angle stage, the differential diagnosis includes the glaucomas associated with angle closure and iris irregularity, such as iridocorneal endothelial syndrome, chronic angle closure glaucoma, chronic inflammation, and old ocular trauma.

CLINICAL MANAGEMENT

Despite the many advances in medical and surgical therapies for glaucoma, the visual prognosis in NVG remains poor. The key to improving patient outcomes is early detection of anterior segment neovascularization and prompt initiation of therapy, targeting the underlying disease process responsible for the rubeosis. Once the IOP becomes markedly elevated, especially in the closed-angle glaucoma stage, the glaucoma is much more difficult to treat and there is a high risk of significant visual loss.

Clinical recommendations for the diagnosis and treatment of NVG may be thought of as Level A (most important to clinical outcome) and Level B (moderately important to clinical outcome) (Table 2). Level A diagnostic recommendations include a high index of suspicion and complete ocular examination, including undilated slit-lamp

Table 2
Recommendations for Diagnosis and Treatment of Neovascular Glaucoma *(1)*

Diagnosis	
1.	Clinicians should maintain a high level of suspicion about neovascularization of the iris or angle, and perform a full ocular examination, including undilated gonioscopy and pupil examination on any eye at risk (A, I)[a].
2.	Iris or angle angiography may be useful to identify neovascularization before it becomes clinically obvious (C, II).
3.	Electroretinography may be useful in estimating the risk of anterior segment neovascularization (C, II).
Treatment	
1.	Complete panretinal photocoagulation, or supplemental panretinal photocoagulation, is indicated as soon as practicable in the eyes with anterior segment neovascularization, if capillary nonperfusion is present (i.e., ischemia of the retina) (A, I).
2.	Treatment of the underlying disease entity responsible for the rubeosis should be undertaken to minimize the risk of subsequent elevated intraocular pressure (A, I).
3.	Medical treatment of both elevated intraocular pressure and any associated ocular inflammation should be initiated promptly (A, I).
4.	Glaucoma surgery is indicated to preserve vision when elevated intraocular pressure is not controlled adequately by medical treatment (B, II).

[a](A, I) Reflects recommendations ratings for importance to the care process (levels A, B, or C) and the strength of evidence from published literature (levels I, II, or III). From ref. *1*, with permission.

biomicroscopy, gonioscopy, and dilated fundus examination. Level A therapeutic recommendations include treatment of the underlying disease process, which usually involves adequate panretinal photocoagulation (PRP), if retinal ischemia is significant, and initial medical control of the IOP and inflammation. Level B recommendations include glaucoma surgery to lower the IOP when medical therapy is unsuccessful.

Retinal Ablation

The initial management of NVG should consist of identification and treatment of the underlying disease process that is responsible for the anterior segment neovascularization, as well as concurrent treatment of the elevated IOP, if necessary. In the majority of patients with NVG, wherein retinal ischemia is the underlying cause, ablation of the peripheral retina is the first line of therapy to counter the angiogenic cascade. In most instances, PRP with an argon laser is the treatment of choice *(55–59)*. Other modalities, such as panretinal cryotherapy, transscleral diode laser retinopexy, and panretinal diathermy, have also been described *(1)*. In the rare instances when the NVG is caused by an underlying inflammatory condition, treatment with antiinflammatory agents is indicated *(60)*, or when ocular neoplasm is the underlying mechanism, treatment of the tumor is required.

Panretinal photocoagulation has been shown to cause regression or elimination of the anterior segment neovascularization *(31,55–57)*. In eyes with PDR, one study showed that treatment with PRP caused regression of rubeosis in 68% of the patients and normalization of the IOP in 42% *(58)*. The importance of adequate PRP treatment was emphasized in one study, wherein 1200 to 1600 laser spots produced regression of rubeosis in 70.4% of diabetic patients, whereas 400 to 650 spots produced regression in only 37.5% *(59)*.

In addition to producing regression of anterior segment neovascularization, PRP has also been demonstrated to prevent the development of rubeosis iridis in eyes with PDR *(61)* and possibly with CRVO *(62,63)*. Even though the efficacy of prophylactic PRP is well documented in patients with diabetic retinopathy, a 10-yr prospective study of eyes with CRVO undergoing PRP, compared with those without PRP, revealed no significant difference in the incidence of subsequent NVG *(64)*. Furthermore, in the CVOS, prophylactic PRP in patients with ischemic CRVO did not completely prevent the development of anterior segment neovascularization, whereas prompt regression of NVI and NVA was more likely to occur when the PRP was performed after early rubeosis became manifest *(65)*. The CVOS investigators also recommended that prompt PRP should be performed when 2 h of NVI or any NVA is observed. Thus, for CRVO, the preferred practice is to follow patients frequently and closely (with undilated slit-lamp examination and gonioscopy) and apply PRP only at the earliest signs of anterior segment neovascularization.

Prophylactic PRP may be indicated when vitrectomy and/or lensectomy is planned in patients with diabetic retinopathy. One study showed that patients with PDR who underwent prophylactic PRP were less likely to develop rubeosis iridis after cataract extraction than those not receiving PRP *(5)*. Furthermore, PRP may reverse IOP elevation in the open-angle stage and in some cases of early-angle-closure NVG *(55,66–68)*. There is also a higher success rate for glaucoma filtering procedures when PRP is performed initially *(69)*.

The mechanism by which PRP influences the neovascularization response is presently not fully known, although it is likely that the ablative procedure decreases retinal oxygen demand, thereby reducing the stimulus for release of the proangiogenic factors *(4)*. This is supported by observations that the photoreceptor-retinal pigment epithelial complex accounts for two-thirds of the total retinal oxygen consumption *(70)*. Another effect of PRP may be the reduction of hypoxia in the anterior ocular segment by reducing the oxygen sink in the posterior segment *(4)*.

Although PRP is the preferred treatment for NVG associated with retinal ischemia, it may be difficult (if not impossible) to perform in patients with media opacities, such as corneal edema, cataract, or hemorrhage, and with poor pupillary dilation. In some situations, PRP may still be applied with the use of an indirect ophthalmoscopic delivery system. When an adequate amount of PRP (at least 1200–1600 laser spots) is not possible, other retinal ablation modalities should be considered, including panretinal cryotherapy and peripheral transscleral retinal diode laser photocoagulation with a contact probe *(1,71–73)*. The latter procedure, which is also known as diode laser retinopexy, has been shown to cause regression of rubeosis *(73–75)* and can be combined with contact diode laser cyclophotocoagulation for IOP control in the treatment of refractory NVG *(73,75)*.

Another surgical option for peripheral retinal ablation is pars plana vitrectomy with laser endophotocoagulation, which can be combined with direct laser coagulation of the ciliary processes if necessary for IOP control *(76,77)*. Concurrent with the vitrectomy, silicone oil tamponade may be employed to prevent or reverse rubeosis iridis by creating a barrier between the anterior segment and posterior segment, thereby reducing the proangiogenic factors and/or the hypoxia in the anterior segment *(76)*. If significant PAS exists, a glaucoma tube shunt may be placed through a pars plana entry site at the time of vitrectomy to control the elevated IOP *(77)*.

All of the previously described retinal ablative procedures are designed to reduce the retinal ischemia and thereby reduce the stimulus for ocular angiogenesis. In some instances, this leads to regression of preexisting NVI and NVA, especially when the neovascularization was present for only a short time interval. Another laser technique, goniophotocoagulation, in which argon laser is applied directly to the new vessels in the angle, was once advocated for the prevention of progressive angle closure *(78)*. It is no longer used, because of poor long-term efficacy and the risk of actually accelerating the angle closure.

Treatment of Elevated IOP

Medical management of NVG is usually required once the IOP begins to rise and is most successful when the disease is still in its open-angle stage. The preferred agents are those that reduce aqueous humor production including the topical β-blockers, topical and oral carbonic anhydrase inhibitors, and the α-2 agonists (which also increase uveoscleral outflow with chronic use) *(1,4)*. Miotics are generally contraindicated because they are not effective when the trabecular meshwork is obstructed by the fibrovascular membrane or synechial closure. In addition, they increase inflammation, worsen synechiae angle closure, and decrease uveoscleral outflow. Prostaglandin analogs also have limited efficacy due to the mechanical obstruction to uveoscleral outflow and may increase inflammation *(1)*.

Topical corticosteroids are often useful because many patients with NVG, regardless of the predisposing condition, will have inflammation and ocular discomfort *(79)*. Cycloplegic agents (e.g., atropine) may be useful in the relief of pain. In a significant percentage of cases, however, medical therapy alone will not adequately control the IOP, and surgical intervention will be required.

One surgical means of controlling elevated IOP in NVG involves cyclodestruction, or partial destruction of the ciliary body, to reduce aqueous humor production. The cyclodestruction may be accomplished with photocoagulation, cryotherapy, or ultrasound destruction. Cyclocryotherapy was once the cyclodestructive procedure of choice for NVG, but has a higher than acceptable failure rate and risk of phthisis, and has been replaced by cyclophotocoagulation *(80)*.

Since the introduction of the first transscleral cyclophotocoagulation procedure with the ruby laser in 1972 *(81)*, photocoagulation has become the cyclodestructive procedure of choice. Since then, the Nd-YAG and diode lasers, using slit-lamp or fiberoptic delivery systems, have been utilized in controlling the IOP in intractable cases of NVG *(82–84)*. Direct visualization and treatment of the ciliary processes with an endoscopic diode laser has also been studied *(85)*. In severe cases of elevated IOP with concurrent florid rubeosis, combined transscleral diode cyclophotocoagulation and diode laser retinopexy may be considered *(73,75)*. However, standardization of a protocol for cyclophotocoagulation in NVG has not been established, and although the IOP can often be controlled, visual results are poor, with long-term visual loss in patients with NVG reaching 46.6% *(82)*.

Glaucoma filtering surgery (e.g., trabeculectomy) in patients with active NVG is rarely successful due to the high incidence of intraoperative bleeding and postoperative progression of the fibrovascular membrane. However, prior application of adequate

PRP may improve the success rates associated with filtering operations by reducing or eliminating the anterior segment neovascularization *(69)*. The adjunctive use of 5-fluorouracil with filtering surgery in patients with NVG who had received prior PRP provided success rates of 67% through the first 2 yr postoperatively, although the success rates fell to 41% and 28% by the fourth and fifth years, respectively *(86)*. Intraoperative application of mitomycin C, a more potent fibroblast inhibitor than 5-fluorouracil, may also increase the success rate *(87)*. Intraocular tissue plasminogen activator has been reported to increase the likelihood of surgical success through its action of decreasing the postoperative fibrin response *(88)*. Modified trabeculectomy procedures have also been described, utilizing either intraocular bipolar cautery of peripheral iris and exposed ciliary processes *(89,90)* or creation of a limbal fistula with the carbon dioxide laser *(91)*. Despite the many modifications to conventional filtering surgery, however, the failure rate of this surgical modality in NVG remains unacceptably high, unless prior PRP was successful in eliminating the active rubeosis.

Aqueous tube shunts have shown promise in the treatment of refractory NVG, including cases in which conventional filtering surgery has failed *(92–94)*. However, the long-term survival with drainage implants is still less than ideal. In a study of 60 eyes with NVG undergoing Molteno tube shunts, IOP control (<21 mmHg) was achieved in only 10.3% at 5 yr. In addition, 48% lost light perception and phthisis occurred in 18% *(92)*. With the Baerveldt shunt implant, 12- and 18-mo survival IOP success rates of 79% and 56%, respectively, were reported in 36 patients with NVG, although 31% lost light perception *(93)*. The Ahmed shunt implant has also been used with some success in the surgical management of refractory NVG *(94)*. Improved success rates have also been reported in some patients with refractory NVG when the drainage tube is implanted through the pars plana, combined with pars plana vitrectomy *(77,95)*. However, as with all surgical modalities for NVG, the visual prognosis is poor, even with successful IOP control, because of the severity of the underlying disease process and the high rate of postoperative complications.

Investigational treatments for NVG have been described in eyes with intractable glaucoma. Surgical retinectomy (to reroute the aqueous drainage through the choroidal circulation) has been performed at the time of pars plana vitrectomy *(96,97)*. Although the IOP was successfully controlled in a majority of patients, long-term ocular complications, including retinal detachment, proliferative vitreoretinopathy, and phthisis, were common. Occlusion of new iris vessels, using photodynamic therapy with verteporfin, without damaging adjacent tissue or normal iris vessels has been postulated, although no results on the progression of rubeosis or NVG have yet been reported *(98)*. Intravitreal injection of crystalline triamcinolone has also been studied as a potential treatment to cause regression of iris neovasculature *(99)*.

Based on an extensive review of the literature *(1)*, a management algorithm has been proposed for the current treatment of patients with rubeosis iridis and angle neovascularization (Fig. 4). For eyes with useful vision, this algorithm focuses on identification and effective treatment of the underlying cause of the neovascularization, as previously discussed. For patients in whom adequate PRP treatment cannot be administered, diode laser retinopexy, panretinal cryotherapy, or vitrectomy with endolaser should be considered. Treatment of the resultant glaucoma may include medical therapy,

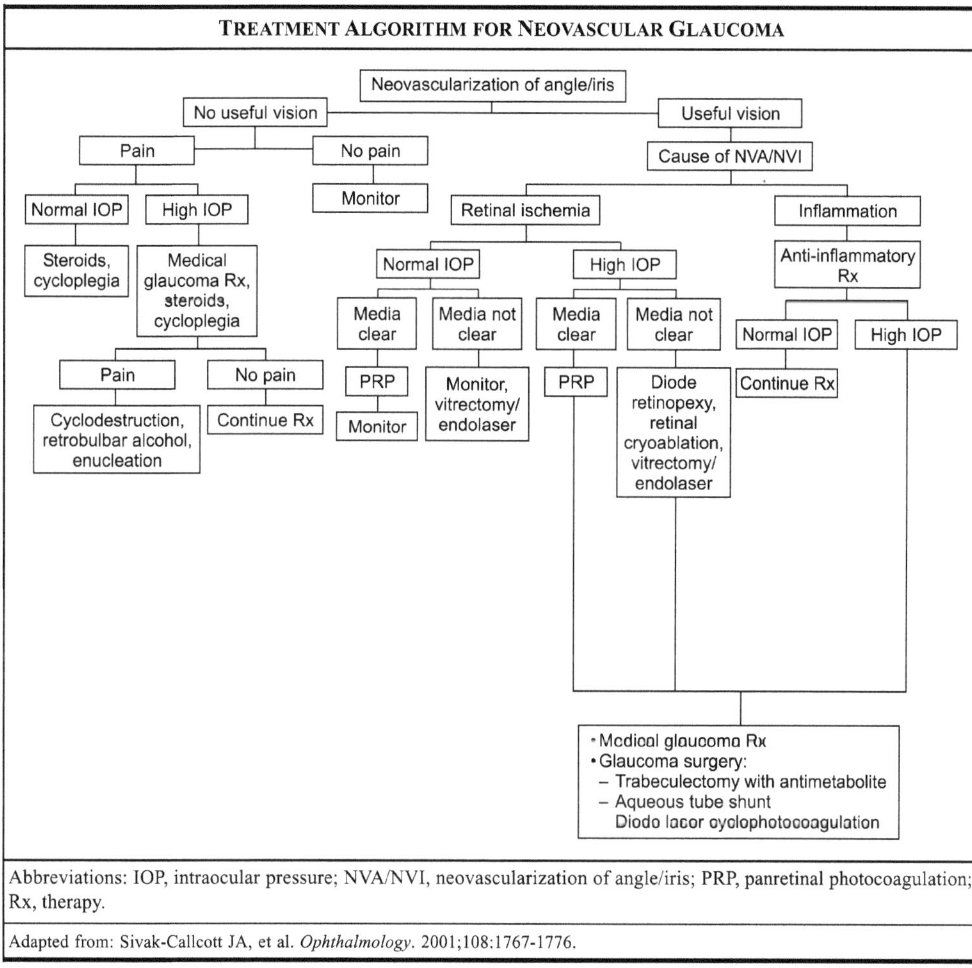

Fig. 4. Treatment algorithm for neovascular glaucoma. (Reprinted with permission from ref. *41*.)

trabeculectomy with an antiproliferative agent, aqueous tube shunt surgery, or diode laser cyclophotocoagulation.

FUTURE THERAPEUTIC OPTIONS

Visual outcome in patients with NVG remains poor, despite advances in the ability to control the IOP with new pharmacological agents and surgical procedures. The optimal approach to the management of NVG lies in the knowledge gained through continued research. Based on an assessment of current literature *(1)*, future research studies that may prove valuable in further refining and improving our management approach are listed in Table 3. More randomized clinical trials are needed to better define the most effective method for retinal ablation and treatments for lowering IOP. In prospective studies, comparing different surgical modalities, success must be defined not only by IOP control but by visual outcome as well.

Table 3
Future Research Studies in Neovascular Glaucoma *(1)*

These should be prospective, randomized clinical studies (if indicated and whenever possible):
Areas in which the current strength of evidence is level I (strong):
Research and development of antivasoproliferative factors
Areas in which the current strength of evidence is level II (substantial):
Efficacy of more aggressive retinal ablation treatment
Efficacy of surgical intervention for retinal ablation in patients with media opacities
Areas in which the current strength of evidence is level II or III (substantial or consensus):
Efficacy and cost-effectiveness of gonioangiography
Indocyanine green vs fluorescein angiography comparison
Comparison of visual outcomes in slit-lamp gonioscopy vs angiography
Determination of the frequency in which gonioscopy should be performed
Study of the pupil examination and its predictive value of neovascularization of angle
Efficacy and cost-effectiveness of electroretinogram
Determination of electroretinogram parameter(s) with highest predictive value of neovascular angle
Evaluation of optimal panretinal photocoagulation treatment protocol
Role of goniophotocoagulation in treatment of neovascular glaucoma
Standardization of parameters for successful retinal ablation when visualization poor
Evaluation of appropriateness of retinectomy in controlling intraocular pressure
Efficacy of glaucoma surgical intervention for elevated intraocular pressure—this should be a randomized, prospective trial comparing cyclodestruction, filtration surgery, and aqueous tube shunts

Future therapeutic approaches will be based increasingly on successful modulation of the angiogenesis cascade. For example, the signal transduction pathway in ocular angiogenesis is not well defined and a better understanding may lead to the development of new pharmacological agents for inhibition of angiogenesis. In animal studies, exposure to 100% oxygen under hyperbaric conditions has been reported to significantly increase the partial pressure of oxygen in the aqueous humor, and may be useful in treating hypoxic diseases of the anterior segment and retina, including rubeosis iridis *(100,101)*. Inhibition of VEGF with neutralizing antibodies has been shown to prevent iris neovascularization in a nonhuman primate model of retinal vein occlusion *(102)*. In another primate model, systemic treatment with α-interferon, a polypeptide that inhibits proliferation and migration of endothelial cells and new vessel growth, resulted in regression of rubeosis iridis *(103)*. In a prospective, randomized, double-masked study of 53 patients with retinal vein occlusion, treatment with troxerutin, which improves microvascular flow by inhibiting platelet and erythrocyte aggregation, increasing erythrocyte deformability, and reducing blood viscosity, significantly improved visual acuity and retinal circulation times, and reduced progressive ischemia *(104)*.

Endogenous angiogenesis inhibitors, particularly those that act broadly at the earliest stages of the angiogenic cascade, could prove to be excellent pharmacological tools in combating neovascularization. To date, an extensive number of antiangiogenic factors have been characterized (Table 4) *(22)*. These molecules are either constitutively

Table 4
Antiangiogenic Factors *(22)*

Constitutive	*Cryptic fragments*
Angiogenin	Angiostatin (38 kDA plasminogen fragment; Kringe 1–4)
Anti-angiogenic anti-thrombin III	Angiotensinogen fragments
Brain angiogenesis inhibitor 1	Arresten (fragment of α1 chain of type IV collagen)
Interferon-α	Canstatin (fragment α2 chain of collagen type IV)
Interferon-inducible protein	Endostatin (20 kDa fragment of XVIII collagen)
Interleukin-12	Fibronectin (20 kDa N-terminal fragment)
PEDF	Fibronectin type 111 peptide
Placental ribonuclease inhibitor	Fibronectin (40 kDa C-terminal fragment)
Plasminogen-activator inhibitor	Heparin hexasaccharide fragment
Proliferin-related protein	Kringle 1–5 (fragment of plasminogen)
Protamine	NC1 domain of type VIII collagen α1
Somatostatin analog octreotide	PEX (metalloproteinase fragment)
SPARC (43 kDa secreted protein acidic and rich in cysteine)	Platelet factor 4 fragment
Thrombospondin-1	Prolactin (16 kDa N-terminal fragment)
Thrombospondin-2	Prolactin fragments
Tissue inhibitors of metalloproteinases 1, 2, and 3	Restin (22 kDa fragment of human collagen XV)
Vasculostatin	Trp-tRMA synthetase splice variant
	Trp-tRNA synthetase C-terminal fragment
	Tumstatin (fragment of α3 chain of type IV)
	Vasostatin (fragment of calreticulin)

expressed in their active form or become active after proteolytic cleavage of larger polypeptides into cryptic fragments.

As previously discussed, PEDF, a potent endogenous angiogenesis inhibitor with neuroprotective properties, shows promise in the future treatment of rubeosis iridis. The molecule has remarkable specificity for causing deterioration of new vessels, with no known deleterious effect on mature vessels *(105)*. Experimental studies have shown that PEDF can be administered therapeutically as a soluble protein or by viral-mediated gene transfer *(22)*. In transgenic mice with expression of VEGF in photoreceptors (rho/VEGF mice) and in wild-type mice with laser-induced choroidal neovascularization, increased in vivo expression of PEDF caused regression of ocular neovascularization *(106)*. Furthermore, in a mouse model of ischemia-induced retinal neovascularization, elevated concentrations of PEDF inhibited VEGF-induced retinal vascular endothelial cell growth and migration and retinal neovascularization *(107)*.

In addition to its proapoptotic effect in vascular endothelial cells, PEDF has apparent neuroprotective effects. Adenoviral vector-mediated intraocular expression of PEDF in rats significantly increased ganglion, inner nuclear, and outer nuclear cell survival after ischemia-reperfusion injury of the retina *(108)*. Although the mechanism by which PEDF exerts this neuroprotective effect is not currently known, possible theories include activation of transcription of antiapoptotic and neuroprotective genes *(109)*.

In this regard, PEDF may have the additional advantage of helping to preserve the integrity of retinal neurons that are damaged from both the underlying retinal ischemia and the resultant elevated IOP in NVG.

SUMMARY

Neovascular glaucoma is the result of a predisposing condition, usually associated with retinal hypoxia, in which anterior segment neovascularization leads to obstruction of aqueous outflow by a fibrovascular membrane. This membrane subsequently contracts, thereby leading to closure of the anterior chamber angle and elevated IOP. The resultant glaucoma is difficult to control, and no currently available medical or surgical treatment has a high success rate.

The most effective treatment to date involves retinal ablation, which reduces the level of retinal hypoxia and retards the subsequent angiogenesis cascade. However, this method is effective only when performed at an early stage of the disease process and has technical limitations. The best hope for preventing the blindness associated with NVG is continued research into the angiogenesis pathway, a better understanding of which will hopefully lead to the development of novel pharmacological agents to prevent and/or reverse the neovascularization process in predisposed patients.

REFERENCES

1. Sivak-Callcott JA, O'Day DM, Gass JDM, Tsai JC. Evidence-based recommendations for the diagnosis and treatment of neovascular glaucoma. Ophthalmology 2001;108:1767–1778.
2. Brown GC, Magargal LE, Schachat A, Shah H. Neovascular glaucoma. Etiologic considerations. Ophthalmology 1984;91:315–320.
3. Krupin T, Kaufman P, Mandell AI, et al. Long-term results of valve implants in filtering surgery for eyes with neovascular glaucoma. Am J Ophthalmol 1983;95:775–782.
4. Shields MB. Textbook of Glaucoma. 4th ed. Williams and Wilkins, Baltimore 1998: 269–278.
5. Aiello LM, Wang M, Liang G. Neovascular glaucoma and vitreous hemorrhage after cataract surgery in patients with diabetes mellitus. Ophthalmology 1983;90:814–820.
6. Rice TA, Michels RG, Maguire MG, Rice EF. The effect of lensectomy on the incidence of iris neovascularization and neovascular glaucoma after vitrectomy for diabetic retinopathy. Am J Ophthalmol 1983;95:1–11.
7. Poliner LS, Christianson DJ, Escoffery RF, et al. Neovascular glaucoma after intracapsular and extracapsular cataract extraction in diabetic patients. Am J Ophthalmol 1985;100:637.
8. Weinreb RN, Wasserstrom JP, Parker W. Neovascular glaucoma following neodymium-YAG laser posterior capsulotomy. Arch Ophthalmol 1986;104:730–731.
9. Hoskins HD Jr. Neovascular glaucoma: current concepts. Trans Am Acad Ophthalmolol Otol 1974;78:330.
10. Duker JS, Sivalingam A, Brown GC, Reber R. A prospective study of acute central retinal artery occlusion. The incidence of secondary ocular neovascularization. Arch Ophthalmol 1991;109:339.
11. Casey R, Li WW. Factors controlling ocular angiogenesis (review). Am J Ophthalmol 1997;124:521–529.
12. Cairns JE. Rationale for therapy in neovascular glaucoma. Trans Ophthalmol Soc UK 1981;101:184, 185.
13. Bresnick GH, DeVenecia G, Myers FL, et al. Retinal ischemia in diabetic retinopathy. Arch Ophthalmol 1975;93:1300–1910.

14. Laatikainen L, Kohner EM. Fluorescein angiography and its prognostic significance in central retinal vein occlusion. Br J Ophthlamol 1976;60:411–418.
15. Aiello LP, Avery RL, Arrigg PG, et al. Vascular endothelial growth factor in ocular fluid of patients with diabetic retinopathy and other retinal disorders. N Engl J Med 1994;331: 1480–1487.
16. Robinson CJ, Stringer SE. The splice variants of vascular endothelial growth factors (VEGF) and their receptors. J Cell Sci 2001;114:853–865.
17. Ferrara N. VEGF and the quest for tumour angiogenesis. Nat Rev Cancer 2002;2:795–803.
18. Giles FJ. The emerging role of angiogenesis inhibitors in hematologic malignancies. Oncology 2002;16:23–29.
19. Tripathi RC, Li J, Tripathi BJ, et al. Increased levels of vascular endothelial growth factor in aqueous humor of patients with neovascular glaucoma. Ophthalmology 1998;105: 232–237.
20. Sone H, Okuda Y, Kawakami Y, et al. Vascular endothelial growth factor level in aqueous humor of diabetic patients with rubeotic glaucoma is markedly elevated (letter). Diabetes Care 1996;19:1306–1307.
21. Tolentino MJ, Miller JW, Gragoudas ES, et al. Vascular endothelial growth factor is sufficient to produce iris neovascularization and neovascular glaucoma in a nonhuman primate. Arch Ophthalmol 1996;114:964–970.
22. Tombran-Tink J, Barnstable CJ. Therapeutic prospects for PEDF: more than a promising angiogenesis inhibitor. Trends Mol Med 2003;9:244–250.
23. Meyer-Schwickerath P, Pfeiffer A, Blum WF, et al. Vitreous levels of insulin-like growth factors I and II, and the insulin-like growth factor binding proteins 2 and 3, increase in neovascular eye diseases. Studies in nondiabetic and diabetic subjects. J Clin Invest 1993;92:2620–2625.
24. Aiello LM, Wand M, Liang G. Neovascular glaucoma and vitreous hemorrhage after cataract surgery in patients with diabetes mellitus. Ophthalmology 1983;90:814–820.
25. Chen KH, Wu CC, Roy S, et al. Increased interleukin-6 in neovascular glaucoma. Invest Ophthalmol Vis Sci 1999;40:2627–2632.
26. Tombran-Tink J, Barnstable CJ. PEDF: a multifaceted neurotrophic factor. Nat Rev 2003;4:1–10.
27. Ogata N, Tombran-Tink J, Jo N, et al. Pigment epithelium-derived factor in the vitreous is low in diabetic retinopathy and high in rhegmatogenous retinal detachment. Am J Ophthalmol 2001;132:378–382.
28. Ogata N, Nishikawa M, Nishimura T, et al. Inverse levels of pigment epithelium-derived factor and vascular endothelial growth factor in the vitreous of eyes with rhegmatogenous retinal detachment and proliferative vitreoretinopathy. Am J Ophthlamol 2002;133: 851–852.
29. Ogata N, Nishikawa M, Nishimura T, et al. Unbalanced vitreous levels of pigment epithelium-derived factor and vascular endothelial growth factor in diabetic retinopathy. Am J Ophthalmol 2002;134:348–353.
30. Stefansson E, Landers MB III, Wolbarsht ML. Oxygenation and vasodilatation in relation to diabetic and other proliferative retinopathies. Ophthalmic Surg 1983;14:209–226.
31. Wand M, Dueker DK, Aiello LM, Grant WM. Effects of panretinal photocoagulation on rubeosis iridis, angle neovascularization, and neovascular glaucoma. Am J Ophthalmol 1978;86:332–339.
32. Henkind P. Ocular neovascularization. Am J Ophthalmol 1978;85:287–301.
33. Nork TM, Tso MO, Duvall J, Hayreh SS. Cellular mechanisms of iris neovascularization secondary to retinal vein occlusion. Arch Ophthalmol 1989;107:581–586.
34. Jocson VL. Microvascular injection studies in rubeosis iridis and neovascular glaucoma. Am J Ophthalmol 1977;83:508–517.

35. Schulze RR. Rubeosis iridis. Am J Ophthalmol 1967;63:487–495.
36. Anderson DM, Morin JD, Hunter WS. Rubeosis iridis. Can J Ophthalmol 1971;6:183–188.
37. Peyman GA, Raichand M, Juarez CP, et al. Hypotony and experimental rubeosis iridis in primate eyes. A clinicopathologic study. Graefes Arch Clin Exp Ophthalmol 1986; 224:435–442.
38. Goldberg MF, Tso MO. Rubeosis iridis and glaucoma associated with sickle cell retinopathy: a light and electron microscopic study. Ophthalmology 1978;85:1028–1041.
39. Ohrt V. The frequency of rubeosis iridis in diabetic patients. Acta Ophthalmol 1971;49: 301–307.
40. John T, Sassani JW, Eagle RC Jr. The myofibroblastic component of rubeosis iridis. Ophthalmology 1983;90:721–728.
41. Tsai JC, Forbes M. Medical Management of Glaucoma, 2nd ed. Professional Communications, West Islip, NY: 2004:222–225.
42. Servais GE, Thompson HS, Hayreh SS. Relative afferent papillary defect in central retinal vein occlusion. Ophthalmology 1986;93:301–303.
43. Bloom PA, Papakostopoulos D, Gogolitsyn Y, et al. Clinical and infrared pupillometry in central retinal vein occlusion. Br J Ophthalmol 1993;77:75–80.
44. Blinder KJ, Friedman SM, Mames RN. Diabetic iris neovascularization. Am J Ophthalmol 1995;120:393–395.
45. Baseline and early natural history report. The Central Vein Occlusion Study. Arch Ophthalmol 1993;11:1087–1095.
46. Browning DJ, Scott AQ, Peterson CB, et al. The risk of missing angle neovascularization by omitting screening gonioscopy in acute central retinal vein occlusion. Ophthalmology 1998;105:776–784.
47. Sanborn GE, Symes DJ, Magargal LE. Fundus-iris fluorescein angiography: evaluation of its use in the diagnosis of rubeosis iridis. Ann Ophthalmol 1986;18:52–58. Erratum in: Ann Ophthalmol 1986;18:155.
48. Ohnishi Y, Ishibashi T, Sagawa T. Fluorescein gonioangiography in diabetic neovascularization. Graefes Arch Clin Exp Ophthalmol 1994;232:199–204.
49. Sabates R, Hirose T, McMeel JW. Electroretinography in the prognosis and classification of central retinal vein occlusion. Arch Ophthalmol 1983;101:232–235.
50. Kaye SB, Harding SP. Early electroretinography in unilateral central retinal vein occlusion as a predictor of rubeosis iridis. Arch Ophthalmol 1988;106:353–356.
51. Breton ME, Quinn GE, Keene SS, et al. Electroretinogram parameters at presentation as predictors of rubeosis in central retinal vein occlusion patients. Ophthalmology 1989;96: 1343–1352.
52. Larsson J, Andreasson S, Bauer B. Cone b-wave implicit time as an early predictor of rubeosis in central retinal vein occlusion. Am J Ophthalmol 1998;125:247–249.
53. Severns ML, Johnson MA. Predicting outcome in central retinal vein occlusion using the flicker electroretinogram. Arch Ophthalmol 1993;111:1123–1130.
54. Johnson MA, McPhee TJ. Electroretinographic findings in iris neovascularization due to acute central retinal vein occlusion. Arch Ophthalmol 1993;111:806–814.
55. Little HL, Rosenthal AR, Dellaporta A, Jacobson DR. The effect of pan-retinal photocoagulation on rubeosis iridis. Am J Ophthalmol 1976;81:804–809.
56. Murphy RP, Egbert PR. Regression of iris neovascularization following panretinal photocoagulation. Arch Ophthalmol 1979;97:700–702.
57. Tasman W, Magargal LE, Augsburger JJ. Effects of argon laser photocoagulation on rubeosis iridis and angle neovascularization. Ophthalmology 1980;87:400–402.
58. Ohnishi Y, Ishibashi T, Sagawa T. Fluorescein gonioangiography in diabetic neovascularization. Graefes Arch Clin Exp Ophthalmol 1994;232:199–204.

59. Striga M, Ivanisevic M. Comparison between efficacy of full- and mild-scatter (panretinal) photocoagulation on the course of diabetic rubeosis iridis. Ophthalmologica 1993;207: 144–147.
60. Rodgin SG. Neovascular glaucoma associated with uveitis. J Am Optom Assoc 1987;58: 499–503.
61. Kaufman SC, Ferris FL III, Swartz M. Intraocular pressure following panretinal photocoagulation for diabetic retinopathy. Diabetic retinopathy report no. 11. Arch Ophthalmol 1987;105:807–809.
62. Magargal LE, Brown GC, Augsburger JJ, Donoso LA. Efficacy of panretinal photocoagulation in preventing neovascular glaucoma following ischemic central retinal vein occlusion. Ophthalmology 1982;89:780–784.
63. Laatikainen L. A prospective follow-up study of panretinal photocoagulation in preventing neovascular glaucoma following ischaemic central retinal vein occlusion. Graefes Arch Clin Exp Ophthalmol 1983;220:236–239.
64. Hayreh SS, Klugman MR, Podhajsky P, et al. Argon laser panretinal photocoagulation in ischemic central retinal vein occlusion. A 10-year prospective study. Graefes Arch Clin Exp Ophthalmol 1990;228:281–296.
65. A randomized clinical trial of early panretinal photocoagulation for ischemic central vein occlusion. The Central Vein Occlusion Study Group N report. Ophthalmology 1995;102: 1434–1444.
66. Laatikainen L. Preliminary report on effect of retinal panphotocoagulation on rubeosis iridis and neovascular glaucoma. Br J Ophthalmol 1977;61:278–284.
67. Teich SA, Walsh JB. A grading system for iris neovascularization. Prognostic implications for treatment. Ophthalmology 1981;88:1102–1106.
68. Jacobson DR, Murphy RP, Rosenthal AR. The treatment of angle neovascularization with panretinal photocoagulation. Ophthalmology 1979;86:1270–1277.
69. Allen RC, Bellows AR, Hutchinson BT, Murphy SD. Filtration surgery in the treatment of neovascular glaucoma. Ophthalmology 1982;89:1181–1187.
70. Weiter JJ, Zuckerman R. The influence of the photoreceptor-RPE complex on the inner retina. An explanation of the beneficial effects of photocoagulation. Ophthalmology 1980;87:1133–1139.
71. May DR, Bergstrom TJ, Parmet AJ, Schwartz JG. Treatment of neovascular glaucoma with transscleral panretinal cryotherapy. Ophthalmology 1980;87:1106–1111.
72. Vernon SA, Cheng H. Panretinal cryotherapy in neovascular disease. Br J Ophthalmol 1988;72:401–405.
73. Flaxel CJ, Larkin GB, Broadway DB, et al. Peripheral transscleral retinal diode laser for rubeosis iridis. Retina 1997;17:421–429.
74. McHugh JDA, Marshall J, Ffytche TJ, et al. Initial clinical experience using a diode laser in the treatment of retinal vascular disease. Eye 1989;3:516–527.
75. Tsai JC, Bloom PA, Franks WA, Khaw PT. Combined transscleral diode laser cyclophotocoagulation and transscleral retinal photocoagulation for refractory neovascular glaucoma. Retina 1996;16:164–166.
76. Bartz-Schmidt KU, Thumann G, Psichias A, et al. Pars plana vitrectomy, endolaser coagulation of the retina and the ciliary body combined with silicone oil endotamponade in the treatment of uncontrolled neovascular glaucoma. Graefes Arch Clin Exp Ophthalmol 1999;237:969–975.
77. Scott IU, Alexandrakis G, Flynn HW Jr, et al. Combined pars plana vitrectomy and glaucoma drainage implant placement for refractory glaucoma. Am J Ophthalmol 2000; 129:334–341.
78. Simmons RJ, Deppermann SR, Dueker DK. The role of gonio-photocoagulation in neovascularization of the anterior chamber angle. Ophthalmology 1980;87:79–82.

79. Drews RC. Corticosteroid management of hemorrhagic glaucoma. Trans Am Acad Ophthalmol Otol 1974;78:334–336.
80. Krupin T, Mitchell KB, Becker B. Cyclocryotherapy in neovascular glaucoma. Am J Ophthalmol 1978;86:24–26.
81. Beckman H, Waeltermann J. Transscleral ruby laser cyclophotocoagulation. Am J Ophthalmol 1984;98:788–795.
82. Shields MB, Shields SE. Noncontact transscleral Nd:YAG cyclophotocoagulation: a long-term follow-up of 500 patients. Trans Am Ophthalmol Soc 1994;92:271–283; discussion 283–287.
83. Bloom PA, Tsai JC, Sharma K, et al. "Cyclodiode." Transscleral diode laser cyclophotocoagulation in the treatment of advanced refractory glaucoma. Ophthalmology 1997;104: 1508–1519; discussion 1519–1520.
84. Oguri A, Takahashi E, Tomita G, et al. Transscleral cyclophotocoagulation with the diode laser for neovascular glaucoma. Ophthalmic Surg Lasers 1998;29:722–727.
85. Uram M. Ophthalmic laser microendoscope ciliary process ablation in the management of neovascular glaucoma. Ophthalmology 1992;99:1823–1828.
86. Tsai JC, Feuer WJ, Parrish RK II, Grajewski AL. 5-Fluorouracil filtering surgery and neovasular glaucoma. Long-term follow-up of the original pilot study. Ophthalmology 1995;102:887–892; discussion 892.
87. Katz GJ, Higginbotham EJ, Lichter PR, et al. Mitomycin C versus 5-fluorouracil in high-risk glaucoma filtering surgery. Extended follow-up. Ophthalmology 1995;102:1263–1269.
88. Lahey JM, Fong DS, Kearney J. Intravitreal tissue plasminogen activator for acute central retinal vein occlusion. Ophthalmic Surg Lasers 1999;30:427–434.
89. Herschler J, Agness D. A modified filtering operation for neovascular glaucoma. Arch Ophthalmol 1979;97:2339–2341.
90. Parrish R, Herschler J. Eyes with end-stage neovascular glaucoma. Natural history following successful modified filtering operation. Arch Ophthalmol 1983;101:745–746.
91. L'Esperance FA Jr, Mittl RN, James WA Jr. Carbon dioxide laser trabeculostomy for the treatment of neovascular glaucoma. Ophthalmology 1983;90:821–829.
92. Mermoud A, Salmon JF, Alexander P, et al. Molteno tube implantation for neovascular glaucoma. Long-term results and factors influencing the outcome. Ophthalmology 1993;100:897–902.
93. Sidoti PA, Dunphy TR, Baerveldt G, et al. Experience with the Baerveldt glaucoma implant in treating neovascular glaucoma. Ophthalmology 1995;102:1107–1118.
94. Tsai JC, Johnson CC, Dietrich MS. The Ahmed shunt versus the Baerveldt shunt for refractory glaucoma: a single-surgeon comparison of outcome. Ophthalmology 2003;110: 1814–1821.
95. Luttrull JK, Avery RL. Pars plana implant and vitrectomy for treatment of neovascular glaucoma. Retina 1995;15:379–387.
96. Kirchhof B. Retinectomy lowers intraocular pressure in otherwise intractable glaucoma: preliminary results. Ophthalmic Surg 1994;25:262–267.
97. Joussen AM, Walter P, Jonescu-Cuypers CP, et al. Retinectomy for treatment of intractable glaucoma: long term results. Br J Ophthalmol 2003;87:1094–1102.
98. Muller VA, Ruokonen P, Schellenbeck M, et al. Treatment of rubeosis iridis with photodynamic therapy with verteporfin—a new therapeutic and prophylactic option for patients with the risk of neovascular glaucoma? Ophthalmic Res 2003;35:1:60–64.
99. Jonas JB, Hayler JK, Sofker A, Panda-Jonas S. Regression of neovascular iris vessels by intravitreal injection of crystalline cortisone. J Glaucoma 2001;10:284–287.
100. Jampol LM. Oxygen therapy and intraocular oxygenation. Trans Am Ophthalmol Soc 1987;85:407–437.

101. Jampol LM, Orlin C, Cohen SB, et al. Hyperbaric and transcorneal delivery of oxygen to the rabbit and monkey anterior segment. Arch Ophthalmol 1988;106:825–829.
102. Adamis AP, Shima DT, Tolentino MJ, et al. Inhibition of vascular endothelial growth factor prevents retinal ischemia-associated iris neovascularization in a nonhuman primate. Arch Ophthalmol 1996;114:66–71.
103. Miller JW, Stinson WG, Folkman J. Regression of experimental iris neovascularization with systemic alpha-interferon. Ophthalmology 1993;100:9–14.
104. Glacet-Bernard A, Coscas G, Chabanel A, et al. A randomized, double-masked study on the treatment of retinal vein occlusion with troxerutin. Am J Ophthalmol 1994;118:421–429.
105. Dawson DW, et al. Pigment epithelium-derived factor: a potent inhibitor of angiogenesis. Science 1999;285:245–248.
106. Mori K, Gehlbach P, Ando A, et al. Regression of ocular neovascularization in response to increased expression of pigment epithelium-derived factor. Invest Ophthalmol Vis Sci 2002;43:2428–2434.
107. Duh EJ, Yang HS, Suzuma I, et al. Pigment epithelium-derived factor suppresses ischemia-induced retinal neovascularization and VEGF-induced migration and growth. Invest Ophthalmol Vis Sci 2002;43:821–829.
108. Takita H, Yoneya S, Gehlbach PL, et al. Retinal neuroprotection against ischemic injury mediated by intraocular gene transfer of pigment epithelium-derived factor. Invest Ophthalmol Vis Sci 2003;44:4497–4504.
109. Yabe T, et al. NF-κβ activation is required for the neuroprotective effects of pigment epithelium-derived factor (PEDF) on cerebellar granule neurons. J Biol Chem 2001;276: 43,313–43,319.

8
Eales' Disease

Jyotirmay Biswas, MD

CONTENTS

INTRODUCTION

Eales' disease was first described by Henry Eales in 1880 *(1)*. The patient presents with retinal perivasculitis predominantly affecting the peripheral retina (inflammatory stage), then sclerosis of retinal veins indicating retinal ischemia (ischemic stage), and finally retinal or optic disk neovascularization, recurrent vitreous hemorrhage with or without retinal detachment (proliferative stage) *(2–4)*.

EPIDEMIOLOGY

The disease is seen more commonly in the Indian subcontinent and the Middle Eastern countries. It commonly affects healthy young males. The predominant age of onset of symptoms is between 20 and 30 yr *(5)*.

CLINICAL FEATURES

Patients are often asymptomatic in the initial stages of retinal perivasculitis. Some patients may develop symptoms such as floaters, blurring of vision, or even gross diminution of vision due to massive vitreous hemorrhage. Vision in these patients can be normal to hand movements or light perception only. Bilaterality is quite common (50–90% of patients) *(2,3)*. Clinical manifestation of this disease is due to three basic pathological

From: *Ophthalmology: Ocular Angiogenesis: Diseases, Mechanisms, and Therapeutics*
Edited by: J. Tombran-Tink and C. J. Barnstable © Humana Press Inc., Totowa, NJ

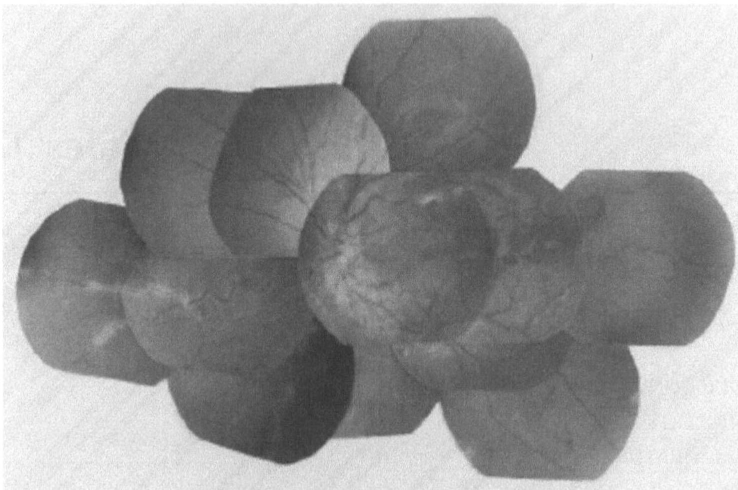

Fig. 1. Montage fundus photograph of a case of Eales' disease showing multiple patches of active retinal periphlebitis. *See* color version on companion CD.

changes: inflammation (peripheral retinal perivasculitis); ischemic changes (peripheral retinal capillary nonperfusion); and neovascularization of the retina or disk, which often leads to vitreous hemorrhage as well as multiple superficial retinal hemorrhages.

Anterior uveitis is uncommon in Eales' disease. However, in the severe active periphlebitis stage, spillover anterior uveitis may occur. Such anterior uveitis is always nongranulomatous. The presence of granulomatous anterior uveitis should lead one to suspect sarcoid uveitis, which mimics Eales' disease. Hypopyon is not seen in Eales' disease, and hypopyon with retinal vasculitis may indicate Behçet's disease *(6)*.

Ophthalmoscopic findings in Eales' disease often vary and depend on the stage of the disease. Arterioles are sometimes affected along with the veins. Typically, active perivasculitis with exudates around the retinal veins is seen involving one or more quadrants. Such exudates are often found to be associated with superficial retinal hemorrhages (Fig. 1).

Healed perivasculitis is often seen as the sheathing of the retinal veins. Other vascular changes includes sclerosed cord of venules, irregularity of vein caliber, pigmentation along venules, kinky venules, abnormal vascular anastomosis, and veins pulled into the vitreous cavity *(2,3,7)*.

Active or healed choroiditis is not seen in Eales' disease. However, a few small chorioretinal atrophic patches close to the retinal vessels are seen *(7)*.

Central retinal periphlebitis is markedly uncommon compared with peripheral retinal periphlebitis *(2,3,8)*. Such central involvement is often limited to one or more venous trunks. This is classified as *central Eales*, a variant of classical Eales' disease *(8)*. Macular changes are relatively uncommon *(9)*. The most common macular change seen is macular edema. Other changes included exudates in the macula and epimacular membrane.

Peripheral retinal neovascularization of the retina is quite frequently seen in Eales' disease *(2,3,7)* (Fig. 2). Optic disk neovascularization is significantly uncommon *(2–4)*. Dense vitritis is uncommon in Eales' disease. However, mild overlying vitreous haze

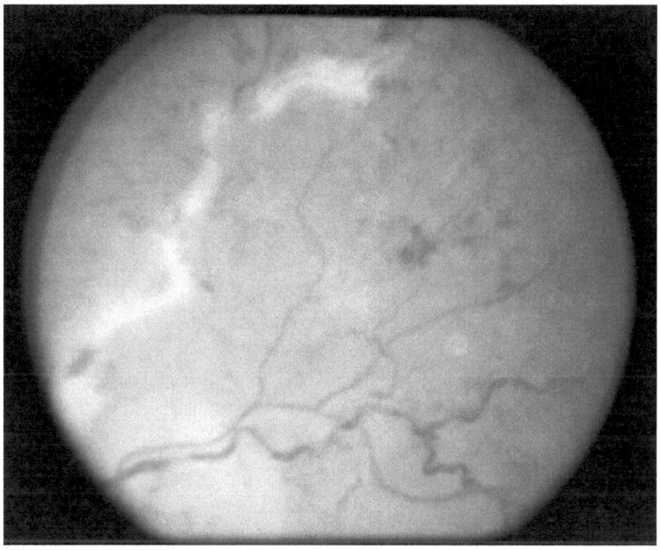

Fig. 2. Fundus photograph of case of Eales' disease in proliferative stage showing neovascular frond in the periphery. *See* color version on companion CD.

can be seen in the area of active retinal vasculitis. Recurrent vitreous hemorrhage is often the hallmark of this disease. The cause of vitreous hemorrhage in such eyes is often bleeding from retinal or disk neovascularization, but it can also occur due to rupture of capillaries or large venules during the active inflammatory stage *(10)*.

DIAGNOSIS

Fundus Fluorescein Angiography

Though not routinely needed to distinguish all cases of Eales' disease, fundus fluorescein angiography (FFA) is particularly beneficial in the ischemic stage to delineate areas of capillary nonperfusion, retinal and/or optic disk neovascularization, and questionable macular edema. In cases of active retinal vasculitis, staining of the veins can be seen in the early venous phase with extravasation of the dye in the late phase. Venous obstruction and venous stasis can be well visualized by FFA, which will show complete nonperfusion, or relative dilation and tortuosity of veins distal to the stasis. Areas of capillary closure, engorged and tortous capillaries, and venovenous shunts can also be seen in the ischemic stage of the disease.

The extent and location of neovascularization can be precisely delineated by FFA. Neovascularization, if present, can be quite characteristic with a sea-fan appearance with intense hyperfluorescence in the early arteriovenous phases of the fundus fluorescein angiogram (Fig. 3). Such neovascularization, when located in the far periphery, can be missed on routine FFA, unless a wide-angle lens is used.

FFA often helps to delineate the location and extent of retinal ischemia and can be of guidance while performing laser photocoagulation. It also helps to evaluate the adequacy of photocoagulation and the need for additional laser photocoagulation, when FFA is repeated on a follow-up visit.

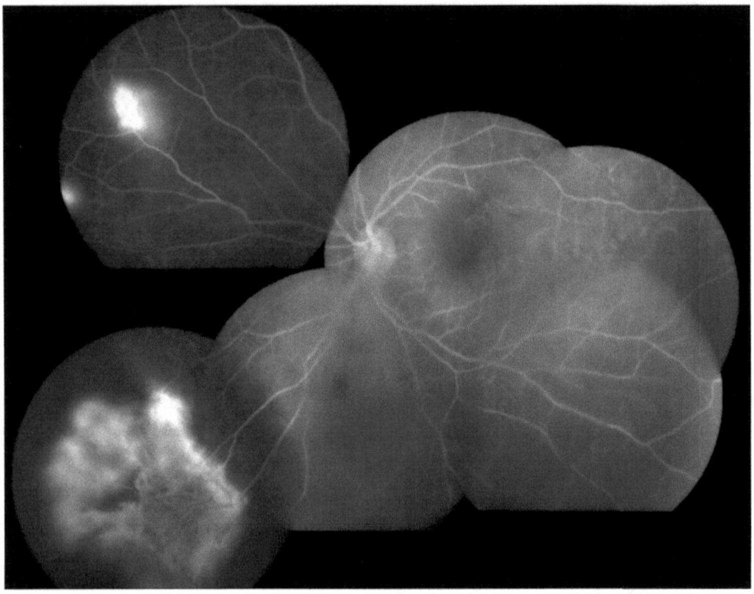

Fig. 3. Montage photograph of fundus fluorescein angiogram showing areas of capillary closure, engorged and tortuous capillaries, venovenous shunts, and leaking neovascular frond in lower nasal quadrant.

Ultrasonography

Ultrasonography (USG) is needed to rule out any associated retinal detachment, either tractional, rhegmatogenous, or combined, in an eye with opaque media. Early vitreous surgery is indicated if such association is demonstrated. USG usually reveals echoes of variable density, depending on the compaction of vitreous hemorrhage. Subhyaloid echoes may also be seen. Both incomplete and complete posterior vitreous detachment with or without tractional retinal detachment can be seen. Membranes in the vitreous cavity, vitreoschisis, and fibrovascular proliferation may be demonstrated. Associated retinal detachment, usually tractional or combined, is sometimes seen.

NATURAL COURSE

The natural course of Eales' disease is quite variable. Classically, an active perivasculitis stage leads to an ischemic stage followed by neovascularization of the retina and subsequent recurrent vitreous hemorrhage. Some patients may lose vision significantly due to recurrent episodes of vitreous hemorrhage, macular changes, and tractional or combined retinal detachment involving macula. In others, a temporary or permanent regression of the disease is noted. Blindness due to Eales' disease is rare *(10)*.

Charmis has classified Eales' disease into four stages *(12)*:

Stage I: Very early in evolution and characterized by mild periphlebitis of small peripheral retinal capillaries, arterioles, and venules detected by ophthalmoscopy.

Stage II: Perivasculitis of the venous capillary system is widespread, larger veins are affected, as are the arterioles lying by the side of affected veins. Vitreous haze is manifested.

Table 1
Systemic Diseases Associated With Eales' Disease

Tuberculosis
Hypersensitivity to tuberculoprotein
Thromboangitis obliterans
Neurological disease
Multiple sclerosis
Acute or subacute myelopathy
Multifocal white matter abnormality
Cerebral stroke
Others
Focal sepsis
Hematological abnormalities
Acanthocytosis
Increased plasma viscosity, erythrocyte rigidity, and erythrocyte aggregation
Hypereosinophilia
Blood coagulation disorder
Impaired oxygen release from blood
Raised fibrinolytic activity
Vestibuloauditory dysfunction
Parasitic infection (amoebiasis, ascariasis)
Others

Stage III: New vessel formation with abundant hemorrhage in the retina and vitreous humor is observed.
Stage IV: End result of massive and recurrent vitreous hemorrhages with retinitis proliferans and traction retinal detachment.

Saxena and Kumar *(51)* have recently proposed a new classification system:
Peripheral disease consists of four stages:

Stage 1 is periphlebitis of small (1a) and large (1b) caliber vessels with superficial retinal hemorrhages.
Stage 2a denotes capillary nonperfusion and 2b neovascularization elsewhere/of the disk.
Stage 3a is classified as fibrovascular proliferation and 3b vitreous hemorrhage.
Stage 4a is traction/combined rhegmatogenous retinal detachment, whereas 4b is rubeosis iridis, neovascular glaucoma, complicated cataract, and optic atrophy (peripheral type).

ETIOPATHOGENESIS

The etiopathogenesis of Eales' disease still remains unclear in spite of several clinical and basic studies. Systemic association with several diseases, in particular tuberculosis, has been described *(7,13–15)*.

The list of the systemic diseases associated with Eales' disease is summarized in Table 1 *(3)*.

BIOCHEMICAL STUDIES

Several biochemical studies have been done on the serum and vitreous samples of patients with Eales' disease. Raised globulins and decreased albumin levels in the serum samples of patients with Eales' disease have been found *(16)*. A distinct protein with molecular weight of around 23 kDa in the serum of Eales' disease patients has been discovered *(17)*. This protein could have angiogenic property.

Oxidative stress has been implicated in the pathogenesis of various diseases. In uveitis, the damage inflicted on the ocular tissues due to reactive oxygen species has been reported *(18,19)*. Elevated lipid peroxides have been found in retinal neovascularization in cases of diabetic retinopathy where there was no inflammation *(20)*.

It has been predicted that in Eales' disease with inflammation and neovascularization, free radicals and lipid peroxide products might accumulate due to oxidant insult overpowering antioxidant defense. Accumulation of thiobarbituric acid reacting substances (TBARS) is an index of the production of excessive oxidants, whereas a deficiency of vitamin C and E is an indication of the weakened antioxidant defense *(21,22)*. Increased accumulation of lipid peroxides and decreased activities of superoxide dismutase and glutathione peroxidase with simultaneous depletion of glutathione in the vitreous of Eales' disease patients have been found. These findings strongly suggest that oxidant stress plays an important role in the pathogenesis of Eales' disease *(23)*. An 88-kDa protein has been identified from the serum and vitreous of Eales' disease patients *(24)*.

DIFFERENTIAL DIAGNOSIS AND INVESTIGATION

Differential diagnosis of Eales' disease depends on the stage of presentation of the disease. Clinical presentation can be one of the following *(25–38)*:

1. Peripheral retinal perivasculitis in one or both the eyes.
2. Neovascular proliferation of the retina or optic disk with peripheral retinal perivasculitis in the same or the other eye.
3. Vitreous hemorrhage with peripheral retinal perivasculitis in the same or the other eye.

In the last two situations, in young healthy adults in the Indian subcontinent, a strong clinical suspicion of Eales' disease is quite justified.

Sarcoidosis can often mimic Eales' disease in the active inflammatory stage. Therefore, investigations for sarcoidosis should be included in the lists of investigations for Eales' disease (*see* Table 2 for complete list). In case of vitreous hemorrhage, the investigations of Eales' disease can be limited to exclusion of diabetes (particularly juvenile diabetes), sickle cell disease, sarcoidosis, and leukemia. Pars planitis patients can have retinal periphlebitis close to pars plana exudates. However, retinal hemorrhages, vascular alteration, and retinal neovascularization (which is often seen in Eales' disease) are absent in pars planitis. Conditions that mimic Eales' disease are listed in Tables 3 and 4.

MANAGEMENT

The management of Eales' disease depends on the stage of the disease. It includes nontreatment with periodic evaluation in the regressed stage of periphlebitis or fresh vitreous hemorrhage, treatment with oral or periocular steroids in the active perivasculitis stage, and laser photocogulation in case of neovascularization of the retina or optic disk, or gross capillary nonperfusion. Vitreous surgery is indicated in nonresolving vitreous hemorrhage (usually more than 3 mo). Any associated retinal detachment will, however,

Table 2
Investigations for Eales' Disease

To rule out leukemia and hemotological disease:
- Hemoglobin (Hb) and hematocrit (polypoidal choroidal vasculopathy)
- Total red blood cell count
- Total white blood cell count and differential count

Other tests:
- Platelet count
- Erythrocyte sedimentation rate
- Reticulocyte count
- Postprandial blood sugar
- Stool analysis
- Mantoux test
- Basic coagulation test
- Bleeding time
- Clotting time
- Clot retraction
- Plasma clotting time
- Sickle cell preparation
- Hemoglobin electrophoresis (sickle cell retinopathy)
- Immunoglobin profile
- VDRL and treponema
- Pallidum hemagglutination test (TPHA)
- Antinuclear antibody (systemic lupus erythematosus and other collagen diseases)
- Serum angiotensin-converting enzyme (sarcoidosis)
- Lysozyme (sarcoidosis)

Radiological tests:
- Chest X-ray (tuberculosis and sarcoidosis)

Table 3
Proliferative Vascular Retinopathy Mimicking Eales' Disease

Systemic	*Ocular*
Diabetes mellitus	Branch retinal vein occlusion
Sarcoidosis	Central retinal vein occlusion
Sickle cell disease	Coats' disease
	Pars planitis
	Dragged disk syndrome *(39)*

warrant early vitreoretinal surgery. The role of anticoagulant hyperbaric oxygen *(40)* and antitubercular therapy remains controversial.

Observation

Patients with inactive retinal vasculitis can be observed periodically at 6-mo to 1-yr intervals. Patients with fresh vitreous hemorrhage also are asked for observation at intervals of 4 to 6 wk if the underlying retina is found, by indirect ophthalmoscopy or by ultrasound, to be attached. Such vitreous hemorrhage often clears by 6 to 8 wk.

Table 4
Retinal Vasculitis Mimicking Eales' Disease

Systemic	*Ocular*
Behçet's disease	Bird-shot choroidopathy
Leukemia	Coats' disease
Chronic myelogenous leukemia	Pars planitis
Lyme borreliosis	Viral retinitis
Multiple sclerosis	IRVAN (idiopathic retinal vasculitis, aneurysms, and neuroretinitis)
Sarcoidosis	Idiopathic central serous chorioretinopathy
Syphilis	Retinal macroaneurysms
Systemic lupus erythematosus	
Toxocariasis	
Toxoplasmosis	
Wegener's granulomatosis	
Large-cell lymphoma	
Acute multifocal hemorrhagic vasculitis	

Medical Therapy

Corticosteroids remain the mainstay of therapy in the active perivasculitis stage of Eales' disease *(41)*. Dosage must be tailored for each patient on the basis of severity of inflammation (quadrants of retina involved). In the majority of cases, oral prednisolone, 1 mg/kg of body weight, is needed. This is tapered to 10 mg/wk over 6 to 8 wk. Some patients may require a maintenance dose of 15 to 20 mg oral prednisolone per day for 1 to 2 mo. In case of associated macular edema, one may add periocular depot steroid injection. Systemic steroids (1 mg/kg of body weight) and posterior subtenon injection of steroid (40 mg/mL triamcinolone acetonide) were found beneficial if there was involvement of three quadrants with cystoid macular edema. Systemic corticosteroids alone were helpful when there was two-quadrant involvement. In the case of one-quadrant involvement, periocular corticosteroids were administered. The need for cyclosporine or other immunosuppressive agents is limited in Eales' disease patients. In patients who do not respond to systemic steroids or have unacceptable side effects due to oral corticosteroids, usage of immunosuppressive agents such as cyclosporine or azathioprine is recommended *(42)*. As many investigators believe that hypersensitivity to tuberculoproteins plays a role in the etiology of Eales' disease, antitubercular treatment (ATT) has been given in Eales' disease empirically. The ATT regimen included two drugs (450 mg rifampicin and 300 mg isonazid once daily) for a period of 9 mo *(43)*. However, the role of ATT drugs in the treatment of this disease remains controversial.

Photocoagulation

Photocoagulation is the mainstay of therapy in the proliferative stage of Eales' disease. In cases of gross capillary nonperfusion, photocoagulation is suggested. Argon green laser is most commonly used, but in cases of significant cataract or mild vitreous hemorrhage, red krypton laser can be used effectively *(44)*. Such a laser can now be delivered through either a slit-lamp delivery system or an indirect ophthalmoscope. Following vitrectomy, an endolaser probe or indirect ophthalmoscope laser can be used for laser delivery on the operating table. The aim of photocoagulation in Eales' disease is to regulate the circulation by diverting blood from hypoxic areas to healthy retina, thereby decreasing the formation of vasoproliferative factors, to obliterate surface neovascularization, and to close leaking intraretinal microvascular abnormalities. Panretinal photocoagulation is necessary when there is optic disk neovascularization. Laser photocoagulation is not advised in the active inflammatory stage, as there is chance of worsening of neovascularization due to several angiogenic factors liberated. Once the inflammation has subsided reasonably with antiinflammatory medications, such as corticosteroids, laser photocoagulation can be done.

Vitreoretinal Surgery

Vitrectomy alone or combined with other vitreoretinal surgical procedures is often required in Eales' disease *(45–47)*. Vitreous hemorrhage occurs quite frequently and is, in fact, the prime cause of visual loss.The vitreous hemorrhage usually clears between 6 and 8 wk. Ultrasonography should always be performed to exclude the presence of an associated retinal detachment. Cases of nonresolving vitreous hemorrhage with obscuration of central vision of 3 mo duration may be subjected to vitrectomy. In the presence of tractional retinal detachment, extensive vitreous membranes, or epimacular membranes, early vitrectomy can be considered. The aim of vitreous surgery is to clear the vitreous opacities and also to evaluate the fundus for any retinal neovascularization. Along with vitrectomy, laser photocoagulation can be performed by endophotocoagulation or indirect laser delivery system. Vitrectomy in Eales' disease is less complicated than in proliferative diabetic retinopathy. A standard three-port pars plana vitrectomy is the method of choice.

Anterior Retinal Cryoablation

Anterior retinal cryoablation (ARC) has been successfully tried in eyes with vitreous hemorrhage caused by proliferative diabetic retinopathy *(48–50)*. Although primary ARC is considered in cases of small undilating pupils, hazy ocular media due to cataract, after cataract, or residual vitreous hemorrhage in Eales' disease, it is usually reserved as an adjunct to photocoagulation in Eales' disease.

REFERENCES

1. Eales H. Retinal haemorrhage associated with epistaxis and constipation. Brim Med Rev 1880;9:262.
2. Atmaca LS, Idli A, Gunduz K. Visualisation of retinal vasculitis in Eales' disease. Ocul Immunol Inflamm 1993;1:41–48.
3. Das T, Biswas J, Kumar A, et al. Eales' disease. Indian J Ophthalmol 1994;42:3–18.
4. Renie WA, Murphy RP, Anderson KC, et al. The evaluation of patients with Eales' disease. Retina 1983;3:243–248.
5. Gadkari SS, Kamdar PA, Jehangir RP, et al. Pars plana vitrectomy in vitreous haemorrhage due to Eales' disease. Indian J Ophthalmol 1992;40:35–37.
6. Stanford MR, Graham EM. Systemic associations of retinal vasculitis. Int Ophthalmol Clin 1991;31:23–33.

7. Abraham C, Baig SM, Badrinath SS. Eales' disease. Proc All India Ophthalmol Soc 1977;33:223–229.
8. Gilbert TW. Periphlebitis and endovasculitis of retinal vessels. Klin Monatsbl Augenheilkd 1935;94:335–349.
9. Biswas J, Mondkar SV, Ahuja VK, et al. Macular involvement in Eales' disease. SNEC Symposium on Macular Diseases, Singapore, 1997.
10. Nagpal PN, Sharma RK, Joshi BS, Patel AM. Management of Eales' disease—analysis of 800 cases (1,214 eyes). Asia Pac J Ophthalmol 1998;10:11–17.
11. Agarwal R, Biswas J. Macular involvement in Eales' disease [abstract]. Amer Acad Ophthalmol New Orleans 1998;118.
12. Charmis J. On the classification and management of the evolutionary course of Eales' disease. Trans Ophthalmol Soc UK 1965;85:157.
13. Ashton N. Pathogenesis and aetiology of Eales' disease. Acta XIX Concilium Ophthalmologicum 1962;2:828.
14. Bonnet P. Recurrent haemorrhage of the vitreous (Eales' disease) and genital tuberculosis. Bull Soc Ophthalmol Fr 1951;7:776.
15. Finnoff WC. Some impressions derived from the study of recurrent haemorrhages into the retina and vitreous of young persons. Trans Am Ophthalmol Soc 1921;19:238.
16. Pratap VB, Mehra MK, Gupta RK. Electrophoretic pattern of serum proteins in Eales' disease. Indian J Ophthalmol 1976;23:14–16.
17. Rengarajan K, Muthukkaruppan VR, Namperumalsamy P. Biochemical analysis of serum proteins from Eales' patients. Curr Eye Res 1989;8:1259–1269.
18. Rao NA, Du GS, Pararajasekaram G. Mechanism of tissue injury in uveitis. Reg Immunol 1994;6:95–100.
19. Rao NA, Sevanian A, Fernandez MA, et al. Role of oxygen radicals in experimental allergic uveitis. Invest Ophthalmol Vis Sci 1987;28:886–892.
20. Armstrong D, Hartnett M, Browne R, et al. Lipid peroxideinduced synthesis of cytokine growth factors during neovascularization in the retina [abstract]. Invest Ophthalmol Vis Sci 1995;36:455.
21. Davies AW, Moore T. Interactions of vitamins A and E. Nature 1941;147:794–796.
22. Moser LA, Simpson DE, Young DD. Retinal macroaneurysms: the natural history in four patients. Optom Vis Sci 1989;66:877–883.
23. Sulochana KN, Biswas J, Ramakrishnan S. Eales' disease: increased oxidation and peroxidation products of membrane constituents chiefly lipids and decreased antioxidant enzymes and reduced glutathione in vitreous. Curr Eye Res 1999;19:254–259.
24. Sulochana KN. Purification and characterization of a novel 88 kDa from serum and vitreous of patients with Eales' disease. Exp Eye Res 2001;73:547–555.
25. Arnold AC, Pepose JS, Hepler RS, Foos RY. Retinal periphlebitis and retinitis in multiple sclerosis. I. Pathologic characteristics. Ophthalmology 1984;91:255–262.
26. Barondes MJ, Fastenberg DM, Schwartz PL, Rosen DA. Peripheral retinal neovascularization in birdshot etinochoroidopathy. Ann Ophthalmol 1989;21:306–308.
27. Blumenkranz MS, Kaplan HJ, Clarkson JG, et al. Acute multifocal hemorrhagic retinal vasculitis. Ophthalmology 1988;95:1663–1672.
28. Dugel PU, Smith RE. Intermediate uveitis (parsplanitis). Ophthalmol Clin North Am 1993;6:29–37.
29. Duker JS, Brown GC, McNamara JA. Proliferative sarcoid retinopathy. Ophthalmology 1988;95:1680–1686.
30. Frank RN, Ryan SJ Jr. Peripheral retinal neovascularization with chronic myelogenous leukemia. Arch Ophthalmol 1972;87:585–589.

31. Gass JD, Little H. Bilateral bullous exudative retinal detachment complicating idiopathic central serous chorioretinopathy during systemic corticosteroid therapy. Ophthalmology 1995;102:737–747.
32. Gaynon MW, Boldrey EE, Strahlman ER, Fine SL. Retinal neovascularization and ocular toxoplasmosis. Am J Ophthalmol 1984;98:585–589.
33. Green WR. Bilateral Coats disease. Massive gliosis of the retina. Arch Ophthalmol 1967;77:378–383.
34. Jabs DA, Fine SL, Hochberg MC, et al. Severe retinal vasoocclusive disease in systemic lupus erythematous. Arch Ophthalmol 1986;104:558–563.
35. Mullaney J, Collum LM. Ocular vasculitis in Behcet's disease. A pathological and immunohistochemical study. Int Ophthalmol 1985;7:183–191.
36. Palmer HE, Zaman AG, Edelsten CE, et al. Systemic morbidity in patients with isolated idiopathic retinal vasculitis. Lancet 1995;346:505, 506.
37. Ridley ME, McDonald HR, Sternberg P Jr, et al. Retinal manifestations of ocular lymphoma (reticulum cell sarcoma). Ophthalmology 1992;99:1153–1160; discussion 1160–1161.
38. Shanmugam MP, Sharma T, Karna SD. Bilateral retinal arteritis with multiple aneurismal dilatations. Indian J Ophthalmol 1999;47:38–39.
39. Barreau E, Cohen SY, Coscas G. Dragged disk syndrome. Review of etiologies. Apropos of a case. J Fr Ophtalmol 1996;19:73–76.
40. Dumitru R. The hyperbaric method in the treatment of diabetic retinopathy, an alternative to laser therapy? Oftalmologia 1993;37:12–16.
41. Howe LJ, Stanford MR, Edelsten C, Graham EM. The efficacy of systemic corticosteroids in sight-threatening retinal vasculitis. Eye 1994;8:443–447.
42. Greenwood AJ, Stanford MR, Graham EM. The role of azathioprine in the management of retinal vasculitis. Eye 1998;12:783–788.
43. Das TP, Namperumalsamy P. Photocoagulation in Eales' disease. Results of prospective randomised clinical study. Presented at XXVI International Congress of Ophthalmology, Singapore, 1990.
44. Atmaca LS, Nagpa PN. Eales' disease medical laser and surgical treatment. Ophthalmol Clin North Am 2000;11:619–626.
45. Namperumalsamy P. Vitrectomy in Eales' disease. Trans Asia-Pacific Acad Ophthalmol 1983;9:457.
46. Namperumalsamy P, Kelkar AR, Das TP. Vitreous surgery in Eales' disease—when and why. Presented at XXVI International Congress of Ophthalmology, Singapore 1990;189.
47. Wang GL, Pang XG. Vitrectomy for non-diabetic vitreous hemorrhage. Chung-Hua Yen Ko Tsa Chih 1991;26:349–351.
48. Benedett R, Olk RJ, Arribas NP, et al. Transconjunctival anterior retinal cryotherapy for proliferative diabetic retinopathy. Ophthalmology 1987;94:612–619.
49. Mosier MA, Dei Piero E, Gheewala SM. Anterior retinal cryotherapy in diabetic vitreous hemorrhage. Am J Ophthalmol 1985;100:440–444.
50. Oosterhuis JA, Bijlmer-Gorter H. Cryotreatment in proliferative diabetic retinopathy. Long-term results. Ophthalmologica 1980;181:81–87.
51. Saxena S, Kumar D. A new staging system for idiopathic retinal periphlebitis. Eur J Ophthalmol 2004;14:236–239.

9

Angiogenesis and Ocular Tumorigenesis

Nader Sheibani, PhD and Daniel M. Albert, MD, MS

CONTENTS

INTRODUCTION

The development of a tumor is dependent on a number of genetic and epigenetic changes. An important step for the propagation and progression of many solid tumors is the induction of a tumor vasculature, i.e., "the angiogenic switch" (*1,2*). This ensures an adequate supply of oxygen and metabolites for tumor growth and metastasis. This switch is activated when the angiogenic balance tips in favor of proangiogenesis; this results in the increased production of proangiogenic factors and/or downregulation of antiangiogenic factors. The angiogenic switch may occur at any stage of tumor progression, depending on the nature of the tumor and the microenvironment. However, tumor angiogenesis differs from physiological angiogenesis in several respects: the vascular structure, the endothelial cell and pericyte interactions, blood flow, increased permeability, and delayed maturation (*3–6*; Table 1).

Tumor blood vessels are typically irregularly shaped, dilated, and tortuous, and can have closed ends. They are not organized into definitive venules, arterioles, or capillaries, and the smooth muscle cells/pericytes are more loosely arranged as compared with normal tissue. This vascular network is consequently often "leaky" and hemorrhagic. These abnormal features are the result of the disproportionate expression of angiogenesis cytokines and inhibitors, which are tumor-dependent and reflect the pathological nature of this process. Therefore, successful targeting of the tumor vasculature in cancer therapy can best be achieved if the phenotypic characteristics of these vessels are adequately addressed. There is a great need for developing reliable methods that would allow for recognition of a tumor's vascular qualities and thus guide antiangiogenic therapies. The potential contribution of the altered expression of anti- and/or proangiogenic factors during the development and progression of ocular tumors remains largely unexplored.

From: *Ophthalmology: Ocular Angiogenesis: Diseases, Mechanisms, and Therapeutics*
Edited by: J. Tombran-Tink and C. J. Barnstable © Humana Press Inc., Totowa, NJ

Table 1
Abnormalities Associated With Tumor Vasculature

Excessive proliferation
Defective structure
Lack of lymphatic system
Lack of local control mechanisms
Aberrant perfusion

ANGIOGENESIS

Angiogenesis, the process of the formation of new blood vessels from preexisting capillaries, is tightly regulated and normally does not occur except during development, wound healing, and the formation of the corpus luteum in the female reproductive cycle. This strict regulation is manifested by a balanced production of positive and negative factors, which keeps angiogenesis in check *(1)*. However, this balance becomes abrogated under various pathological conditions, such as cancer development, resulting in the growth of new vessels. It is now well accepted that the progressive growth and metastasis of many solid tumors are dependent on the growth of new vessels. Therefore, there has been great interest in understanding the molecular and cellular mechanisms that go awry during tumorigenesis, resulting in the acquisition of an angiogenic phenotype. In addition, this knowledge has been exploited in the development of agents that can inhibit angiogenesis as a means of stopping tumorigenesis dead in its tracks.

There has been great progress in understanding the process of angiogenesis and the identification of many factors that have pro- or antiangiogenic activity. Although proangiogenic factors were believed to be involved in promoting angiogenesis for quite some time, it was not until the early 1990s that the potential contribution of antiangiogenic factors to this process began to be appreciated *(7)*. There is now a growing list of naturally occurring inhibitors of angiogenesis whose altered expression is shown to contribute to the angiogenic phenotypes of a variety of tumors (Table 2). One of the first of these to be identified was thrombospondin-1 (TSP1), whose expression was downregulated during malignant transformation *(7,8)*. TSP1 expression was subsequently demonstrated to be downregulated in a variety of tumors, perhaps through inactivation of tumor suppressor genes such as p53. In addition, reexpression of TSP1 in these tumors suppresses their aggressive growth and metastasis *(7,8)*. This is believed to be mediated through the antiangiogenic activity of TSP1.

TSP1 inhibits angiogenesis in vivo and endothelial cell proliferation and migration in vitro *(7,8)*. These activities of TSP1 are mediated through its interaction with CD36, a scavenger receptor expressed on the surface of microvascular endothelial cells *(8)*. TSP1 promotes apoptosis of endothelial cells through the activation of caspases and Jun N-terminal kinase (JNK) signaling pathways, as well as downregulation of bcl-2 expression in vivo and in vitro *(8)*. TSP1 has been shown to be an important regulator of the endothelial cell phenotype, and its expression promotes the quiescent, differentiated phenotype of the endothelium *(7)*. In fact, TSP1-deficient mice exhibit increased retinal vascular density from a defect in vascular pruning and remodeling during later stages of vascular development *(9)*. The regression of hyaloid vessels is also delayed in

Table 2
Endogenous Regulators of Angiogenesis

Activators	*Inhibitors*
Vascular endothelial growth factors	Thrombospondin-1
Fibroblast growth factors	Angiostatin
Platelet-derived growth factor B	Endostatin
Epidermal growth factor	Capstatin
Lysophosphatidic acid	Tumstatin
Interleukin-8	Capsaicin
Tumor necrosis factor-α	PEDF
Angiogenin	PF4
Hepatocyte growth factor	Interferon-α
Placental growth factor	Interferon-β
Transforming growth factor (TGF)-α	Maspin
TGF-β	Vasostatin

TSP1-deficient mice. Therefore, the tightly regulated, balanced expression of anti-angiogenic factors, such as TSP1, along with that of proangiogenic factors, such as vascular endothelial growth factor (VEGF), play an important role in ocular vascular development and angiogenesis. A better understanding of the potential mechanisms that may contribute to acquisition of an angiogenic phenotype during progression and metastasis of ocular tumors will provide further insight into how these tumors develop and lead to alternative modalities in treating them.

Angiogenesis as a Biological Target for Cancer Therapy

For three decades, Judah Folkman has believed that attacking the growth of blood vessels that feed growing tumors would be an effective therapeutic strategy. A key finding in the development of this idea was the discovery that an essential step in the progression of a tumor from the benign to the malignant state is the "angiogenic switch" discussed above *(10)*. This switch, as previously noted, turns on the production or activation of angiogenic factors by the tumor cells and in many cases also turns off production of inhibitors of angiogenesis *(11)*. A different version of this switch is found in tumors that inhibit growth of their own metastases by release or activation of angiogenic inhibitors such as angiostatin and endostatin *(12,13)*. These are fragments of plasminogen and collagen XVIII, respectively. Even though their mechanisms of action remain largely undefined, they establish the principle of angiostatic therapy as an effective means of controlling the growth of tumors. As long as the inhibitors circulate, metastases seeded in distant organs remain dormant, and grow and become readily detected only after resection of the primary tumor mass. In a different approach, Brooks and colleagues found that the $\alpha_V\beta_3$ integrin is preferentially expressed on angiogenic vessels, and the blockade of the RGD binding site of the integrin with a monoclonal antibody or peptides could inhibit vascularization of tumors, the retina, and arthritic disease *(14–16)*. Several small-molecule inhibitors and humanized anti-$\alpha_V\beta_3$ are in clinical trials as cancer therapies.

The development of tumor vasculature is dependent on the proliferation and migration of endothelial cells to provide nutrients and oxygen to the tumor. Therefore, tumor endothelial cells have become an important target in the development of antiangiogenesis drugs. Targeting these cells that support tumor growth offers several unique advantages over conventional cytotoxic chemotherapy. The early recruitment of endothelial cells during tumor angiogenesis provides an opportunity to inhibit tumor vessel growth early. Endothelial cells are genetically stable and are less likely to accumulate mutations that enable them to acquire a drug-resistant phenotype. They are also easily accessible through the bloodstream, allowing optimal delivery and homogeneous distribution of the drug within the tumor. In addition, the loss of even a small number of capillaries within the tumor may amplify an antiangiogenic effect *(3–6)*. These potentially therapeutic advantages have inspired the development of additional new angiogenesis inhibitors that target a variety of endothelial cell effector molecules, which work together to mediate specific steps in the angiogenesis process. A number of such molecules have been shown to effectively inhibit tumor growth in various animal models and are at various stages of clinical trials *(17)*. These include various protease inhibitors, including marimastat (a synthetic MMP1 inhibitor), which is in phase III clinical trials for breast cancer, lung cancer, pancreatic cancer, and glioma. Other inhibitors of angiogenesis include direct inhibitors of endothelial cell proliferation and migration, such as TNP470, endostatin, and angiostatin. Antagonists of angiogenic growth factors, such as VEGF antibody, angiozyme (a ribozyme that attenuates VEGF receptors' mRNA), and SU6668 (which blocks growth factor receptor signaling) are all at different stages of clinical trials and showing good efficacy *(17)*. The significance of these findings is clear: Angiostatic therapy is feasible and within our reach. Given the devastating impact of angiogenesis-dependent diseases, the diversity of their origin and etiology, and the early stage of this promising approach for treatment, it seems prudent to pursue all sensible leads toward the goal of identifying and testing candidates for angiostatic therapy. The list of compounds with antiangiogenic activity is growing rapidly. In view of the heterogeneity of tumors and their different mechanisms of development, combination therapy may be more effective than monotherapy. However, the success of these modalities is highly dependent on a complete understanding of the drugs' mechanisms of action and the stage of angiogenesis at which they are most effective.

Angiogenesis and Ocular Tumors

Uveal melanoma and retinoblastoma, which occur in the eyes of adults and children, have been a major focus for research in ocular oncology. Although the role of angiogenesis has been extensively studied and is utilized as a means of therapy in many types of tumors, its contribution to the development and progression of ocular tumors has been specifically studied only in the past several years. Recent investigations indicate that angiogenesis plays an integral role in the progression and metastasis of these ocular tumors, and antiangiogenic therapy may provide an additional alternative in the treatments of these cancers *(18–25)*.

Uveal Melanoma

Uveal melanoma is the most common primary intraocular tumor in humans, and it occurs in a nonhereditary, sporadic manner *(26)*. The majority of uveal melanomas occur in the choroid and/or ciliary body, whereas a lower percentage occurs in the iris. The lack of a hereditary pattern or association with an inherited condition has greatly hampered the search for causative genes in uveal melanoma. This is in contrast to retinoblastoma, where the hereditary pattern led to discovery of the first tumor suppressor gene *(27)*. Therefore, a major effort is being made to identify the cytogenetic changes and mutations that may contribute to the development and progression of uveal melanoma. A variety of new techniques, including differential display, serial analysis of gene expression (SAGE), and DNA array analysis, has been employed in this endeavor *(28)*. These studies will provide further insight into the development and progression of uveal melanoma and will enhance the ability to manage and treat this disease.

Uveal melanomas are treated with enucleation, radiotherapy, transpupillary thermotherapy, laser photocoagulation, intravenous chemotherapy, immunotherapy, local tumor resection, or a combination of these treatments *(29)*. There is a range in mortality rates depending on the cell type and on the size and location of the tumor. The major site of metastasis is the liver. Although acquisition of an angiogenic phenotype is essential for the malignant progression of a variety of solid tumors, its role in uveal melanoma development and progression requires further delineation. Polans and colleagues have demonstrated that a number of genes, including those with important roles in angiogenesis, are differentially expressed in melanoma cells with a more metastatic and migratory phenotype *(28,30)*.

These studies suggest that an angiogenic switch may occur in uveal melanomas. In animal studies, removal of the primary tumor by enucleation is stated to promote metastatic diseases *(31)*. Therefore, in these models ocular tumors may produce antiangiogenic factors, such as angiostatin, which normally keep metastasis in check by counterbalancing the activity of potential proangiogenic factors such as VEGF. Indeed, some animal models of uveal melanomas produce angiostatin and appear to suppress metastasis *(31)*. However, it is not known whether this mechanism is operative in humans and whether angiostatin therapy would be beneficial to uveal melanoma patients at high risk for metastasis. Further studies are required to identify potential changes in the expression of other antiangiogenic factors in uveal melanoma and to test their efficacy in metastatic disease. The availability of animal models more closely related to human tumors and human tumor cell lines *(28,32)* would be helpful.

Another recently identified characteristic of uveal melanoma cells is their apparent ability to form vascular networks in the absence of endothelial cells, a phenomenon referred to as "vascular mimicry." These vascular networks have been stated to be devoid of endothelial cells and are formed by more aggressive and metastatic cells *(33)*. However, recent gene array analyses indicate that these cells exhibit many characteristics of angiogenic endothelial cells. They express VE-cadherin (an endothelial cell-specific marker), as well as the VEGF receptor, and have increased metalloproteinase activity *(34)*. However, it is not clear whether aberrant expression of these genes is essential for the formation of vascular networks or tumor metastases. Further characterization of the mechanisms and factors involved in the formation of these vascular structures may provide alternative methods to inhibit and/or interfere with the formation of these networks and block tumor growth and metastasis.

No single method has been shown to significantly alter the course of uveal melanomas, prevent metastasis, or increase long-term survival. A range of therapeutic options is currently available in the management of uveal melanomas *(29)*. Although methods and indications vary, a trend toward the usage of eye-sparing techniques whenever possible has emerged. However, only limited progress in the management of the systemic disease has been achieved. A greater understanding of the biological events associated with extraocular and systemic metastases is required. Therefore, delineation of these pathways will allow the development of more effective therapies that might move us closer to achieving all the goals of treatment, including curing the intraocular tumor, preventing extraocular disease, and preserving the eye and vision. Understanding the pathogenesis of intraocular pigmented tumors in transgenic mice should provide further insights into the growth and metastatic properties of these tumors and lead to the development of more effective treatments.

Retinoblastoma

Retinoblastoma is the most common primary intraocular tumor in children *(35,36)*. In the United States, this tumor presents most frequently as unilateral, usually sporadic tumors, and less frequently as bilateral hereditary tumors. If left untreated, retinoblastoma is generally fatal. However, this childhood cancer has a high percentage of survival—more than 95% in the United States and Western Europe *(36)*. The extent of invasion of the retinoblastoma into ocular coats and the optic nerve is a major risk factor. Many small tumors, if detected early, can be treated effectively using laser therapy or cryotherapy. Unfortunately, many tumors are not detected until they are larger and visible, which generally necessitates removal by enucleation of the affected eye. Radiotherapy and chemotherapy are also used to treat more advanced disease *(36)*. However, these treatments, which are mutagenic, may increase the likelihood that the surviving child will develop additional malignancies later in life. The prognosis for patients who develop metastatic disease is generally poor. Metastases can occur directly by expansion and invasive growth of tumor cells along the optic nerve to the brain, nasopharynx, or cranium, or may occur through the bloodstream or lymphatics. Development of metastases is dependent on angiogenesis *(23)*.

The primary goal of retinoblastoma treatment is to ensure the survival of these children, as well as the retention of their eyes and of useful vision. Another goal is prevention of facial bony deformities and other physical changes that can affect functional well-being. Enucleation historically has been the most commonly employed technique for treating retinoblastoma *(36)*. External-beam radiation therapy is usually employed to preserve the vision of children with small tumors located within the macula. The most serious complication is an increased risk of secondary nonocular tumors in children with the genetic form of retinoblastoma. Therefore, focal treatments such as cryotherapy and photocoagulation provide a desirable alternative.

Transgenic mouse models have been instrumental not only in the study of the molecular genetics of retinoblastoma, but also in the in vivo evaluation of novel therapeutic approaches *(37–39)*. LH beta-Tag mice, in particular, are extensively used for evaluating a wide range of therapeutic approaches for the treatment of retinoblastoma, including delivery of standard chemotherapeutic agents, external-beam radiation, a variety of combined modality approaches, and several novel anticancer agents, some with potential antiangiogenic activity *(39)*. However, the contribution of angiogenesis to the progression and metastasis of retinoblastoma has not been well documented.

The presence of calcification as a consistent feature of spontaneously cured or regressed retinoblastoma has led to the hypothesis that vitamin D analogs may have activity as chemotherapeutic agents in this tumor type. Systemic administration of vitamin D_3 to LH beta-Tag mice inhibits the growth and local extension of tumors in a dose-dependent manner *(40–42)* and has been further demonstrated to inhibit angiogenesis in this model *(41)*. However, calcitriol or vitamin D_2 treatment is associated with significant toxicity, including hypercalcemia, weight loss, and death *(39)*. In recent years, a number of vitamin D analogs have been developed, several of which appear to have greater antitumor activity with reduced side-effect toxicity. Two such analogs, 1,25-dihydroxy-16-ene-23-yne-vitamin D_3 and 1-α-hydroxyvitamin D_2, have also been evaluated in LH beta-Tag mice, and these compounds showed comparable antitumor activity with significant reduced systemic toxicity *(39)* compared with vitamin D_3. Other vitamin D analogs with much-reduced calcium toxicity are under development, and some have shown significant activity against retinoblastoma. Although the primary mechanism of action of vitamin D compounds against retinoblastoma appears to be apoptosis, the molecular and cellular mechanisms that lead to cell death remain largely unexplored. Although tumors treated with vitamin D also show reduced vascular density, it is not clearly demonstrated that these effects are due to vitamin D's antiangiogenic activity. However, in vitro and in vivo studies have demonstrated that vitamin D can directly affect endothelial cell activity and inhibit angiogenesis *(43–45)*.

The potential contribution of the angiogenic switch to the development and progression of retinoblastoma requires further investigation. Many retinoblastomas initially develop near major retinal vessels and perhaps co-opt these as a source of nutrition and oxygen. However, as the tumor grows, this need increases, resulting in extensive necrosis of the tumor. Recent studies indicate that the more invasive retinoblastomas are more vascularized *(25)*. Therefore, gaining an angiogenic phenotype may be essential for the expansion and distant metastasis of retinoblastoma. In fact, as noted above, treatment of mice bearing retinoblastomas with vitamin D analogs affects their vasculature, which may contribute to inhibition of tumor growth *(41)*. Therefore, there has been an effort to better determine whether the inhibition of tumor growth is secondary to the inhibition of angiogenesis. The expression of TSP1 and of pigment epithelium-derived factor (PEDF), two proteins with antiangiogenic activity, has recently been examined in Y79 retinoblastoma cells. Although Y79 cells produce significant amounts of PEDF, they express little or no TSP1 (Fig. 1A). In addition, incubation of Y79 cells with vitamin D resulted in increased expression of the cell cycle inhibitor P21 (Fig. 1B) but did not significantly affect expression of TSP1. These results are consistent with potential in vivo mechanisms of vitamin D action in xenograft models of human retinoblastoma *(42)*.

One hypothesis is that downregulation of TSP1 contributes to the malignant transformation and progression of retinoblastoma. In fact, it has recently been observed that reexpression of TSP1 in Y79 retinoblastoma cells has an adverse effect on their proliferation in vitro and their tumor formation in vivo. Figure 2 shows that the tumor formed

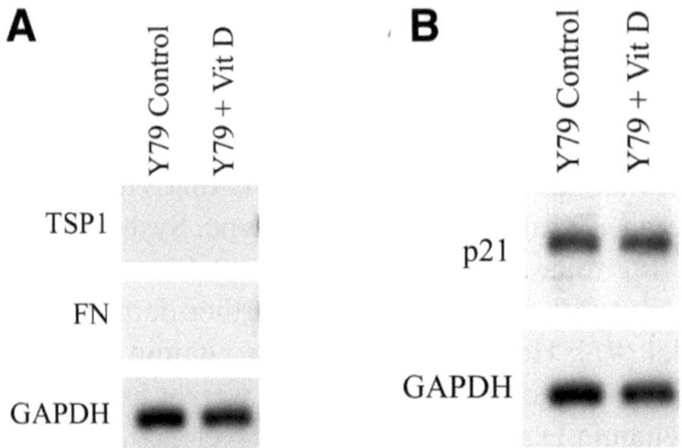

Fig. 1. Northern blot analysis of mRNA prepared from Y79 cells incubated with solvent control or vitamin D for 3 d (10^{-7}M). Five μg of Poly A^+ RNA were run on a 1.2% formaldehyde/agarose gel, transferred to Zeta-probe membrane, and probed with specific cDNA for thrombospondin (TSP)1 (**A**) or p21 (**B**). Blot was also probed with GAPDH to control for loading. Please note lack of TSP1 expression in Y79 cells and increased expression of p21 relative to GAPDH.

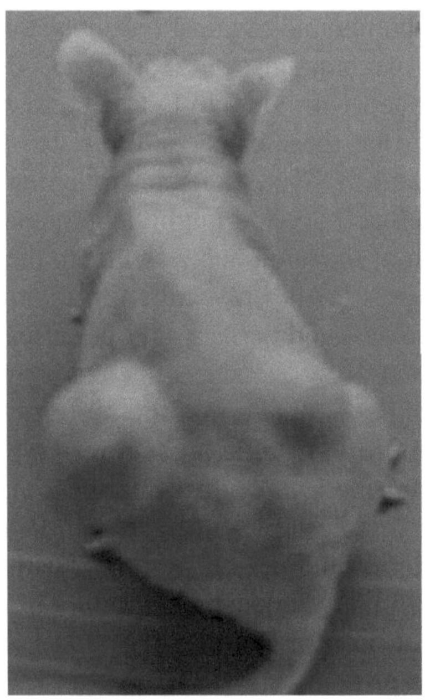

Fig. 2. Tumor formation by Y79 retinoblastoma cells in nude mice. Vector- or thrombospondin (TSP)1-transfected Y79 cells (5×10^6/0.25 mL) were injected into the hind flank of nude mice and tumor volumes were evaluated 3 wk after injection. Please note the increased volume of the tumor formed by vector control cells (left) compared with TSP1-expressing cells (right).

by Y79 cells that express TSP1 has reduced in volume approximately fivefold during 3 wk of growth. The effects of TSP1 expression on Y79 cells were dramatic and prohibited their further characterization in culture. Therefore, downregulation of TSP1 expression, a naturally occurring inhibitor of angiogenesis, may contribute to the aggressive, proliferative, and angiogenic phenotype of Y79 cells. However, a better understanding of the role TSP1 plays in modulation of the Y79 cell phenotype will require a tightly regulated expression system that allows inducible expression of TSP1 in these cells at will, along with assessment of its effect on growth and differentiation in culture and tumor formation in vivo.

Inhibition of angiogenesis has been the focus of many recent studies to inhibit tumor growth and metastasis. Extensive efforts are under way to develop and test agents that have antiangiogenic activity and that can be utilized to treat a variety of diseases with a neovascular component *(46)*. As noted above, a better understanding of the molecular and cellular mechanisms that lead to acquisition of the angiogenic phenotype in uveal melanoma and retinoblastoma may provide further insight to the development of better treatment modalities for these cancers.

Other Ocular Tumors

There are additional ocular tumors, mostly benign, that are less common and as a result have not been extensively studied. These include medulloepithelioma, astrocytic hamartoma, combined hamartoma, and retinal capillary hemangiomas. Little is known about the contribution of angiogenesis to the development and progression of these tumors. Here, too, the development of animal models and cell lines for these tumors will help to further delineate the contribution of angiogenesis to the progression and metastasis of these tumors and enable the use of antiangiogenic factors for their treatment.

LIMITATIONS AND FUTURE DIRECTIONS

The failure of some antiangiogenesis therapies in recent years has led to a realization that developing clinically useful antiangiogenic therapy is more challenging than originally thought. This reflects our limited understanding of tumor vessel biology and of how tumor cells "cross-talk" with tumor-associated endothelial cells. We need to know more about the redundancy of angiogenic factors. It is important to know what is unique about tumor vessels compared to normal vessels. It is obvious that targeting one of many potentially significant factors in tumor development may have a limited effect. The unique gene expression profiles in tumor vessels should help to alleviate this concern. The heterogeneity found in different types of tumors may affect the tumor vasculature in dissimilar ways. A better understanding of how angiogenesis inhibitors affect their target, and the consequences to surrounding tumor and stromal cells, is necessary for successful translation into clinically relevant treatment. The most highly anticipated outcome of this line of research is the identification of specific molecular changes that contribute to the angiogenic switch and the consequent development of specific, more effective antiangiogenic therapy.

REFERENCES

1. Carmeliet P. Angiogenesis in health and disease. Nat Med 2003;9:653–660.
2. Bergers G, Benjamin LE. Tumorigenesis and the angiogenic switch. Nat Revs 2003;3: 401–410.
3. McDonald DM, Foss AJE. Endothelial cells of tumor vessels: Abnormal but not absent. Canc Metast Revs 2000;19:109–120.
4. Sivridis E, Giatromanolaki A, Koukourakis MI. The vascular network of tumours—what is it not for? J Pathol 2003;201:173–180.

5. Dvorak HF. How tumors make bad blood vessels and stroma. Am J Pathol 2003;162: 1747–1757.
6. Gee MS, Procopio WN, Makonnen S, Feldman MD, Yeilding NM, Lee WMF. Tumor vessel development and maturation impose limits on the effectiveness of anti-vascular therapy. Am J Pathol 2003;162:183–193.
7. Sheibani N, Frazier WA. Thrombospondin-1, PECAM-1, and regulation of angiogenesis. Histol Histopathol 1999;14:285–294.
8. Volpert OV. Modulation of endothelial cell survival by an inhibitor of angiogenesis thrombospondin-1: a dynamic balance. Cancer Metas Revs 2000;19:87–92.
9. Wang S, Zhifeng W, Sorenson CM, Lawler J, Sheibani N. Thrombospondin-1-deficient mice exhibit increased vascular density during retinal vascular development and are less sensitive to hyperoxia-mediated vessel obliteration. Dev Dyn 2003;228:630–642.
10. Folkman J, Watson K, Ingber D, Hanahan D. Induction of angiogenesis during the transition from hyperplasia to neoplasia. Nature 1989;339:58–61.
11. Rastinejad F, Polverini PJ, Bouck NP. Regulation of the activity of a new inhibitor of angiogenesis by a cancer suppressor gene. Cell 1989;56:345–355.
12. O'Reilly MS, Holmgren L, Shing Y, et al. Angiostatin: a novel angiogenesis inhibitor that mediates the suppression of metastases by a Lewis lung carcinoma. Cell 1994;79:315–328.
13. O'Reilly MS, Boehm T, Shing Y, et al. Endostatin: an endogenous inhibitor of angiogenesis and tumor growth. Cell 1997;88:277–285.
14. Brooks PC, Clark RAF, Cheresh DA. Requirement of vascular integrin $\alpha_v\beta_3$ for angiogenesis. Science 1994;264:569–571.
15. Brooks PC, Montgomery AMP, Rosenfeld M, et al. Integrin $\alpha_v\beta_3$ antagonists promote tumor regression by inducing apoptosis of angiogenic blood vessels. Cell 1994;79:1157–1164.
16. Storgard CM, Stupack DG, Jonczyk A, Goodman S, Fox RI, Cheresh DA. Decreased angiogenesis and arthritic disease in rabbits treated with an $\alpha_v\beta_3$ antagonist. J Clin Invest 1999;103:47–54.
17. Davis DW, McConkey DJ, Zhang W, Herbst RS. Antiangiogenic tumor therapy. BioTechniques 2003;34:1048–1063.
18. Foss AJE, Cree IA, Dolin PJ, Hungerford JL. Modelling uveal melanoma. Br J Ophthalmol 1999;83:588–594.
19. Sheidow TG, Hooper PL, Crukley C, Young J, Heathcote JG. Expression of vascular endothelial growth factor in uveal melanoma and its correlation with metastasis. Br J Ophthalmol 2000;84:750–756.
20. Dithmar S, Rusciano D, Lynn MJ, Lawson DH, Armstrong CA, Grossniklaus HE. Neoadjuvant interferon alfa-2b treatment in a murine model for metastatic ocular melanoma. Arch Ophthalmol 2000;118:1085–1089.
21. Boyd SR, Tan DSW, de Souza L, et al. Uveal melanomas express vascular endothelial growth factor and basic fibroblast growth factor and support endothelial cell growth. Br J Ophthalmol 2002;86:440–447.
22. Stitt AW, Gardiner TA. Anti-angiogenic therapy for uveal melanoma—more haste, less speed. Br J Ophthalmol 2002;86:368, 369.
23. Marback EF, Arias VEA, Paranhos Jr A, Soares FA, Murphree AL, Erwenne CM. Tumor angiogenesis as a prognostic factor for disease dissemination in retinoblastoma. Br J Ophthalmol 2003;87:1224–1228.
24. van der Velden PA, Zuidervaart W, Hurks MHMH, et al. Expression profiling reveals that methylation of TIMP3 is involved in uveal melanoma development. Int J Cancer 2003;106:472–479.
25. Rössler J, Dietrich T, Pavlakovic H, et al. Higher vessel densities in retinoblastoma with local invasive growth and metastasis. Am J Pathol 2004;164:391–394.

26. Harbour JW. Clinical overview of uveal melanoma: introduction to tumors of the eye. In: Ocular Oncology, Albert DM, Polans A, eds. Marcel Dekker, New York: 2003:1–18.
27. Shields JA, Shields CL. Clinical overview: retinoblastoma. In: Ocular Oncology, Albert DM, Polans A, eds. Marcel Dekker, New York: 2003:19–34.
28. van Ginkel PR. Structural alterations and gene expression in the pathogenesis of uveal melanoma. In: Ocular Oncology, Albert DM, Polans A, eds. Marcel Dekker, New York: 2003:81–102.
29. Gombos DS, Mieler WF. Therapy of uveal melanoma: methods and risk factors associated with treatment. In: Ocular Oncology, Albert DM, Polans A, eds. Marcel Dekker, New York: 2003:321–352.
30. van Ginkel PR, Gee RL, Shearer RL, et al. Expression of the receptor tyrosine kinase Axl promotes ocular melanoma cell survival. Cancer Res 2004;64:128–134.
31. Apte RS, Niederkorn JY, Mayhew E, Alizadeh H. Angiostatin produced by certain primary uveal melanoma cell lines impedes the development of liver metastases. Arch Ophthalmol 2001;119:1805–1809.
32. Dithmar S, Grossniklaus HE. Models of uveal melanoma: characterization of transgenic mice and other animal models for melanoma. In: Ocular Oncology, Albert DM, Polans A, eds. Marcel Dekker, New York: 2003:269–296.
33. Folberg R, Hendrix MJC, Maniotis AJ. Vasculogenic mimicry and tumor angiogenesis. Am J Pathol 2000;156:361–381.
34. Hendrix MJC, Seftor EA, Meltzer PS, et al. Expression and functional significance of VE-cadherin in aggressive human melanoma cells: Role in vasculogenic mimicry. Proc Natl Acad Sci USA 2001;98:8018–8023.
35. Albert DM. Historic review of retinoblastoma. Opthalmology 1987;94:654–662.
36. Abramson DH, Schefler AC. The treatment of retinoblastoma. In: Ocular Oncology, Albert DM, Polans A, eds. Marcel Dekker, New York: 2003:353–376.
37. Windle JJ, Albert DM, O'Brien JM, et al. Retinoblastoma in transgenic mice. Nature 1990;343:665–669.
38. Chávez-Barrios P, Hurwitz MY, Louie K, et al. Metastic and nonmetastic models of retinoblastoma. Am J Pathol 2000;157:1405–1412.
39. Windle JJ, Albert DM. Genetically engineered mouse models of retinoblastoma. In: Ocular Oncology, Albert DM, Polans A, eds. Marcel Dekker, New York: 2003:465–487.
40. Saulenas AM, Cohen SM, Key LL, Winter C, Albert DM. Vitamin D and retinoblastoma. Arch Ophthalmol 1988;106:533–535.
41. Shokravi MT, Marcus DM, Alroy J, Egan K, Saornil MA, Albert DM. Vitamin D inhibits angiogenesis in transgenic murine retinoblastoma. Invest Ophthal Vis Sci 1995;36:83–87.
42. Audo I, Darjatmoko SR, Schlamp CL, et al. Vitamin D analogues increase p53, p21, and apoptosis in a xenograft model of human retinoblastoma. Invest Ophthalmol Vis Sci 2003;44:4192–4199.
43. Suzuki T, Sano Y, Kinoshita S. Effects of 1α,25-dihydroxyvitamin D_3 on langerhans cell migration and corneal neovascularization in mice. Invest Ophthalmol Vis Sci 2000;41:154–158.
44. Mantell DJ, Owens PE, Bundred NJ, Mawer EB, Canfield AE. 1α,25-dihydroxyvitamin D_3 inhibits angiogenesis in vitro and in vivo. Circ Res 2000;87:214–220.
45. Bernardi RJ, Johnson CS, Modzelewski RA, Trump DL. Antiproliferative effects of 1α,25-dihydroxyvitamin D_3 and vitamin D analogs on tumor-derived endothelial cells. Endocrinology 2002;143:2508–2514.
46. Tosetti F, Ferrari N, De Flora S, Albini A. "Angioprevention": angiogenesis is a common and key target for cancer chemopreventive agents. FASEB J 2002;16:2–14.

10
Genetics of Ocular Vascular Disease

Jacquie Greenberg, PhD, **Ari Ziskind,** MSc(Eng), BSc(Med), MB ChB, FCS(SA)(Ophth.), **and Stephen P. Daiger,** PhD

CONTENTS

OCULAR ANGIOGENESIS: MORE COMMON INHERITED DISEASES AND MECHANISMS

Genetic Basis of Degenerative Aging Diseases

In considering inherited disease, one important distinction is between diseases with a clear, unequivocal genetic cause and other diseases whose occurrence is influenced by genetic factors, but whose causes are multifactorial. The first type, simple or Mendelian inherited diseases, typically have a distinct mode of inheritance—autosomal dominant, autosomal recessive or X-linked—and are the result of rare, pathogenic mutations with high penetrance (presence of the mutation or mutations has a high likelihood of causing disease). Examples of Mendelian diseases that include neovascularization are X-linked Norrie's disease *(1)* and autosomal dominant glaucoma caused by mutations in myocilin *(2)*. Even "simple" inherited diseases are genetically complicated, as mutations in different genes may cause the same disease, and different mutations in the same gene may cause different diseases. However, it is reasonable to assume that the cause of a Mendelian disease in a given individual and family is one mutation only (or two, if recessive) in a specific gene.

In contrast, complex multifactorial diseases, such as the more commonly seen age-related macular degeneration (AMD) and primary open-angle glaucoma (POAG), are the result of interactions among genetic, environmental, and stochastic factors. Genetic differences—that is, allelic differences—may play a role in increasing or decreasing lifetime risk, or in determining clinical details, but the predisposing alleles may have low to moderate penetrance; that is, the presence of a "mutation" is neither necessary nor sufficient to cause disease in a specific affected individual. The contributing factors

From: *Ophthalmology: Ocular Angiogenesis: Diseases, Mechanisms, and Therapeutics*
Edited by: J. Tombran-Tink and C. J. Barnstable © Humana Press Inc., Totowa, NJ

in a given individual may be multiple; more than one factor may segregate in a family; and multiple genes and alleles may be involved in a collection of affected individuals.

In practice, there may be a continuum between simple and complex inherited diseases. For example, digenic and triallelic forms of Mendelian retinal diseases are known *(3–5)*. Also, high-penetrance alleles may account for a fraction of AMD and POAG cases. However, the distinction is useful because methods for finding mutations causing simple inherited diseases are currently much more effective than methods focused on complex diseases, and the implications for affected individuals and families are very different.

The differences between simple and complex genetic diseases have important methodological consequences. Methods for identifying simple disease genes and mutations are highly developed. These include gene mapping in families, positional gene cloning, and mutation screening of known disease genes. More than 150 genes causing inherited retinal diseases have been identified by these methods *(6)*, and at least a dozen genes causing glaucoma have been found *(7)*. For broad categories of inherited retinal disease, such as retinitis pigmentosa or Leber congenital amaurosis, sequencing of known disease genes can detect pathogenic mutations in at least 50% of affected individuals *(8,9)*.

Methods for identifying genes and alleles contributing to complex diseases are currently less effective. There are basically two approaches: linkage mapping or other methods for observing segregation, and evaluation of candidate genes in affected individuals. Both approaches have been applied to large patient cohorts, with all the problems attendant to such studies: inconsistent clinical definitions, age and environmental factors as cofactors, population heterogeneity, and the like. For mapping methods, the goal is to find alleles, typically common alleles, that segregate with disease in siblings or small nuclear families. A positive result may identify the chromosomal location of a causative gene, but not the actual gene among, perhaps, scores of genes in the same region. For candidate gene screening, the goal is to find *either* common alleles that influence risk *or* rare, pathogenic mutations that, in aggregate, are common. Although efforts to identify genetic factors associated with complex diseases such as AMD and POAG have met with limited success to date, there are a number of notable, suggestive associations, as discussed subsequently.

Despite the differences between simple and complex inherited diseases, investigation of Mendelian diseases contributes directly to research on complex disorders, for several reasons. First, Mendelian diseases serve as clinical models for complex diseases. For example, a dominantly inherited form of macular degeneration, ARMD1, which maps to chromosome 1q, is clinically similar to AMD *(10)*, and several mapped forms of inherited glaucoma are similar to POAG *(7)*. Second, genes causing Mendelian diseases are excellent candidates for genes affecting complex traits. For example, variants of the hemicentin 1 gene, the probable cause of ARMD1, may be associated with AMD *(11)*. These candidate genes are relevant to both linkage mapping and gene screening.

Third, in any large cohort of patients with complex diseases, a subset of individuals will have a Mendelian disease, even though family history may be insufficient to establish the mode of inheritance. For these individuals, the recurrence risk may be much higher than for individuals with complex disorders.

Finally, identification of rare, Mendelian disease-causing genes contributes to understanding normal biology, which, in turn, applies to complex diseases. Any recent review of ocular genetics proves this point.

Age-Related Macular Degeneration

Age-related macular degeneration also known as age-related maculopathy, is the leading cause of legal blindness among individuals over the age of 65 in the Western world *(12)*. It has been estimated to affect 1% of individuals in the 65- to 74-yr age group and 11% of individuals over 85 yr of age in the United States. It has been predicted that by 2030, 42 million Americans will have AMD or will be at risk of developing it. It is currently more common than Alzheimer's disease or Parkinson's disease.

Several studies suggest that the cause of AMD in a proportion of patients may result from a genetic predisposition. The molecular genetic analysis of AMD is hampered by it being a late-onset disorder and often parents of an affected individual are deceased, whereas the children have yet to manifest the clinical manifestations. Clinically, AMD is a complex degenerative disorder involving the retinal pigment epithelium (RPE), choriocapillaris, and retina and affects primarily, but not exclusively, the macular region of the eye. Symptoms include central vision loss, metamorphopsia, and impaired light adaptation.

Clinically, there are two forms of AMD:

1. An exudative or "wet" form, which is characterized by detachment of the RPE and/or development of subretinal choroidal neovascular membranes. This form results in the most damage and can result in blindness overnight from hemorrhaging, under the retina, which originates from blood vessels that have aberrantly entered this area after crossing Bruch's membrane and the RPE. No genes have as yet been found to be associated with "wet" AMD.
2. A "dry" form, which is associated with drusen, within or beneath the RPE, and includes mottling of the RPE and/or geographic atrophy.

There are other known genetic forms of macular degeneration, such as Stargardt disease (STGD) *(13)*, which has some similarity to dry AMD, and Sorsby fundus dystrophy (SFD) *(14)*, where the clinical picture is similar to the wet form of macular degeneration. These macular degeneration diseases manifest clinical symptoms at an early age and are therefore more amenable to genetic studies. More importantly, these macular dystrophies share some similarities in their clinical and histopathological phenotypes and it could therefore be expected that genetic and molecular investigations of these conditions would contribute to the understanding of AMD.

Stargardt Disease

Stargardt disease is the most common hereditary macular dystrophy (MD) affecting children; the prevalence is estimated to be about 1 in 10,000 *(15)*. The condition is characterized by central visual loss and atrophy of the RPE, and in the early stages of the disease there may actually be a significant accumulation of lipofuscin-like material within the macular RPE in a significant percentage of patients. This resembles a "beaten bronze" appearance and has a distribution of ill-defined orange-yellow flecks around the macula and/or the mid-periphery of the retina *(13)*. STGD is predominantly inherited as an autosomal recessive trait. The first genetic locus for STGD, also the first mapped recessive form of MD, was localized to the short arm of chromosome 1 (1p21–p13) *(16)*. This was achieved by linkage analysis using eight families initially. Shortly thereafter, more families with a clinical phenotype consistent with STGD and fundus flavimaculatus were also mapped to the same genetic locus *(13)*. These studies provided further supporting evidence for the hypothesis that a mutation in a single gene was underlying STGD/fundus flavimaculatus. Four years after the publication of this genetic localization, the disease-causing gene was identified as *ABCR* (retina-specific ABC transporter), which was later renamed *ABCA4* *(17)*. *ABCA4* was fully characterized in 1998 *(18–20)* and its genomic organization revealed that it is a typical representation of the ATP-binding cassette (ABC) transporter superfamily of genes.

Numerous studies using mutation analyses of *ABCA4* have provided evidence suggesting that it is perhaps the most polymorphic retinal gene studied to date *(21,58)*. More than 200 disease-causing mutations, ranging from single base substitutions to deletions of several exons, have been identified in *ABCA4* and the majority of reported changes are missense mutations *(22–25)*. Disease-causing mutations in *ABCA4* account for 66 to 80% of STGD-associated chromosomes investigated *(26)*.

Genes Causing Mendelian Forms of Macular Degeneration and Other Mendelian Retinal Diseases with Angiogenesis

ABCA4 has been implicated in several clinical distinct retinal phenotypes, which include:

1. Autosomal recessive STGD *(17)*.
2. Autosomal recessive retinitis pigmentosa (RP), RP19 *(27)*.
3. Autosomal recessive cone-rod dystrophy (CRD) *(28)*.
4. Age-related macular degeneration *(29)*.

Two surveys suggest an association between AMD and common allelic variants at the ABCA4 locus *(17,29,30)*. However, as stated previously, the ABCA4 locus harbors an astonishing number of polymorphic variants in human populations *(31)*, so it is very difficult to detect an association, if any, between these variants and a common disorder such as AMD. Indeed, other studies do not support an association *(32)*. This question is therefore still under investigation and there is still a great deal of controversy around the reports of this association between ABCA4 and AMD *(33)*.

Table 1 lists genes known to cause Mendelian forms of macular degeneration or macular diseases with clinical features in common with AMD. As has been discussed above for ABCA4, for several genes, different mutations in the same gene may cause different disorders. For example, mutations in the RDS gene, on 6p, may cause dominant retinitis pigmentosa, macular dystrophy, or pattern dystrophies, or may contribute to digenic disease *(3,4)*. Thus some genes listed in Table 1 have multiple entries in the disease(s) column. Undoubtedly, further molecular investigation of these genes may provide information about the understanding of macular degeneration, specifically the complex multifactorial ARMD.

Table 2 lists genes known to cause Mendelian forms of disease that include retinal angiogenesis among their symptoms. As with genes causing macular degeneration, multiple diseases may be associated with one gene.

Table 1
Genes Causing Mendelian Forms of Macular Degeneration (MD)

Symbol *Location*	*Protein*	*Disease(s)*	*References*
ABCA4 1p22.1	ATP-binding cassette transporter—retinal	1. Recessive Stargardt disease, juvenile and late onset 2. Recessive MD 3. Recessive retinitis pigmentosa (RP) 4. Recessive fundus flavimaculatus 5. Recessive cone-rod dystrophy	*17* *28* *16* *27* *49* *50* *51* *52*
ARMD1 1q31.1	Hemicentin 1	Dominant MD, age-related	*10* *11*
EFEMP1 2p16.1	Epidermal growth factor-containing fibrillin-like extracellular matrix protein 1	1. Dominant radial, macular drusen 2. Dominant Doyne honeycomb retinal degeneration (Malattia Leventinese)	*53* *54* *40*
STGD 4p	Unknown	Dominant MD, Stargardt-like	*55*
MCDR3 5p15.33–p13.1	Unknown	Dominant MD	*56*
BSMD 5q21.2–q33.2	Unknown	Dominant MD, butterfly-shaped	*57*
RDS 6p21.2	Peripherin 2	1. Dominant RP 2. Dominant MD 3. Digenic RP with ROM1 4. Dominant MD, adult vitelliform type	*58* *59* *60* *61* *3* *4*
BCMAD 6p12.3–q16	Unknown	Dominant MD, benign concentric annular	*62*
MCDR1 6q14–q16.2	Unknown	1. Dominant MD, North Carolina type 2. Dominant progressive bifocal chorioretinal atrophy	*63* *64*
ELOVL4 6q14.1	Elongation of very long fatty acids protein	Dominant MD, Stargardt-like	*65* *66* *67*
MDDC 7p21–p15		Dominant MD, cystoid	*68* *69*
VMD2 11q12.3	Bestrophin	Dominant MD, Best type	*70* *71* *72*
C1QTNF5 11q23.3	C1q and tumor necrosis-related protein 5 collagen	Dominant MD, late onset	*73*

(Continued)

Table 1 *(Continued)*

Symbol *Location*	*Protein*	*Disease(s)*	*References*
TIMP3 22q12.3	Tissue inhibitor of metalloproteinases-3	Dominant MD, Sorsby's fundus dystrophy	*74* *75* *76* *14*
RPGR Xp11.4	Retinitis pigmentosa GTPase regulator	1. Recessive X-linked RP	*77*
		2. Dominant X-linked RP	*78*
		3. Dominant X-linked congenital stationary night blindness	*79*
		4. X-linked cone dystrophy 1	*80*
		5. Recessive X-linked atrophic MD	*81* *82* *83*

From these lists it is clear that the two approaches to finding genes contributing to AMD, linkage mapping and candidate gene screening, have implicated several genes. Numerous genome-wide linkage studies have identified chromosomal sites that are likely to harbor AMD-related genes *(34–38)*. The reports are discouraging, in one sense, because each independent study identified a different set of possible linked locations. However, two locations, 1q31 and 10q26, show significant association with AMD in three or more studies. Of these, the potential AMD gene on 10q is not known but the 1q gene may have been found.

The chromosome 1 site linked to AMD overlaps with the Mendelian ARMD1 locus *(10)*. Recent evidence suggests that the gene causing ARMD1 produces hemicentin 1, a retinal-expressed extracellular matrix protein of unknown function. Rare missense changes in hemicentin 1 have also been found in AMD patients *(11)*. This association is supported by linkage evidence *(35)* but not by subsequent sequencing studies *(34)*. In summary, it is likely that a major gene influencing AMD maps to 1q31 at or near the ARMD1 locus, the ARMD1 gene may also be the AMD gene, and mutations in hemicentin 1 are the probable cause of ARMD1.

Essentially all the potential candidate genes in Table 1 have been tested in AMD patients, by both linkage mapping and sequencing. Most are not associated with AMD, although individuals with rare pathogenic, high-penetrance mutations at any of these loci may be among the AMD patients.

Recently, a gene not yet known to cause Mendelian disease, fibulin 5, has been associated with AMD *(39)*. The fibulin 5 gene (FBLN5) maps to human chromosome 14q32, a region not previously implicated by linkage mapping. The fibulin 5 protein is similar to fibulin 3 (EFEMP1 on 2p), mutations that cause Doyne honeycomb retinal dystrophy, a Mendelian disorder with similarities to AMD *(40)*. Screening the FBLN5 gene in patients and controls revealed apparent dominant-acting missense mutations in 1.7% of AMD patients.

If supported by subsequent studies, FBLN5 joins other possible AMD genes that affect few patients per gene, but account for larger numbers in aggregate. This model

Table 2
Genes Causing Mendelian Retinal Diseases with Angiogenesis

Symbol *Location*	*Protein*	*Disease(s)*	*References*
COL11A1 1p21.1	Collagen, type XI, α 1	1. Dominant Stickler syndrome, type II 2. Dominant Marshall syndrome	*84* *85*
CRB1 1q31.3	Crumbs homology 1	1. Recessive RP with para-arteriolar preservation of the RPE (PPRPE) 2. Recessive RP 3. Recessive Leber congenital amaurosis	*86* *87* *88* *89* *90* *91* *92*
CRV 3p21.3–p21.1		Dominant hereditary vascular retinopathy with Raynaud phenomenon and migraine	*93* *94* *95*
WGN1 5q13–q14		Dominant Wagner disease and erosive vitreoretinopathy	*96* *97*
EVR3 11p13–p12		Dominant familial exudative vitreoretinopathy	*47*
FZD4 11q14.2	Frizzled-4 Wnt receptor homolog	Dominant familial exudative vitreoretinopathy	*98* *99* *49*
VRNI 11q13		Dominant neovascular inflammatory vitreoretinopathy	*100*
LRP5 11q13.2	Low-density lipoprotein receptor-related protein 5	1. Dominant familial exudative vitreoretinopathy 2. Dominant high bone mass trait 3. Recessive osteoporosis-pseudoglioma syndrome 4. Recessive FEVR	*101* *102* *103*
COL2A1 12q13.11	Collagen, type II, α 1	1. Dominant Stickler syndrome, type I 2. Dominant Wagner syndrome 3. Dominant epiphyseal dysplasia	*104* *105* *106*
ABCC6 16p13.11	ATP-binding casette, subfamily C, member 6	1. Recessive pseudoxanthoma elasticum 2. Dominant pseudoxanthoma elasticum	*107* *108* *109* *110* *111*
NDP Xp11.3	Norrie disease protein	1. Norrie's disease 2. Familial exudative vitreoretinopathy 3. Coats' disease	*112* *113* *114,115* *116* *117*

CSNB, congenital stationary night blindness; FEVR, familial exudative vitreoretinopathy; MD, macular degeneration; RP, retinitis pigmentosa; RPE, retinal pigment epithelium.

is distinct from the possibility of common polymorphic alleles at a locus affecting lifetime risk, a possibility that linkage mapping should reveal. Thus linkage mapping, gene screening, and identification of genes causing Mendelian diseases offer complementary, but distinct, methods for finding genes associated with AMD.

The association between these particular genes and well-recognized degenerative diseases of aging does not imply that environmental factors should now be considered less important. This knowledge may eventually help to provide individuals with a risk profile, so that they can avoid the particular environmental factors that are likely to have a negative impact on their genetic inheritance. Caution should be exercised with genomic profiling, however, as it has become evident that many initial gene–disease associations have, on follow-up, been found to be spurious or weaker than previously reported or predicted. The premature use of presymptomatic genetic testing based on this type of gene–disease associations and prophylactic interventions of as yet unknown value could in fact do more harm than good to the public as well as to the field of genomic medicine. As Susanne Haga et al. state *(41)*, "Genomic profiling to promote a healthy lifestyle: not ready for prime time."

RARER BUT IMPORTANT GENETIC FORMS OF OCULAR VASCULAR DISEASE

Norrie's Disease

Norrie's disease is a rare X-linked recessive condition characterized by progressive bilateral congenital blindness that is usually associated with mental retardation and cochlear deafness. The congenital blindness is secondary to retinal dysplasia caused by failure of the retina to develop normally during embryonic life. This may result in detachment of the retina, vitreous hemorrhage, and the ultimate formation of a white retrolental mass that may be complicated by the formation of a secondary cataract. Norrie's disease was linked to a locus on the X chromosome, and the disease gene has since been cloned and the protein product shown to have a tertiary structure similar to transforming growth factor β. This would suggest that the gene may have a role in retinal cell differentiation and proliferation *(42)*.

Although at the end stage of the disease the condition can be confused with retinopathy of prematurity (ROP), the pathogenesis of the conditions are considered to be fairly distinct, with ROP developing in response to the production of VEGF by the relatively ischemic peripheral retina of premature, low-birth-weight infants. In some infants with ROP the condition progresses inexorably to the very severe end-stage form in spite of intensive therapy, but in the majority it regresses. Mutations in the Norrie's disease gene have been implicated as a risk factor for progression in these infants, but this is controversial and has not been noted in other studies *(43)*.

Von Hippel-Lindau Syndrome

Von Hippel-Lindau syndrome (VHL) is classified as one of the phakomatoses, a group of complex multisystem disorders that some authors have defined as neuroculocutaneous syndromes with autosomal dominant inheritance *(44)*. VHL syndrome itself is also a multisystem disorder, and is characterized by retinal capillary hemangiomas, central nervous system (CNS) hemangioblastomas, various solid and cystic hamartomas, and malignant neoplasms, including renal cell carcinomas and phaeochromocytomas. Capillary hemangiomas of the retina are usually the earliest detectable manifestation, with CNS manifestations presenting a little later, whereas renal cell carcinomas develop substantially later. The fact that the renal cell carcinoma presents in more than 60% of individuals makes early diagnosis and monitoring of the condition absolutely crucial, and protocols for managing these individuals have been developed.

Not every patient with a retinal capillary hemangioma has VHL, but the presence of two or more of these lesions increases the likelihood of the syndrome dramatically. Identification of the gene for VHL syndrome on chromosome 3p26 has now made it possible for suspected individuals to undergo genetic testing with a high degree of accuracy, thereby avoiding the necessity of patients without the syndrome being exposed to lifelong screening programs *(45)*.

The VHL gene acts as a tumor suppressor gene of the retinoblastoma type, as tumors develop when there is inactivation or loss of the normal wild-type allele in a susceptible cell *(46)*. In normal cells VEGF is regulated by multiple factors, including hypoxia. In contrast, the VHL gene is induced under normoxic conditions and, working via as yet incompletely characterized pathways, results in reduced expression of VEGF in this situation. In the case of mutant VHL, however, this inhibition of VEGF in normoxic conditions does not occur and inappropriate overexpression of VEGF occurs, resulting in the development of localized angiomatous proliferation.

Familial Exudative Vitreoretinopathy

Familial exudative vitreoretinopathy (FEVR) is a genetic eye disease charaterized by a failure of peripheral retinal vascularization. It is caused by an abrupt cessation of growth of peripheral capillaries, which may ultimately lead to retinal neovascularization as compensation for the growth loss, and could then result in exudative leakage, bleeding, and eventually retinal detachment. Early diagnosis is thus essential to prevent unnecessary severe and irreversible damage. To date, a few FEVR genetic loci have been mapped to chromosome 11q13-23, Xp11.4 and 11p13-12 *(47)*. More recently, a mutation in a gene for autosomal dominant FEVR was identified as being in the development gene, frizzled-4 (FSD4) *(48)*.

THERAPEUTIC MODALITIES FOR GENETIC FORMS OF OCULAR VASCULAR DISEASE

The exponential increase in our understanding of genetic diseases has led to increasing expectations of direct benefit to individual patients or their families. Although this topic is receiving a great deal of attention and human trials of a limited nature have already begun for some inherited conditions, such as cystic fibrosis, this enthusiasm should be tempered with the realization that the road ahead is still strewn with difficulties. The chances of effective therapies in the short to medium term, specifically for the retinal degenerations, are still rather slim. Although each group of genetic conditions is likely to benefit from experience gained in managing genetic disease in other organs, such as the lung, each site is likely to present its own unique difficulties.

One of the obvious benefits for individuals and families with genetic retinal degenerative disease is accurate diagnosis, prognosis, and genetic counseling. A major problem with ophthalmic genetic conditions and future therapies arises because of the enormous molecular heterogeneity of the majority of these diseases. There are many instances in which different mutations in the same gene have been shown to cause different degrees of vision loss. In addition, different mutations in the same gene could also cause different diseases (e.g., *ABCA4* and STGD, RP, CRD, and ARMD). It is therefore possible that therapies may have to be tailored to such a degree of individuality that although solutions may be possible in theory, gene therapy may not be economically feasible. We know that there are more than 150 genes known to be associated with retinal degeneration with many different mutations in some of these genes. We ultimately need to know more about the mechanism behind the degeneration before we are going to be able to cure the conditions. Much has been learned from animal models and transgenic mice, and the RCS rat has taught us great deal in the past few years.

A direct benefit of the new genetic knowledge about the actual genes that are causative of some forms of inherited blindness is the fact that many of them can be grouped by function; this then also allows insight into the disease process. Potential therapies can therefore now be tested in subgroups of patients with defects in the same (similar function) genes or pathways.

REFERENCES

1. Berger W, Ropers H-H. Norrie disease, in The Metabolic and Molecular Bases of Inherited Disease, 8th edition, Eds Scriver CR, Beaudet AL, Sly WS, Valle D, McGraw Hill, New York, 2001, 5977–5986.
2. Fingert JH, Stone EM, Sheffield VC, Alward WL. Myocilin glaucoma. Surv Ophthalmol 2002;47:547–561.
3. Kajiwara K, Hahn LB, Mukai S, Travis GH, Berson EL, Dryja,TP. Mutations in the human retinal degeneration slow gene in autosomal dominant retinitis pigmentosa. Nature 1991;354:480–483.
4. Kajiwara K, Berson EL, Dryja TP. Digenic retinitis pigmentosa due to mutations at the unlinked peripherin/RDS and ROM1 loci. Science 1994;264:1604–1608.
5. Katsanis N, Ansley SJ, Badano JL, et al. Triallelic inheritance in Bardet-Biedl syndrome, a Mendelian recessive disorder. Science 2001;293:2256–2259.
6. RetNet, Retinal Information Network, http://www.sph.uth.tmc.edu/RetNet, copyright 2004, University of Texas Health Science Center at Houston.
7. Sheffield VC, Alward WLM, Stone EM. The glaucomas. In: The Metabolic and Molecular Bases of Inherited Disease, 8th ed. Scriver CR, Beaudet AL, Sly WS, Valle D, eds. McGraw Hill, New York: 2001:6063–6076.
8. Daiger SP. Identifying retinal disease genes: how far have we come, how far do we have to go? Novartis Found Symp 2004;255:17–27; discussion 27–36, 177–178.
9. Hanein S, Perrault I, Gerber S, et al. Leber congenital amaurosis: comprehensive survey of the genetic heterogeneity, refinement of the clinical definition, and genotype-phenotype correlations as a strategy for molecular diagnosis. Hum Mutat 2004;23:306–317.
10. Klein ML, Schultz DW, Edwards A, et al. Age-related macular degeneration. Clinical features in a large family and linkage to chromosome 1q. Arch Ophthalmol 1998;116:1082–1088.
11. Schultz DW, Klein ML, Humpert AJ, et al. Analysis of the ARMD1 locus: Evidence that a mutation in HEMICENTIN-1 is associated with age-related macular degeneration in a large family. Hum Mol Genet 2003;12:3315–3123.

12. van Driel MA, Maugeri A, Klevering BJ, Hoyng CB, Cremers FP. ABCR unites what ophthalmologists divide(s) Ophthalmic Genet 1998;19:117–122.
13. Anderson KL, Baird L, Lewis RA, et al. A. YAC contig encompassing the recessive Stargardt disease gene (STGD) on chromosome 1p. Am J Hum Genet 1995;57: 1351–1363.
14. Peters A, Greenberg J. Sorsby's Fundus Dystrophy: A South African family with a point mutation on the tissue inhibitor of Metalloproteinases-3 gene on chromosome 22. Retina 1995;15,480–15,485.
15. Papaioannou M, Ocaka L, Bessant D, et al. An analysis of ABCR mutations in British patients with recessive retinal dystrophies. Invest Ophthalmol Vis Sci 2000;41:16–19.
16. Kaplan J, Gerber S, Larget-Piet D, et al. A gene for Stargardt's disease (fundus flavimaculatus) maps to the short arm of chromosome 1. Nature Genet 1993;5:308–311.
17. Allikmets R, Singh N, Sun H, et al. A photoreceptor cell-specific ATP-binding transporter gene (ABCR) is mutated in recessive Stargardt macular dystrophy. Nature Genet 1997;15:236–246.
18. Allikmets R, Wasserman WW, Hutchinson A, et al. Organization of the ABCR gene: analysis of promoter and splice junction sequences. Gene 1998;215:111–122.
19. Gerber S, Rozet JM, van de Pol TJ, et al. Complete exon-intron structure of the retina-specific ATP binding transporter gene (ABCR) allows the identification of novel mutations underlying Stargardt disease. Genomics 1998;48:139–142.
20. Azarian SM, Megarity CF, Weng J, Horvath DH, Travis GH. The human photoreceptor rim protein gene (ABCR): genomic structure and primer set information for mutation analysis. Hum Genet 1998;102:699–705.
21. Schmidt S, Postel EA, Agarwal A, et al. Detailed analysis of allelic variation in the ABCA4 gene in age-related maculopathy. Invest Ophthalmol Vis Sci 2003;44: 2868–2875.
22. Rivera A, White K, Stohr H, et al. A comprehensive survey of sequence variation in the ABCA4 (ABCR) gene in Stargardt disease and age-related macular degeneration. Am J Hum Genet 2000;67:800–813.
23. Briggs CE, Rucinski D, Rosenfeld PJ, Hirose T, Berson EL, Dryja TP. Mutations in ABCR (ABCA4) in patients with Stargardt macular degeneration or cone-rod degeneration. Invest Ophthalmol Vis Sci 2001;42:2229–2236.
24. Yatsenko AN, Shroyer NF, Lewis RA, Lupski JR. Late-onset Stargardt disease is associated with missense mutations that map outside known functional regions of ABCR (ABCA4). Hum Genet 2001;108:346–355.
25. Gerth C, Andrassi-Darida M, Bock M, Preising MN, Weber BH, Lorenz B. Phenotypes of 16 Stargardt macular dystrophy/fundus flavimaculatus patients with known ABCA4 mutations and evaluation of genotype-phenotype correlation. Arch Clin Exp Ophthalmol 2002;240:628–638.
26. Yatsenko AN, Shroyer NF, Lewis RA, Lupski JR. An ABCA4 genomic deletion in patients with Stargardt disease. Hum Mutat 2003;21:636–644.
27. Martinez-Mir A, Paloma E, Allikmets R, et al. Retinitis. pigmentosa caused by a homozygous mutation in the Stargardt disease gene ABCR. Nature Genet 1998;18:11, 12.
28. Cremers FP, van de Pol DJ, van Driel M, et al. Autosomal. recessive retinitis pigmentosa and cone-rod dystrophy caused by splice site mutations in the Stargardt's disease gene ABCR. Hum Mol Genet 1998;7:355–362.
29. Allikmets R, Shroyer NF, Singh N, et al. Mutation of the Stargardt disease gene (ABCR) in age-related macular degeneration. Science 1997;277:1805–1807.
30. Allikmets R. Further evidence for an association of ABCR alleles with age-related macular degeneration. The International ABCR Screening Consortium. Am J Hum Genet 2000;67:487–491.

31. Webster AR, Heon E, Lotery AJ, et al. An analysis of allelic variation in the ABCA4 gene. Invest Ophthalmol Vis Sci 2001;42:1179–1189.
32. Stone EM, Webster AR, Vandenburgh K, et al. Allelic variation in ABCR associated with Stargardt disease but not age-related macular degeneration. Nature Genet 1998;20: 328, 329.
33. September A. The molecular investigation of Stargardt disease in South Africa. Ph.D. thesis. University of Cape Town, South Africa.
34. Abecasis GR, Yashar BM, Zhao Y, et al. Age-related macular degeneration: a high-resolution genome scan for susceptibility loci in a population enriched for late-stage disease. Am J Hum Genet 2004;74:482–494.
35. Iyengar SK, Song D, Klein BE, et al. Dissection of genomewide-scan data in extended families reveals a major locus and oligogenic susceptibility for age-related macular degeneration. Am J Hum Genet 2004;74:20–39.
36. Kenealy SJ, Schmidt S, Agarwal A, et al. Linkage analysis for age-related macular degeneration supports a gene on chromosome 10q26. Mol Vis 2004;10:57–61.
37. Schick JH, Iyengar SK, Klein BE, et al. A whole-genome screen of a quantitative trait of age-related maculopathy in sibships from the Beaver Dam Eye Study. Am J Hum Genet 2003;72:1412–1424.
38. Weeks DE, Conley YP, Tsai HJ, et al. Age-related maculopathy: a genomewide scan with continued evidence of susceptibility loci within the 1q31, 10q26, and 17q25 regions. Am J Hum Genet 2004;75:174–189.
39. Stone EM, Braun TA, Russell SR, et al. Missense variations in the fibulin 5 gene and age-related macular degeneration. N Engl J Med 2004;351:346–353.
40. Stone EM, Lotery AJ, Munier FL, et al. A single *EFEMP1* mutation associated with both Malattia Leventinese and Doyne honeycomb retinal dystrophy. Nature Genet 1999;22: 199–202.
41. Haga SB, Khoury M, Burke W. Genomic profiling to promote a healthy lifestyle: not ready for prime time. Nat Genet 2003;34:347–350.
42. Haider MZ, Devarajan LV, Al-Essa M, Kumar H. A C597—>A polymorphism in the Norrie disease gene is associated with advanced retinopathy of prematurity in premature Kuwaiti infants. J Biomed Sci 2002;9:365–370.
43. Kim JH, Yu YS, Kim J, Park SS. Mutations of the Norrie gene in Korean ROP infants. Korean J Ophthalmol 2002;16:93–96.
44. Couch V, Lindor NM, Karnes PS, Michels VV. Von Hippel-Lindau disease. Mayo Clin Proc 2000;75:265–272.
45. Wijnhoven BP, Lindstedt EW, Abbou M, et al. Rotterdam Esophageal Tumor Study Group. Molecular genetic analysis of the von Hippel-Lindau and human peroxisome proliferator-activated receptor gamma tumor-suppressor genes in adenocarcinomas of the gastroesophageal junction. Int J Cancer 2001;94:891–895.
46. Morris MR, Maina E, Morgan NV, et al. Molecular genetic analysis of FIH-1, FH, and SDHB candidate tumour suppressor genes in renal cell carcinoma. J Clin Pathol 2004;57:706–711.
47. Downey LM, Keen TJ, Roberts E, Mansfield DC, Bamashmus M, Inglehearn CF. A new locus for autosomal dominant familial exudative vitreoretinopathy maps to chromosome 11p12-13. Am J Hum Genet 2001;68:778–781.
48. Robitaille J, MacDonald ML, Kaykas A, et al. Mutant frizzled-4 disrupts retinal angiogenesis in familial exudative vitreoretinopathy. Nat Genet 2002;32:326–330.
49. Nasonkin I, Illing M, Koehler MR, Schmid M, Molday RS, Weber BH. Mapping of the rod photoreceptor ABC transporter (ABCR) to 1p21-p22.1 and identification of novel mutations in Stargardt's disease. Hum Genet 1998;102:21–26.
50. Rozet JM, Gerber S, Souied E, et al. Spectrum of ABCR gene mutations in autosomal recessive macular dystrophies. Eur J Hum Genet 1998;6:291–295.

51. Zhang K, Kniazeva M, Hutchinson A, Han M, Dean M, Allikmets R. The ABCR gene in recessive and dominant Stargardt diseases: a genetic pathway in macular degeneration. Genomics 1999;60:234–237.
52. September AV, Vorster AA, Ramesar RS, Greenberg LJ. Mutation Spectrum and Founder Chromosomes for the *ABCA4* gene in South African Stargardt disease patients. Invest Ophthalmol Vis Sci 2004;45:1705–1711.
53. Héon E, Piguet B, Munier F, et al. Linkage of autosomal dominant radial drusen (malattia leventinese) to chromosome 2p16-21. Arch Ophthalmol 1996;114:193–198.
54. Gregory CY, Evans K, Wijesuriya SD, et al. The gene for autosomal dominant Doyn's honeycomb retinal dystrophy (DHRD) maps to chromosome 2p16. Hum Mol Genet 1996;7:1055–1059.
55. Kniazeva M, Chiang MF, Morgan B, et al. A new locus for autosomal dominant Stargardt-like disease maps to chromosome 4. Am J Hum Genet 1999;64:1394–1399.
56. Michaelides M, Johnson S, Tekriwal AK, et al. An early-onset autosomal dominant macular dystrophy (MCDR3) resembling North Carolina macular dystrophy maps to chromosome 5. Invest Ophthalmol Vis Sci 2003;44:2178–2183.
57. den Hollander AI, van Lith-Verhoeven JJC, Kersten FF, et al. Identification of novel locus for autosomal dominant butterfly shaped macular dystrophy on 5q21.2-q33.2. J Med Genet 2004;41:699–702.
58. Dryja TP, Hahn LB, Kajiwara K, Berson EL. Dominant and digenic mutations in the peripherin/RDS and ROM1 genes in retinitis pigmentosa. Invest Ophthalmol Vis Sci 1997;18:1972–1982.
59. Farrar GJ, Jordan SA, Kenna P, et al. Autosomal dominant retinitis pigmentosa: localization of a disease gene (RP6) to the short arm of chromosome 6. Genomics 1991;11:870–874.
60. Felbor U, Schilling H, Weber BHF. Adult vitelliform macular dystrophy is frequently associated with mutations in the peripherin/RDS gene. Hum Mutat 1997;10:301–309.
61. Jordan SA, Farrar GJ, Kumar-Singh R, et al. Autosomal dominant retinitis pigmentosa (adRP; RP6): cosegregation of RP6 and the peripherin-RDS locus in a late-onset family of Irish origin. Am J Hum Genet 1992;50:634–639.
62. van Lith-Verhoeven JJC, Hoyng CB, van den Helm B, et al. The benign concentric annular macular dystrophy locus maps to 6p12.3-q16. Invest Ophthalmol Vis Sci 2004;45:30–35.
63. Small KW, Weber JL, Roses A, Lennon F, Vance JM, Pericak-Vance MA. North Carolina macular dystrophy is assigned to chromosome 6. Genomics 1992;13:681–685.
64. Small KW, Puech B, Mullen L, Yelchits S. North Carolina macular dystrophy phenotype in France maps to the MCDR1 locus. Mol Vis 1997;3:1.
65. Edwards AO, Donoso LA, Ritter III R. A novel gene for autosomal dominant Stargardt-like macular dystrophy with homology to the SUR4 protein family. Invest Ophthalmol Vis Sci 2001;42:2652–2663.
66. Kniazeva M, Traboulsi EI, Yu Z, et al. A new locus for dominant drusen and macular degeneration maps to chromosome 6q14. Am J Ophthalmol 2000;130:197–202.
67. Zhang K, Kniazeva M, Han M, et al. A 5-bp deletion in ELOVL4 is associated with two related forms of autosomal dominant macular dystrophy. Nature Genet 2001;27:89–93.
68. Inglehearn CF, Keen TJ, Al-Maghtheh M, Bhattacharya SS. Loci for autosomal dominant retinitis pigmentosa and cystoid macular dystrophy on chromosome 7q are not allelic. Am J Hum Genet 1994;55:581, 582.
69. Kremer H, Pinckers A, van den Helm B, Deutman AF, Ropers HH, Mariman ECM. Localization of the gene for dominant cystoid macular dystrophy on chromosome 7p. Hum Mol Genet 1994;3:299–302.
70. Marquardt A, Stöhr H, Passmore LA, Krämer F, Rivera A, Weber BHF. Mutations in a novel gene, VMD2, encoding a protein of unknown properties cause juvenile-onset vitelliform macular dystrophy (Best's disease). Hum Mol Genet 1998;7:1517–1525.

71. Petrukhin J, Koisti MJ, Bakall B, et al. Identification of the gene responsible for Best macular dystrophy. Nat Genet 1998;19:241–247.
72. Stone EM, Nichols BE, Streb LM, Kimura AE, Sheffield VC. Genetic linkage of vitelliform macular degeneration (Best's disease) to chromosome 11q13. Nat Genet 1992;1: 246–250.
73. Hayward C, Shu X, Cideciyan AV, et al. Mutation in a short-chain collagen gene, CTRP5, results in extracellular deposit formation in late-onset retinal degeneration—a genetic model for age-related macular degeneration. Hum Mol Genet 2003;12:2657–2667.
74. Felbor U, Suvanto EA, Forsius HR, Eriksson AW, Weber BHF. Autosomal recessive Sorsby fundus dystrophy revisited: molecular evidence for dominant inheritance. Am J Hum Genet 1997;60:57–62.
75. Weber BHF, Vogt G, Pruett RC, Stöhr H, Felbor U. Mutations in the tissue inhibitor of metalloproteinases-3 (TIMP3) in patients with Sorsby's fundus dystrophy. Nat Genet 1994;8:352–355.
76. Weber BHF, Vogt G, Wolz W, Ives EJ, Ewing CC. Sorsby's fundus dystrophy is genetically linked to chromosome 22q13-qter. Nat Genet 1994;7:158–161.
77. Ayyagari RF, Demirci FY, Liu J, et al. X-linked recessive atrophic macular degeneration from RPGR mutation. Genomics 2002;80:166–171.
78. Hermann K, Meindl A, Apfelstedt-Sylla E, et al. RPGR mutation analysis in patients with retinitis pigmentosa and congenital stationary night blindness. Am J Hum Genet 1996;59:A263.
79. Meindl A, Dry K, Herrmann K, et al. A gene (RPGR) with homology to the RCC1 guanine nucleotide exchange factor is mutated in X-linked retinitis pigmentosa (RP3). Nat Genet 1996;13:35–42.
80. Musarella MA, Anson-Cartwright L, Leal SM, et al. Multipoint linkage analysis and heterogeneity testing in 20 X-linked retinitis pigmentosa families. Genomics 1990;8: 286–296.
81. Ott J, Bhattacharya S, Chen JD, et al. Localizing multiple X chromosome-linked retinitis pigmentosa loci using multilocus homogeneity tests. Proc Natl Acad Sci USA 1990; 87:701–704.
82. Roepman R, van Duijnhoven G, Rosenberg T, et al. Positional cloning of the gene for X-linked retinitis pigmentosa 3: homology with the guaninine-nucleotide-exchange factor RCC1. Hum Mol Genet 1996;5:1035–1041.
83. Rozet JM, Perrault I, Gigarel N, et al. Dominant X linked retinitis pigmentosa is frequently accounted for by truncating mutations in exon ORF15 of the *RPGR* gene. J Med Genet 2002;39:284, 285.
84. Annunen S, Korkko J, Czarny M, et al. Splicing mutations of 54-bp exons in the COL11A1 gene cause Marshall syndrome, but other mutations cause overlapping Marshall/Stickler phenotypes. Am J Hum Genet 1999;65:974–983.
85. Richards AJ, Yates JRW, Williams R, et al. A family with Stickler syndrome type 2 has a mutation in the COL11A1 gene resulting in the substitution of glycine 97 by valine in alpha-1(XI) collagen. Hum Mol Genet 1996;5:1339–1343.
86. den Hollander AI, ten Brink JB, de Kok YJM, et al. Mutations in a human homologue of Drosophila crumbs cause retinitis pigmentosa (RP12). Nat Genet 1999;23:217–221.
87. den Hollander AI, Heckenlively JR, van den Born LI, et al. Leber congenital amaurosis and retinitis pigmentosa with Coats-like exudative vasculopathy are associated with mutations in the crumbs homologue 1 (*CRB1*) gene. Am J Hum Genet 2001;69:198–203.
88. Heckenlively JR. Preserved para-arteriole retinal pigment epithelium (PPRPE) in retinitis pigmentosa. Br J Ophthalmol 1982;66:26–30.
89. Leutelt J, Oehlmann R. Autosomal recessive retinitis pigmentosa locus maps on chromosome 1q in a large consanguineous family from Pakistan. Clin Genet 1995;47:122–124.

90. Lotery AJ, Jacobson SG, Fishman GA, et al. Mutations in the CRB1 gene cause Leber congenital amaurosis. Arch Ophthalmol 2001;119:415–420.
91. Lotery AJ, Malik A, Shami SA, et al. CRB1 mutations may result in retinitis pigmentosa without para-arteriolar RPE preservation. Ophthal Genet 2001;22:163–169.
92. van Soest S, van den Born LI, Gal A, et al. Assignment of a gene for autosomal dominant recessive retinitis pigmentosa (RP12) to chromosome 1q31-q32.1 in an inbred and genetically heterogeneous disease population. Genomics 1994;20:499–504.
93. Grand MG, Kaine J, Fulling K, et al. Cerebroretinal vasculopathy. A new hereditary syndrome. Ophthalmology 1988;95:649–659.
94. Jen J, Cohen AH, Yue Q, et al. Hereditary endotheliopathy with retinopathy, nephropathy, and stroke (HERNS). Neurology 1997;49:1322–1330.
95. Ophoff RA, J DeYoung, SK Service, et al. Hereditary vascular retinopathy, cerebroretinal vasculopathy, and hereditary endotheliopathy with retinopathy, nephropathy, and stroke map to a single locus on chromosome 3p21.1-p21.3. Am J Hum Genet 2001;69:447–453.
96. Black GCM, Perveen R, Wiszniewski W, Dodd CL, Donnai D, McLeod D. A novel hereditary developmental vitreoretinopathy with multiple ocular abnormalities localizing to a 5-cM region of chromosome 5q13-q14. Ophthalmology 1999;106:2074–2081.
97. Brown DM, Graemiger RA, Hergersberg M, et al. Genetic linkage of Wagner disease and erosive vitreoretinopathy to chromosome 5q13-14. Arch Ophthalmology 1995;113: 671–675.
98. Li Y, Fuhrmann C, Schwinger E, Gal A, Laqua H. The gene for autosomal dominant familial exudative vitreoretinopathy (Criswick-Schepens) on the long arm of chromosome 11. Am J Ophthalmol 1992;113:712, 713.
99. Li Y, Müller B, Fuhrmann C, et al. The autosomal dominant familial exudative vitreoretinopathy locus maps on 11q and is closely linked to D11S533. Am J Hum Genet 1992;51:749–754.
100. Stone EM, Kimura AE, Folk JC, et al. Genetic linkage of autosomal dominant neovascular inflammatory vitreoretinopathy to chromosome 11q13. Hum Mol Genet 1992;1:685–689.
101. Jiao X, Ventruto V, Trese MT, Shastry BS, Hejtmancik JF. Autosomal recessive familial exudative vitreoretinopathy is associated with mutations in *LRP5*. Am J Hum Genet 2004;75:878–884.
102. Price SM, Periam N, Humphries A, Woodruff G, Trembath RC. Familial exudative vitreoretinopathy linked to D11S533 in a large Asian family with consanguinity. Ophthal Genet 1996;17:53–57.
103. Toomes C, Bottomley HM, Jackson RM, et al. Inglehearn Mutations in *LRP5* or *FZD4* underlie the common familial exudative vitreoretinopathy locus on chromosome 11q. Am J Hum Genet 2004;74:721–730.
104. Francomano CA, Liberfarb RM, Hirose T, et al. The Stickler syndrome: evidence for close linkage to the structural gene for type II collagen. Genomics 1987;1:293–296.
105. Go SL, Maugeri A, Mulder JJS, van Driel MA, Cremers FPM, Hoyng CB. Autosomal dominant rhegmatogenous retinal detachment associated with an Arg453Ter mutation in the *COL2A1* gene. Invest Ophthalmol Vis Sci 2003;44:4035–4043.
106. Lee B, Vissing H, Ramirez F, Rogers D, Rimoin D. Identification of the molecular defect in a family with spondyloepiphyseal dysplasia. Science 1989;244:978–980.
107. Bergen AAB, Plomp AS, Schuurman ES, et al. Mutations in ABCC6 cause pseudoxanthoma elasticum. Nat Genet 2000;25:228–231.
108. Le Saux O, Urban Z, Tschuch C, et al. Mutations in a gene encoding an ABC transporter cause pseudoxanthoma elasticum. Nat Genet 2000;25:223–227.
109. Ringpfeil F, Lebwohl MG, Christiano AM, Uitto J. Pseudoxanthoma elasticum: mutations in the *MRP6* gene encoding a transmembrane ATP-binding cassette (ABC) transporter. Proc Natl Acad Sci USA 2000;97:6001–6006.

110. Struk B, Neldner KH, Rao VS, St Jean P, Lindpaintner K. Mapping of both autosomal recessive and dominant variants of pseudoxanthoma elasticum to chromosome 16p13.1. Hum Mol Genet 1997;6:1823–1828.
111. van Soest S, Swart J, Tijmes N, Sandkuijl LA, Rommers J, Bergen AAB. A locus for autosomal recessive pseudoxanthoma elasticum, with penetrance of vascular symptoms in carriers, maps to chromosome 16p13.1. Genome Res 1997;7:830–834.
112. Berger W, Meindl A, van de Pol TJ, et al. Isolation of a candidate gene for Norrie disease by positional cloning. Nat Genet 1992;1:199–203.
113. Black GCM, Perveen R, Bonshek R, et al. Coats' disease of the retina (unilateral retinal telangiectasis) caused by somatic mutation in the NDP gene: a role for norrin in retinal angiogenesis. Hum Mol Genet 1999;11:2021–2035.
114. Chen ZY, Hendriks RW, Jobling MA, et al. Isolation and characterization of a candidate gene for Norrie disease. Nat Genet 1992;1:204–208.
115. Chen ZY, Battinelli EM, Fiedler A, et al. A mutation in the Norrie disease gene (NDP) associated with X-linked familial exudative vitreoretinopathy. Nat Genet 1993;5:180–182.
116. Gal A, Stolzenberger C, Wienker T, et al. Norrie's disease: close linkage with genetic markers from the proximal short arm of the X chromosome. Clin Genet 1985;27:282, 283.
117. Rehm HL, Gutiérrez-Espeleta GA, Garcia R, et al. Norrie disease gene mutation in a large Costa Rican kindred with a novel phenotype including venous insufficiency. Hum Mutat 1997;9:402–408.

II

Endogenous Promoters and Inhibitors of Angiogenesis

11
Vascular Endothelial Growth Factor and Retinal Diseases

Sam Dahr, MD and Karl G. Csaky, MD, PhD

CONTENTS

VEGF BACKGROUND

VEGF Isoforms

In humans, the vascular endothelial growth factor (VEGF) gene resides on chromosome 6p21.3 *(1)*. Northern blot and primer extension analysis have shown that the human VEGF gene has a single major transcription start site, 1038 bp upstream from the ATG initiation codon. This start site is located near a cluster of potential Sp1 factor binding sites, and the promoter contains potential binding sites for the transcription factors AP-1 and AP-2 *(2)*. A hypoxia response element located upstream of the VEGF genes can bind hypoxia-inducible factor (HIF)-1 and may act as an enhancer *(3,4)*. Hypoxia can also increase the half-life of VEGF mRNA, which is intrinsically labile. Binding of HuR, a hypoxia-induced stability factor that is a member of the Elav-like protein family, to an AU-rich element in the 3′-UTR of VEGF mRNA increases the half-life of VEGF mRNA by three- to eightfold *(5)*.

VEGF, a disulfide linked homodimer composed of two 23-kDa subunits, was first purified by Gospodarowicz et al. *(6)* and Ferrara and Henzel *(7)* from pituitary-derived bovine folliculostellate cells. Initial characterization of the mRNA forms in fetal human vascular smooth muscle cells suggested a VEGF coding region of eight exons with three forms of the protein formed by alternative exon splicing. The initial three transcripts were found to be 5.5, 4.4, and 3.7 kb, corresponding to 189, 165, and 121 amino acid proteins, respectively. The coding sequence contains seven introns. The alternative splicing involves exons 6 and 7 (Fig. 1). $VEGF_{165}$ lacks exon 6, whereas $VEGF_{121}$ lacks

From: *Ophthalmology: Ocular Angiogenesis: Diseases, Mechanisms, and Therapeutics*
Edited by: J. Tombran-Tink and C. J. Barnstable © Humana Press Inc., Totowa, NJ

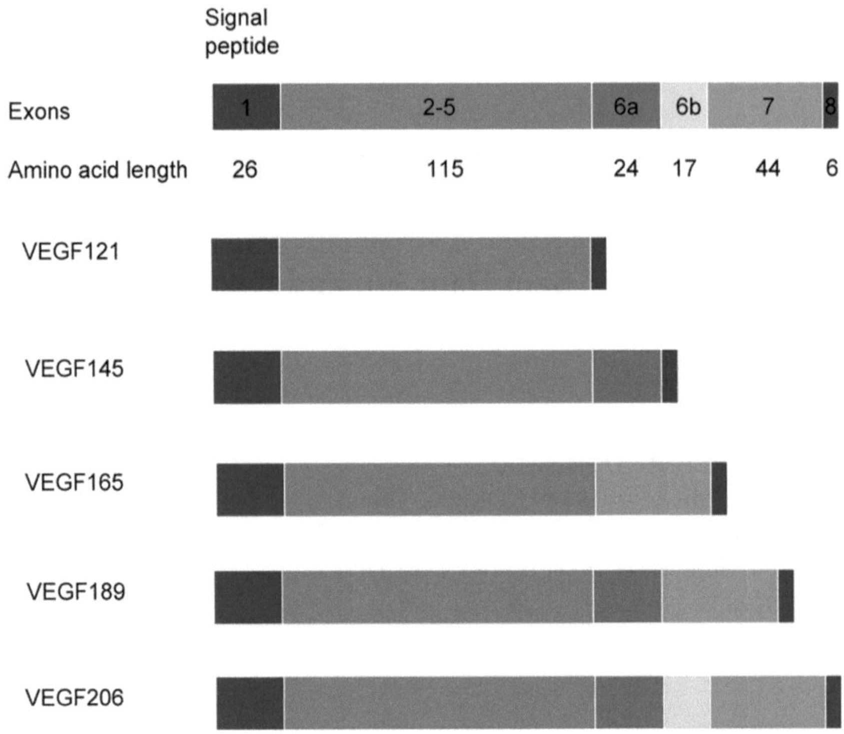

Fig. 1. Splice variants of the vascular endothelial growth factor gene.

exons 6 and 7. Exon 7 codes a 44 amino acid sequence rich in arginine and lysine residues, conferring a basic nature to the segment. Exon 6 codes a 24-amino-acid segment that is also quite basic, with 12 lysine and arginine residues. Additional isoforms include $VEGF_{145}$, $VEGF_{183}$, $VEGF_{189}$, and $VEGF_{206}$ *(1)*. $VEGF_{145}$ and $VEGF_{206}$ appear to be restricted to cells of placental origin.

The bioavailability of VEGF can be regulated at the RNA level, through alternate splicing, and at the protein level, through proteolysis. To determine secretion properties, various forms of VEGF cDNA were cloned into human embryonic kidney cells (CEN4 cells). Although little or no $VEGF_{189}$ was found in a freely soluble form in the tissue culture medium, $VEGF_{165}$ and $VEGF_{121}$ were found freely soluble in the medium. Upon addition of suramin (a compound known to interfere with the binding of growth factors to receptors) and anti-VEGF mAb, sodium dodecyl sulfate-polyacrylamide gel electrophoresis (SDS-PAGE) analysis of the immunoprecipitate showed the presence of $VEGF_{189}$. Interestingly, adding heparin to CEN4 culture also induced the release of $VEGF_{189}$ and $VEGF_{165}$ into the culture medium, whereas $VEGF_{121}$ levels were unaffected. These results suggested that $VEGF_{189}$, $VEGF_{165}$, and $VEGF_{121}$ behave differently as secreted factors: $VEGF_{121}$ is entirely soluble, $VEGF_{189}$ is virtually all bound to extracellular sites containing heparin-associated proteoglycans, and $VEGF_{165}$ shows intermediary behavior, with 50 to 70% bound *(8)*. In comparison with $VEGF_{121}$, $VEGF_{165}$ contains 44 additional amino acids at its carboxy terminal end; these amino acids convert $VEGF_{165}$ to a basic protein that can bind heparin. $VEGF_{189}$ contains an additional 24 highly basic amino acids. Heparin-containing proteoglycans are components of the extracellular matrix. The extracellular matrix may bind $VEGF_{165}$ and $VEGF_{189}$ and act as a reservoir for those growth factors *(8)*. Plasmin or other proteases released during angiogenesis may cleave the basic proteins at the carboxy terminus of $VEGF_{165}$ and $VEGF_{189}$ and liberate those angiogenic agents.

VEGF Receptors

Through an elegant series of experiments, Gille and associates characterized the different signaling properties of VEGF receptors VEGFR-2 and VEGFR-1 *(9)*. VEGFR-2 selective $VEGF_{165}$ mutants activated p38 MAP kinase to phosphorylate ERK1 and ERK2 in human vascular endothelial cells, to an extent indistinguishable from that obtained using wild-type $VEGF_{165}$. VEGFR-1 selective $VEGF_{165}$ mutants resulted in only minimal phosphorylation of ERK2. Wild-type and VEGFR-2 selective $VEGF_{165}$ mutants stimulated phosphorylation of PLCγ and PI3K, whereas VEGFR-1 selective $VEGF_{165}$ mutants did not. In a Boyden chamber cell migration assay, VEGFR-2 selective $VEGF_{165}$ mutants and wild-type $VEGF_{165}$ promoted human umbilical vein endothelial cell (HUVEC) migration to an equal extent, whereas VEGFR-1 selective $VEGF_{165}$ mutants did not increase cell migration over background levels. To assess in vivo angiogenesis, hydron pellets containing 200 ng of the growth factor variants were implanted into rat corneas and the angiogenic areas were evaluated at 1 wk. Pellets containing VEGFR-2 selective $VEGF_{165}$ mutants were as effective as wild-type VEGF-implanted pellets in inducing corneal angiogenesis. VEGFR-1 selective $VEGF_{165}$ mutants did not stimulate angiogenesis over control levels. In addition, vascular permeability of these $VEGF_{165}$ variants was assessed. VEGFR-2 selective $VEGF_{165}$ mutants induced vascular permeability to a comparable extent as wild-type $VEGF_{165}$, whereas VEGFR-1 selective $VEGF_{165}$ mutants caused essentially no leakage. These findings suggest that VEGFR-2 alone is capable of mediating VEGF-induced endothelial cell intracellular signaling, migration, angiogenesis, and permeability. Interestingly, in endothelial cells, $VEGF_{165}$ shows a more potent ability to stimulate phosphorylation and activation of VEGFR-2 than does $VEGF_{121}$. The Kd of $VEGF_{165}$ for VEGFR-2 is 760 p*M*, approx 45 times greater than for VEGFR-1 (16 p*M*) *(10)*.

Neurophilin-1 (Npn-1) and neurophilin-2 (Npn-2) are also receptors that bind $VEGF_{165}$. Neither binds $VEGF_{121}$. In COS-1 cells coexpressing VEGFR-2 and Npn-1, a VEGFR-2 specific antibody not only precipitated VEGFR-2, but SDS-PAGE analysis also showed a band that ran at the predicted size for Npn-1 crosslinked to $VEGF_{165}$. Conversely, an Npn-1-specific antibody coprecipitated VEGFR-2. This complex did not, however, show increased binding affinity for $VEGF_{165}$. Blocking $VEGF_{165}$–Npn-1 binding with a specific Npn-1-binding antagonist did reduce the signaling potency of $VEGF_{165}$ in HUVEC. Use of that same Npn-1 antagonist in the presence of $VEGF_{121}$ did not alter the signaling potency of $VEGF_{121}$. These results suggested that the ability of $VEGF_{165}$ to bind the VEGFR-2–Npn-1 complex may explain the enhanced ability of $VEGF_{165}$ vs $VEGF_{121}$ to stimulate VEGFR-2 *(11)*.

Downstream Receptor Signaling (Fig. 2)

It is thought that protein tyrosine kinase (PTK) receptors such as VEGFR-1 and VEGFR-2 "autophosphorylate" when receptor dimerization occurs with ligand binding

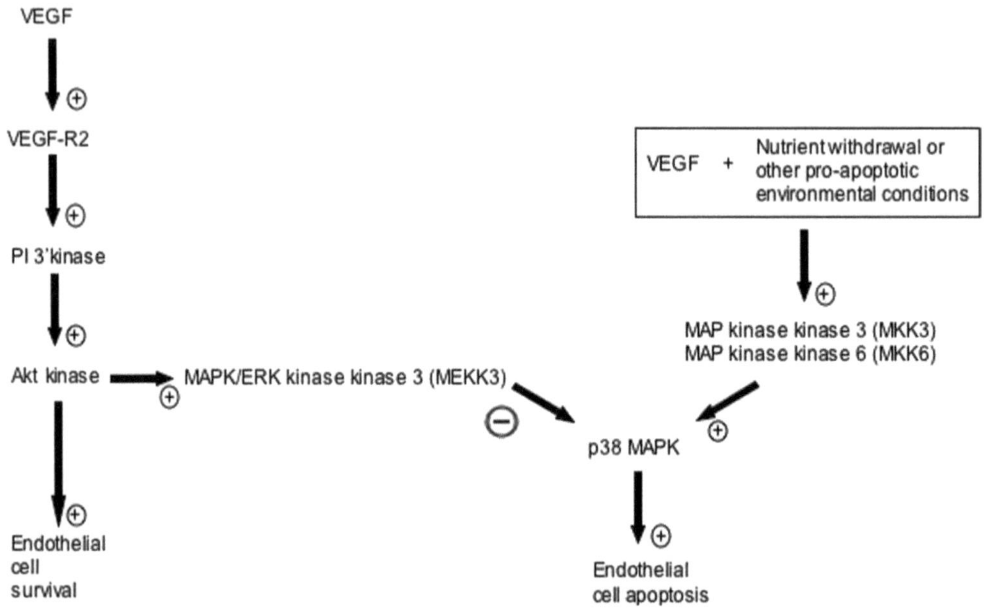

Fig. 2. Crosstalk between the PI3-kinase/Akt signal pathway (prosurvival, antiapoptosis) and the p38 MAPK pathway (proapoptosis). Akt-mediated phosphorylation of MEKK3 may account for decreased p38 MAPK activity. (Data from ref. *25.*)

and one receptor transphosphorylates its dimerized partner *(12)*. The phosphorylated tyrosine residues of the intracystolic portion of the receptor may then bind intracellular signaling molecules.

The phosphatidylinositol 3´-kinase (PI3-kinase)/Akt signal transduction pathway is known to mediate the survival signal of various growth factors and cytokines *(13–22)*. Gerber and associates *(23)* have provided evidence that VEGF may also possess antipoptotic activities in endothelial cells most likely mediated through VEGF stimulation of PI3-kinase. VEGFR-2 selective $VEGF_{165}$ mutants exerted a similar survival activity as wild-type $VEGF_{165}$, whereas VEGFR-1 selective $VEGF_{165}$ mutants did not. Both wild-type and VEGFR-2 selective $VEGF_{165}$ increased Akt phosphorylation, whereas VEGFR-1 selective $VEGF_{165}$ mutants did not. VEGF-induced survival was seen only in the presence of wild-type Akt but not when endothelial cells were transfected with expression vectors coding for mutant inactive Akt. In summary, then, VEGF mediates an antiapoptotic/prosurvival signal in cells via VEGFR-2and the PI3-kinase/Akt signal transduction pathway. Akt likely delivers its antiapoptotic signal through blocking the proteolytic events of apoptosis mediated by the caspase pathways *(18,24)*.

VEGF may also mediate a proapoptotic signal predominately through the p38 family of MAP kinases. Gratton and associates *(25)* treated endothelial cells with a PI3-kinase inhibitor and showed a significant increase in p38 phosphorylation, whereas phosphorylation of Akt was concomitantly reduced. This PI3-kinase inhibition enhanced apoptosis, correlating with the increase in p38 phosphorylation. In addition, VEGF treatment in the presence of a PI3-kinase inhibitor blunted the antiapoptotic actions of VEGF. However, in the presence of a p38 inhibitor, the level of apoptosis was reduced.

In summary then VEGF can deliver pro- and antiapoptotic signals in endothelial cells, and that crosstalk occurs between the PI3-kinase/Akt (antiapoptotic, pro-cell survival) and the p38 pathway (proapoptotic).

VEGF and Retinal Development

Transgenic mice expressing single VEGF isoforms have been produced and have demonstrated that overexpression of $VEGF_{165}$ in mice is consistent with normal retinal vascular development, whereas overexpression of $VEGF_{189}$ resulted in the development of venules and capillaries but only half the normal number of arterioles. $VEGF_{120}$-overexpressing mice displayed impaired arteriolar and venular development. The capillaries that did develop were fragile, with numerous hemorrhages *(26)*.

VEGFR-1 may also play a role in neural retina development. In developing mice, VEGFR-1 mRNA is first detected on postnatal day 7 in the developing ganglion cell layer and inner nuclear layer of the avascular retina. At day 12 expression is detected in the photoreceptor layer, consistent with the pattern of Müller cell development. From postnatal days 4 to 33, VEGFR-1 mRNA increases 14-fold in whole retina *(27)*.

At postnatal day 5, VEGFR-2 mRNA is first detected, localized to the inner retina layers. At day 15, VEGFR-2 mRNA is detected in the photoreceptor layer. From days 17 to 33, VEGFR-2 mRNA starts to localize to blood vessels, but is still observed outside blood vessels in the nerve fiber, ganglion cell, and inner nuclear layers. This pattern appears to be consistent with expression in Müller cell processes, astrocytes, and/or ganglion cells. VEGFR-2 mRNA decreases threefold in whole retina from early development to postnatal day 33 (adult) *(27)*.

Treatment with SU5416, an antagonist of VEGFR-1 and VEGFR-2, from days 0 to 9 caused loss of thickness of the inner nuclear, inner plexiform, and ganglion cell layers in avascular undeveloped retina compared with controls *(27)*.

VEGF and Inflammation

VEGF appears to be proinflammatory. VEGF can induce leukocyte adherence, ICAM-1, VCAM-1, and E-selectin expression *(28)* and retinal barrier breakdown. However, these effects may be isoform-dependent. For example, in a rat model of diabetes, $VEGF_{120}$ and $VEGF_{164}$ demonstrated different potencies in inducing these proinflammatory activities *(28,29)*. $VEGF_{165}$ appears to be more potent in recruitment of CD45-positive leukocytes than $VEGF_{120}$, as well as in inducing ICAM expression. One possible explanation for the increased potency of $VEGF_{164}$ may be explained by Npn-1 binding of the exon 7 encoded domain of $VEGF_{164/165}$, a domain lacking in $VEGF_{120/121}$. Further evidence suggests that the effect of $VEGF_{165}$ on leukocyte migration may be mediated through VEGFR-1, whereas the effect of $VEGF_{165}$ on endothelial ICAM-1 expression may be mediated through VEGFR-2 *(30)*.

VEGF and Retinal Neovascularization

In physiological neovascularization during retinal development, new vessels grow from the optic disk outward toward the peripheral avascular retina. During pathological neovascularization, the new vessels grow into the vitreous cavity. Interestingly, the ratio of $VEGF_{165}$ to $VEGF_{121}$ may be critical in these different processes *(29)*. For example, in physiologically developing retinas this ratio is 2.2 vs 25.3 ± 8.7 in eyes with proliferative retinopathy and pathological neovascularization. Transgenic mice in which the rhodopsin promoter is connected to a VEGF sequence immunohistochemically show increased VEGF expression in the photoreceptor layer; these same mice develop intraretinal and subretinal neovascularization *(31)*.

There also appears to be a link between ocular neovascularization and inflammation. Leukocytes associate with incipient pathological neovascular fronds in an animal model of proliferative retinopathy, whereas eyes undergoing physiologic postnatal retinal vascular development do not show leukocytes at the leading edge of vascularization. Immunohistochemistry demonstrated that these adherent leukocytes were CD8 and CD25 (IL-2 receptor) positive, suggesting the presence of T lymphocytes as well. $VEGF_{165}$ blockade inhibits leukocyte adhesion and pathological neovascularization in proliferative retinopathy but has no effect on physiological vascular development. However, when all VEGF isoforms are inhibited, suppression of both pathological and physiological neovascularization occurs.

When monocytes, which express VEGFR-2 and are known to be recruited by VEGF *(32)*, are depleted, suppression of pathological neovascularization also occurs *(33)*.

Neuroprotection

Neurogenesis is the process by which precursor cells differentiate into a mature neuronal phenotype. Multiple studies have demonstrated that VEGF may be involved in this process through the activity of VEGFR-2 *(34–37)*. Specifically, VEGF may play a role in the differentiation and protection of cortical neurons, astrocytes *(34,36)*, and Schwann cells *(35)*. This may be especially important in cases of ischemia-induced neuronal damage *(38)*.

VEGF may also be important in retinal neuronal differentiation and survival especially for photoreceptor and amacrine cells *(39)*.

VEGF AND RETINAL DISEASE

Diabetes

In analysis of retinal tissues, VEGF has been found to be normally expressed in glial cells *(40)* and has been shown to be elevated in the vitreous of patients with both active and inactive PDR *(41)* with the predominant form found being $VEGF_{121}$. $VEGF_{165}$ and 189 have also been found, as well as VEGFR-1, VEGFR-2, and Npn-1. However, no evidence of vitreous levels of $VEGF_{145}$ or $VEGF_{206}$ have been detected.

Age-Related Macular Degeneration

In the 1990s, immunohistochemical evidence came to light suggesting that VEGF plays a pathogenic role in exudative age-related macular degeneration (AMD). The endothelial cells and interstitial fibroblasts of surgically excised choroidal neovascular membranes (CNVMs) showed positive immunohistochemical staining for VEGF *(42,43)*, as have the macrophages *(44)*. Although retinal pigment epithelium (RPE) cells and choriocapillary endothelial cells in CNVMs from patients with AMD immunostained for VEGF, regions of normal retina did not stain *(45)*.

In situ hybridization studies in CNV animal models also support a role for VEGF. In a laser-induced model of choroidal neovascularization in rats, *in situ* hybridization showed VEGF and VEGFR-2 (KDR) mRNA expression in the retinal pigment epithelium (RPE)-like cells, fibroblasts, and endothelial cells of CNV *(46,47)*. In an primate model of laser-induced CNV, choroidal vascular endothelial cells migrated into the subretinal space through the laser-induced defect in Bruch's membrane, leading to the development of new vessels 7 to 14 d after injury; *in situ* hybridization demonstrated increased VEGF mRNA levels in the accumulating macrophages, RPE cells, and Müller cells 3 to 7 d after laser injury *(48)*.

Molecular models also support a role for VEGF in the development of ocular neovascularization. After injection of an adenovirus vector encoding VEGF into the subretinal space of rats, subsequent fluorescein angiography and histopathological examination showed the development of choroidal neovascularization with growth through Bruch's membrane *(49–51)*. In one study, transgenic mice consisting of a murine RPE promoter (RPE 65) coupled to murine VEGF (164) cDNA were constructed. Histopathological examination showed choroidal neovascularization that did not penetrate the intact Bruch's membrane. The authors suggested that additional insults to Bruch's membrane are needed for VEGF-driven choroidal neovascularization to penetrate Bruch's and grow into the subretinal space *(52)*. VEGF production by human RPE cells is polarized, with two- to sevenfold more production basolaterally than apically. This polarized relationship appears to be consistent with a paracrine relationship between the RPE and choriocapillaris *(53)*.

VEGF, due to its strong permeability effects, may play a critical role in macular edema formation. Optical coherence tomography (OCT) has shown that in the context of retinal elevation on funduscopic exam and exudative CNV on fluorescein angiography, what in the past was often presumed to be "subretinal fluid" is often intraretinal fluid. Interestingly, VEGF released by endothelial cells may play a role not only by increasing retinal vascular permeability, but also by diminishing the barrier function of the RPE monolayer *(54)*.

In the context of neovascularization, other molecules may interact with VEGF. Tissue inhibitor of metalloproteinases-3 (TIMP-3) has been shown to have inhibitory effects on angiogenesis and has been shown to block the binding of VEGF to VEGF receptor-2 *(55)*. VEGF also appears to upregulate angiopoietin-1, a protein involved in vascular maturation and stability *(56)*, in CNVMs *(57)*.

Other Conditions

In von Hippel-Lindau disease, disruption of VEGF regulation may contribute to the development of vascular tumors such as central nervous system, retinal hemangioblastomas, and renal cell carcinoma as well as tumor associated edema and cysts *(58)*. VEGF upregulation may also contribute to the development of macular edema in other disorders including uveitis. Fine et al. found that uveitis patients with cystoid macular edema have higher aqueous VEGF levels than uveitis patients without cystoid macular edema *(59)*.

ANTI-VEGF MEDICATIONS IN CLINICAL TRIALS

Ranibizumab

Ranibizumab (also known as rhuFab or Lucentis) is an antigen-binding fragment of a recombinant humanized monoclonal antibody directed toward VEGF. A primate model of laser-induced CNV showed that intravitreal injections of this compound inhibited choroidal neovascularization (CNV) *(60)* and has promoted the further study of this compound in clinical trials. The Anti-VEGF Antibody for the Treatment of Predominantly Classic Choroidal Neovascularization in AMD (ANCHOR) trial is a phase III clinical trial currently evaluating the safety and efficacy of ranibizumab intravitreal injections versus photodynamic therapy with verteporforin in predominantly classic subfoveal lesions whereas the MARINA trial is evaluating the safety and efficacy of ranibizumab injections in the context of occult and minimally classic lesions.

Pegaptanib

Pegaptanib (also known as Macugen) is an anti-$VEGF_{165}$ pegylated aptamer. This aptamer is a 28-base oligonucleotide that binds to the exon 7-encoded domain of human $VEGF_{165}$ with high specificity and affinity (200 p*M*). To increase its half-life, the oligonucleotide is conjugated to a 40-kDa PEG moiety. Pegaptanib does not bind $VEGF_{120/121}$ *(28)*. A phase IA single ascending dose study of intravitreal injections of pegaptanib performed in 15 patients with subfoveal choroidal neovascularization secondary to exudative AMD showed no significant safety issues related to the drug *(61)*.

In a phase II multiple injection safety study, 21 patients were treated with intravitreal injection with and without photodynamic therapy. Of patients who received the anti-VEGF aptamer alone, 87.5% showed stabilized or improved vision 3 mo after treatment and 25% of those eyes demonstrated a 3-line or greater improvement in vision. Of patients who received pegaptanib and photodynamic therapy, 60% experienced a 3-line gain at 3-mo *(62)*. However, several patients within the trial suffered possibly associated systemic adverse events, including mortality, prompting a word of caution in its use in older patients due to the systemic absorption following an intravitreal injection *(63)*. Pegaptanib is currently in domestic and international Phase II/III clinical trials.

Ruboxistaurin

Because of its prominent role in VEGF signaling, PKC β inhibition is a candidate for therapy. For example, it has been shown that an intravitreal injection of VEGF in animal models increased retinal vascular permeability through activation of the PKC β isoform and that inhibition of PKC β blocked this activity *(64,65)*. PKC β-isoform inhibition with ruboxistaurin (LY333531) has been shown to ameliorate the decreased retinal blood flow and increased oxidative stress seen in the retinas of diabetic rats *(4)*. Ruboxistaurin has also been shown to have potential beneficial effects for diabetic nephropathy in animal models *(66)*. The potential therapeutic benefit of PKC β inhibition may be the result of its interaction with other molecules. For example, hyperglycemia increases expression of endothelin-1, a vasoconstrictor. In bovine retinal endothelial cells and pericytes, hyperglycemia increases membranous protein kinase C activity and ET-1 in parallel, and inhibition of protein kinase C β and δ isoforms blocks this glucose-induced ET-1 upregulation *(67,68)*. Another potential affected molecule may be nitrous oxide. Hyperglycemia abolishes nitrous oxide-mediated vasodilation. In rats pretreated with ruboxistaurin, there was a preservation of nitrous oxide-mediated vasodilation under hyperglycemic conditions *(69–71)*. In humans, hyperglycemia reduces vasodilation normally induced by the endothelium releasing nitrous oxide.

Healthy humans given ruboxistaurin did not experience reduced forearm blood flow in response to hyperglycemia in contrast to humans fed placebo *(72)*.

The initial results of a phase II/III study of ruboxistaurin treatment of diabetic macular edema were presented at the American Academy of Ophthalmology meeting in November 2003. Six hundred eighty-six patients with diabetic macular edema greater than 300 μm from the center of the macula and no previous laser photocoagulation were randomized to one of four arms: placebo, ruboxistaurin 4 mg/d, ruboxistaurin 16 mg/d, or ruboxistaurin 32 mg/d. The primary endpoint was the delay of DME progression to the center of the macula or the delay of photocoagulation for DME. Patients were treated and followed for at least 2.5 yr. Treatment with ruboxistaurin did not demonstrate a statistically significant effect on the primary study outcome of progression of DME or application of photocoagulation.

PKC412

PKC412 (n-benzoyl staurosporine) inhibits VEGF receptor kinase as well as PKC. PKC412 decreased VEGF-induced breakdown of the blood retinal barrier in a mouse model *(73)*. In a porcine model of laser-induced choroidal neovascularization, periocular injection of PKC412-containing microspheres resulted in a smaller total area of CNV at sites of rupture of Bruch's membrane in comparison with control injections *(74)*.

In a recent randomized double-masked placebo-controlled study of 141 subjects with diabetic macular edema, subjects received PKC412 at 50, 100, or 150 mg/d or placebo for up to 3 mo. The 100 mg and 150 mg doses showed a statistically significant reduction in retinal thickening as assessed with OCT. The 100 mg group also showed a statistically significant 4 letter (EDTRS chart) improvement in acuity at 3 mo. Side effects included nausea, diarrhea, vomiting, and liver enzyme abnormalities *(75)*.

ANTI-VEGF THERAPIES IN DEVELOPMENT

VEGF Trap

The VEGF trap is a decoy soluble VEGF receptor engineered by fusing the ligand-binding elements of the VEGF receptor to an immunoglobulin-constant region *(76)*. Intravitreal injections of VEGF trap in a mouse model of laser-induced choroidal neovascularization inhibited CNV *(77)* as well as reducing VEGF-induced breakdown of the blood retinal barrier in a mouse model *(77)*.

siRNA

Small interfering RNAs (siRNAs) are small fragments of nucleotide that have the purported activity of permanently downregulating specific RNAs. In a mouse model of laser-induced CNV, subretinal injection *(78)* or intravitreal injection *(79)* of siRNAs against murine VEGF inhibited CNV development.

Gene Transfer

In a mouse model of CNV, intravitreal or periocular injection of an adenoviral vector encoding soluble VEGF receptor-1 suppressed choroidal neovascularization at the rupture sites in Bruch's membrane. In a mouse model for diabetes, periocular injection of the same vector reduced VEGF-induced breakdown of the blood–retinal barrier, but failed to inhibit ischemia-induced retinal neovascularization *(80)*.

In a transgenic mouse model of VEGF-induced breakdown of the blood–retinal barrier, subretinal injection of adenoviral vectors expressing endostatin, a collagen XVIII fragment, reduced VEGF-induced vascular permeability. Endostatin also appeared to reduce retinal neovascularization associated with prolonged exposure to increased VEGF levels *(81)*.

POTENTIAL SIDE EFFECTS OF ANTI-VEGF THERAPY

Even local anti-VEGF therapy could potentially cause serious systemic side effects, particularly in patients with ischemic heart disease *(63)*. At extremely low concentrations of 0.16 to 1.3 n*M*, pegaptanib, for example, can block 50% (IC_{50}) of VEGF-induced cell proliferation, and at a concentration of 10 n*M* will block all VEGF binding and activity *(63,82)*. This has relevance even to local delivery to the eye because systemic absorption can occur. For example, in the intravitreal trials of pegaptanib, the serum concentrations ranged from 0.5 to 21 n*M* *(62)*. Patients with ischemic heart disease, who are in the same demographic as AMD and many diabetes patients, may be dependent on VEGF-driven cardiac angiogenesis and collateral blood vessel development or on VEGF-mediated coronary artery vasodilation, and suppression of this therapeutic activity of VEGF may have serious consequences.

REFERENCES

1. Robinson CJ, Stringer SE. The splice variants of vascular endothelial growth factor (VEGF) and their receptors. J Cell Sci 2001;114:853–865.
2. Tischer E, Mitchell R, Hartman T, et al. The human gene for vascular endothelial growth factor. Multiple protein forms are encoded through alternative exon splicing. J Biol Chem 1991;266:11,947–11,954.
3. Levy AP, Levy NS, Wegner S, Goldberg MA. Transcriptional regulation of the rat vascular endothelial growth factor gene by hypoxia. J Biol Chem 1995;270:13,333–13,340.
4. Abiko T, Abiko A, Clermont AC, et al. Characterization of retinal leukostasis and hemodynamics in insulin resistance and diabetes: role of oxidants and protein kinase-C activation. Diabetes 2003;52:829–837.
5. Levy NS, Chung S, Furneaux H, Levy AP. Hypoxic stabilization of vascular endothelial growth factor mRNA by the RNA-binding protein HuR. J Biol Chem 1998;273:6417–6423.
6. Gospodarowicz D, Abraham JA, Schilling J. Isolation and characterization of a vascular endothelial cell mitogen produced by pituitary-derived folliculo stellate cells. Proc Natl Acad Sci USA 1989;86:7311–7315.
7. Ferrara N, Henzel WJ. Pituitary follicular cells secrete a novel heparin-binding growth factor specific for vascular endothelial cells. Biochem Biophys Res Commun 1989;161:851–858.
8. Houck KA, Leung DW, Rowland AM, et al. Dual regulation of vascular endothelial growth factor bioavailability by genetic and proteolytic mechanisms. J Biol Chem 1992;267: 26,031–26,037.
9. Gille H, Kowalski J, Li B, et al. Analysis of biological effects and signaling properties of Flt-1 (VEGFR-1) and KDR (VEGFR-2). A reassessment using novel receptor-specific vascular endothelial growth factor mutants. J Biol Chem 2001;276:3222–3230.
10. Waltenberger J, Claesson-Welsh L, Siegbahn A, et al. Different signal transduction properties of KDR and Flt1, two receptors for vascular endothelial growth factor. J Biol Chem 1994; 269:26,988–26,995.

11. Whitaker GB, Limberg BJ, Rosenbaum JS. Vascular endothelial growth factor receptor-2 and neuropilin-1 form a receptor complex that is responsible for the differential signaling potency of VEGF(165) and VEGF(121). J Biol Chem 2001;276:25,520–25,531.
12. Zachary I. Vascular endothelial growth factor: how it transmits its signal. Exp Nephrol 1998;6:480–487.
13. Minshall C, Arkins S, Freund GG, Kelley KW. Requirement for phosphatidylinositol 3′-kinase to protect hemopoietic progenitors against apoptosis depends upon the extracellular survival factor. J Immunol 1996;156:939–947.
14. Dudek H, Datta SR, Franke TF, et al. Regulation of neuronal survival by the serine-threonine protein kinase Akt. Science 1997;275:661–665.
15. Yao R, Cooper GM. Requirement for phosphatidylinositol-3 kinase in the prevention of apoptosis by nerve growth factor. Science 1995;267:2003–2006.
16. Yao R, Cooper GM. Growth factor-dependent survival of rodent fibroblasts requires phosphatidylinositol 3-kinase but is independent of pp70S6K activity. Oncogene 1996;13: 343–351.
17. Datta SR, Dudek H, Tao X, et al. Akt phosphorylation of BAD couples survival signals to the cell-intrinsic death machinery. Cell 1997;91:231–241.
18. Kennedy SG, Wagner AJ, Conzen SD, et al. The PI 3-kinase/Akt signaling pathway delivers an anti-apoptotic signal. Genes Dev 1997;11:701–713.
19. Franke TF, Kaplan DR, Cantley LC. PI3K: downstream AKTion blocks apoptosis. Cell 1997;88:435–437.
20. Franke TF, Kaplan DR, Cantley LC, Toker A. Direct regulation of the Akt proto-oncogene product by phosphatidylinositol-3, 4-bisphosphate. Science 1997;275:665–668.
21. Fulton D, Gratton JP, McCabe TJ, et al. Regulation of endothelium-derived nitric oxide production by the protein kinase Akt. Nature 1999;399:597–601.
22. Songyang Z, Baltimore D, Cantley LC, et al. Interleukin 3-dependent survival by the Akt protein kinase. Proc Natl Acad Sci USA 1997;94:11,345–11,350.
23. Gerber HP, McMurtrey A, Kowalski J, et al. Vascular endothelial growth factor regulates endothelial cell survival through the phosphatidylinositol 3(-kinase/Akt signal transduction pathway. Requirement for Flk-1/KDR activation. J Biol Chem 1998;273: 30,336–30,343.
24. Miller DK. The role of the Caspase family of cysteine proteases in apoptosis. Semin Immunol 1997;9:35–49.
25. Gratton JP, Morales-Ruiz M, Kureishi Y, et al. Akt down-regulation of p38 signaling provides a novel mechanism of vascular endothelial growth factor-mediated cytoprotection in endothelial cells. J Biol Chem 2001;276:30,359–30,365.
26. Stalmans I, Ng YS, Rohan R, et al. Arteriolar and venular patterning in retinas of mice selectively expressing VEGF isoforms. J Clin Invest 2002;109:327–336.
27. Robinson GS, Ju M, Shih SC, et al. Nonvascular role for VEGF: VEGFR-1, 2 activity is critical for neural retinal development. FASEB J 2001;15:1215–1217.
28. Ishida S, et al. VEGF164 is proinflammatory in the diabetic retina. Invest Ophthalmol Vis Sci 2003;44:2155–2162.
29. Ishida S, Usui T, Yamashiro K, et al. VEGF164-mediated inflammation is required for pathological, but not physiological, ischemia-induced retinal neovascularization. J Exp Med 2003;198:483–489.
30. Usui T, Ishida S, Yamashiro K, et al. VEGF164(165) as the pathological isoform: differential leukocyte and endothelial responses through VEGFR1 and VEGFR2. Invest Ophthalmol Vis Sci 2004;45:368–374.
31. Okamoto N, Tobe T, Hackett SF, et al. Transgenic mice with increased expression of vascular endothelial growth factor in the retina: a new model of intraretinal and subretinal neovascularization. Am J Pathol 1997;151:281–291.

32. Clauss M, Pipp F, Issbrucker K, et al. Dissection of monocyte and endothelial activities by using VEGF-receptor specific ligands. Adv Exp Med Biol 2003;522:75–82.
33. Espinosa-Heidmann DG, Suner IJ, Hernandez EP, et al. Macrophage depletion diminishes lesion size and severity in experimental choroidal neovascularization. Invest Ophthalmol Vis Sci 2003;44:3586–3592.
34. Jin K, Zhu Y, Sun Y, et al. Vascular endothelial growth factor (VEGF) stimulates neurogenesis in vitro and in vivo. Proc Natl Acad Sci USA 2002;99:11,946–11,950.
35. Sondell M, Lundborg G, Kanje M. Vascular endothelial growth factor has neurotrophic activity and stimulates axonal outgrowth, enhancing cell survival and Schwann cell proliferation in the peripheral nervous system. J Neurosci 1999;19:5731–5740.
36. Krum JM, Mani N, Rosenstein JM. Angiogenic and astroglial responses to vascular endothelial growth factor administration in adult rat brain. Neuroscience 2002;110: 589–604.
37. Jin KL, Mao XO, Greenberg DA. Vascular endothelial growth factor: direct neuroprotective effect in in vitro ischemia. Proc Natl Acad Sci USA 2000;97:10,242–10,247.
38. Sun Y, Jin K, Xie L, et al. VEGF-induced neuroprotection, neurogenesis, and angiogenesis after focal cerebral ischemia. J Clin Invest 2003;111:1843–1851.
39. Yourey PA, Gohari S, Su JL, Alderson RF. Vascular endothelial cell growth factors promote the in vitro development of rat photoreceptor cells. J Neurosci 2000;20:6781–6788.
40. Amin RH, Frank RN, Kennedy A, et al. Vascular endothelial growth factor is present in glial cells of the retina and optic nerve of human subjects with nonproliferative diabetic retinopathy. Invest Ophthalmol Vis Sci 1997;38:36–47.
41. Duh EJ, Yang HS, Haller JA, et al. Vitreous levels of pigment epithelium-derived factor and vascular endothelial growth factor: implications for ocular angiogenesis. Am J Ophthalmol 2004;137:668–674.
42. Asayama N, Shimada H, Yuzawa M. Correlation of indocyanine green angiography findings and expression of vascular endothelial growth factor in surgically excised age-related macular degeneration-related choroidal neovascular membranes. Nippon Ganka Gakkai Zasshi 2000;104:390–395.
43. Kvanta A, Algvere PV, Berglin L, Seregard S. Subfoveal fibrovascular membranes in age-related macular degeneration express vascular endothelial growth factor. Invest Ophthalmol Vis Sci 1996;37:1929–1934.
44. Grossniklaus HE, Ling JX, Wallace TM, et al. Macrophage and retinal pigment epithelium expression of angiogenic cytokines in choroidal neovascularization. Mol Vis 2002;8: 119–126.
45. Frank RN. Growth factors in age-related macular degeneration: pathogenic and therapeutic implications. Ophthalmic Res 1997;29:341–353.
46. Wada M, Ogata N, Otsuji T, Uyama M. Expression of vascular endothelial growth factor and its receptor (KDR/flk-1) mRNA in experimental choroidal neovascularization. Curr Eye Res 1999;18:203–213.
47. Yi X, Ogata N, Komada M, et al. Vascular endothelial growth factor expression in choroidal neovascularization in rats. Graefes Arch Clin Exp Ophthalmol 1997;235:313–319.
48. Ishibashi T, Hata Y, Yoshikawa H, et al. Expression of vascular endothelial growth factor in experimental choroidal neovascularization. Graefes Arch Clin Exp Ophthalmol 1997;235: 159–167.
49. Baffi J, Byrnes G, Chan CC, Csaky KG. Choroidal neovascularization in the rat induced by adenovirus mediated expression of vascular endothelial growth factor. Invest Ophthalmol Vis Sci 2000;41:3582–3589.
50. Yu MJ, Shen WY, Lai MC, et al. Generation and characterization of a recombinant adenovirus expressing vascular endothelial growth factor for studies of neovascularization in the eye. Aust N Z J Ophthalmol 1999;27:250–253.

51. Spilsbury K, Garrett KL, Shen WY, et al. Overexpression of vascular endothelial growth factor (VEGF) in the retinal pigment epithelium leads to the development of choroidal neovascularization. Am J Pathol 2000;157:135–144.
52. Schwesinger C, Yee C, Rohan RM, et al. Intrachoroidal neovascularization in transgenic mice overexpressing vascular endothelial growth factor in the retinal pigment epithelium. Am J Pathol 2001;158:1161–1172.
53. Blaauwgeers HG, Holtkamp GM, Rutten H, et al. Polarized vascular endothelial growth factor secretion by human retinal pigment epithelium and localization of vascular endothelial growth factor receptors on the inner choriocapillaris. Evidence for a trophic paracrine relation. Am J Pathol 1999;155:421–428.
54. Hartnett ME, Lappas A, Darland D, et al. Retinal pigment epithelium and endothelial cell interaction causes retinal pigment epithelial barrier dysfunction via a soluble VEGF-dependent mechanism. Exp Eye Res 2003;77:593–599.
55. Qi JH, Ebrahem Q, Moore N, et al. A novel function for tissue inhibitor of metalloproteinases-3 (TIMP3): inhibition of angiogenesis by blockage of VEGF binding to VEGF receptor-2. Nat Med 2003;9:407–415.
56. Jones PF. Not just angiogenesis—wider roles for the angiopoietins. J Pathol 2003;201:515–527.
57. Hangai M, Murata T, Miyawaki N, et al. Angiopoietin-1 upregulation by vascular endothelial growth factor in human retinal pigment epithelial cells. Invest Ophthalmol Vis Sci 2001;42:1617–1625.
58. Lonser RR, Glenn GM, Walther M, et al. von Hippel-Lindau disease. Lancet 2003;361: 2059–2067.
59. Fine HF, Baffi J, Reed GF, et al. Aqueous humor and plasma vascular endothelial growth factor in uveitis-associated cystoid macular edema. Am J Ophthalmol 2001;132:794–796.
60. Krzystolik MG, Afshari MA, Adamis AP, et al. Prevention of experimental choroidal neovascularization with intravitreal anti-vascular endothelial growth factor antibody fragment. Arch Ophthalmol 2002;120:338–346.
61. Eyetech Study Group. Preclinical and phase 1A clinical evaluation of an anti-VEGF pegylated aptamer (EYE001) for the treatment of exudative age-related macular degeneration. Retina 2002;22:143–152.
62. Eyetech Study Group. Anti-vascular endothelial growth factor therapy for subfoveal choroidal neovascularization secondary to age-related macular degeneration: phase II study results. Ophthalmology 2003;110:979–986.
63. Csaky K. Anti-vascular endothelial growth factor therapy for neovascular age-related macular degeneration: promises and pitfalls. Ophthalmology 2003;110:879–881.
64. Aiello LP, Bursell SE, Clermont A, et al. Vascular endothelial growth factor-induced retinal permeability is mediated by protein kinase C in vivo and suppressed by an orally effective beta-isoform-selective inhibitor. Diabetes 1997;46:1473–1480.
65. Aiello LP. The potential role of PKC beta in diabetic retinopathy and macular edema. Surv Ophthalmol 2002;47 Suppl 2:S263–S269.
66. Tuttle KR, Anderson PW. A novel potential therapy for diabetic nephropathy and vascular complications: protein kinase C beta inhibition. Am J Kidney Dis 2003;42:456–465.
67. Park JY, Takahara N, Gabriele A, et al. Induction of endothelin-1 expression by glucose: an effect of protein kinase C activation. Diabetes 2000;49:1239–1248.
68. Yokota T, Ma RC, Park JY, et al. Role of protein kinase C on the expression of platelet-derived growth factor and endothelin-1 in the retina of diabetic rats and cultured retinal capillary pericytes. Diabetes 2003;52:838–845.
69. Bohlen HG, Nase GP. Arteriolar nitric oxide concentration is decreased during hyperglycemia-induced betaII PKC activation. Am J Physiol Heart Circ Physiol 2001;280: H621–H627.
70. Bohlen HG. Protein kinase betaII in Zucker obese rats compromises oxygen and flow-mediated regulation of nitric oxide formation. Am J Physiol Heart Circ Physiol 2004;286:H492–H497.

71. Cotter MA, Jack AM, Cameron NE. Effects of the protein kinase C beta inhibitor LY333531 on neural and vascular function in rats with streptozotocin-induced diabetes. Clin Sci (Lond) 2002;103:311–321.
72. Beckman JA, Goldfine AB, Gordon MB, et al. Inhibition of protein kinase Cbeta prevents impaired endothelium-dependent vasodilation caused by hyperglycemia in humans. Circ Res 2002;90:107–111.
73. Saishin Y, Takahashi K, Melia M, et al. Inhibition of protein kinase C decreases prostaglandin-induced breakdown of the blood-retinal barrier. J Cell Physiol 2003;195: 210–219.
74. Saishin Y, Silva RL, Callahan K, et al. Periocular injection of microspheres containing PKC412 inhibits choroidal neovascularization in a porcine model. Invest Ophthalmol Vis Sci 2003;44:4989–4993.
75. Campochiaro PA. Reduction of diabetic macular edema by oral administration of the kinase inhibitor PKC412. Invest Ophthalmol Vis Sci 2004;45:922–931.
76. Holash J, Davis S, Papadopoulos N, et al. VEGF-Trap: a VEGF blocker with potent antitumor effects. Proc Natl Acad Sci USA 2002;99:11,393–11,398.
77. Saishin Y, Takahashi K, Lima e Silva R, et al. VEGF-TRAP(R1R2) suppresses choroidal neovascularization and VEGF-induced breakdown of the blood-retinal barrier. J Cell Physiol 2003;195:241–248.
78. Reich SJ, Fosnot J, Kuroki A, et al. Small interfering RNA (siRNA) targeting VEGF effectively inhibits ocular neovascularization in a mouse model. Mol Vis 2003;9:210–216.
79. Tolentino MJ, Brucker AJ, Fosnot J, et al. Intravitreal injection of vascular endothelial growth factor small interfering RNA inhibits growth and leakage in a nonhuman primate, laser-induced model of choroidal neovascularization. Retina 2004;24:132–138.
80. Gehlbach P, Demetriades AM, Yamamoto S, et al. Periocular gene transfer of sFlt-1 suppresses ocular neovascularization and vascular endothelial growth factor-induced breakdown of the blood-retinal barrier. Hum Gene Ther 2003;14:129–141.
81. Takahashi K, Saishin Y, Silva RL, et al. Intraocular expression of endostatin reduces VEGF-induced retinal vascular permeability, neovascularization, and retinal detachment. FASEB J 2003;17:896–898.
82. Bell C, Lynam E, Landfair DJ, et al. Oligonucleotide NX1838 inhibits VEGF165-mediated cellular responses in vitro. In Vitro Cell Dev Biol Anim 1999;35:533–542.

12
The Role of Fibroblast Growth Factors in Ocular Angiogenesis

Andreas Bikfalvi, MD, PhD and Sophie Javerzat

CONTENTS

INTRODUCTION

The eye is a highly vascularized organ that possesses two vascular networks in the adult, the retinal vessels and the choroid vessels, as well as a transitory vascular system, the hyaloid vessels, which regress in vertebrates after birth. Abnormal vessel growth is observed in a number of ocular pathologies such as retinopathy or age-related macular dystrophy. Studies on the molecular mechanisms of eye vascularization have demonstrated a central role of vascular endothelial growth factor (VEGF) family members in these processes *(1–5)*. Other molecular players, such as angiopoietins, seem to be implicated in the remodeling of retinal vessels *(6)*.

Fibroblast growth factors (FGFs) stimulate growth, survival, and/or differentiation of a number of mesenchyme-derived cells and neurons *(7–9)*. Most of these functions have been demonstrated both in cultured cells and in transgenic mice *(7–9)*. It has long been known that exogenous FGFs are very potent inducers of capillary formation in vitro and in vivo *(7–9)*. FGFs stimulate endothelial cell proliferation, migration, tubulogenesis, and also angiogenesis in a variety of in vivo and ex vivo systems such as in the developing chicken chorioallantoid membrane, in the aortic ring assay, or in matrigel plugs in mice *(8,9)*. These effects are mediated through the activation of many signal transduction molecules, such as the mitogen-activated protein (MAP) kinase pathway or the PI-3 kinase pathway *(8–10)*. Furthermore, FGFs regulate the expression of cellular matrix receptors such as integrin $\alpha_4\beta_1$, $\alpha_5\beta_1$, or $\alpha_v\beta_3$, or proteolytic enzyme systems (plasminogen

From: *Ophthalmology: Ocular Angiogenesis: Diseases, Mechanisms, and Therapeutics*
Edited by: J. Tombran-Tink and C. J. Barnstable © Humana Press Inc., Totowa, NJ

activators, matrix metalloproteinases) that are implicated in the morphogenic effects induced by FGFs *(11–13)*.

FGFs and their receptors are widely expressed in the eye and participate in lens differentiation, photoreceptor survival, or retinal pigment epithelium (RPE) function and survival *(14–17)*. However, the contribution of FGFs to normal and pathological vascular development in the eye has been questioned until recently.

In this article, we will give a brief overview about the molecular mechanisms of eye vascularization and describe recent findings that indicate that FGFs indeed participate directly or indirectly in vascular developmental processes.

GENERAL MECHANISMS OF VASCULARIZATION IN THE EYE

The vertebrate eye possesses two vascular networks that develop asynchronously. Choroid vessels furnish the outer blood supply and are formed during the fetal period. Retinal blood vessels emerge from the optic disk and form a primary vascular layer that is remodeled and gives rise to the inner and outer vascular plexus of the retina. This latter process occurs during the postnatal period in mice.

The choroid is the most densely vascularized tissue in the body. Choroid vessels are formed by a combination of vasculogenesis and angiogenesis. Retinal blood vessels seem to be formed by an angiogenesis-dependent mechanism *(1–3,18)*. A concept for the formation of retinal blood vessels has been proposed, designated as contact spanning *(1,2)*. Astrocytes migrate into the retina and are organized into a trabecular scaffold. Endothelial cells follow the forming scaffold and become organized into tubular structures. VEGF has been identified as one of the key molecules responsible for endothelial cell migration and tubulogenesis during retinal angiogenesis *(1–4)*. Its mechanism has been recently refined by the identification of the guidance tip-cell that clusters VEGF receptors at the leading edge and in the filipodia and senses a VEGF gradient *(19)*. The heparin-binding VEGF-A isoforms seem to be implicated in this process, because they are able to associate with the extracellular matrix through the heparin-binding domain, thus permitting gradient formation *(4)*. One of the driving forces of VEGF expression is hypoxia, which acts by regulating the proline hydroxylases (PHDs) and the hypoxia-inducible factor (HIF)-1α system *(20–22)*. Besides VEGFs, other molecules, such as neuronal guidance molecules, are also possibly involved in vessel network formation.

A vasculogenesis-dependent mechanism in the formation of retinal blood vessels has also been proposed *(23,24)*. This is convincingly supported by a recent publication describing the incorporation of lineage-negative hematopoietic cells into retinal vessels *(24)*.

Vascular remodeling is a critical step in retinal vascular development. Recent genetic evidence indicates that angiopoietin-1 (Ang1) is involved in this process *(6)*.

Ocular neoangiogenesis can occur in pathological conditions (retinopathy, age-related macular dystrophy) or can be induced experimentally in the retina (retinopathy of prematurity model in mice), the choroid (laser-induced choroidal neovascularization), and the cornea (implantation of pellets containing angiogenesis factors). The VEGF system, again, has been recognized as a major molecular player in these conditions *(5)*.

Besides VEGF and angiopoietin-1, which constitute useful paradigms to explain vascular development in the eye or neoangiogenesis, other growth factor systems such as FGFs may play a role in physiological and pathological eye vascularization as well. Evidence for this is outlined below.

EXPRESSION OF FGF FAMILY MEMBERS IN OCULAR TISSUE AND RELATIONSHIP TO VASCULATURE

Many cell types in the eye express FGF molecules or FGF receptors. In the RPE, FGF prototypes are expressed, including FGF-1, FGF-2, FGF-4, or FGF-9, which all are potential candidates for a role in vascular development *(25–27)*. FGF-2 may be induced in the RPE by reactive oxygen species (ROS) and is also expressed in the newt iris *(28,29)*. FGF-2 is also found in neurons, photoreceptors, and macroglia (Müller cells, astrocytes) *(30)*. During experimentally induced choroidal neovascularization, FGF-2 is significantly upregulated together with pigment epithelium-derived factor (PEDF), neurophilin-2, angiopoietin-1 and 2 (Ang-1, Ang-2), ephrin A7 (EphA7), and VEGF receptor-1 (VEGFR-1) *(31)*.

Expression of FGF receptors (FGFRs) is also widespread, and different receptor types and spliced variants may exist. In the RPE, for example, FGFs may activate either FGFR2IIIc or FGFR3IIIc *(27)*. Photoreceptors express FGFR1 and FGFR4, which are critical for their development *(32)*. FGFR1 is prominent in the cytoplasm of photoreceptors and in their axon terminals, where it is closely associated with synaptic vesicles *(33)*. In the vascular compartment, FGF receptor expression has been detected in choroidal endothelial cells and seem to activate the FGFR1IIIc isoform *(34)*. FGFs can also bind to retinal vessels and activate signaling molecules such as PKB/Akt *(35)*. However, the specific FGF receptor variant expressed in retinal vessels is not known.

The existence of FGFs and their receptors in different cell types in the eye, including the vasculature, suggests direct and indirect mechanisms for FGFs in ocular angiogenesis. For example, the RPE expresses FGF prototypes that may interact with FGF receptors localized on the RPE, providing an autocrine regulatory loop that induces secondary angiogenesis factors such as VEGF. FGF released from the RPE may also act on the choroidal blood vessels localized in the vicinity, which express FGF receptors (Fig. 1).

ROLE OF FGFs IN EYE VASCULARIZATION?

FGFs are among the most powerful endothelial mitogens and are able to induce vessel formation in a number of in vitro and in vivo models *(8,9)*. Furthermore, blockade of FGF signalling in cultured embryonic day 9 mice leads to abnormal vasculature in both the embryo and extraembryonic structures *(36)*. This strongly supports a role for FGF as an endogenous angiogenic factor.

A number of arguments support a role for FGFs in angiogenesis processes in the eye. When applied through a catheter by external perfusion, exogenous FGF stimulates angiogenesis in the choroid *(27)*. Furthermore, recently, Cao et al. have reported that the combination of FGF-2 with platelet-derived growth factor (PDGF) strongly synergizes in the stimulation of corneal blood vessel growth *(38)*. These vessels seem to be structured, remodeled, and perfectly hierarchically organized. Most surprisingly, after withdrawal of growth factors, vessels continue to grow. This synergism is not observed with VEGF, which leads only to the formation of leaky and aberrant vessels. FGF family members are also expressed in cells that are localized in vicinity

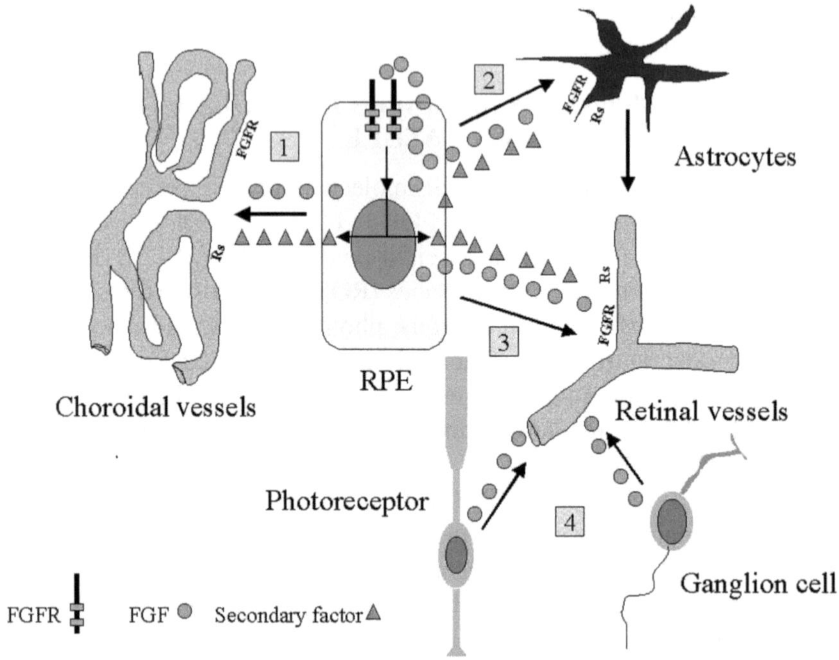

Fig. 1. Potential roles of FGF in choroidal and retinal vascularization induced by the RPE. Both direct and indirect mechanisms may be involved. For both the choroid (1) and the retina (3), FGF may control angiogenesis either directly by activating FGF receptors on endothelial cells or indirectly by autocrine stimulation of secondary angiogenesis factors. For the retina, it is more likely that FGF stimulates the formation of the astrocyte scaffold (2), which in turn favors endothelial cell migration and tubulogenesis. FGFs may also be produced by other cell types (4) such as photoreceptors or ganglion cells to control angiogenesis. FGFR, fibroblast growth factor receptors; Rs, receptors of secondary angiogenesis factors; RPE, retinal pigment epithelium. *See* color version on companion CD.

of blood vessels, such as in the RPE, and could therefore be involved in eye vascularization. Finally, like VEGF, FGF prototypes, in general, have a high affinity for heparan sulfate proteoglycans and could be involved in gradient formation in the retina.

However, results from FGF knockout studies have been rather disappointing. For example, FGF-2 knockout mice did not reveal vascular phenotypes during normal developmental choroidal or retinal angiogenesis or after laser-induced neoangiogenesis *(39)* (Table 1). On the other hand, FGF receptor knockouts are early embryonic lethal and thus not informative *(8,9,40)*.

To gain better insights of FGF effects on the vasculature, we have chosen to target the mouse RPE with a truncated FGF receptor (FGFR1-DN) that acts as an dominant-negative molecule *(41,42)*. For targeting, we used a promoter derived from the melanogenic enzyme tyrosinase-related protein-1 (tyrp1) gene. Eyes from homozygous mice at 1 mo of age were greatly reduced in size and displayed irregular shapes and cataracts. Furthermore, the choroid was thinned and the neural retina was convoluted, with numerous rosettes seen in different regions of the eye. Hemizygous mice also

Table 1
Vascular Phenotypes in Eye in Mouse Models for FGF Misregulation

FGF-1 –/–	Viable, absence of gross phenotype, detailed analysis of eyes not performed
FGF-2 –/–	Viable, absence of ocular phenotype
FGF-1–/– / FGF-2 –/–	Viable, absence of gross phenotype, detailed analysis of eyes not performed
Tyrp1 FGFR1-DN	Thinned choroid, decrease of vessels, effect of vessel branching, absence of retinal blood vessels, compensatory retinal angiogenesis from the hyaloid vessels
Tyrp1 Tag/Tyrp1 FGFR1-DN	Inhibition of tumor development and angiogenesis in primary and secondary tumors
Rho FGF-2	Latent phenotype revealed after injury (photo laser)

FGF, fibroblast growth factor; FGFR1-DN, dominant negative FGF receptor-1; Tyrp1, tyrosinase-related protein-1; Tag, T antigen; Rho, rhodopsin.

showed a number of phenotypic abnormalities, although less severe than in homozygous animals, the constant feature being a thinned choroid. Apical microvilli in transgenic retinas did not diplay the tight contacts with photoreceptor outer segments. When the choroidal vasculature was analyzed by corrosion casting, we found atrophy of some of the long ciliary arteries that did not reach the limbus. The size of the branching arteries and tributaries to the vortex veins were reduced. At the capillary level, vessel number was severely decreased and branching was reduced.

Using a specific immunostaining of eye vessels with *Bandeira simplicifolia* isolectin (BS-1), we next demonstrated that the effects on the vasculature were seen before birth, and thus preceded the neuronal defects. Flat mounts of choroids from transgenic mice between embryonic day 15.5 and 17.5 showed that the capillary bed was much less developed and branched than in wild-type control embryos. Thus, the phenotype observed in transgenic animals is a true developmental defect due to arrested development of choroid vessels rather than to vessel regression after birth. Surprisingly, retinal vascularization was also abnormal in transgenic animals. In transgenic retinas, numerous BS-1-positive single cells were present between day 0.5 and 3.5 postnatal (pn) but no vascular structures were seen. At later stages, the BS-1-positive single cells gradually disappeared, but no retinal vascular structures were observed. Furthermore, astrocyte migration seemed to be abnormal. A reduced amount of glial fibrillar acidic protein (GFAP)-positive astrocytes was observed in early retinas and no GFAP-positive network was detected in later-stage retinas. These observations indicate that FGF is also involved in the formation of the retinal vasculature, possibly through an indirect effect on astrocyte differentiation or patterning.

A persistence of the hyaloid vessels was observed after birth. Hyaloid vessels vascularize the retina with neovessels growing perpendicular deep into the retina. Hyaloid vessel persistence may be explained by compensation for the absence of retinal vessels.

This phenotype is similar to the angiopoietin-2 (Ang2) –/– mouse, which also shows a compensatory persistence of hyaloid vessels *(43)*.

Taken together, these observations suggest that FGF is a key component of the blood vessel development system in the eye. Possible mechanisms are depicted in Fig. 1.

What are the signaling mechanisms induced by FGFs in the eye vasculature?

FGF-2 induces a strong activation of MEK1, ERK1/2, and P90(RSK) in choriodal endothelial cells (CECs) *(44)*. Blockade of Ras, MEK1, and ERK1/2 by pharmacological agents significantly inhibited FGF2-induced cell proliferation, although not completely *(44)*. Furthermore, FGF2 stimulates the activation of the PI 3-K, P70(S6K) and Akt *(44)*. Blockade of PI 3-kinase also significantly decreased CEC proliferation *(44)*. This indicates that FGF signaling in CECs is dependent on both the MAP kinase and PI3 kinase pathways *(44)*. These effects seem to be more pronounced for FGFs than for VEGF *(44)*.

Are FGFs implicated in pathological angiogenesis processes in the eye? It is possible that FGFs may contribute to choroidal neovascularization. Indeed, laser photocoagulation at low intensity in transgenic mice that overexpress FGF in photoreceptors (rhodopsin promoter-FGF-2 mice) unmasks a latent proangiogenic phenotype *(45)*. Thus, under certain circumstances, such as retinal injury, FGFs may be released from cells or matrices and induce neovascularization. Another possible involvement of FGF in pathological angiogenesis is malignant ocular disease. To test this hypothesis, we created a bigenic mouse model that expresses both FGFR1-DN and the T antigen (Tag) under the control of the tyrp-1 promoter *(46)*. Monogenic tyrp1-Tag mice gave rise to ocular tumors that started to develop from the RPE before birth at the anterior part of the eye (ora serrata) and later grew at the median part and the posterior pole. The tumor then filled the eye and invaded the optic nerve and the brain. Tumors from bigenic mice demonstrated a significant reduction of size, a decrease of vessel density, and an increase in the apoptotic rate. Furthermore, invasion into the neural tissue was significantly inhibited. This effect is related to an inhibition of angiogenesis, as cocultures from RPE cells derived from bigenic mice with capillary endothelial cells did not show an induction of capillary morphogenesis, in contrast to RPE cells derived from tyrp1-Tag tumors.

Hypoxia is one of the driving forces in ocular angiogenesis, especially in the retina. Despite evidence of hypoxia regulation of FGF expression during branching morphogenesis in the fly, FGF does not seem to be controlled, in mammals, by hypoxia-regulated systems *(47)*.

However, it has been recently demonstrated that FGF receptor activity in endothelial cells can be controlled by the HIF system *(48)*. Li et al. have demonstrated that two enzymes important for the biosynthesis of heparan-sulfate proteoglycans (HSPGs) are hypoxia-regulated and induced a significant increase in the synthesis of HSPGs *(48)*. HSPGs are important coreceptors required for FGF receptor activity, and their increase enhances FGF receptor activity. It is not yet established whether this type of regulation is also operating in retinal or choroid blood vessels.

CONCLUSION

Fibroblast growth factors and their receptors are widely distributed in the ocular tissue and exert pleiotropic effects. Recently, a number of observation have demonstrated that FGFs are implicated in ocular angiogenesis as well:

- FGFs are strong angiogenesis factors and induce a highly hierarchically ordered mature vascular network in the cornea. This effect is synergistic with PDGFs.
- Inhibition of FGF receptor activity in transgenic mice in the eye gives rise to vascular defects in the choroid and the retina. The choroid is poorly vascularized, thinned, and shows a vessel branching defect. The formation of retinal vessels is completely inhibited. These are developmental defects that appear prior to birth.
- FGFs also seem to play a role in neoangiogenesis processes in the eye. Laser-induced injury reveals a latent proangiogenic phenotype in FGF-transgenic mice. Furthermore, inhibition of FGF activity in transgenic mice expressing the T antigen in the RPE demonstrated impaired tumor growth and a decrease in angiogenesis.
- FGFs are able to elicit specific signaling events in endothelial cells derived from the eye vasculature. For example, FGF-2 stimulates the MAP kinase and PI-3 kinase pathways in choroidal endothelial cells. This effect seems to be stronger than that of VEGF.

How FGFs are integrated in a signaling network with other players and precisely regulate vascular development in the eye in a coordinated fashion remains to be determined.

ACKNOWLEDGMENTS

The authors would like to thank Dr. Anne Eichmann (INSERM U36, Collège de France, Paris) for her critical reading of the manuscript. The work from our laboratory described in this article has been supported by grants from Retina France and the Ligue Contre le Cancer (Equipe Labellisée) and the Conseil Régional d'Aquitaine.

Credits to EC: Supported by grants from the European Union FP6, LSHC-CT-2003-503233, STROMA; this publication reflects only the authors' view. The European Commission is not liable for any use that may be made of the information contained herein.

REFERENCES

1. Gariano RF. Cellular mechanisms in retinal vascular development. Prog Retin Eye Res 2003;22:295–306.
2. Provis JM. Development of the primate retinal vasculature. Prog Retin Eye Res 2001;20:799–821.
3. Provis JM, Leech J, Diaz CM, Penfold PL, Stone J, Keshet E. Development of the human retinal vasculature: cellular relations and VEGF expression. Exp Eye Res 1997;65:555–568.
4. Stalmans I, Ng YS, Rohan R, et al. Arteriolar and venular patterning in retinas of mice selectively expressing VEGF isoforms. J Clin Invest 2002;109:327–336.
5. Campochiaro PA, Hackett SF. Ocular neovascularization: a valuable model system. Oncogene 2003;22:6537–6548.
6. Uemura A, Ogawa M, Hirashima M, et al. Recombinant angiopoietin-1 restores higher-order architecture of growing blood vessels in mice in the absence of mural cells. J Clin Invest 2002;110:1619–1628.
7. Bikfalvi A, Klein S, Pintucci G, Rifkin DB. Biological roles of fibroblast growth factor-2. Endocr Rev 1997;18:26–45.
8. Javerzat S, Auguste P, Bikfalvi A. The role of fibroblast growth factors in vascular development. Trends Mol Med 2002;8:483–489.
9. Auguste P, Javerzat S, Bikfalvi A. Regulation of vascular development by fibroblast growth factors. Cell Tissue Res 2003;314:157–166.
10. Gerwins P, Skoldenberg E, Claesson-Welsh L. Function of fibroblast growth factors and vascular endothelial growth factors and their receptors in angiogenesis. Crit Rev Oncol Hematol 2000;34:185–194.

11. Klein S, Bikfalvi A, Birkenmeier TM, Giancotti FG, Rifkin DB. Integrin regulation by endogenous expression of 18-kDa fibroblast growth factor-2. J Biol Chem 1996;271:22,583–22,590.
12. Hood JD, Frausto R, Kiosses WB, Schwartz MA, Cheresh DA. Differential alphav integrin-mediated Ras-ERK signaling during two pathways of angiogenesis. J Cell Biol 2003;162: 933–943.
13. Pepper MS. Extracellular proteolysis and angiogenesis. Thromb Haemost 2001;86:346–355.
14. Counis MF, Chaudun E, Arruti C, et al. Analysis of nuclear degradation during lens cell differentiation. Cell Death Differ 1998;5:251–261.
15. Bryckaert M, Guillonneau X, Hecquet C, Perani P, Courtois Y, Mascarelli F. Regulation of proliferation-survival decisions is controlled by FGF1 secretion in retinal pigmented epithelial cells. Oncogene 2000;19:4917–4929.
16. Russell C. The roles of hedgehogs and fibroblast growth factors in eye development and retinal cell rescue. Vision Res 2003;43:899–912.
17. Chaum E. Retinal neuroprotection by growth factors: a mechanistic perspective. J Cell Biochem 2003;88:57–75.
18. Fruttiger M. Development of the mouse retinal vasculature: angiogenesis versus vasculogenesis. Invest Ophthalmol Vis Sci 2002;43:522–527.
19. Gerhardt H, Golding M, Fruttiger M, et al. VEGF guides angiogenic sprouting utilizing endothelial tip cell filopodia. J Cell Biol 2003;161:1163–1177.
20. Semenza G. Signal transduction to hypoxia-inducible factor 1. Biochem Pharmacol 2002;64:993–998.
21. Masson N, Ratcliffe PJ. HIF prolyl and asparaginyl hydroxylases in the biological response to intracellular O(2) levels. J Cell Sci 2003;116:3041–3049.
22. Stone J, Itin A, Alon T, et al. Development of retinal vasculature is mediated by hypoxia-induced vascular endothelial growth factor (VEGF) expression by neuroglia. J Neurosci 1995;15:4738–4747.
23. Chan-Ling T, McLeod DS, Hughes S, et al. Astrocyte-endothelial cell relationships during human retinal vascular development. Invest Ophthalmol Vis Sci 2004;45:2020–2032.
24. Otani A, Kinder K, Ewalt K, Otero FJ, Schimmel P, Friedlander M. Bone marrow-derived stem cells target retinal astrocytes and can promote or inhibit retinal angiogenesis. Nat Med 2002;8:1004–1010.
25. Guillonneau X, Bryckaert M, Launay-Longo C, Courtois Y. Endogenous FGF1-induced activation and synthesis of extracellular signal-regulated kinase 2 reduce cell apoptosis in retinal-pigmented epithelial cells. J Biol Chem 1998;273:22,367–22,373.
26. Mousa SA, Lorelli W, Campochiaro PA. Role of hypoxia and extracellular matrix-integrin binding in the modulation of angiogenic growth factors secretion by retinal pigmented epithelial cells. J Cell Biochem 1999;74:135–143.
27. Alizadeh M, Miyamura N, Handa JT, Hjelmeland LM. Human RPE cells express the FGFR2IIIc and FGFR3IIIc splice variants and FGF9 as a potential high affinity ligand. Exp Eye Res 2003;76:249–256.
28. Hayashi T, Mizuno N, Ueda Y, Okamoto M, Kondoh H. FGF2 triggers iris-derived lens regeneration in newt eye. Mech Dev 2004;121:519–526.
29. Wada M, Gelfman CM, Matsunaga H, et al. Density-dependent expression of FGF-2 in response to oxidative stress in RPE cells in vitro. Curr Eye Res 2001;23:226–231.
30. Walsh N, Valter K, Stone J. Cellular and subcellular patterns of expression of bFGF and CNTF in the normal and light stressed adult rat retina. Exp Eye Res 2001;72:495–501.
31. Martin G, Schlunck G, Hansen LL, Agostini HT. Differential expression of angioregulatory factors in normal and CNV-derived human retinal pigment epithelium. Graefes Arch Clin Exp Ophthalmol 2004;242:321–326.

32. Zhang L, El-Hodiri HM, Ma HF, et al. Targeted expression of the dominant-negative FGFR4a in the eye using Xrx1A regulatory sequences interferes with normal retinal development. Development 2003;130:4177–4186.
33. Valter K, van Driel D, Bisti S, Stone J. FGFR1 expression and FGFR1-FGF-2 colocalisation in rat retina: sites of FGF-2 action on rat photoreceptors. Growth Factors 2002;20: 177–188.
34. Matsushima M, Ogata N, Takada Y, et al. FGF receptor 1 expression in experimental choroidal neovascularization. Jpn J Ophthalmol 1996;40:329–338.
35. Gu X, El-Remessy AB, Brooks SE, Al-Shabrawey M, Tsai NT, Caldwell RB. Hyperoxia induces retinal vascular endothelial cell apoptosis through formation of peroxynitrite. Am J Physiol Cell Physiol 2003;285:546–554.
36. Lee SH, Schloss DJ, Swain JL. Maintenance of vascular integrity in the embryo requires signaling through the fibroblast growth factor receptor. J Biol Chem 2000;275:33,679–33,687.
37. Soubrane G, Cohen SY, Delayre T, et al. Basic fibroblast growth factor experimentally induced choroidal angiogenesis in the minipig. Curr Eye Res 1994;13:183–195.
38. Cao R, Brakenhielm E, Pawliuk R, et al. Angiogenic synergism, vascular stability and improvement of hind-limb ischemia by a combination of PDGF-BB and FGF-2. Nat Med 2003;9:604–613.
39. Tobe T, Ortega S, Luna JD, et al. Targeted disruption of the FGF2 gene does not prevent choroidal neovascularization in a murine model. Am J Pathol 1998;15:1641–1666.
40. Ornitz DM, Itoh N. Fibroblast growth factors. Genome Biol 2, REVIEWS3005.
41. Rousseau B, Dubayle D, Sennlaub F, et al. Neural and angiogenic defects in eyes of transgenic mice expressing a dominant-negative FGF receptor in the pigmented cells. Exp Eye Res 2000;71:395–404.
42. Rousseau B, Larrieu-Lahargue F, Bikfalvi A, Javerzat S. Involvement of fibroblast growth factors in choroidal angiogenesis and retinal vascularization. Exp Eye Res 2003;77:147–156.
43. Hackett SF, Wiegand S, Yancopoulos G, Campochiaro PA. Angiopoietin-2 plays an important role in retinal angiogenesis. J Cell Physiol 2002;192:182–187.
44. Zubilewicz A, Hecquet C, Jeanny JC, Soubrane G, Courtois Y, Mascarelli F. Two distinct signalling pathways are involved in FGF2-stimulated proliferation of choriocapillary endothelial cells: a comparative study with VEGF. Oncogene 2001;20:1403–1413.
45. Yamada H, Yamada E, Kwak N, et al. Cell injury unmasks a latent proangiogenic phenotype in mice with increased expression of FGF2 in the retina. J Cell Physiol 2000;185:135–142.
46. Rousseau B, Larrieu-Lahargue F, Javerzat S, Guilhem-Ducleon F, Beermann F, Bikfalvi A. The tyrp1-Tag/tyrp1-FGFR1-DN bigenic mouse: a model for selective inhibition of tumor development, angiogenesis, and invasion into the neural tissue by blockade of fibroblast growth factor receptor activity. Cancer Res 2004;64:2490–2495.
47. Lubarsky B, Krasnow MA. Tube morphogenesis: making and shaping biological tubes. Cell 2003;112:19–28.
48. Li J, Shworak NW, Simons M. Increased responsiveness of hypoxic endothelial cells to FGF2 is mediated by HIF-1alpha-dependent regulation of enzymes involved in synthesis of heparan sulfate FGF2-binding sites. J Cell Sci 2002;115:1951–1959.

13

Control of Neovascularization and Cell Survival in the Eye by PEDF

Joyce Tombran-Tink, PhD and Colin J. Barnstable, DPhil

CONTENTS

INTRODUCTION

Pathological angiogenesis is by far the most common aspect of eye diseases. Corneal lesions and inflammatory ocular diseases have a strong angiogenesis component and are the most common causes of visits to ophthalmologists. Proliferative diabetic retinopathy (PDR) and age-related macular degeneration (AMD) affect more than 7 million people in the United States alone. As described elsewhere in this volume, pathological angiogenesis is also an important component of many other diseases of the eye. Controlling blood vessel growth, therefore, offers a unique opportunity to affect a wide spectrum of physiological and pathological functions.

The vasculature of most tissues is held in a state of quiescence through a finely tuned balance between pro- and antiangiogenic factors. Normal tissue repair, reproductive cycles, and wound healing represent a few adult processes that require neovascularization and stimulate physiological angiogenesis *(1,2)*. Abnormal blood vessels can be generated in response to numerous pathological stimuli as well. These are often leaky and underlie the progression of most tumors, many inflammatory conditions, and a wide range of human disorders *(3)*.

Dozens of pro- and antiangiogenic factors that are essential to maintain vascular quiescence in the adults have been identified. Some of the more well-characterized factors are listed in Table 1. This group of molecules can be divided into two classes: those that

From: *Ophthalmology: Ocular Angiogenesis: Diseases, Mechanisms, and Therapeutics*
Edited by: J. Tombran-Tink and C. J. Barnstable © Humana Press Inc., Totowa, NJ

Table 1
Pro- and Antiangiogenic Factors Currently Identified

Proangiogenic factors

Constitutive	*Cryptic fragments*
Angiogenin	Collagen type IV (proteolytic fragment)
Angiopoietin 1	Laminin (SIKVAV sequence)
Epidermal growth factor (EGF)	SPARC (proteolytic fragment)
Fibroblast growth factor family (e.g., FGF-1 and FGF-2)	
Follistatin	
Granulocyte colony-stimulating factor (G-CSF)	
Hepatocyte growth factor (HGF)	
Insulin growth factor 1 (IGF-1)	
Interleukin-8 (IL-8)	
Leptin	
Matrix metalloproteinases (MMPs)	
Midkine	
Placental growth factor (PIGF)	
Platelet activating factor (PAF)	
Platelet-derived endothelial cell growth factor (PD-ECGF)	
Platelet-derived growth factor (PDGF)	
Pleiotrophin	
Proliferin	
Transforming growth factors (TGF-α and TGF-β)	
Tumor necrosis factor (TNF-α)	
Vascular endothelial growth factors (VEGF-A,B,C,D)	

Antiangiogenic factors

Constitutive	*Cryptic fragments*
Angiogenin	Angiostatin (38-kDa plasminogen fragment; Kringle 1–4)
Antiangiogenic antithrombin III (aaATIII)	Angiotensinogen fragments
Brain angiogenesis inhibitor-1 (BAI-1)	Arresten (fragment of α1 chain of type IV collagen)
Interferon α (IFNα)	Canstatin (fragment α2 chain of type IV collagen)
Interferon inducible protein	Endostatin (20-kDa fragment of XVIII collagen)
Interleukin-12	Fibronectin—29-kDa N-terminal fragment
Pigment epithelium-derived factor (PEDF)	Fibronectin type 111 peptide
Placental ribonuclease inhibitor	Fibronectin—40-kDa C-terminal fragment
Plasminogen activator inhibitor	Heparin hexasaccharide fragment
Proliferin-related protein	Kringle 1–5 (fragment of plasminogen)
Protamine	NC1 domain of type VIII collagen α1
Somatostatin analogue octreotide	PEX (metalloproteinase fragment)
SPARC (43 kDa secreted protein acidic and rich in cystein/osteonectin/BM-40)	Platelet factor 4 fragment (PF4)
	Prolactin—16-kDa N-terminal fragment
Thrombospondin-1 (TSP-1)	Prolactin fragments
Thrombospondin-2 (TSP-2)	Restin (22-kDa fragment of human collagen XV)

Antiangiogenic factors (Continued)	
Constitutive	*Cryptic fragments*
Tissue inhibitors of metalloproteinases—TIMP 1	Tryp-tRNA synthetase (TrpRS) splice variant
Tissue inhibitors of metalloproteinases—TIMP 2	Tryp-tRNA synthetase C-terminal fragment
Tissue inhibitors of metalloproteinases—TIMP 3	Tumstatin (fragment of $\alpha 3$ chain of type IV)
	Vasostatin (fragment of calreticulin)
Vasculostatin	

Note that different fragments cause some molecules to appear in both categories.

are constitutively found in their active form and those that become active only after they are released by proteolytic cleavage of larger polypeptides. These molecules are the players in key processes that stimulate endothelial cell growth, facilitate endothelial cell migration, alter cell adhesive properties, permit tube formation, and promote stability of the newly formed vessel. Knowing whether these factors act independently, hierarchically, or cooperatively is a prerequisite for developing decisive targeting strategies against one or a few to promote pleiotropic effects on the others. Gene knockout and transgenic animal studies implicate vascular endothelial growth factor (VEGF) as one of the major initiators of both normal and pathological angiogenesis *(5,6)*. In this chapter, we will discuss the growing evidence that one of the key factors that prevent abnormal blood vessel growth, possibly by directly interfering with VEGF's activity, is pigment epithelium-derived factor (PEDF).

PEDF EXPRESSION

PEDF was first identified as a neurotrophic factor in conditioned medium obtained from fetal human RPE cell cultures. The purified 50-kDa protein effectively switched Y79 retinoblastoma cells from an actively growing suspension cell line to nonproliferating cells that attached to a substrate, extended neurites, and increased expression of molecules associated with differentiated neurons at concentrations as low as 1 n*M (7,8)*.

The interphotoreceptor space is a major reservoir for the PEDF secreted by the RPE cells in vivo. The vitreous contains a significant amount of PEDF as well, possibly from sources such as the retinal ganglion cells, several cell types in the cornea, and the ciliary epithelial cells, which have all been shown to synthesize the protein (Fig. 1). Detection of PEDF in cultured Müller cells suggests that other types of retinal cells can also be induced to express this protein *(10)*.

PEDF is found in most regions of the brain *(11)*. Ependymal cells are responsible for some of the PEDF detected in the cerebrospinal fluid, but a variety of neurons also express this protein. In the spinal cord, the protein is localized to motor neurons of the ventral horn and some neurons in the dorsal horn. Like the retina, much of the brain and spinal cord are bathed in this neurotrophic factor. Several nonneural tissues, including skeletal muscle, bone, heart, placenta, and liver, also synthesize PEDF, but its function in these organs is not yet elucidated *(10–12)*.

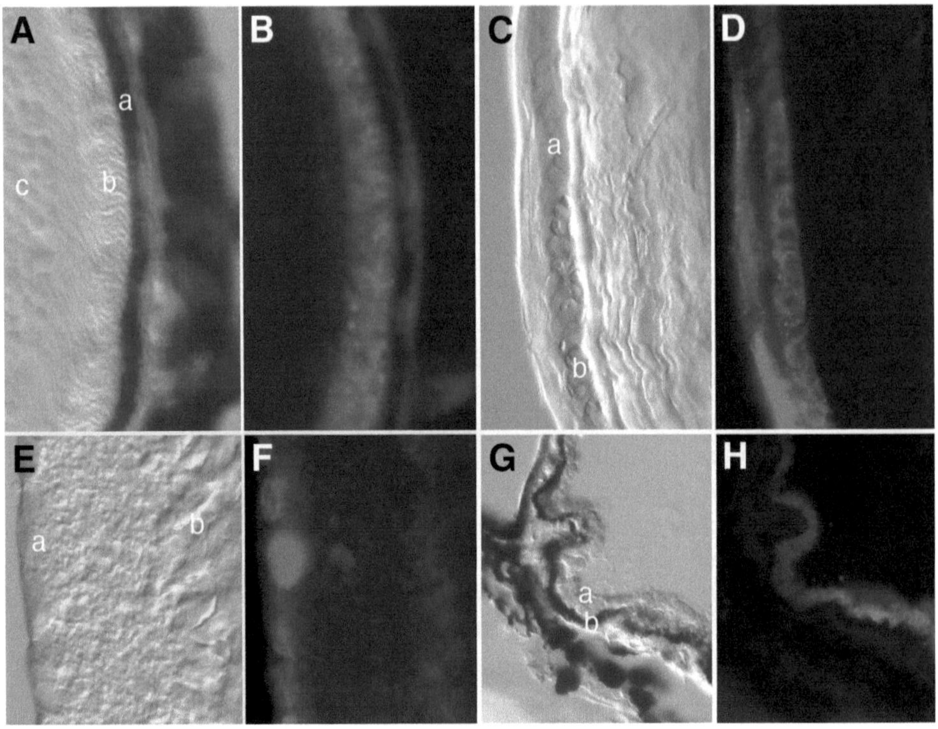

Fig. 1. Detection of pigment epithelium-derived factor (PEDF) expression in the mouse eye by indirect immunofluorescence. **(A,B)** PEDF is expressed in the RPE cells (a) and collects in the interphotoreceptor matrix surrounding photoreceptor outer segments (b). No fluorescence is detectable over the photoreceptor cell bodies of the outer nuclear layer (c). **(C,D)** PEDF is expressed by corneal epithelial cells (a) with more intense labeling in the limbal region (b). **(E,F)** In the inner retina labeling can be found in cells of the ganglion cell layer (a) but very little in the inner nuclear layer (b). **(G,H)** In the ciliary epithelium strong labeling is observed in the nonpigmented layer (a) but none in the pigmented layer (b). **(A,C,E,G)** Nomarski images; **(B,D,F,H)** Fluorescence images. (Adapted from ref. *9*.) *See* color version on companion CD.

PEDF AND ANGIOGENESIS

An antiangiogenic role for PEDF in the retina emerged when Dawson et al. *(13)* showed that PEDF inhibited angiogenic processes and was more effective than the well-studied angiogenesis inhibitor angiostatin. PEDF inhibited endothelial cell migration even in the presence of proangiogenic factors such as FGF-1, FGF-2, VEGF, interleukin-8, and lysophosphatic acid. This finding is not entirely surprising, as PEDF is present in high concentrations in avascular regions of the eye.

PEDF is detected early in human and mouse development *(14,15)*. The embryonic expression of PEDF suggests that it may play a role in early vasculogenesis, although there is currently little information on the ways in which antiangiogenic factors, such as PEDF, can regulate this process. As a factor that can bind to specific extracellular matrix components (*see* "Structure–Function Relationships of PEDF"), PEDF could promote the spatial definition of developing vessel pathways. Such a role has been postulated for PEDF in the hypophyseal plate of bone and the uterine endometrium *(16,17)*.

This could also be true in the eye, where the concentration of PEDF in the limbal region of the cornea may be part of the barrier that keeps the cornea avascular.

PEDF Inhibits Growth of New Blood Vessels

Pharmacological approaches to treat neovascular diseases can be divided into attempts to block the actions of proangiogenic factors or to enhance the actions of antiangiogenic factors. So far, VEGF has been a major target in ophthalmology to ameliorate neovascularization in PDR and AMD. Although antagonists of VEGF show promising results, VEGF therapy alone is unlikely to be sufficient to fully counteract angiogenesis because of endothelial cell diversity, regional variation in tissue expression of VEGF, the complexity of the VEGF family, isoforms and receptors, and the growth-stimulating contribution of dozens of other factors in the angiogenic cascade. Antiangiogenic therapies alone will not counteract the damaging effects of angiogenesis on various retinal cell types. The alternative approach of augmenting both antiangiogenic and neuroprotective molecules in the body is critical to effective treatments and is just beginning to be explored in detail. The following discussion will be limited to the possible use of PEDF as both a therapeutic antiangiogenic and a neuroprotective factor.

There is strong evidence that PEDF reduces blood vessel growth in the eye using viral-mediated gene transfer approaches (*see* Chapter 20, this volume). Ocular injection of an adenoviral construct containing the PEDF gene inhibits the formation of both retinal and choroidal neovascularization in mouse models of ocular angiogenesis. Even more important, PEDF causes regression of neovascularization already under way *(18,19)*. In other studies in which mice are placed in hyperoxic conditions, intraocular application of an adeno-associated virus (AAV)-PEDF vector results in high levels of PEDF expression in the eye over extended periods and a significant correlation with reduced development of ocular vessels *(20,21)*. Choroidal neovascularization arising from laser-induced damage to Bruch's membrane can also be inhibited by both intravitreous and subretinal injections of AAV-PEDF *(22)*. These studies are convincing and indicate that PEDF establishes specific mechanisms of interference that mitigate vascular growth-propelling signals.

In addition to the growth of new vessels, many ocular problems arise because of increased vessel permeability. One of the earliest activities observed for VEGF was increased permeability of blood vessels *(23)*. Recently, it has been shown that PEDF cancels VEGF-induced increases in vascular permeability *(24)*. Coinjection of PEDF with VEGF into mouse eyes results in much lower fluorescein leakage than in eyes injected with VEGF alone. More than 95% of the VEGF-induced permeability can be abolished by PEDF as determined by quantitative assays using Evans blue. This additional activity of PEDF strengthens the argument for its use as a major component of any ocular neovascular disease therapy.

PEDF and VEGF Strike Balance in Angiogenesis

As mentioned earlier, there are many pro- and antiangiogenic factors capable of modulating vessel growth, although not all play an equal role in this process. There is increasing evidence that, at least in the eye, the balance between the proangiogenic factor VEGF and the antiangiogenic factor PEDF appears to determine new vessel formation *(25)*.

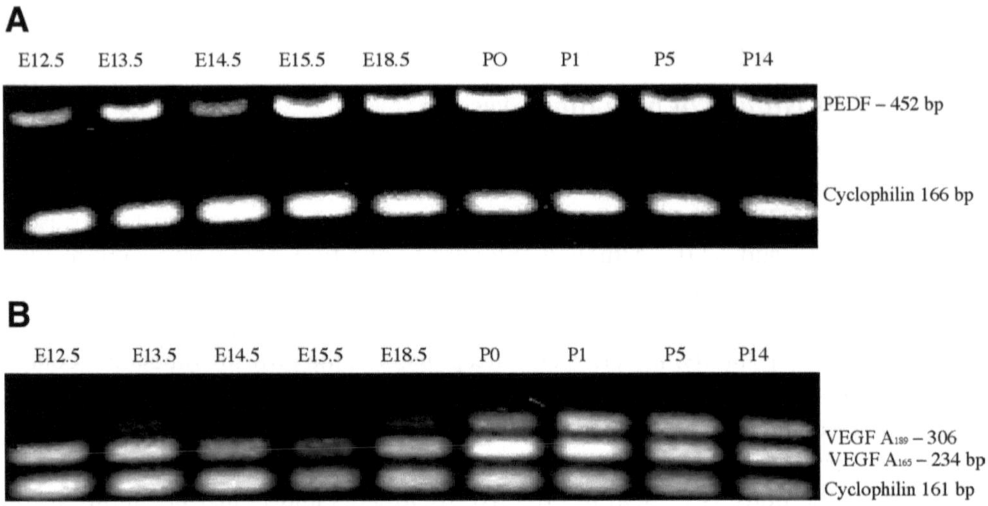

Fig. 2. Detection of pigment epithelium-derived factor (PEDF) and vascular endothelial growth factor (VEGF)-A expression in developing mouse liver by reverse transcription-polymerase chain reaction (RT-PCR). PEDF mRNA is expressed at all developmental stages of mouse liver. However, it increases at E15.5 and is maintained throughout the remaining stages of liver development. VEGF-A_{165} is expressed at early stages in all developmental stages of mouse liver but shows a marked increase at postnatal day 0. There are undetectable levels of VEGF-A_{189} during early liver development but this isoform is expressed at high levels in the liver at all postnatal days studied. Cyclophilin is used as internal control in each PCR reaction. (Data from ref. *26*.)

Both factors are expressed very early in embryological development. For example, in the highly vascularized liver, PEDF and VEGF are coexpressed, although there is differential expression of the VEGF isoforms during development (Fig. 2) *(26)*. In the adult eye, VEGF levels increase and PEDF levels decrease in several angiogenic diseases. For example, an inverse relationship is noted between these two factors in the vitreous of patients with PDR and AMD, suggesting an underlying cooperative relationship between these proteins in maintaining vascular quiescence. Analogous observations that PEDF levels are lower in the vitreous of active compared with inactive forms of diabetic retinopathy further support this theory *(27–31)*. Both PEDF and VEGF are detected in choroidal neovascular membranes and polypoidal choroidal vasculopathy, with decreased expression of both in new vessels where fibrosis is present *(32)*.

Although it is attractive to envisage a direct and unique relationship between PEDF and VEGF, there is currently no evidence to support this at the molecular level. We have shown that PEDF does not alter VEGF transcription in either basal or hypoxia-stimulated conditions, and that VEGF does not alter the level of PEDF transcripts in vitro *(33)*. Thus effects on the levels of each factor may occur at the level of protein secretion or degradation. However, there is growing evidence that PEDF blocks the actions of VEGF on blood vessel sprouting. We have shown that although PEDF does not alter VEGF levels, it reduces the transcription of VEGFR-2 (Flk-1) receptor, suggesting that one way in which PEDF might antagonize VEGF is by reducing the availability of key VEGF receptors *(33)*.

Another way in which PEDF can inhibit VEGF activity to maintain a normal balance in angiogenesis is by reducing the activation of the VEGFR-2 receptor. Our preliminary data show that PEDF decreases phosphorylation of VEGFR-2 in human umbilical vein endothelial cells (HUVECs) and alters the growth promoting signals triggered by VEGF. In addition, VEGF-induced survival of endothelial cells is blocked by PEDF in a caspase-dependent manner. The survival of HUVEC cells is thought to be contingent on the activation of one or more specific signaling molecules including AKT, Erk1/2, P38, and JNK. PEDF inhibits VEGF activation of AKT and Erk1/2 *(34)* and enhances VEGF stimulation of P38 and JNK. When we interrupt these signals with specific pharmacological inhibitors, we found that PEDF-induced death of HUVECs is predominantly mediated through PI3 kinase and P38 MAPK. In addition, PEDF can regulate the MAPK pathway by altering ERK1/2 phosphorylation in retinal endothelial cells and by decreasing the expression of MAPKK *(34)*. The modulation of ERK1/2 phosphorylation by PEDF varies according to the growth conditions under which cells are exposed *(34)*.

Antiangiogenic signals are also generated by PEDF through activation of the Fas/FasL death cascade in endothelial cells *(35)*. However, because PEDF inhibits ocular angiogenesis in mice deficient in Fas or FasL as well, it presumably has additional inhibitory actions independent of the Fas/FasL cascade on endothelial cells *(36)*.

Interference with activation of caspase 8 and 3, two essential transducers of the Fas/FasL cascade, blocks PEDF-induced apoptotic signals on endothelial cells. PEDF's control of apoptotic signals in these cells may be linked to its regulation of Flip 1, an inhibitor of caspase 8 and a key mediator of cell death. Flip 1 is expressed above physiological levels when VEGF activates NFkB in endothelial cells *(37)*. PEDF can restore physiological levels of Flip1 in the presence of VEGF in endothelial cells and thus may restore the caspase 8 executioner pathway. Similarly, recent studies have shown that VEGF-induced activation of the transcription factor NFAT can lead to increased Flip1 expression, and that this too is blocked by PEDF *(38)*.

Overlaid on this dynamic equilibrium of PEDF and VEGF levels is the interesting finding that there is an age-related decrease in PEDF expression in a number of cell types *(14)*, and that this decline can be reset in cloned animals *(39)*. Perhaps many age-related neovascular diseases occur because the amount or activity of angiogenic inhibitors such as PEDF has become attenuated.

Some factors can initiate the key first step of angiogenesis by causing an activation and proliferation of endothelial cells that set in motion a complex cascade of interrelated events among cells, soluble factors, second messengers, and extracellular matrix components. Molecules influencing early events in this cascade are likely to be stronger regulators of angiogenesis and thus better growth-limiting targets.

PEDF Inhibits Tumor Angiogenesis and Cell Differentiation

The antiangiogenic activities of PEDF are not limited to neovascular eye diseases. There is now evidence that the action of PEDF on tumor regression is twofold: partly from its antiangiogenic activity and partly from cell differentiation effects. The original identification of PEDF was directly related to a measure of its differentiation and antiproliferative activity on human retinoblastoma cells *(1,2)*. This differentiation activity is also noticed in primitive neuroblastoma, which, when treated with the protein, is converted into the less malignant ganglionic or other cell types, which, in turn, produce more PEDF *(40)*. In support of this biological activity, it has been shown that PEDF expression is lost in metastatic subclones of some tumors, and that there is allelic loss of the PEDF gene in others *(41,42)*. In addition, others have shown that mouse lung cancer cells infected with a PEDF adenovirus construct have less tumor burden, and that the proliferation rates decrease in melanoma cells transfected to express PEDF *(43,44)*. Studies of human melanoma cells in mice have suggested that PEDF can inhibit both migration and survival of melanoma cells and thus reduce metastases *(45)*.

In many tumor studies it is difficult to separate direct antitumor effects of PEDF from its powerful antiangiogenic activity. In numerous models, including lung carcinoma, hepatocellular carcinoma, and melanoma, elevating the levels of PEDF reduces the growth of blood vessels into the tumor, thereby reducing the tumor mass *(44–47)*. These experimental studies are supported by clinical observations that patients whose tumors have higher levels of PEDF expression show fewer metastases and have a better prognosis *(48)*.

These actions of PEDF on cell proliferation and blood vessel growth are further confirmed in a PEDF knockout mouse strain *(49)* where a lack of PEDF expression results in hyperplasia of organs such as the prostate and increased microvasculature in several tissues, including the retina. Based on these findings, it could be argued that PEDF contributes to vascular quiescence by maintaining the differentiated state of endothelial cells and by inhibiting growth promoting signals that lead to the aberrant proliferation of these cells in neovascular diseases.

PEDF AND NEUROPROTECTION

Although the aberrant growth of blood vessels is a major factor contributing to the progression of neovascular eye disease, it is the damage that it does to surrounding tissues that ultimately leads to visual loss or progression of the disease. In the retina, invading leaky choroidal vessels contribute to the degeneration of the retinal pigment epithelium (RPE) and photoreceptor cells as seen in the wet form of age-related macular degeneration. In this condition, controlling neovascularization alone does not eliminate the degeneration already in progress unless there is very early diagnosis. Thus, it is important that neuroprotective factors are an essential component of therapeutic strategies for these pathologies.

In addition to its antiangiogenic properties, PEDF is an effective neuroprotective factor in many parts of the nervous system. In the eye, PEDF reduces apoptosis induced by H_2O_2 or light damage in rat photoreceptors *(50,51)*, preserves the spatial organization, morphology, and function of photoreceptors after RPE detachment in a *Xenopus* model of retinal degeneration *(52)*, and protects retinal neurons from injuries caused by increased intraocular pressure from transient ischemic reperfusion *(53)*. In cells of other parts of the nervous system, such as cerebellar granule cells, hippocampal neurons and spinal cord motor neurons, nanogram amounts of PEDF provide protection from the damaging effects of glutamate toxicity *(54–56)*. These protective effects add to the value of PEDF as a therapeutic factor, as neurodegeneration is a common result of neovascular disease.

The conclusion that PEDF exerts neuroprotective effects in the nervous system and apoptosis in endothelial cells appears contradictory. How does PEDF intercept growth-promoting signals, accelerate cell death cascades, and prolong cellular life span? Does it use multiple receptors? Are there buried fragments within the PEDF protein that contain different biological activities? Does PEDF activate or permit crosstalk with parallel transduction cascades? Are there differential responses to activation of a single pathway? Could cellular diversity account for variation in response to PEDF? Are there developmentally regulated PEDF signals and responses? Are there developmentally regulated cues that would influence these signals and responses?

Unfortunately, a receptor for PEDF has not yet been identified to allow us to clearly address these questions. An 80-kDa PEDF binding protein has been detected on Y79, cerebellar granule cells, and the retina but whether this is a receptor for PEDF or an associated regulatory protein is still not clear *(57)*.

Although we are far from a comprehensive picture of how PEDF controls neuroprotective, differentiation, and cell death signals, examination of the molecules PEDF activates suggests three possible signaling modules: NFκB/AKT module, which is linked to neuroprotective signaling; the MAP kinase module, which is associated with cell differentiation and proliferation; and the caspase executioner module. In cerebellar granule cells, PEDF stimulates phosphorylation of IκB, leading to activation and translocation of NFκB to the nucleus. This results in a chain of sequential events that link the NFκB pathway to a defined extracellular signal and transcription of antiapoptotic and neuroprotective genes *(58)*. Whether the same pathways, or combination of pathways, are responsible for both the antiangiogenic and neuroprotective actions of PEDF has yet to be established.

It is worth noting that NFκB can also promote apoptosis by inducing FasL through binding regulatory motifs on FasL promoter and that VEGF can activate NFκB to promote cell survival by reducing caspase 8 death-promoting signals. The available data suggest that NFκB is a primary intracellular junction molecule used by PEDF (Fig. 3). However, cellular diversity and other extracellular signals may allow signal crosstalk between the NFκB cascade and other transduction pathways, or for cell-type specific gene activation responses.

The hierarchy of PEDF's action and signaling diversity could be influenced by other factors, such as lateral complementation through cooperative signaling ligands, receptors, pathways, and codes that cells use to generate diversity, as well as duration and intensity of the signal. In addition, different cell types may use various combinations of these mechanisms. Understanding how PEDF inhibits angiogenesis will certainly be labor-intensive but potentially rewarding, as it could elucidate upstream mechanisms of abnormal vessel growth in the eye and uncover other clinically relevant biological targets for ocular angiogenesis.

Summarizing the data presented above, we can conclude that PEDF facilitates cell movement into a quiescent phase of the cell cycle, aids in differentiation, protects neurons from damage, and blocks angiogenesis. It is possible that these actions reflect activation of a few key signaling molecules that receive input from a wide spectrum of normal and pathological stimuli.

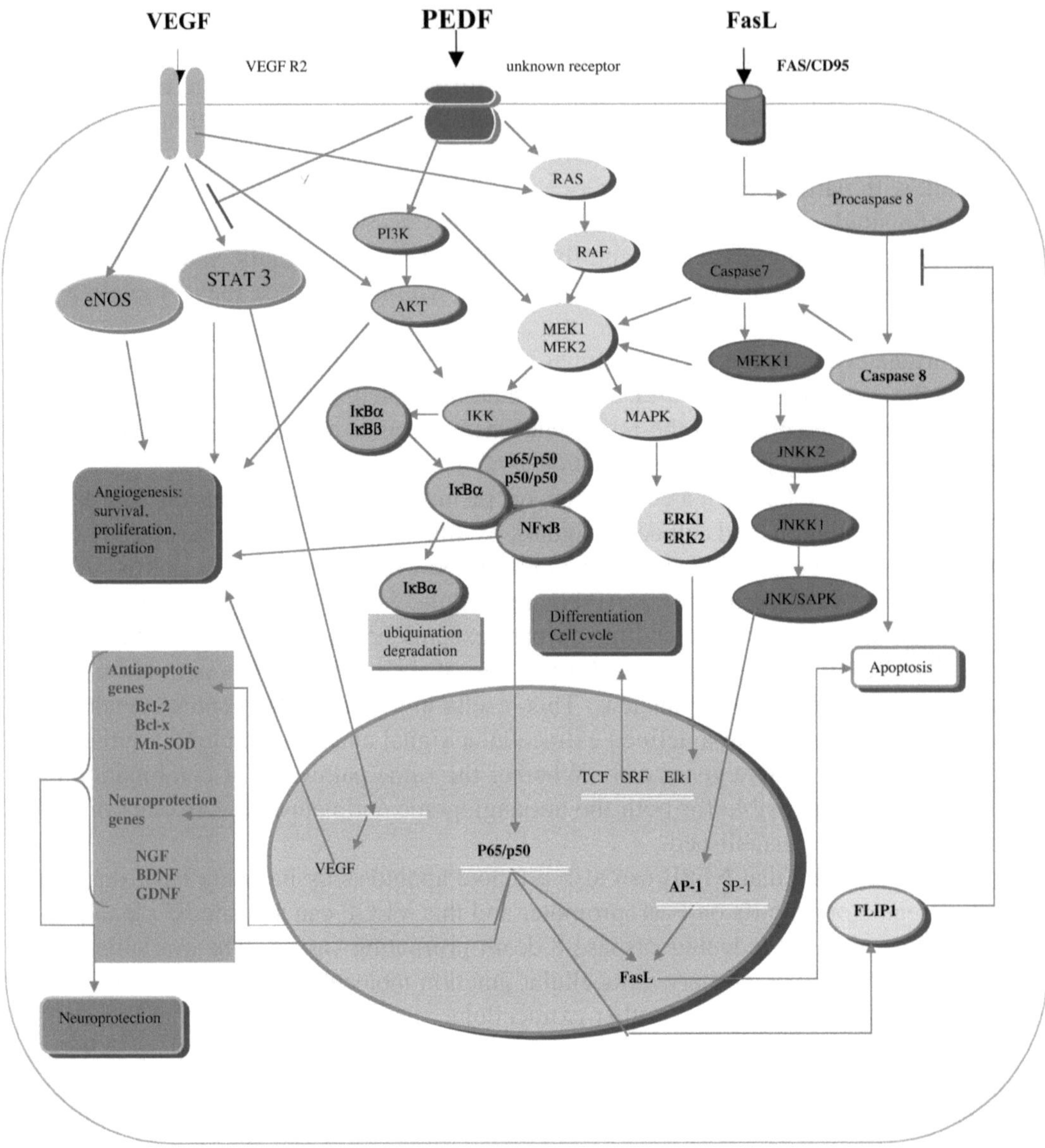

Fig. 3. Intracellular transduction pathways activated by pigment epithelium-derived factor (PEDF) and vascular endothelial growth factor (VEGF). *See* color version on companion CD.

STRUCTURE–FUNCTION RELATIONSHIPS OF PEDF

Our detailed knowledge of the structure of PEDF provides explanations for some of its observed properties and allows a rational design of PEDF-derived therapeutics.

We have recently identified the PEDFs from an additional eight species, bringing the total to 13 *(59)*. Alignment of all these sequences, which represent approx 300 million years of evolution, shows that PEDF has a highly conserved hydrophobic signal sequence and a single carbohydrate side chain, suggesting that its biological activity is tightly linked to its secretion and critical to life throughout evolution.

Based on the crystal structure of the 418 amino acid human PEDF protein *(59)*, we have identified several exposed peptides that are being tested for candidacy as strong PEDF mimetics. In the future, the chemistries of these peptides could be structurally altered to improve function and therapeutic delivery to replace the use of the entire protein.

There are two sites on PEDF for interactions with extracellular matrix molecules that may contribute to both the neurotrophic and antiangiogenic actions of PEDF. There is a concentration of aspartic and glutamic acid side chains in the N-terminal portion of the protein, which promote binding with high affinity to type I collagen and with lower affinity to type III collagen *(61,62)*. Low-affinity interactions between PEDF and heparin and other glycosaminoglycans have been found as well. These are probably mediated by a large surface rich in the basic amino acids, lysine and arginine *(60,63)*. Binding to heparin is critical for the activation and function of some serpins such as antithrombin *(64)* and interaction with other extracellular matrix components is important to the function of factors, such as the fibroblast growth factor (FGF) gene family.

PEDF is a member of the serpin gene family; its heparin-binding domain could be important to its antiangiogenic activity, especially because endothelial cells contain a significant amount of heparin sulfate on their surface. Whether these interactions with extracellular matrix components modulate the activity of PEDF or provide a local reservoir of functional PEDF that could be released under specific normal or pathological conditions is currently an area of research focus. Another possible mechanism of regulating PEDF activity is suggested by a recent report that extracellular phosphorylation of PEDF plays a key role in controlling both the antiangiogenic and the neuroprotective activities of PEDF *(65)*. Whether phosphorylation of the serine residues is a regulated process and responsive to pathogenic stimuli has yet to be shown.

The reactive center loop (RCL) of inhibitory serpins is an important structure of these proteins. It is known to interact and inactivate specific serine proteases, thereby controlling processes like inflammation, blood coagulation, and conformational diseases such as Parkinson's and Alzheimer's disease *(66,67)*. The PEDF RCL is conserved in evolution and is a prominent structure that extends from the molecule. Although its function is not yet elucidated, it is a prime target for interactions with diffusible factors and matrix molecules that could augment its function.

THERAPEUTIC POTENTIAL OF PEDF IN NEOVASCULAR EYE DISEASES

The development of effective antiangiogenic therapies must also take into consideration specificity of vascular targeting so that only new vessels deteriorate, while existing ones remain intact. Undesirable side effects such as hemorrhaging from existing vessels or inappropriate degradation of extracellular matrix surrounding normal tissues should be minimized. PEDF meets this criterion, as it has no known deleterious effect on mature vessels *(13)*.

One advantage to using endogenous antiangiogenic molecules, such as PEDF, to target new sprouting vessels is that they would not be expected to activate drug-resistance genes and thus may offer some of the most promising breakthroughs for effective long-term angiogenesis therapy. A further advantage of these molecules is that they are tolerated in the body and are unlikely to elicit an immunological response or produce the toxic side effects of synthetic inhibitors.

PEDF has the additional advantage of preserving neurons that are often damaged in vascular diseases of the nervous system. Its differentiation effect on cancer cells could also produce less-aggressive tumors and should be of additional therapeutic benefit in the treatment of neural malignancies.

The concentration of PEDF in the eye is near therapeutic levels *(14,28,31,68)*. Providing additional amounts of PEDF, however, is clearly beneficial in many of the disease models discussed above. It is possible that much of the PEDF detected in the eye is not available because it is present in an inactive conformation or bound to other molecules. Thus, therapeutic application of PEDF requires increasing its availability. There are three ways of doing this: increasing endogenous synthesis, supplying PEDF by gene transfer, and supplying PEDF protein or small peptides derived from it.

The expression of PEDF in the nervous system can be controlled by injury or oxygen tension, but the molecular mechanisms responsible for this are unknown. Müller cell PEDF secretion can be altered by hypoxia intraocular injection, which by itself is known to increase the levels of PEDF *(69,70)*. This has made interpretation of some studies problematic to interpret where other factors have been injected. An alternative approach is to use small molecules such as retinoic acid and dexamethasone, which can increase the expression of PEDF in a number of cell types *(10)*. It is possible that these, or related, molecules can be applied to the eye in noninvasive ways that increase endogenous PEDF expression. The PEDF promoter contains sites for other potential regulatory mechanisms, and it is likely that future work will identify additional ways of manipulating the transcription, translation, or secretion of this protein. One of the major sources of ocular PEDF is the ciliary epithelium. Many drugs used to control intraocular pressure are applied as eyedrops and can regulate ciliary epithelial function. Thus it is possible that compounds regulating PEDF expression in the ciliary epithelium could also be delivered as eyedrops.

As described above, and more fully in Chapter 20, PEDF DNA-mediated gene transfer experiments show short-term attenuation of up to 50% growth of blood vessels. Certain problems and risks to the individual are often encountered using current DNA-mediated gene transfer strategies. These include obtaining clinically effective viral titers, toxicity and immunogenicity due to the expression of viral genes, stable transgene expression in individuals requiring long-term treatment, and insertional mutagenesis by random viral integration into the host genome. Although continued development of improved viral vectors and better control of gene expression levels will overcome some of these problems, it is not clear that this is the most effective approach for long-term conditions with intermittent flare-up such as diabetic retinopathy or macular degeneration.

The problem with using the PEDF molecule as a therapeutic agent is that it is a 50-kDa protein. This creates difficulty in getting effective doses into the eye and in maintaining therapeutic levels over extended periods. There is growing evidence that peptide fragments of PEDF have substantial biological activity. Current evidence using peptide fragments suggests that separate regions of PEDF may carry out neuroprotective and antiangiogenic functions. Systematic mapping of functional regions of the PEDF molecule has not been completed and the minimal size of active peptides is not yet defined.

It may be possible to use small peptides as therapeutic agents; these could be formulated in slow release devises to provide protection over extended periods of time (*see* Chapter 22, this volume). The isolation of potent small PEDF peptides will also be important in defining the biology of responses initiated by PEDF and identifying other possible targets for antiangiogenic therapies.

With continued improvement in long-term ocular drug delivery systems, active mixtures of PEDF peptides offer a viable, and possibly better, approach to controlling chronic diseases that have neovascular episodes. It is likely that a truly effective antiangiogenic therapy will require a mixture of agents and adjunct strategies. Because of the potency and multifaceted properties of PEDF it is likely to become one of the key elements in any such cocktail.

Finally, although this article focuses on the utilization of PEDF to block angiogenesis, there are pathological conditions, such as ischemia-related heart diseases, where an increase in blood vessel growth may be desirable. Antagonists of PEDF would be more valuable, and possibly more subtle, than the strong promoters of angiogenesis currently being tested.

CONCLUSION

Naturally occuring antiangiogenic and neuroprotective factors will play a pivotal role in combating vascular diseases. The properties of PEDF make it a strong candidate gene to be tested in ocular antiangiogenic strategies. More important, the widespread tissue expression of PEDF suggests that it should also be tested against a wider range of angiogenic diseases, including tumors. It is crucial that we understand the biochemical pathways with which PEDF interacts so that we can maximize the therapeutic potential of this protein or its derivatives. With the increasing focus on PEDF activity in many tissues, its signaling mechanisms, structure–function analysis of the molecule, and the initiation of clinical trials, we should soon have a better understanding of the multifaceted nature of this protein and its application in neovascular eye diseases.

REFERENCES

1. Folkman J, D'Amore PA. Blood vessel formation: what is its molecular basis? Cell 1996;87:1153–1155.
2. Bikfalvi A, Bicknell R. Recent advances in angiogenesis, anti-angiogenesis and vascular targeting. Trends Pharmacol Sci 2002;23:576–582.
3. Folkman J. Role of angiogenesis in tumor growth and metastasis. Sem Oncol 2002;29:15–18.
4. Tombran-Tink J, Barnstable CJ. Therapeutic prospects for PEDF: more than a promising angiogenesis inhibitor. Trends Mol Med 2003;9:244–250.
5. Stalmans I, Ng YS, Rohan R, et al. Arteriolar and venular patterning in retinas of mice selectively expressing VEGF isoforms. J Clin Invest 2002;109:327–336.
6. Ishida S, Usui T, Yamashiro K, et al. VEGF164-mediated inflammation is required for pathological, but not physiological, ischemia-induced retinal neovascularization. J Exp Med 2003;198:483–489.
7. Tombran-Tink J, Johnson LV. Neuronal differentiation of retinoblastoma cells induced by medium conditioned by human RPE cells. Invest Opthalmol Vis Sci 1989;30:1700–1707.
8. Tombran-Tink J, Chader GG, Johnson LV. PEDF: a pigment epithelium derived factor with potent neuronal differentiative activity. Exp Eye Res 1991;53:411–414.

9. Tombran-Tink J, Barnstable CJ. PEDF: A multifaceted neurotrophic factor. Nat Rev Neurosci 2003;4:628–636.
10. Tombran-Tink J, Lara N, Apricio SE, et al. Retinoic acid and dexamethasone regulate the expression of PEDF in proliferating cells. Exp Eye Res 2004;78:945–955.
11. Tombran-Tink J, Mazaruk K, Chung D, Linker T, Chader GJ, Rodriguez I. Organization, evolutionary conservation, expression and unusual Alu density of the human gene for pigment epithelium-derived factor, a unique neurotrophic serpin. Mol Vis 1996;2:11.
12. Tombran-Tink J, Barnstable CJ. Osteoblasts and osteoclasts express PEDF, VEGF-A isoforms, and VEGF receptors: possible mediators of angiogenesis and matrix remodeling in the bone. Biochem Biophys Res Comm 2004;316:573–579.
13. Dawson DW, Volpert OV, Gillis P, et al. Pigment epithelium-derived factor: a potent inhibitor of angiogenesis. Science 1999;285:245–248.
14. Tombran-Tink J, Shivaram SM, Chader GJ, Johnson LV, Bok D. Expression,. secretion and age-related down regulation of pigment epithelium-derived factor, a serpin with neurotrophic activity. J Neurosci 1995;15:4992–5003.
15. Karakousis PC, John SK, Behling KC, et al. Localization of pigment epithelium derived factor (PEDF) in developing and adult human ocular tissues. Mol Vis 2001;7:154–163.
16. Quan GM, Ojaimi J, Nadesapillai AP, Zhou H, Choong PF. Resistance of epiphyseal cartilage to invasion by osteosarcoma is likely to be due to expression of antiangiogenic factors. Pathobiology 2002;70:361–367.
17. Palmieri D, Watson JM, Rinehart CA. Age-related expression of PEDF/EPC-1 in human endometrial stromal fibroblasts: implications for interactive senescence. Exp Cell Res 1999;247:142–147.
18. Mori K, Duh E, Gehlbach P, et al. Pigment epithelium-derived factor inhibits retinal and choroidal neovascularization. J Cell Physiol 2001;188:253–263.
19. Mori K, Gehlbach P, Ando A, McVey D, Wei L, Campochiaro PA. Regression of ocular neovascularization in response to increased expression of pigment epithelium-derived factor. Invest Ophthalmol Vis Sci 2002;43:2428–2434.
20. Raisler BJ, Berns KI, Grant MB, Beliaev D, Hauswirth WW. Adeno-associated virus type-2 expression of pigmented epithelium-derived factor or Kringles 1-3 of angiostatin reduce retinal neovascularization. Proc Natl Acad Sci USA 2002;99:8909–8914.
21. Auricchio A, Behling KC, Maguire AM, et al. Inhibition of retinal neovascularization by intraocular viral-mediated delivery of anti-angiogenic agents. Mol Ther 2002;6:490–494.
22. Mori K, Gehlbach P, Yamamoto S, et al. AAV-mediated gene transfer of pigment epithelium-derived factor inhibits choroidal neovascularization. Invest Ophthalmol Vis Sci 2002;43: 1994–2000.
23. Senger DR, Galli SJ, Dvorak AM, Perruzzi CA, Harvey VS, Dvorak HF. Tumor cells secrete a vascular permeability factor that promotes accumulation of ascites fluid. Science 1983;219:983–985.
24. Liu H, Ren JG, Cooper WL, Hawkins CE, Cowan MR, Tong PY. Identification of the antivasopermeability effect of pigment epithelium-derived factor and its active site. Proc Natl Acad Sci USA 2004;101:6605–6610.
25. Ohno-Matsui K, Morita I, Tombran-Tink J, et al. Novel mechanism for age-related macular degeneration: an equilibrium shift between the angiogenesis factors VEGF and PEDF. J Cell Physiol 2001;189:323–333.
26. Sawant S, Aparicio S, Tink AR, Lara N, Barnstable CJ, Tombran-Tink J. Regulation of factors controlling angiogenesis in liver development: a role for PEDF in the formation and maintenance of normal vasculature. Biochem Biophys Res Commun 2004;325:408–413.
27. Ogata N, Tombran-Tink J, Nishikawa M, et al. Pigment epithelium-derived factor in the vitreous is low in diabetic retinopathy and high in rhegmatogenous retinal detachment. Am J Ophthalmol 2001;132:378–382.

28. Spranger J, Osterhoff M, Reimann M, et al. Loss of the antiangiogenic pigment epithelium-derived factor in patients with angiogenic eye disease. Diabetes 2001;50:2641–2645.
29. Ogata N, Nishikawa M, Nishimura T, Mitsuma Y, Matsumura M. Inverse levels of pigment epithelium-derived factor and vascular endothelial growth factor in the vitreous of eyes with rhegmatogenous retinal detachment and proliferative vitreoretinopathy. Am J Ophthalmol 2002;133:851–852.
30. Holekamp NM, Bouck N, Volpert O. Pigment epithelium-derived factor is deficient in the vitreous of patients with choroidal neovascularization due to age-related macular degeneration. Am J Ophthalmol 2002;134:220–227.
31. Ogata N, Nishikawa M, Nishimura T, Mitsuma Y, Matsumura M. Unbalanced vitreous levels of pigment epithelium-derived factor and vascular endothelial growth factor in diabetic retinopathy. Am J Ophthalmol 2002;134:348–353.
32. Matsuoka M, Ogata N, Otsuji T, Nishimura T, Takahashi K, Matsumura M. Expression of pigment epithelium derived factor and vascular endothelial growth factor in choroidal neovascular membranes and polypoidal choroidal vasculopathy. Br J Ophthalmol 2004;88:809–815.
33. Lara N, Aparicio S, Sawant S, et al. PEDF regulates expression of VEGF-R2 and VEGF-R3 in the retina: A possible mechanism for controlling angiogenesis in the eye. (Submitted).
34. Hutchings H, Maitre-Boube M, Tombran-Tink J, Plouet J. Pigment epithelium-derived factor exerts opposite effects on endothelial cells of different phenotypes. Biochem Biophys Res Commun 2002;294:764–769.
35. Volpert OV, Zaichuk T, Zhou W, et al. Inducer-stimulated Fas targets activated endothelium for destruction by anti-angiogenic thrombospondin-1 and pigment epithelium-derived factor. Nat Med 2002;8:349–357.
36. Barreiro R, Schadlu R, Herndon J, et al. The role of Fas–FasL in the development and treatment of ischemic retinopathy. Invest Ophthalmol Vis Sci 2003;44:1282–1286.
37. Kataoka T, Budd RC, Holler N, et al. The caspase-8 inhibitor FLIP promotes activation of NF-κB and Erk signaling pathways. Curr Biol 2000;10:640–648.
38. Zaichuk TA, Shroff EH, Emmanuel R, Filleur S, Nelius T, Volpert OV. Nuclear factor of activated T cells balances angiogenesis activation and inhibition. J Exp Med 2004;199: 1513–1522.
39. Lanza RP, Cibelli JB, Blackwell C, et al. Extension of cell life-span and telomere length in animals cloned from senescent somatic cells. Science 2000;288:665–669.
40. Crawford SE, Stellmach V, Ranalli M, et al. Pigment epithelium-derived factor (PEDF) in neuroblastoma: a multifunctional mediator of Schwann cell antitumor activity. J Cell Sci 2001;114:4421–4428.
41. Li S, Chen Y, Wei H. Muscle pigment epithelium-derived factor gene associating with tumorigenesis of B16 melanoma. Chinese J Pathol 2001;30:281–284.
42. Guan M, Yam HF, Su B, et al. Loss of pigment epithelium derived factor expression in glioma progression. J Clin Pathol 2003;56:277–282.
43. Mahtabifard A, Merritt RE, Yamada RE, Crystal RG, Korst RJ. In vivo gene transfer of pigment epithelium-derived factor inhibits tumor growth in syngeneic murine models of thoracic malignancies. J Thorac Cardiovasc Surg 2003;126:28–38.
44. Abe R, Shimizu T, Yamagishi S, et al. Overexpression of pigment epithelium-derived factor decreases angiogenesis and inhibits the growth of human malignant melanoma cells in vivo. Am J Pathol 2004;164:1225–1232.
45. Garcia M, Fernandez-Garcia NI, Rivas V, et al. Inhibition of xenografted human melanoma growth and prevention of metastasis development by dual antiangiogenic/antitumor activities of pigment epithelium-derived factor. Cancer Res 2004;64:5632–5642.
46. Wang L, Schmitz V, Perez-Mediavilla A, Izal I, Prieto J, Qian C. Suppression of angiogenesis and tumor growth by adenoviral-mediated gene transfer of pigment epithelium-derived factor. Mol Ther 2003;8:72–79.

47. Matsumoto K, Ishikawa H, Nishimura D, Hamasaki K, Nakao K, Eguchi K. Antiangiogenic property of pigment epithelium-derived factor in hepatocellular carcinoma. Hepatology 2004;40:252–259.
48. Uehara H, Miyamoto M, Kato K, et al. Expression of pigment epithelium-derived factor decreases liver metastasis and correlates with favorable prognosis for patients with ductal pancreatic adenocarcinoma. Cancer Res 2004;64:3533–3537.
49. Doll JA, Stellmach VM, Bouck NP, et al. Pigment epithelium-derived factor regulates the vasculature and mass of the prostate and pancreas. Nat Med 2003;9:774–780.
50. Cao W, Tombran-Tink J, Chen W, Mrazek D, Elias R, McGinnis JF. Pigment epithelium-derived factor protects cultured retinal neurons against hydrogen peroxide-induced cell death. J Neurosci Res 1999;57:789–800.
51. Cao W, Tombran-Tink J, Elias R, Sezate S, Mrazek D, McGinnis JF. In vivo protection of photoreceptors from light damage by pigment epithelium-derived factor. Invest Ophthalmol Vis Sci 2001;42:1646–1652.
52. Jablonski MM, Tombran-Tink J, Mrazek DA, Iannaccone A. Pigment epithelium-derived factor supports normal development of photoreceptor neurons and opsin expression after retinal pigment epithelium removal. J Neurosci 2000;20:7149–7157.
53. Ogata N, Wang L, Jo N, et al. Pigment epithelium derived factor as a neuroprotective agent against ischemic retinal injury Curr Eye Res 2001;22:245–252.
54. Taniwaki T, Hirashima N, Becerra SP, Chader GJ, Etcheberrigaray R, Schwartz JP. Pigment epithelium-derived factor protects cultured cerebellar granule cells against glutamate-induced neurotoxicity. J Neurochem 1997;68:26–32.
55. DeCoster MA, Schabelman E, Tombran-Tink J, Bazan NG. Neuroprotection by pigment epithelial-derived factor against glutamate toxicity in developing primary hippocampal neurons. J Neurosci Res 1999;56:604–610.
56. Bilak MM, Corse AM, Bilak SR, Lehar M, Tombran-Tink J, Kuncl RW. Pigment epithelium-derived factor (PEDF) protects motor neurons from chronic glutamate-mediated neurodegeneration. J Neuropathol Exp Neurol 1999;58:719–728.
57. Alberdi E, Aymerich MS, Becerra SP. Binding of pigment epithelium-derived factor (PEDF) to retinoblastoma cells and cerebellar granule neurons. Evidence for a PEDF receptor. J Biol Chem 1999;274:31,605–31,612.
58. Yabe T, Wilson D, Schwartz JP. NFkappaB activation is required for the neuroprotective effects of pigment epithelium-derived factor (PEDF) on cerebellar granule neurons. J Biol Chem 2001;276:43,313–43,319.
59. Tombran-Tink J, Aparicio S, Xu X, et al. PEDF and the serpins: phylogeny, sequence conservation, and functional domains. J Structural Biol 2005;151:130–150.
60. Simonovic M, Gettins PG, Volz K. Crystal structure of human PEDF, a potent anti-angiogenic and neurite growth-promoting factor. Proc Natl Acad Sci USA 2001;98:11,131–11,135.
61. Kozaki K, Miyaishi O, Koiwai O, et al. Isolation, purification, and characterization of a collagen-associated serpin, caspin, produced by murine colon adenocarcinoma cells. J Biol Chem 1998;273:15,125–15,130.
62. Meyer C, Notari L, Becerra SP. Mapping the type I collagen-binding site on pigment epithelium-derived factor. Implications for its antiangiogenic activity. J Biol Chem 2002;277:45,400–45,407.
63. Alberdi E, Hyde CC, Becerra SP. Pigment epithelium-derived factor (PEDF) binds to glycosaminoglycans: analysis of the binding site. Biochemistry 1998;37:10,643–10,652.
64. Whisstock JC, Pike RN, Jin L, et al. Conformational changes in serpins: II. The mechanism of activation of antithrombin by heparin. J Mol Biol 2000;301:1287–1305.
65. Maik-Rachline G, Shaltiel S, Seger R. Extracellular phosphorylation converts pigment epithelium-derived factor from a neurotrophic to an antiangiogenic factor. Blood 2005;105:670–678.

66. Pike RN, Bottomley SP, Irving JA, Bird PI, Whisstock JC. Serpins: finely balanced conformational traps. IUBMB Life 2002;54:1–7.
67. Lomas DA, Carrell RW. Serpinopathies and the conformational dementias. Nat Rev Genet 2004;3:759–768.
68. Wu YQ, Becerra SP. Proteolytic activity directed toward pigment epithelium-derived factor in vitreous of bovine eyes. Implications of proteolytic processing. Invest Ophthalmol Vis Sci 1996;37:1984–1993.
69. Eichler W, Yafai Y, Wiedemann P, Reichenbach A. Angiogenesis-related factors derived from retinal glial (Muller) cells in hypoxia. Neuroreport 2004;15:1633–1637.
70. Stitt AW, Graham D, Gardiner TA. Ocular wounding prevents pre-retinal neovascularization and upregulates PEDF expression in the inner retina. Mol Vis 2004;10:432–438.

14
Thrombospondin
Guarding the Clear View

Arin Aurora and Olga V. Volpert, PhD

CONTENTS

INTRODUCTION

A number of isolated studies clearly point to the contribution of thrombospondin-1 and related proteins to the regulation of angiogenesis in disparate eye compartments. Surprisingly there has been no attempt to systematically review this information and to summarize these proteins' role in ocular angiogenesis. The goal of this chapter is to provide a unified view of their function as a part of complex defense mechanism protecting vascular stasis in the eye.

THROMBOSPONDINS: STRUCTURE, FUNCTION, MECHANISMS

The thrombospondin (TSP) family encompasses five proteins, TSPs 1 through 5, with TSP5 frequently called cartilage oligomeric protein (COMP). TSPs are multimeric multidomain glycoproteins; they function at the cell surface and as matrix components (matricellular proteins). The complexity of TSPs is striking: Multiple functions conferred by their structurally diverse domains dictate an extremely complex biology.

TSPs are divided in two subfamilies: A includes trimers TSP1 and 2 *(1–3)* and B encompasses pentameric TSPs 3–5, whose members lack the procollagen homology region and type 1 repeats but have unique N-terminal regions *(2–5)* (Fig. 1).

Main Structural Determinants

TSP sequences are most homologous in the type 2 and 3 repeats and the C-terminal domain, the hallmark of TSPs (Fig. 1) (82% identity in group A and 60% identity between the groups). The type 1 (properdin) repeats, on the other hand, are found

From: *Ophthalmology: Ocular Angiogenesis: Diseases, Mechanisms, and Therapeutics*
Edited by: J. Tombran-Tink and C. J. Barnstable © Humana Press Inc., Totowa, NJ

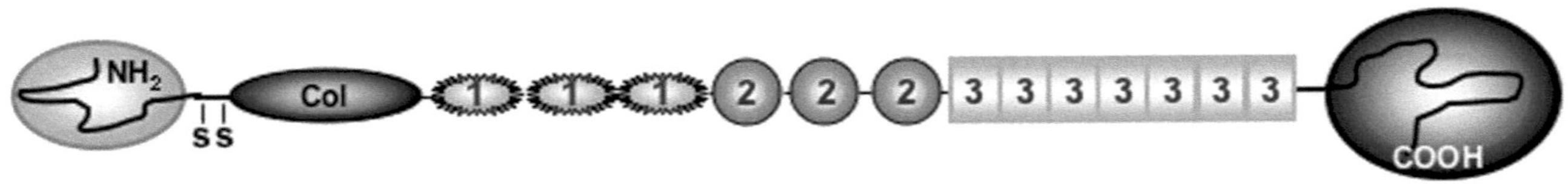

Domain	N-ter	O proCollagen	Type 1 repeats (TSR)	Type 2 repeats	Type 3 repeats	Ca binding domain
Motifs	BBXB	GVITRIR	GVITRIR CSVTCG KRFK		RGD	RFYMVVWK
Interactions	Decorin Fibrinogen Syndecan/HSPG LRP Integrin $\alpha_3\beta_1$	Oligomerization	Collagen V Fibronectin TGF-β Laminin MMP2 CD36 HSPG	Plasminogen Fibrinogen β1 integrins	Ca^{2+} Cathepsin D Elastase Integrin $\alpha_V\beta_3$ Integrin $\alpha_{II}\beta_3$	CD47 105/80kDa
Function	Cell attachment Cell spreading Cell migration Proliferation Disassembly of focal adhesions Platelet aggregation Endocytosis		Cell attachment Cell-matrix interations Neurite outgrowth Endothelial functions: Inhibit migration, proliferation, angiogenesis Induces apoptosis Immune deviation		Cell attachment Cell spreading Protease inhibition	Cell attachment Cell proliferation Smooth muscle cell proliferation T-cell activation Platelet aggregation Immune deviation

Fig. 1. Thrombospondin (TSP)1 structural elements, their partners, receptors, and functional importance. *See* color version on companion CD.

in evolutionarily and structurally diverse proteins unified into the thrombospondin type 1 repeat (TSR) superfamily, which likely emerged late in evolution by exon shuffling in group A (reviewed in ref. *6*).

N- and C-terminal globular TSP domains are connected by a flexible stalk *(7–10)*, which stretches upon calcium depletion *(11)*. The procollagen region is involved in trimer assembly and folds as a compact monomer stabilized by disulfide bonds *(12)*. In type 1 repeats, antiparallel β-sheets form ellipsoids *(13)*, type 2 (EGF) repeats are globular *(14)*, and type 3 repeats form a rod unit *(15)*. In TSP1 the type 3 repeats form a common globular structure with the C-terminal domain *(11)*.

Type 3 repeats recruit multiple Ca^{2+} ions *(2)*, an average of 35 Ca^{2+} per TSP1 molecule *(16)*. Calcium binding confers conformational changes, which alter physical properties, sensitivity to proteolysis, and adhesion potency of TSPs. TSPs bind heparin *(7)* via a high-affinity heparin-binding motif BBXB in the N-terminal domain and the lower affinity sites in type 1 repeats, which vary between the differentially glycosylated forms *(17,18)*.

General Functions

Attachment

TSP binds to the matrix components, proteases, cytokines, and growth factors (Fig. 1). For some of these interactions critical motifs have been mapped in TSP1 domains and repeats. TSP1 binding frequently modifies the behavior of binding partners, e.g., it lowers activities of thrombin, plasmin, cathepsin G, and elastase, and improves the activity of plasminogen activator inhibitor *(19)*.

TSPs support cell attachment in a Ca^{2+}-dependent manner: All four regions of the 180-kDa TSP1 subunit carry interaction motifs for distinct adhesion receptors (Fig. 1). The repertoire of TSP1 adhesion receptors, which combine and cooperate to stabilize attachment, spreading, and cytoskeletal reorganizations, ultimately determines cell fate (motility, proliferation, and survival) *(20,21)*. For instance, endothelial cell attachment is mediated by the RGD motif, whose availability is determined by the disulfide bond pattern in the type 3 repeats, which, in turn, is regulated by protein disulfide isomerase (PDI) *(22)*. Thus only PDI-secreting cells are capable of RGD-dependent attachment on TSP1 and 2 *(20)*.

Development

The essential functions of TSP1 and TSP2 appear nonredundant. Mice null for TSP1 or TSP2 show normal development and fertility and only partial overlap in their respective sets of abnormalities *(23,24)*. TSP1 knockouts display higher embryonal lethality, spinal lordosis, early pneumonia, and increase in circulating monocytes. TSP2 nulls have lax tendons, fragile skin, and high bone density. Both TSP1 and TSP2 nulls show higher vascularization in select tissues and altered wound healing *(24,25)*.

Angiogenesis

TSP1 was the first identified natural protein inhibitor of angiogenesis *(26)*, with this activity shared by TSP2 *(27)*. Studies of the knockout mice revealed no major changes in the vascular development; however, TSP1 and TSP2 null mice show increased vascularity in the nonidentical sets of tissues *(23,24,28)*. In contrast, both proteins are important in wound healing: angiogenesis is increased in skin wounds of both TSP1 and TSP2 nulls, while vascularization of the granulation tissue is delayed *(24,25)*. TSP1 transgene targeted to the basal skin keratinocytes causes healing delays of the full-thickness excision wounds owing to the impaired endothelial cell proliferation and migration toward the granulation site. TSP1 overexpression also disrupts the normal increase in vessel size/density in healing wounds *(29)*.

Tumor Growth

Forced reintroduction of TSP1 or TSP2 inhibits the growth of diverse tumors—a secondary effect due to the angiogenesis blockade *(30–34)*. TSP decreases both the size and number of tumor capillaries. TSP1 and TSP2 affect different stages of angiogenesis: TSP1 is more effective in blocking endothelial cell migration and corneal angiogenesis *(27)*, whereas TSP2 is more potent at inhibiting tumor growth in the mouse model. The combination of TSP1 and TSP2 completely inhibits tumor growth *(30)*, also pointing to distinct molecular targets.

TSP Molecular Pathways

TSP1 conformational flexibility, variability of the expression profiles, and activity of the TSP1 receptors cause a staggering complexity of the cell-type specificity of functional effects and cell surface interactions. TSP1 molecular mechanisms have been defined for specific cell types and the deductions for other cell types could be made only with caution.

Active Motifs

Complexity of TSP organization impedes the search for active epitopes conferring antiangiogenic activity. Antiangiogenic TSP1 and TSP2 share N-terminal heparin-binding domain (HBD) *(35)*, a coiled-coil that dictates trimer assembly and contains cysteines that form the internal disulfide bonds; a cysteine-rich procollagen-like sequence, 3 type I (TSR or properdin) repeats similar to domains of complement proteins C6-9 and ADAM-TS proteases; 3 type II (EGF) repeats; 7 calcium-binding type III repeats; and a C-terminal globular domain *(1,6)* (Fig. 1). TSP1 stalk, a 50/70-kDa proteolytic fragment, contains procollagen domain, the type I and II repeats, and is sufficient to inhibit angiogenesis *(36)*. Recombinant TSP1 type I repeats block epithelial cell (EC) proliferation and angiogenesis, whereas recombinant HBD interferes with the endothelial cell proliferation *(37,38)*. In contrast, TSP1 N- and C-terminal domains stimulate EC migration and angiogenesis *(39–41)*.

Screening of synthetic peptides detected inhibitory activity in the TSP1 procollagen domain and in the type I repeats *(36)* (Fig. 1). CSVTCG motif in type 1 repeats has been shown to bind to CD36, a molecule deemed as a TSP1 antiangiogenic receptor. Further studies implicated an adjacent motif, GVITRIR also present in the antiangiogenic procollagen domain, as a true active region, and CSVTCG as a sequence complementing its activity *(42,43)*. WXXWXXW, another antiangiogenic sequence in type 1 repeats, blocks only basic fibroplast growth factor (bFGF)-induced vascularization, whereas GVITRIR inhibits angiogenesis by multiple stimuli *(44)*. D-enantiomers of the peptides containing GVITRIR motif, with increased conformational stability are especially potent *(45–47)*.

Receptors and Binding Proteins (summarized in Fig. 1)

The best-characterized receptor for TSP antiangiogenic signals is CD36, a member of the scavenger receptor B family *(48,49)*. TSP1 inhibitory peptides and fragments bind recombinant CD36, and CD36 neutralizing antibodies and soluble fragments block angiosuppresion by TSP1 *(43)*. Stimulatory antibodies and other CD36 ligands mimic TSP1 effects on EC. CD36-negative EC and CD36-null mice are refractory to the angiosuppression by TSP1, whereas cell sensitivity is restored by CD36 reexpression *(43,50)*. The plasma protein, histidine-rich glycoprotein (HRGP), binds TSP1 at the same site as CD36, and sequesters TSP1 from CD36 interaction *(51)*. Thus HRGP may attenuate TSP1 activity in the pathological situations, where plasma leakage is common. The outcomes of systemic TSP treatments may also depend on HRGP levels in circulation.

TSP1 also directly binds and sequesters bFGF, thus neutralizing its proangiogenic activity *(52)*. TSP1 and TSP2 blockade of bFGF prosurvival activity is poroportional to bFGF sequestration. However, VEGF receptor activation is not TSP-sensitive *(53)*.

TSP binds and activates TGF-β1, another angiogenesis mediator: the WSXW motif binds latent precursor protein, whereas the KRFK sequence between the first and second type I repeats is necessary for the activation *(54)*. TSP2 contains the WSXW motif but not the KRFK sequence, and thus binds but not activates TGF-β1 in vitro *(55)*. Again, the complexity of TGF-β1 role in angiogenesis renders accurate predictions regarding the TSP/TGF interactions nearly impossible.

TSP1 and TSP2 binding to serine proteases and matrix metalloproteinases (MMPs) may affect the proteolytic events in angiogenesis, basement membrane degradation, growth factor mobilization, and release of the cryptic fragments of matrix components. TSP2 binds and directs MMP2 to the endocytosis receptor, LRP1 *(56)*. Lack of TSP2 causes excess MMP2, thus decreasing adhesion. MMP2 attenuation by TSP2 may also block angiogenesis; as MMP2 deficiency impairs angiogenesis in healing wounds and in tumor xenografts *(57)*. In TSP2-null mice, increased vascularity of sponge implants is concomitant with MMP2 increase *(58)*. TSP1 blockade of MMP9 opposes the release of matrix-bound VEGF *(59)*.

Other endothelial receptors may participate in the angiosuppression by TSP1 and 2. Type III repeats contain RGD motif required for the binding to the integrin $\alpha_v\beta_3$, which supports endothelial cell adhesion to TSP1 *(24)*. Although the role of TSP1–$\alpha_v\beta_3$ interaction in angiostasis is not proven, it is feasible, as $\alpha_v\beta_3$ engagement by another angiogenesis inhibitor, tumstatin, causes endothelial cell apoptosis *(60)*.

Some of the TSP1 receptors are proangiogenic. Unlike soluble TSP1, immobilized TSP1 stimulates proliferation of bovine aortic endothelial cells. This activity maps to the N-terminal amino acids 190–201, which bind integrin $\alpha_3\beta_1$ *(61)*. Another site (amino acids 17–31), binds cell surface calreticulin, and might prime endothelial cell migration by disrupting focal contacts *(62,63)*. The TSP1 N-terminal 25-kDa fragment contains both these sites, and promotes endothelial migration and corneal angiogenesis via a nonspecified receptor *(41)*.

Finally, C-terminal domains of TSP1 and TSP2 contain binding sites for the integrin-associated protein IAP/CD47, a G protein-coupled receptor, which associates with $\alpha_v\beta_3$ and $\alpha_2\beta_1$ integrins. The IAP binding site of TSP1 (4N1K) can be both stimulatory and inhibitory. It inhibits tube formation but not proliferation of immortalized mouse

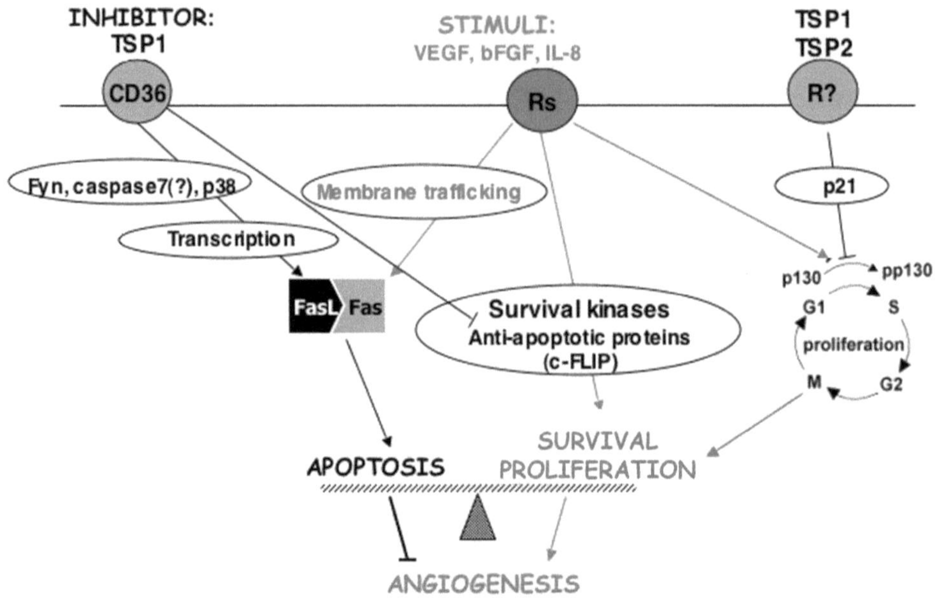

Fig. 2. Thrombospondin signaling pathways in quiescent and active endothelium. *See* color version on companion CD.

brain endothelium *(64)*. The same peptide stimulates EC adhesion and migration and proangiogenic effect of high TSP1 concentrations has been attributed to the low-affinity IAP binding *(39)*.

TSP1 activates TGF-β1 via the KRFK epitope. This TSP1 function determines similarities between TGF-β1 and TSP1-null mice including pneumonia and abnormal vascularization of the lung and pancreas *(64a)*. Treatment with KRFK peptide increases TGF-β1 activity and largely restores TSP1 knockouts to the wild-type phenotype. Conversely, treatment of the wild-type mice with LSKL, a peptide from TGF-β1 latent active peptide, which disrupts TGF-β1 activation, causes lung abnormalities similar to those in TSP1-nulls *(65)*. Thus TSP1 serves as a dominant activator of TGF-β1, and therefore a modifier of the epithelial homeostasis and immune response.

Signaling Events

Multiple studies implicated TSP1/CD36 complexes in the killing of the microvascular endothelium, and delineate the ensuing signaling pathways (Fig. 1). TSP1 binding promotes recruitment of the Src kinase p59fyn to CD36 *(50)* and subsequent phosphorylation of p38 and Jun N-terminal kinases (JNKs). Both JNK and p38 are required for the apoptosis by TSP1 *(50,66)*. p38 activation enhances transcription of the cell surface proapoptotic molecule CD95(Fas)L, which ligates CD95(Fas) death receptor to activate caspases, DNA fragmentation, and apoptosis *(67)* (Fig. 2).

Several studies demonstrate that TSP1, its fragments, and its peptides induce apoptosis in the activated EC *(45,50,68)*. Recent studies show that although they are protective at high concentrations, several growth factors at low concentration range render endothelial cells susceptible to apoptosis by TSP1 *(53,67)*. Low doses of growth factors (vascular endothelial growth factor [VEGF], bFGF and interleukin-8 [IL-8]) potentiate TSP1-dependent endothelial apoptosis by inducing CD95 translocation from the intracellular pool in Golgi complexes to the cell surface. Caspase inhibitors relieve TSP1 inhibition of angiogenesis, pointing to an essential role of apoptosis in this process *(50)*.

Recent findings identify the divergence between TSP proapoptotic and antiproliferative mechanisms (Fig. 2). Protective levels of the angiogenic stimuli, including VEGF, fail to restore proliferation of the endothelial cells arrested at G1/S transition by TSP1 or TSP2. Not surprisingly, cell cycle arrest due to TSP is not relieved by broad spectrum caspase inhibitor *(53)*. Antiproliferative events by TSP1 and TSP2 include p21-driven inhibition of Rb and homolog p130 phosphorylation by the proangiogenic VEGF *(69)*.

Mechanosensitive Signaling

TSP1 is a unique function mechanosensitive death mediator. Vascular endothelium undergoes apoptosis in the absence of flow (cessation of hemodynamic force)—a mechanism for the removal of irrelevant vasculature *(70)*. Mechanical stimuli and apoptosis are linked via an autocrine loop between TSP1 and $\alpha_v\beta_3$ integrin/IAP receptor complex *(71,72)*. The lack of flow causes a concomitant increase in secreted TSP1 and surface IAP by confluent endothelial monolayer, whereas $\alpha_v\beta_3$ is expressed constitutively, regardless of the flow conditions. An RGD motif binds to the $\alpha_v\beta_3$, whereas another motif, CBD, recruits IAP and the resulting ternary complex initiates an apoptotic cascade *(71)*. TSP1, the only known protein carrying both RGD and CBD, is therefore a sole mediator of the vascular remodeling in response to flow conditions.

GUARDING OCULAR FUNCTION

Angiogenesis in Eye Pathology

The role of TSPs in the eye is controversial and has not been systematically pursued. However, several interesting leads have emerged in the past decades.

Proper eye function, reception, and transmission of the visual signals determine stringent control of the vascular patterning in this complex tissue. It is obvious that the light-transmitting areas, the cornea and the lens, have to remain free of capillaries. Wound repair is normally dependent on the vasculature of the damaged tissue. However, the transparent structures of the eye (e.g., central cornea, lens, vitreous) remain avascular during repair and fibrosis. Even ophthalmic scars in the cornea remain avascular.

In contrast, the light-receiving retina contains photoreceptor neurons whose viability is impossible without proper nutrition and oxygenation ensured by an adequate vascular supply. However, an extremely complex cellular architecture of the retina with its multiple layers of cells with distinct and mutually dependent functions cannot be disrupted by erratic capillary expansion. Thus intraretinal and subretinal (choroidal) capillaries, albeit necessary, should remain in stasis. Undesired expansion of the vasculature in the retina and choroid is linked to multiple vision disorders, such as retinopathies, vitreopathies, macular degeneration, and glaucoma *(73–75)*.

Positive and Negative Angiogenic Mediators in the Eye

Steady-state angiogenesis, as that described in the eye, requires tight regulation via multiple, possibly redundant, control elements.

Vascular expansion in the developing eye is dependent on VEGF, a ubiquitous and multifunctional inducer of angiogenesis *(75)*. In the adult eye the presence of stimulatory VEGF supports the viability of existing endothelium as well as vascular integrity: Exposure to hyperoxia decreases VEGF in adult mouse retina while increasing endothelial cell apoptosis and causing irreversible damage to the retinal vasculature *(76)*. Increased VEGF production has been documented in the majority of patients with retinopathies and macular degeneration *(77,78)*.

The molecule mainly vaunted as a VEGF antiangiogenic counterpart is pigment epithelium-derived factor (PEDF). Depletion of PEDF from the cornea, corneal extracts, and vitreous fluid reveals underlying proangiogenic activity, which is largely due to VEGF *(79,80)*. The disturbances of the VEGF/PEDF ratio, rather than each of these factors alone, seem to determine the course of vascular abnormalities in the eye *(81–83)*.

In the embryonic eye retina PEDF expression is low at the early, prevascular stages of eye development; it increases gradually and reaches maximum when the vasculature is fully developed *(80)*. VEGF, on the other hand, appears to decrease once the vasculature has been formed *(75)*. Thus, again, in eye development the ratio between proangiogenic VEGF and its antiangiogenic partner, PEDF, appears to balance the fate and pattern of vascular formation *(84)*.

Nevertheless, the spectrum of the angiogenesis inhibitors and stimuli in the eye is not limited to VEGF and PEDF; the angiogenic balance in the eye is considerably more complex. Multiple effectors of angiogenesis have been detected in ocular fluids and tissues. The inducers include, but are not limited to, stimulatory (IL-6), IL-8, insulin-like growth factor (IGF)-1, IGF-2, and bFGF *(85–91)* and inhibitory secreted protein acidic and rich in cysteine (SPARC), cryptic angioinhibitory fragments angiostatin and endostatin, and multiple thrombospondins *(92–95)*. Although none of these has been explored in the same depth as was the VEGF/PEDF equation, their presence is consistent with the idea of multiple and at least partially redundant mechanisms controlling proper vascularization of the ocular tissues.

Thrombospondin Expression Pattern

TSP is expressed by multiple cell types in the eye (Fig. 3A), including ocular pigment epithelial cells, corneal endothelium, and stromal fibroblasts. It is constitutively found at high levels in the aqueous humor *(96,97)*. TSP1 immunoreactivity localizes to the epithelial basement membrane, posterior Descemet's membrane, and endothelium of human and bovine cornea. In normal corneal endothelium TSP1 staining is localized to the basement membrane in a characteristic punctate pattern. After a circular freeze injury the epithelial cells (ECs) surrounding the injury zone express significantly higher TSP1 levels for at least 48 h. TSP1 is also localized at the tracks of EC migration into the wound site, where it is thought to assist migration along the natural basement membrane *(98)*.

The bulk of the corneal stroma, stromal fibroblasts (keratocytes), and the anterior part of Descemet's membrane are devoid of TSP1. Consistent with TSP1's role in attachment, immunogold labeling shows focal TSP1 deposits on the membranes of corneal EC and basal epithelial cells *(99)*. Reverse transcription-polymerase chain reaction (RT-PCR)

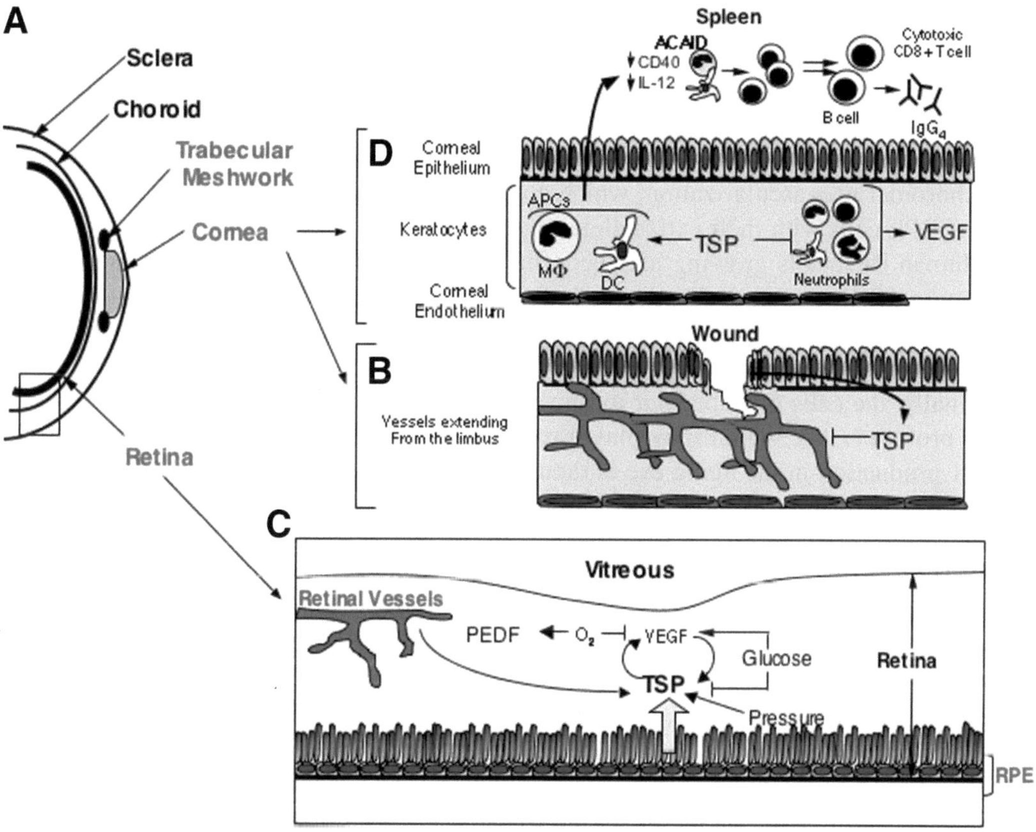

Fig. 3. Thrombospondin (TSP) in the eye, the role and regulation. **(A)** Schematic representation of the eye tissues. The tissues and compartment where TSP affects angiogenesis are shown. **(B)** Thrombospondin protects corneal angiostasis: Wounded (proliferating) corneal epithelium secretes increased TSP1 levels, thus preventing vascularization of the cornea. **(C)** Thrombospondin: the sources and regulatory influences in the retina. TSP generated by the retinal pigment epithelium (RPE) cells ensures angiostasis in adult retina. Its expression is linked with vascular endothelial growth factor (VEGF) via positive feedback loop: hypoxia-driven VEGF increase upregulates TSP1 levels, which compensate for the downregulation of antiangiogenic pigment epithelium-derived factor (PEDF). TSP-dependent delay in vascularization augments ischemia, which contributes to the VEGF production. TSP is negatively regulated by glucose levels, possible contributing to the progression of diabetic retinopathy. TSP is increased by increased pressure; this increase may reduce cellularity of the trabecular meshwork in glaucoma patients. **(D)** The role of thrombospondin in immune privilege of the cornea: TSP1 tethers and activates TGF-β on the antigen-presenting cells (APCs) by binding CD36 and latent transforming growth factor-β precursor via GVITRIR and KRFK sequences. Both APCs and T cells express another TSP1 receptor, CD47, which diverts them from a normal immune response. FasL increase on corneal endothelium due toTSP1 expedites elimination of the infiltrating T cells. *See* color version on companion CD.

analysis revealed the mRNA for TSP1, TSP2, and TSP3 but not for TSP4 or TSP5 in keratocytes of the healing corneal wounds. Normal cornea contains mRNA for TSP1 but not for other family members; however, the keratocytes stain positive for TSP1, TSP2, and TSP3 only in repairing, and not in the normal adult human cornea *(100,101)*.

The retinal pigment epithelium (RPE) is a monolayer of polarized cells localized between retinal photoreceptors and blood vessels of the choroid. The basal surface of the RPE cells rests on Bruch's membrane, a complex extracellular matrix structure, involved in several disease processes, including age-related macular degeneration (AMD). Ruptures or abnormalities in Bruch's membrane are frequently accompanied by choroidal neovascularization, which could be aggravated by disturbed interactions of the RPE cells with their extracellular matrix.

Human RPE cells growing in subconfluent monolayers express TSP1 message and maintain TSP1 secretion. Human retinal tissue strongly stains for TSP1 in the RPE and patchily on some parts of Bruch's membrane, whereas the neuroretina, choroid, and sclera are TSP1-negative *(97)*.

Finally, the cells of trabecular meshwork express a thrombospondin-like cytoadhesion protein *(102)*, which may play a role in cell attachment at this site. Decreased TSP1 production in the aging eye is thought to contribute to a decreased cellularity of trabecular meshwork as a result of poor attachment *(103)*.

Function in the Cornea

The roles of TSP1 and TSP2, both abundant in the cornea and in the iris stroma, appear nonredundant when it comes to the control of physiological angiogenesis in the cornea *(104)*. Ectopic TSP1 is more potent in blocking bFGF-induced angiogenesis in the rat and mouse cornea *(27,104)*. Apparently, TSPs 1 and 2 are nonessential for the establishing of the corneal angiogenic privilege, as the corneas of mice null for both TSP1 and TSP2 are normal and avascular. On the other hand, the lack of TSP1 and TSP2 increases vessel incidence in the iris stroma. Both TSPs are important in suppressing postdevelopmental angiogenesis in the cornea: Angiogenesis induced by suturing is greater in TSP nulls than in wild-type animals. Consistent with the differences in TSP1 and TSP2 signaling mechanisms, their roles appear to be only partly redundant: Constitutive angiogenesis in the iris is greater in TSP2 nulls, whereas suture-induced, inflammatory angiogenesis is more prominent in TSP1 knockouts *(27,104)*. Thus it is possible that during development vascular privilege of the cornea relies on PEDF, whereas thrombospondins are crucial components of the maintenance system, which ensures the avascularity of the adult cornea.

In skin wounds TSP1 comes exclusively from the platelet α-granules. In the corneal wounds, where platelet availability is limited by the lack of vascularization, TSP1 is generated locally, by the corneal epithelium *(105)*. TSP1 expression is enhanced in the cornea, wounded either by abrasion or by laser treatment *(106)*. The increase is detectable on the wounded surface as early as 30 min postabrasion and persists until reepithelialization is complete. The TSP1 mRNA level is increased in the wounded corneas as much as three-fold compared with background control *(107)*. TSP1 increase in the corneal epithelial wounds is probably responsible for the vascular privilege in adults. The expression of TSP1 in the wounded area also has an indirect angioinhibitory effect by promoting reepithelialization and thus reducing the duration of inflammatory response and inflammation-associated angiogenesis (Fig. 3B).

Interestingly, avascular wound healing in the cornea may become a disadvantage as it contributes to ophthalmic fibrosis (scarring), which may ultimately lead to blindness.

Thus TSP1 production in the healing cornea has yet to be carefully gauged to determine levels optimal for the balance between scarring and avascularity.

Consistent with its role in the repair of corneal epithelium, TSP1 levels are altered in the patients with pseudoexfoliation (PEX) syndrome, a common but little-known degenerative condition *(108)*. TSP1 expression is increased in keratocytes of the corneas from patients with PEX, but not of age-matched normal corneas *(109)*. Not incidentally, the density of the corneal endothelium is lower in patients with PEX compared with the non-PEX patients *(110)*, likely reflecting increased TSP1-induced endothelial cell apoptosis.

Studies of the strain-related differences in the inducer-stimulated corneal angiogenic response revealed the weakest response in C57BL/6J and the strongest in 129S3/SvIM mouse strains. Limbal vasculature surrounding the vascular area of the cornea was also most prominent in 129S3/SvIM animals. When relative (normalized to Ang-2) message level for the two angiogenesis inhibitors, PEDF and TSP1, was compared between strains, PEDF levels were similar, whereas TSP1 expression was significantly lower in the cornea of 129S3/SvIM *(111)*, suggesting that the differences in endogenous TSP1 determine the appearance of the limbal vessels during quiescence. On the other hand, because corneal neoangiognesis originates at the limbus, TSP1 and TSP2 levels may determine and predict the extent of corneal angiogenesis in response to injury, inflammation, or angiogenic stimuli.

In the Retina

In cultured RPE cells TSP1 treatment causes dramatic alterations of the secretory pattern, namely an increase in proangiogenic factors, VEGF and bFGF. RPE grown on TSP1-coated surfaces also shows increase in secreted VEGF, but not bFGF. Unexpectedly, TSP1-dependent VEGF upregulation occurs regardless of oxygen content, thus suggesting that hypoxia-inducible factor (HIF) is not involved. This increase in secreted angiogenic stimuli is partially blocked with the antibodies against integrins $\alpha_5\beta_1$, $\alpha_v\beta_3$, and $\alpha_v\beta_5$, suggesting the role for integrins as TSP1 receptors. However, it is unclear if TSP1 contributes to the excessive choroidal neovascularization as TSP localization to the Bruch's membrane is, at best, patchy *(112)*. On the other hand, the ability of TSP1 to activate metalloproteases is likely to contribute to the RPE detachment form Bruch's membrane *(113)*.

In mouse model of retinal neovascularization, TSP1 mRNA is increased from postnatal day 13 (P13), with a maximum three-fold increase on P15, corresponding to the time of development of retinal neovascularization. TSP1 expression is especially prominent in neovascular cells, particularly those adjacent to the area of nonperfusion. Quite unexpectedly, this increase in TSP1 is VEGF-driven: In bovine retinal microcapillary endothelial cells VEGF changed TSP1 expression in a biphasic manner with an early 1.4-fold decrease at 4 h, and a late three-fold increase at 24 h. As VEGF-induced endothelial cell proliferation can be completely inhibited by exogenous TSP1 and increased with TSP1-neutralizing antibody, it seems probable that in the ischemic retina, increased TSP1 expression in the neovessels in response to VEGF upregulation constitutes a part of the protective response, which halts endothelial proliferation and angiogenesis *(114)* (Fig. 3C).

Retinal neurons interact with TSP via integrins containing the α_v or β_1 subunits *(115)*. Retinal glial (Müller) cells play a major role in vascular eye diseases as a source of proaniogenic VEGF under hypoxic conditions due to ischemia. The same cells release significant amounts of the antiangiogenic factors TGF-β2, PEDF, and TSP1. Unlike PEDF, TSP1 is not downregulated by hypoxia. On the contrary, whereas in human (MIO-M1) and guinea-pig Müller cells hypoxia causes a decrease in secreted TGF-β2 and PEDF, TSP1 secretion is considerably elevated. This increase may be akin to the VEGF-dependent TSP upregulation in retinal endothelium *(114)*: The mix of VEGF with antiangiogenic factors at ratios found in Müller cell secretions cultured under either normoxic or hypoxic conditions failed to induce the proliferative response of the retinal endothelial cells. However, antibodies to either one of the three angiogenesis inhibitors relieved this proliferation blockade, indicating that Müller cells may perpetuate antiproliferative conditions for the retinal endothelial cells. Apparently, under hypoxic conditions the loss of inhibitory TGF-β2 and PEDF is counterbalanced by increased TSP1 *(116)* (Fig. 3C).

These findings are supported by more general observations in TSP1 knockout mice, where retinal vascular density is increased compared with the wild-type controls. This relief in control of the retinal vascular density reflects significantly higher numbers of retinal endothelial cells, which in turn may be explained by the lack of TSP1-dependent endothelial cell apoptosis. During oxygen-induced ischemic retinopathy, the developing retinal vasculature of TSP1-null mice is less sensitive to vessel obliteration due to hyperoxia. However, the return to normoxia induces a similar level of neovascularization to that induced in wild-type mice. It is likely that low VEGF levels in hyperoxic conditions sensitize retinal endothelium to TSP1-induced apoptosis *(67)*. The regression of ocular embryonic (hyaloid) and the newly formed retinal vessels during oxygen-induced ischemic retinopathy in TSP1-null mice is also delayed *(117)*.

Treatment with exogenous TSP1 and its peptides containing tryptophan-rich heparin-binding sequences and TGF-β1 activating sequence KRFK block retinal angiogenesis in two independent models: a retinal explant assay and a rat model of the retinopathy of prematurity. It is possible that heparin-binding sequences are acting indirectly, by sequestering proangigoenic VEGF and bFGF *(41)*. Peptides from the native TSP-1 sequence, with both the tryptophan-rich repeat and the TGF-β1 activation motif, were most potent in the retinal explant assay, whereas heparin-binding sequence alone was more active in blocking the retinopathy of prematurity. Thus TSP1 TSRs contain two subdomains that may independently block neovascularization and could be independently used for the treatment of retinal angiogenesis *(118)*.

Thus TSP1 is an important modulator of vascular homeostasis in the eye, essential for appropriate remodeling and maturation of the retinal vasculature.

TSP1 regulation is also linked to vascular malformations in diabetes: TSP1 or its functional antiangiogenic fragment, gp140, are detectable in considerable quantities in vitreous samples from normal human, rat, and bovine eyes, in contrast with the vitreous and aqueous humor samples from the diabetic rat eyes, which are virtually TSP1-negative. Microvascular cells secrete TSP1 in vivo and in culture: TSP1 expression in vitro is decreased in response to hyperglycemia. Decreased TSP1 levels correlate with the nonuniform, tortuous, and dilated appearance of the blood vessels in diabetic animals, again underscoring TSP1 contribution to the vascular homeostasis in the retina and its importance for preventing vascular dysfunctions and malformations associated with diabetes *(96)* (Fig. 3B).

Recent studies in rat glomerular mesangial cells provide a possible mechanistic explanation for these observations: In these cells glucose upregulates TSP1 at the mRNA level. This regulation requires an 18-bp sequence within the –1172 to –878 region of the human TSP1 promoter, which specifically binds nuclear proteins upstream stimulatory factors (USFs) 1 and 2. USFs themselves accumulate in the presence of glucose via the protein kinase C, p38 MAPK, and Erk kinase pathways. Activation of the cGMP-dependent protein kinase completely abolishes USF1 and USF2 binding to the recombinant or endogenous TSP1 promoter due to hypergycemia. It appears that PKG downregulates both USF2 levels and DNA binding activity under high-glucose conditions, causing TSP1 downregulation *(119)*. The same players may be involved in the TSP1 regulation in diabetic vasculature.

In Epiretinal Membranes

The role of TSP1 in the eye is not one-dimensional—there are some indications of its unfavorable contribution to eye disease. Epiretinal and subretinal membranes (ERM and SRM) are fibrocellular proliferations, which form on the surfaces of the neuroretina as a sequel to a variety of ocular diseases. When these proliferations complicate rhegmatogenous retinal detachment (a condition known as proliferative vitreoretinopathy [PVR]), the membranes often contain numerous RPE cells and a variety of extracellular proteins. In ERM, TSP1 codistributes with vitronectin and SPARC, and may play a role in the assembly of the extracellular matrix, which constitutes the bulk of the membranes *(120)*. In this context TSP1 and SPARC are likely to reduce RPE adhesion and thus permit their migration and shape change during periretinal membrane development. Furthermore, in a cocktail containing metalloproteinases, growth factors such as hepatocyte growth factor, TSP1and SPARC may facilitate RPE cell dissociation from Bruch's membrane, an early harbinger of PVR *(121)*. Migratory subsets of RPE cells show positive immunoreactivity for TSP1 and SPARC; hence these two proteins may become possible therapeutic targets in the management of ERM *(113)*.

TSP1, Immune Privilege, and Ocular Angiogenesis

The eye is one of the few tissues in the body characterized by immune privilege, a condition associated with delayed graft rejection. Immune privilege is manifested by the lack of MHC class II and reduced MHC class I expression in the cornea and in the resident antigen-presenting cells (APCs) *(122,123)*. As a result of a deficiency in MHC-presenting APCs in the transplanted tissue, the recipient alloreactive T cells fail to recognize donor APCs in the draining lymph nodes, and, to capture donor antigens, are forced to invade transplanted tissue. Additional delay occurs when the new lymphatics have to emerge from the graft bed for the trafficking of recipient APC (reviewed in ref. *124*).

Once foreign antigens reach the draining lymph nodes, the immune privilege is maintained by tolerance induction, via anterior-associated immune deviation (ACAID), a pathway existing solely in the eye, with exclusive formation of noncomplement fixing antibodies and a CD8+ T-cell response *(125–128)*. CD4+/CD8+ T-cell response is attenuated by the regulatory T cells in the spleen and eye. In ACAID, antigen-primed APCs are trafficking from the eye into the spleen where multicellular clusters of antigen-bearing APCs from the eye interact with NKT and splenic B cells (reviewed in ref. *129*).

The final barrier upholding the eye immune privilege is held by the soluble immunosuppressive factors in the intraocular fluid and the cell surface molecules of the ocular parenchyma *(130)*. Constitutive expression of CD95L in the corneal endothelium causes infiltrating T cells to apoptose, while complement-binding surface molecules CD46, CD55, and CD59 prevent tissue destruction by complement fixation/activation.

TSP1 holds an important place among soluble factors suppressing the innate and adaptive immune responses *(131–133)* (Fig. 3C). ACAID is supported by several of the antiinflammatory factors in the aqueous humor. APCs exposed to aqueous humor in vitro confer ACAID when returned to the eye, owing to the presence of TGF-β2, a TGF isoform exclusive to the eye *(128)*. Complex changes in the cytokine expression profile of the APCs in the eye were found to be ultimately dependent on TSP1, whose expression is elevated in response to TGF-β2. The mechanism by which TSP1 promotes ACAID is not completely understood but entails a decrease in IL-12 and CD40. TSP1 was proposed to tether and then activate TGF-β on the APC surface via sequences binding CD36 (GVITRIR) and latent TGF-β precursor (KRFK). Both APCs and T cells also express another TSP1 receptor, CD47, which is thought to divert them from a normal immune response (reviewed in ref. *124*). Finally, the increased FasL due to TSP1 *(67)* may expedite the elimination of infiltrating T cells.

Inflammation and inflammatory disease are tightly linked to angiogenesis. Angiogenic stimuli secreted or released from the matrix by immune cells into inflamed tissue cause angiogenesis, which augments the existing pathology *(134–138)*. Angiogenesis and inflammation are controlled by the same soluble factors—T cells activated by hypoxia secrete VEGF, but are also VEGFR-2-positive and differentiate in response to VEGF *(139)*. Conversely, inflammatory cytokines induce angiogenesis by acting directly on endothelial cells *(140)* and indirectly, by stimulating leukocytes to release angiogenic factors *(141)*. Thus it is not entirely unexpected that the same controls maintain immune privilege and angiogenesis blockade in the eye.

In addition to its role in ACAID, TSP also exerts direct immunosuppression of dendritic cells and macrophages *(142–144)*. It is likely that immunosuppression by TSP, including its pivotal role in ACAID, helps to maintain ocular angiostasis by subduing the inflammatory response and its angiogenic potential. The significance of the ocular immune privilege established by TSP in blocking inflammatory angiogenesis can be clearly appreciated in cases in which this barrier is perturbed. For instance, in patients with choroidal neovascularization, ocular macrophages express VEGF and tumor necrosis factor (TNF)-α, which in turn stimulate VEGF production by RPE cells *(145–147)*. Similarly, in corneas vascularized as a result of ocular disease, stroma and vasculature are invaded by T cells and macrophages positive for proangiogenic TGFα, TGF-β1, and VEGF *(148)*. Postischemic inflammation causes an influx of macrophage-derived TNF-α, which induces angiogenesis directly and by inducing production of MCP-1, IL-8, and bFGF by retinal glia *(149)*. Corneal dendritic cells, which express VEGFR-3 in the normal eye, may play a role in ocular lymphangiogenesis, as they can produce

VEGF-C in response to inflammation induced by cauterization of the corneal surface *(150)*. Circulating polymorphonuclear neutrophils have also been shown to be necessary for angiogenesis in a mouse model of FGF-2-induced corneal neovascularization *(151)*. Finally, ocular angiogenesis induced by herpes simplex virus infection in the eye is dependent on MMP9 produced by neutrophils invading the cornea *(152)*.

Thus the immune response can be a potent stimulator of ocular angiogenesis and the central role of TSP1 in the maintenance of ocular immune privilege is equally central in the maintenance of angiostasis.

CONCLUSION

In conclusion, the contribution of TSP(s) in ocular angiogenesis is beyond doubt. Unfortunately, comparative studies evaluating and matching the input of multiple endogenous angiogenesis inhibitors, including PEDF, SPARC, angiostatin, endostatin, thrombospondins, and others are still deficient. There are isolated studies in which a decrease in one angiogenesis inhibitor is followed by an increase in another (*see* PEDF and TSP1), pointing to a likelihood of a compensatory mechanism(s). Compilation analysis indicates that the functions of multiple angiosuppressive proteins in the eye are at least partially redundant and that they may replace each other in the event of a deficit. It is intuitively clear that such important function as visual perception has to be rigorously protected via multiple lines of defense, but the cooperation between such defense systems is yet to be unraveled. Undoubtedly, thrombospondins hold an important place among these cooperating controlling elements. They contribute directly to the maintenance of angiosuppression in the cornea, vitreous, and aqueous humor, as well as in steady-state angiostasis of the existing vasculature in the vitreous and choroids. Thrombospondin and its receptors are instrumental in upholding ocular immune privilege and therefore indirectly contribute to ocular angiostasis by keeping inflammation-related angiogenesis at bay. Finally, TSP's unique function as a mechanosensitive angiogenesis inhibitor marks it as a player and possible therapeutic target in the management of glaucoma. The role of TSP1 in diabetes is not fully understood. It is possible that it is decreased concomitantly with PEDF due to hyperglycemia: Elimination of the two main angiosuppressive proteins leads to drastic vascular malformations and leakage, causing blindness, one of the devastating complications in diabetes.

Thus the role of TSP1 in the eye warrants further scrutiny, and its antiangiogenic derivatives may become promising investigative drugs to be used for the treatment of multiple angiogenesis-related ocular diseases.

REFERENCES

1. Bornstein P. Thrombospondins: structure and regulation of expression. FASEB J 1992;6:3290–3299.
2. Lawler J, Hynes RO. The structure of human thrombospondin, an adhesive glycoprotein with multiple calcium-binding sites and homologies with several different proteins. J Cell Biol 1986;103:1635–1648.
3. O'Rourke KM, Laherty CD, Dixit VM. Thrombospondin 1 and thrombospondin 2 are expressed as both homo- and heterotrimers. J Biol Chem 1992;267:24,921–24,924.
4. Bornstein P, Devarayalu S, Edelhoff S, Disteche CM. Isolation and characterization of the mouse thrombospondin 3 (Thbs3) gene. Genomics 1993;15:607–613.

5. Vos HL, Devarayalu S, de Vries Y, Bornstein P. Thrombospondin 3 (Thbs3), a new member of the thrombospondin gene family. J Biol Chem 1992;267:12,192–12,196.
6. Adams JC, Tucker RP. The thrombospondin type 1 repeat (TSR) superfamily: diverse proteins with related roles in neuronal development. Dev Dyn 2000;218:280–299.
7. Chen H, Herndon ME, Lawler J. The cell biology of thrombospondin-1. Matrix Biol 2000;19:597–614.
8. Lawler J, McHenry K, Duquette M, Derick L. Characterization of human thrombospondin-4. J Biol Chem 1995;270:2809–2814.
9. Morgelin M, Heinegard D, Engel J, Paulsson M. Electron microscopy of native cartilage oligomeric matrix protein purified from the Swarm rat chondrosarcoma reveals a five-armed structure. J Biol Chem 1992;267:6137–6141.
10. Qabar A, Derick L, Lawler J, Dixit V. Thrombospondin 3 is a pentameric molecule held together by interchain disulfide linkage involving two cysteine residues. J Biol Chem 1995;270:12,725–12,729.
11. Lawler J, Derick LH, Connolly JE, Chen JH, Chao FC. The structure of human platelet thrombospondin. J Biol Chem 1985;260:3762–3772.
12. Misenheimer TM, Huwiler KG, Annis DS, Mosher DF. Physical characterization of the procollagen module of human thrombospondin 1 expressed in insect cells. J Biol Chem 2000;275:40,938–40,945.
13. Kilpelainen I, Kaksonen M, Avikainen H, et al. Heparin-binding growth-associated molecule contains two heparin-binding beta -sheet domains that are homologous to the thrombospondin type I repeat. J Biol Chem 2000;275:13,564–13,570.
14. Baron M, Norman DG, Harvey TS, et al. The three-dimensional structure of the first EGF-like module of human factor IX: comparison with EGF and TGF-alpha. Protein Sci 1992;1:81–90.
15. Maddox BK, Mokashi A, Keene DR, Bachinger HP. A cartilage oligomeric matrix protein mutation associated with pseudoachondroplasia changes the structural and functional properties of the type 3 domain. J Biol Chem 2000;275:11,412–11,417.
16. Misenheimer TM, Mosher DF. Calcium ion binding to thrombospondin 1. J Biol Chem 1995;270:1729–1733.
17. Hofsteenge J, Huwiler KG, Macek B, et al. C-mannosylation and O-fucosylation of the thrombospondin type 1 module. J Biol Chem 2001;276:6485–6498.
18. Lawler J, Ferro P, Duquette M. Expression and mutagenesis of thrombospondin. Biochemistry 1992;31:1173–1180.
19. Hogg PJ. Thrombospondin 1 as an enzyme inhibitor. Thromb Haemost 1994;72:787–792.
20. Adams JC, Lawler J. Diverse mechanisms for cell attachment to platelet thrombospondin. J Cell Sci 1993;104(Pt 4):1061–1071.
21. Adams JC. Characterization of cell-matrix adhesion requirements for the formation of fascin microspikes. Mol Biol Cell 1997;8:2345–2363.
22. Hotchkiss KA, Matthias LJ, Hogg PJ. Corrigendum to: "Exposure of the cryptic arg-gly-Asp sequence in thrombospondin-1 by protein disulfide isomerase." Biochim Biophys Acta 1999;1434:210.
23. Kyriakides TR, Zhu YH, Smith LT, et al. Mice that lack thrombospondin 2 display connective tissue abnormalities that are associated with disordered collagen fibrillogenesis, an increased vascular density, and a bleeding diathesis. J Cell Biol 1998;140:419–430.
24. Lawler J, Sunday M, Thibert V, et al. Thrombospondin-1 is required for normal murine pulmonary homeostasis and its absence causes pneumonia. J Clin Invest 1998;101: 982–992.
25. Kyriakides TR, Leach KJ, Hoffman AS, Ratner BD, Bornstein P. Mice that lack the angiogenesis inhibitor, thrombospondin 2, mount an altered foreign body reaction characterized by increased vascularity. Proc Natl Acad Sci USA 1999;96:4449–4454.

26. Good DJ, Polverini PJ, Rastinejad F, et al. A tumor suppressor-dependent inhibitor of angiogenesis is immunologically and functionally indistinguishable from a fragment of thrombospondin. Proc Natl Acad Sci USA 1990;87:6624–6628.
27. Volpert OV, Tolsma SS, Pellerin S, et al. Inhibition of angiogenesis by thrombospondin-2. Biochem Biophys Res Commun 1995;217:326–332.
28. Stellmach V, Volpert OV, Crawford SE, Lawler J, Hynes RO, Bouck N. Tumour suppressor genes and angiogenesis: the role of TP53 in fibroblasts. Eur J Cancer 1996;32A:2394–2400.
29. Streit M, Velasco P, Riccardi L, et al. Thrombospondin-1 suppresses wound healing and granulation tissue formation in the skin of transgenic mice. EMBO J 2000;19:3272–3282.
30. Streit M, Riccardi L, Velasco P, et al. Thrombospondin-2: a potent endogenous inhibitor of tumor growth and angiogenesis. Proc Natl Acad Sci USA 1999;96:14,888–14,893.
31. Streit M, Velasco P, Brown LF, et al. Overexpression of thrombospondin-1 decreases angiogenesis and inhibits the growth of human cutaneous squamous cell carcinomas. Am J Pathol 1999;155:441–452.
32. Weinstat-Saslow DL, Zabrenetzky VS, VanHoutte K, Frazier WA, Roberts DD, Steeg PS. Transfection of thrombospondin 1 complementary DNA into a human breast carcinoma cell line reduces primary tumor growth, metastatic potential, and angiogenesis. Cancer Res 1994;54:6504–6511.
33. Volpert OV, Lawler J, Bouck NP. A human fibrosarcoma inhibits systemic angiogenesis and the growth of experimental metastases via thrombospondin-1. Proc Natl Acad Sci USA 1998;95:6343–6348.
34. Bleuel K, Popp S, Fusenig NE, Stanbridge EJ, Boukamp P. Tumor suppression in human skin carcinoma cells by chromosome 15 transfer or thrombospondin-1 overexpression through halted tumor vascularization. Proc Natl Acad Sci USA 1999;96:2065–2070.
35. Yu H, Tyrrell D, Cashel J, et al. Specificities of heparin-binding sites from the amino-terminus and type 1 repeats of thrombospondin-1. Arch Biochem Biophys 2000;374:13–23.
36. Tolsma SS, Volpert OV, Good DJ, Frazier WA, Polverini PJ, Bouck N. Peptides derived from two separate domains of the matrix protein thrombospondin-1 have anti-angiogenic activity. J Cell Biol 1993;122:497–511.
37. Vogel T, Guo NH, Krutzsch HC, et al. Modulation of endothelial cell proliferation, adhesion, and motility by recombinant heparin-binding domain and synthetic peptides from the type I repeats of thrombospondin. J Cell Biochem 1993;53:74–84.
38. Iruela-Arispe ML, Vazquez F, Ortega MA. Antiangiogenic domains shared by thrombospondins and metallospondins, a new family of angiogenic inhibitors. Ann N Y Acad Sci 1999;886:58–66.
39. Gao AG, Lindberg FP, Dimitry JM, Brown EJ, Frazier WA. Thrombospondin modulates alpha v beta 3 function through integrin-associated protein. J Cell Biol 1996;135:533–544.
40. Chandrasekaran S, Guo NH, Rodrigues RG, Kaiser J, Roberts DD. Pro-adhesive and chemotactic activities of thrombospondin-1 for breast carcinoma cells are mediated by alpha3beta1 integrin and regulated by insulin-like growth factor-1 and CD98. J Biol Chem 1999;274:11,408–11,416.
41. Taraboletti G, Morbidelli L, Donnini S, et al. The heparin binding 25 kDa fragment of thrombospondin-1 promotes angiogenesis and modulates gelatinase and TIMP-2 production in endothelial cells. FASEB J 2000;14:1674–1676.
42. Silverstein RL. The face of TSR revealed: an extracellular signaling domain is exposed. J Cell Biol 2002;159:203–206.
43. Dawson DW, Pearce SF, Zhong R, Silverstein RL, Frazier WA, Bouck NP. CD36 mediates the In vitro inhibitory effects of thrombospondin-1 on endothelial cells. J Cell Biol 1997;138:707–717.
44. Iruela-Arispe ML, Luque A, Lee N. Thrombospondin modules and angiogenesis. Int J Biochem Cell Biol 2004;36:1070–1078.

45. Guo N, Krutzsch HC, Inman JK, Roberts DD. Thrombospondin 1 and type I repeat peptides of thrombospondin 1 specifically induce apoptosis of endothelial cells. Cancer Res 1997;57:1735–1742.
46. Dawson DW, Volpert OV, Pearce SF, et al. Three distinct D-amino acid substitutions confer potent antiangiogenic activity on an inactive peptide derived from a thrombospondin-1 type 1 repeat. Mol Pharmacol 1999;55:332–338.
47. Reiher FK, Volpert OV, Jimenez B, et al. Inhibition of tumor growth by systemic treatment with thrombospondin-1 peptide mimetics. Int J Cancer 2002;98:682–689.
48. Febbraio M, Hajjar DP, Silverstein RL. CD36: a class B scavenger receptor involved in angiogenesis, atherosclerosis, inflammation, and lipid metabolism. J Clin Invest 2001; 108:785–791.
49. Simantov R, Silverstein RL. CD36: a critical anti-angiogenic receptor. Front Biosci 2003;8:S874–S882.
50. Jimenez B, Volpert OV, Crawford SE, Febbraio M, Silverstein RL, Bouck N. Signals leading to apoptosis-dependent inhibition of neovascularization by thrombospondin-1. Nat Med 2000;6:41–48.
51. Simantov R, Febbraio M, Crombie R, Asch AS, Nachman RL, Silverstein RL. Histidine-rich glycoprotein inhibits the antiangiogenic effect of thrombospondin-1. J Clin Invest 2001;107:45–52.
52. Taraboletti G, Belotti D, Borsotti P, et al. The 140-kilodalton antiangiogenic fragment of thrombospondin-1 binds to basic fibroblast growth factor. Cell Growth Differ 1997; 8:471–479.
53. Armstrong LC, Bjorkblom B, Hankenson KD, Siadak AW, Stiles CE, Bornstein P. Thrombospondin 2 inhibits microvascular endothelial cell proliferation by a caspase-independent mechanism. Mol Biol Cell 2002;13:1893–1905.
54. Murphy-Ullrich JE, Poczatek M. Activation of latent TGF-beta by thrombospondin-1: mechanisms and physiology. Cytokine Growth Factor Rev 2000;11:59–69.
55. Schultz-Cherry S, Chen H, Mosher DF, et al. Regulation of transforming growth factor-beta activation by discrete sequences of thrombospondin 1. J Biol Chem 1995;270: 7304–7310.
56. Yang Z, Strickland DK, Bornstein P. Extracellular matrix metalloproteinase 2 levels are regulated by the low density lipoprotein-related scavenger receptor and thrombospondin 2. J Biol Chem 2001;276:8403–8408.
57. Itoh Y, Ito A, Iwata K, Tanzawa K, Mori Y, Nagase H. Plasma membrane-bound tissue inhibitor of metalloproteinases (TIMP)-2 specifically inhibits matrix metalloproteinase 2 (gelatinase A) activated on the cell surface. J Biol Chem 1998;273:24,360–24,367.
58. Kyriakides TR, Zhu YH, Yang Z, Huynh G, Bornstein P. Altered extracellular matrix remodeling and angiogenesis in sponge granulomas of thrombospondin 2-null mice. Am J Pathol 2001;159:1255–1262.
59. Rodriguez-Manzaneque JC, Lane TF, Ortega MA, Hynes RO, Lawler J, Iruela-Arispe ML. Thrombospondin-1 suppresses spontaneous tumor growth and inhibits activation of matrix metalloproteinase-9 and mobilization of vascular endothelial growth factor. Proc Natl Acad Sci USA 2001;98:12,485–12,490.
60. Maeshima Y, Sudhakar A, Lively JC, et al. Tumstatin, an endothelial cell-specific inhibitor of protein synthesis. Science 2002;295:140–143.
61. Chandrasekaran L, He CZ, Al-Barazi H, Krutzsch HC, Iruela-Arispe ML, Roberts DD. Cell contact-dependent activation of alpha3beta1 integrin modulates endothelial cell responses to thrombospondin-1. Mol Biol Cell 2000;11:2885–2900.
62. Orr AW, Pedraza CE, Pallero MA, et al. Low density lipoprotein receptor-related protein is a calreticulin coreceptor that signals focal adhesion disassembly. J Cell Biol 2003;161: 1179–1189.

63. Goicoechea S, Orr AW, Pallero MA, Eggleton P, Murphy-Ullrich JE. Thrombospondin mediates focal adhesion disassembly through interactions with cell surface calreticulin. J Biol Chem 2000;275:36,358–36,368.
64. Kanda S, Shono T, Tomasini-Johansson B, Klint P, Saito Y. Role of thrombospondin-1-derived peptide, 4N1K, in FGF-2-induced angiogenesis. Exp Cell Res 1999;252:262–272.
64a. Shull MM, Ormsby I, Kier AB, et al. Targeted disruption of the mouse transforming growth factor-beta 1 gene results in multifocal inflammatory disease. Nature 1992;359:693–699.
65. Crawford SE, Stellmach V, Murphy-Ullrich JE, et al. Thrombospondin-1 is a major activator of TGF-beta1 in vivo. Cell 1998;93:1159–1170.
66. Jimenez B, Volpert OV, Reiher F, et al. c-Jun N-terminal kinase activation is required for the inhibition of neovascularization by thrombospondin-1. Oncogene 2001;20:3443–3448.
67. Volpert OV, Zaichuk T, Zhou W, et al. Inducer-stimulated Fas targets activated endothelium for destruction by anti-angiogenic thrombospondin-1 and pigment epithelium-derived factor. Nat Med 2002;8:349–357.
68. Nor JE, Mitra RS, Sutorik MM, Mooney DJ, Castle VP, Polverini PJ. Thrombospondin-1 induces endothelial cell apoptosis and inhibits angiogenesis by activating the caspase death pathway. J Vasc Res 2000;37:209–218.
69. Armstrong LC, Bornstein P. Thrombospondins 1 and 2 function as inhibitors of angiogenesis. Matrix Biol 2003;22:63–71.
70. Kaiser HJ, Schoetzau A, Stumpfig D, Flammer J. Blood-flow velocities of the extraocular vessels in patients with high-tension and normal-tension primary open-angle glaucoma. Am J Ophthalmol 1997;123:320–327.
71. Freyberg MA, Kaiser D, Graf R, Vischer P, Friedl P. Integrin-associated protein and thrombospondin-1 as endothelial mechanosensitive death mediators. Biochem Biophys Res Commun 2000;271:584–588.
72. Kaiser D, Freyberg MA, Schrimpf G, Friedl P. Apoptosis induced by lack of hemodynamic forces is a general endothelial feature even occuring in immortalized cell lines. Endothelium 1999;6:325–334.
73. Aiello LP. Vascular endothelial growth factor and the eye. Past, present and future. Arch Ophthalmol 1996;114:1252–1254.
74. Aiello LP. Keeping in touch with angiogenesis. Nat Med 2000;6:379–381.
75. Ferrara N. Vascular endothelial growth factor: basic science and clinical progress. Endocr Rev 2004;25:581–611.
76. Yamada H, Yamada E, Hackett SF, Ozaki H, Okamoto N, Campochiaro PA. Hyperoxia causes decreased expression of vascular endothelial growth factor and endothelial cell apoptosis in adult retina. J Cell Physiol 1999;179:149–156.
77. Ferrara N, Gerber HP, LeCouter J. The biology of VEGF and its receptors. Nat Med 2003;9:669–676.
78. Miller JW, Adamis AP, Aiello LP. Vascular endothelial growth factor in ocular neovascularization and proliferative diabetic retinopathy. Diabetes Metab Rev 1997;13:37–50.
79. Boehm BO, Lang G, Feldmann B, et al. Proliferative diabetic retinopathy is associated with a low level of the natural ocular anti-angiogenic agent pigment epithelium-derived factor (PEDF) in aqueous humor. a pilot study. Horm Metab Res 2003;35:382–386.
80. Dawson DW, Volpert OV, Gillis P, et al. Pigment epithelium-derived factor: a potent inhibitor of angiogenesis. Science 1999;285:245–248.
81. Boehm BO, Lang G, Volpert O, et al. Low content of the natural ocular anti-angiogenic agent pigment epithelium-derived factor (PEDF) in aqueous humor predicts progression of diabetic retinopathy. Diabetologia 2003;46:394–400.
82. Holekamp NM, Bouck N, Volpert O. Pigment epithelium-derived factor is deficient in the vitreous of patients with choroidal neovascularization due to age-related macular degeneration. Am J Ophthalmol 2002;134:220–227.

83. Gao G, Li Y, Zhang D, Gee S, Crosson C, Ma J. Unbalanced expression of VEGF and PEDF in ischemia-induced retinal neovascularization. FEBS Lett 2001;489:270–276.
84. Bouck N. PEDF: anti-angiogenic guardian of ocular function. Trends Mol Med 2002;8: 330–334.
85. Wong CG, Rich KA, Liaw LH, Hsu HT, Berns MW. Intravitreal VEGF and bFGF produce florid retinal neovascularization and hemorrhage in the rabbit. Curr Eye Res 2001;22: 140–147.
86. Hyatt GA, Beebe DC. Regulation of lens cell growth and polarity by an embryo-specific growth factor and by inhibitors of lens cell proliferation and differentiation. Development 1993;117:701–709.
87. Grant MB, Guay C, Marsh R. Insulin-like growth factor I stimulates proliferation, migration, and plasminogen activator release by human retinal pigment epithelial cells. Curr Eye Res 1990;9:323–335.
88. Simo R, Lecube A, Segura RM, Garcia Arumi J, Hernandez C. Free insulin growth factor-I and vascular endothelial growth factor in the vitreous fluid of patients with proliferative diabetic retinopathy. Am J Ophthalmol 2002;134:376–382.
89. Ruberte J, Ayuso E, Navarro M, et al. Increased ocular levels of IGF-1 in transgenic mice lead to diabetes-like eye disease. J Clin Invest 2004;113:1149–1157.
90. Strieter RM, Kunkel SL, Elner VM, et al. Interleukin-8. A corneal factor that induces neovascularization. Am J Pathol 1992;141:1279–1284.
91. Funatsu H, Yamashita H, Noma H, Mimura T, Yamashita T, Hori S. Increased levels of vascular endothelial growth factor and interleukin-6 in the aqueous humor of diabetics with macular edema. Am J Ophthalmol 2002;133:70–77.
92. Funatsu H, Yamashita H, Noma H, Shimizu E, Yamashita T, Hori S. Stimulation and inhibition of angiogenesis in diabetic retinopathy. Jpn J Ophthalmol 2001;45:577–584.
93. Marneros AG, Keene DR, Hansen U, et al. Collagen XVIII/endostatin is essential for vision and retinal pigment epithelial function. EMBO J 2004;23:89–99.
94. Sack RA, Beaton AR, Sathe S. Diurnal variations in angiostatin in human tear fluid: a possible role in prevention of corneal neovascularization. Curr Eye Res 1999;18: 186–193.
95. Rhee DJ, Fariss RN, Brekken R, Sage EH, Russell P. The matricellular protein SPARC is expressed in human trabecular meshwork. Exp Eye Res 2003;77:601–607.
96. Sheibani N, Sorenson CM, Cornelius LA, Frazier WA. Thrombospondin-1, a natural inhibitor of angiogenesis, is present in vitreous and aqueous humor and is modulated by hyperglycemia. Biochem Biophys Res Commun 2000;267:257–261.
97. Miyajima-Uchida H, Hayashi H, Beppu R, et al. Production and accumulation of thrombospondin-1 in human retinal pigment epithelial cells. Invest Ophthalmol Vis Sci 2000;41:561–567.
98. Munjal ID, Crawford DR, Blake DA, Sabet MD, Gordon SR. Thrombospondin: biosynthesis, distribution, and changes associated with wound repair in corneal endothelium. Eur J Cell Biol 1990;52:252–263.
99. Hiscott P, Seitz B, Schlotzer-Schrehardt U, Naumann GO. Immunolocalisation of thrombospondin 1 in human, bovine and rabbit cornea. Cell Tissue Res 1997;289:307–310.
100. Armstrong DJ, Hiscott P, Batterbury M, Kaye S. Keratocyte matrix interactions and thrombospondin 2. Mol Vis 2003;9:74–79.
101. Armstrong DJ, Hiscott P, Batterbury M, Kaye S. Corneal stromal cells (keratocytes) express thrombospondins 2 and 3 in wound repair phenotype. Int J Biochem Cell Biol 2002;34:588–593.
102. Tripathi BJ, Tripathi RC, Yang C, Millard CB, Dixit VM. Synthesis of a thrombospondin-like cytoadhesion molecule by cells of the trabecular meshwork. Invest Ophthalmol Vis Sci 1991;32:181–188.

103. Tripathi BJ, Li T, Li J, Tran L, Tripathi RC. Age-related changes in trabecular cells in vitro. Exp Eye Res 1997;64:57–66.
104. Cursiefen C, Masli S, Ng TF, et al. Roles of thrombospondin-1 and -2 in regulating corneal and iris angiogenesis. Invest Ophthalmol Vis Sci 2004;45:1117–1124.
105. Hiscott P, Armstrong D, Batterbury M, Kaye S. Repair in avascular tissues: fibrosis in the transparent structures of the eye and thrombospondin 1. Histol Histopathol 1999;14: 1309–1320.
106. Cao Z, Wu HK, Bruce A, Wollenberg K, Panjwani N. Detection of differentially expressed genes in healing mouse corneas, using cDNA microarrays. Invest Ophthalmol Vis Sci 2002;43:2897–2904.
107. Uno K, Hayashi H, Kuroki M, Uchida H, Yamauchi Y, Oshima K. Thrombospondin-1 accelerates wound healing of corneal epithelia. Biochem Biophys Res Commun 2004; 315:928–934.
108. Sowka J. Pseudoexfoliation syndrome and pseudoexfoliative glaucoma. Optometry 2004; 75:245–250.
109. Hiscott P, Schlotzer-Schrehardt U, Naumann GO. Unexpected expression of thrombospondin 1 by corneal and iris fibroblasts in the pseudoexfoliation syndrome. Hum Pathol 1996;27:1255–1258.
110. Inoue K, Okugawa K, Oshika T, Amano S. Morphological study of corneal endothelium and corneal thickness in pseudoexfoliation syndrome. Jpn J Ophthalmol 2003; 47:235–239.
111. Chan CK, Pham LN, Chinn C, et al. Mouse strain-dependent heterogeneity of resting limbal vasculature. Invest Ophthalmol Vis Sci 2004;45:441–447.
112. Mousa SA, Lorelli W, Campochiaro PA. Role of hypoxia and extracellular matrix-integrin binding in the modulation of angiogenic growth factors secretion by retinal pigmented epithelial cells. J Cell Biochem 1999;74:135–143.
113. Sheridan CM, Magee RM, Hiscott PS, et al. The role of matricellular proteins thrombospondin-1 and osteonectin during RPE cell migration in proliferative vitreoretinopathy. Curr Eye Res 2002;25:279–285.
114. Suzuma K, Takagi H, Otani A, Oh H, Honda Y. Expression of thrombospondin-1 in ischemia-induced retinal neovascularization. Am J Pathol 1999;154:343–354.
115. Neugebauer KM, Emmett CJ, Venstrom KA, Reichardt LF. Vitronectin and thrombospondin promote retinal neurite outgrowth: developmental regulation and role of integrins. Neuron 1991;6:345–358.
116. Eichler W, Yafai Y, Wiedemann P, Reichenbach A. Angiogenesis-related factors derived from retinal glial (Muller) cells in hypoxia. Neuroreport 2004;15:1633–1637.
117. Wang S, Wu Z, Sorenson CM, Lawler J, Sheibani N. Thrombospondin-1-deficient mice exhibit increased vascular density during retinal vascular development and are less sensitive to hyperoxia-mediated vessel obliteration. Dev Dyn 2003;228:630–642.
118. Shafiee A, Penn JS, Krutzsch HC, Inman JK, Roberts DD, Blake DA. Inhibition of retinal angiogenesis by peptides derived from thrombospondin-1. Invest Ophthalmol Vis Sci 2000;41:2378–2388.
119. Wang S, Skorczewski J, Feng X, Mei L, Murphy-Ullrich JE. Glucose up-regulates thrombospondin 1 gene transcription and transforming growth factor-beta activity through antagonism of cGMP-dependent protein kinase repression via upstream stimulatory factor 2. J Biol Chem 2004;279:34,311–34,322.
120. Hiscott P, Larkin G, Robey HL, Orr G, Grierson I. Thrombospondin as a component of the extracellular matrix of epiretinal membranes: comparisons with cellular fibronectin. Eye 1992;6(Pt 6):566–569.
121. Hiscott P, Hagan S, Heathcote L, et al. Pathobiology of epiretinal and subretinal membranes: possible roles for the matricellular proteins thrombospondin 1 and osteonectin (SPARC). Eye 2002;16:393–403.

122. Abi-Hanna D, Wakefield D, Watkins S. HLA antigens in ocular tissues. I. In vivo expression in human eyes. Transplantation 1988;45:610–613.
123. Wang HM, Kaplan HJ, Chan WC, Johnson M. The distribution and ontogeny of MHC antigens in murine ocular tissue. Invest Ophthalmol Vis Sci 1987;28:1383–1389.
124. Streilein JW. Ocular immune privilege: the eye takes a dim but practical view of immunity and inflammation. J Leukoc Biol 2003;74:179–185.
125. Kaplan HJ, Streilein JW. Analysis of immunologic privilege within the anterior chamber of the eye. Transplant Proc 1977;9:1193–1195.
126. Streilein JW, Niederkorn JY, Shadduck JA. Systemic immune unresponsiveness induced in adult mice by anterior chamber presentation of minor histocompatibility antigens. J Exp Med 1980;152:1121–1125.
127. Ksander BR, Streilein JW. Immune privilege to MHC-disparate tumor grafts in the anterior chamber of the eye. I. Quantitative analysis of intraocular tumor growth and the corresponding delayed hypersensitivity response. Transplantation 1989;47:661–667.
128. Wilbanks GA, Streilein JW. Characterization of suppressor cells in anterior chamber-associated immune deviation (ACAID) induced by soluble antigen. Evidence of two functionally and phenotypically distinct T-suppressor cell populations. Immunology 1990;71:383–389.
129. Streilein JW, Ma N, Wenkel H, Ng TF, Zamiri P. Immunobiology and privilege of neuronal retina and pigment epithelium transplants. Vision Res 2002;42:487–495.
130. Streilein JW. Regional immunity and ocular immune privilege. Chem Immunol 1999; 73:11–38.
131. Streilein JW, Stein-Streilein J. Does innate immune privilege exist? J Leukoc Biol 2000; 67:479–487.
132. Kaiser CJ, Ksander BR, Streilein JW. Inhibition of lymphocyte proliferation by aqueous humor. Reg Immunol 1989;2:42–49.
133. Taylor AW, Streilein JW, Cousins SW. Immunoreactive vasoactive intestinal peptide contributes to the immunosuppressive activity of normal aqueous humor. J Immunol 1994;153:1080–1086.
134. Kasama T, Shiozawa F, Kobayashi K, et al. Vascular endothelial growth factor expression by activated synovial leukocytes in rheumatoid arthritis: critical involvement of the interaction with synovial fibroblasts. Arthritis Rheum 2001;44:2512–2524.
135. Koch AE, Volin MV, Woods JM, et al. Regulation of angiogenesis by the C-X-C chemokines interleukin-8 and epithelial neutrophil activating peptide 78 in the rheumatoid joint. Arthritis Rheum 2001;44:31–40.
136. Coussens LM, Raymond WW, Bergers G, et al. Inflammatory mast cells up-regulate angiogenesis during squamous epithelial carcinogenesis. Genes Dev 1999;13:1382–1397.
137. Brenchley PE. Angiogenesis in inflammatory joint disease: a target for therapeutic intervention. Clin Exp Immunol 2000;121:426–429.
138. Schioppa T, Uranchimeg B, Saccani A, et al. Regulation of the chemokine receptor CXCR4 by hypoxia. J Exp Med 2003;198:1391–1402.
139. Mor F, Quintana FJ, Cohen IR. Angiogenesis-inflammation cross-talk: vascular endothelial growth factor is secreted by activated T cells and induces Th1 polarization. J Immunol 2004;172:4618–4623.
140. Romagnani P, Lasagni L, Annunziato F, Serio M, Romagnani S. CXC chemokines: the regulatory link between inflammation and angiogenesis. Trends Immunol 2004; 25:201–209.
141. Scapini P, Morini M, Tecchio C, et al. CXCL1/macrophage inflammatory protein-2-induced angiogenesis in vivo is mediated by neutrophil-derived vascular endothelial growth factor-A. J Immunol 2004;172:5034–5040.

142. Johansson U, Higginbottom K, Londei M. CD47 ligation induces a rapid caspase-independent apoptosis-like cell death in human monocytes and dendritic cells. Scand J Immunol 2004; 59:40–49.
143. Johansson U, Londei M. Ligation of CD47 during monocyte differentiation into dendritic cells results in reduced capacity for interleukin-12 production. Scand J Immunol 2004; 59:50–57.
144. Doyen V, Rubio M, Braun D, et al. Thrombospondin 1 is an autocrine negative regulator of human dendritic cell activation. J Exp Med 2003;198:1277–1283.
145. Otani A, Takagi H, Oh H, Koyama S, Matsumura M, Honda Y. Expressions of angiopoietins and Tie2 in human choroidal neovascular membranes. Invest Ophthalmol Vis Sci 1999;40:1912–1920.
146. Oh H, Takagi H, Takagi C, et al. The potential angiogenic role of macrophages in the formation of choroidal neovascular membranes. Invest Ophthalmol Vis Sci 1999;40:1891–1898.
147. Grossniklaus HE, Ling JX, Wallace TM, et al. Macrophage and retinal pigment epithelium expression of angiogenic cytokines in choroidal neovascularization. Mol Vis 2002; 8:119–126.
148. Cursiefen C, Rummelt C, Kuchle M. Immunohistochemical localization of vascular endothelial growth factor, transforming growth factor alpha, and transforming growth factor beta1 in human corneas with neovascularization. Cornea 2000;19:526–533.
149. Yoshida S, Yoshida A, Ishibashi T. Induction of IL-8, MCP-1, and bFGF by TNF-alpha in retinal glial cells: implications for retinal neovascularization during post-ischemic inflammation. Graefes Arch Clin Exp Ophthalmol 2004;242:409–413.
150. Hamrah P, Chen L, Zhang Q, Dana MR. Novel expression of vascular endothelial growth factor receptor (VEGFR)-3 and VEGF-C on corneal dendritic cells. Am J Pathol 2003;163:57–68.
151. Shaw JP, Chuang N, Yee H, Shamamian P. Polymorphonuclear neutrophils promote rFGF-2-induced angiogenesis in vivo. J Surg Res 2003;109:37–42.
152. Deshpande SP, Zheng M, Lee S, Rouse BT. Mechanisms of pathogenesis in herpetic immunoinflammatory ocular lesions. Vet Microbiol 2002;86:17–26.

15

Regulation of Ocular Angiogenesis by Matrix Proteases and Tissue Inhibitors of Metalloproteinases

Bela Anand-Apte, MBBS, PhD

CONTENTS

INTRODUCTION

Angiogenesis, the sprouting of new capillaries from preexisting blood vessels, is a multistep process requiring the degradation of the basement membrane, endothelial cell migration, capillary tube formation, and endothelial cell proliferation. Until recently, this was considered to be the sole mechanism of neovascularization in postnatal life. However, recent studies have altered this dogma with emerging evidence that bone marrow-derived endothelial, hematopoietic stem, and progenitor cells contribute significantly to postnatal neovascularization. Precise spatial and temporal regulation of extracellular proteolytic activity mediated by matrix-degrading enzymes appears to be important in the initial process of endothelial cell invasion into the extracellular matrix (ECM) *(1)*, as well as in the recruitment of progenitor cells to the angiogenic site. Endogenous inhibitors of these proteases have been postulated to play a key role in maintaining the physiological quiescence of blood vessels in adults. Here, we review the potential roles and mechanisms of action of matrix proteases and tissue inhibitors of metalloproteinases (TIMPs) in angiogenesis.

MATRIX-DEGRADING ENZYMES AS REGULATORS OF NEOVASCULARIZATION

Extracellular proteolysis is mediated for the most part by three families of enzymes (Table 1): the matrix metalloproteinases (MMPs), the **a** **d**isintegrin **a**nd **m**etalloprotease

From: *Ophthalmology: Ocular Angiogenesis: Diseases, Mechanisms, and Therapeutics*
Edited by: J. Tombran-Tink and C. J. Barnstable © Humana Press Inc., Totowa, NJ

Table 1
Expression of Matrix Proteases in Retina

Enzyme	*MMP*	*Expression in normal retina*	*Retinal vascular disease*	*Experimental model of ocular neovascularization*
Collagenases				
Interstitial collagenase; collagenase 1	MMP-1	Inner and outer nuclear and plexiform layers *(26)*; IPM and vitreous *(27)*; perivascular microglia of optical nerve head *(28)*; Bruch's membrane *(29)*	PDR membrane *(26)*	
Gelatinases				
Gelatinase A	MMP-2	IPM, vitreous, and RPE *(27,30,31)*; Müller cells *(32)*; perivascular microglia of optical nerve head *(28)*; Bruch's membrane/choroid *(29)*	Increased expression in IPM *(33)* and surrounding vessels *(34)* in AMD; Increased expression in PDR membranes *(26,35)*	Increased expression in laser induced CNV *(36)* and hyperoxia *(37)*. Reduced CNV formation in MMP-2 deficient mice *(38)*
Gelatinase B	MMP-9	IPM, vitreous, and RPE *(27,30,31)*; Müller cells *(32)*; Bruch's membrane/ choroid *(29)*	Increased expression in AMD *(34)* Increased expression in PDR membranes *(39)*	Laser-induced CNV reduced in MMP-9-deficient mice *(40)*
Stromelysins				
Stromelysin 1	MMP-3	Bruch's membrane; perivascular microglia of optical nerve head *(28)*	?	?
Membrane-type MMPs				
Transmembrane MT1-MMP	MMP-14	Sclera, cornea, lens, choroid, RPE, and retina *(41)*; perivascular microglia of optical nerve head *(28)*	?	?
ADAMs				
ADAM15		Retinal capillaries	?	Reduced neovascularization in *adam15*$^{-/-}$ in a mouse model of ROP *(20)*

MMP, matrix metalloproteinase; PDR, proliferative diabetic retinopathy; IPM, interphotoreceptor matrix; RPE, retinal pigment epithelium; AMD, age-related macular degeneration; CNV, choroidal neovascularization; ADAM, a distintegrin and a metalloproteinase; ROP, retinopathy of prematurity.

domain (ADAM) family and the **a d**isintegrin-like **a**nd **m**etalloprotease domain (reprolysin type) with **t**hrombo**s**pondin type I repeats (ADAMTS) family. MMPs (e.g., collagenases; gelatinases A, 72 kDa, and B, 92 kDa; and stromelysins) are a family of zinc-binding, Ca^{2+}-dependent neutral endopeptidases that can act together or in concert with other enzymes to degrade most components of the ECM *(2,3)*. These enzymes have been implicated in invasive cell behavior; recent studies have indicated that MMPs play an important role in the regulation of angiogenesis *(4–8)*. MMP-2, the most widely distributed MMP is localized on the surface of angiogenic blood vessels *(9)*. Shedding of MMP-containing vesicles by activated endothelial cells may be a mechanism for regulating focal proteolytic activity vital for invasive and morphogenic events during angiogenesis *(10)*. Mice deficient in MMP-2, MMP-9, or MMP-14 exhibit reduced angiogenesis in vivo *(11–13)*. In contrast, ADAMTS-1 has been shown to sequester vascular endothelial growth factor (VEGF) and prevent binding to its receptor *(14)*, resulting in potent antiangiogenic properties *(15)*.

A number of mechanisms by which remodeling of the ECM by MMPs and other proteases can regulate angiogenesis have been proposed (Fig. 1) *(8,16)*. Because MMPs degrade proteins in the ECM, their primary function has been considered to be the breakdown of the capillary basement membrane to allow the migration of endothelial cells into the surrounding matrix. MMP-2 interacts with $\alpha_v\beta_3$ on the surface of angiogenic blood vessels *(17)*, which can be blocked by PEX (a noncatalytic C-terminal hemopexin-like domainfragment of MMP-2) resulting in angiogenesis inhibition *(18)*. More recently, additional ectodomain shedding and release of matrix-bound angiogenic factors, cytokine receptors, and adhesion molecules, mediated by MMPs *(19)* and ADAMs *(20,21)*, has been suggested to contribute to this process. In addition, MMPs are capable of disengaging cryptic domains of basement membrane proteins to expose integrin binding sites and angiogenesis regulatory sequences *(18,22)*. Endostatin, arrestin, canstatin, and tumstatin are examples of novel basement membrane-derived fragments that are endogenous inhibitors of angiogenesis *(23)*. Mobilization of bone marrow-derived endothelial progenitor cells (EPCs) to an angiogenic site is regulated by chemokines/cytokines. Recent evidence suggests that MMP-9-mediated Kit ligand (stem cell factor) processing is essential for the mobilization of EPCs *(24)*. Survival of angiogenic endothelial cells and perhaps EPCs is also regulated by cooperation between growth factor receptors and integrins, which are governed by the composition of the local ECM *(25)*. Thus, MMPs can play both a proangiogenic role, by breaking down capillary basement membrane as well as releasing matrix-bound angiogenic factors as well as an antiangiogenic role by generating ECM fragments with antiangiogenic properties. The precise balance between these two functions is likely important in the determination of the angiogenic state of a tissue.

MATRIX PROTEASES IN NORMAL RETINA AND RETINAL NEOVASCULAR DISEASES

MMP-1, MMP-2, MMP-3, MMP-9, MMP-13, and MMP-14 are expressed in the human retina (Table 1). However, detailed spatial and temporal expression patterns of the active forms of these enzymes has not been determined. Interestingly, expression of active MMP-2 exclusively in the peripheral retina and its distinct absence from the macula *(29)* suggests active remodeling in the periphery and provides clues to the pathogenesis of macular disease. A complex pattern of MMP and ADAM gene expression

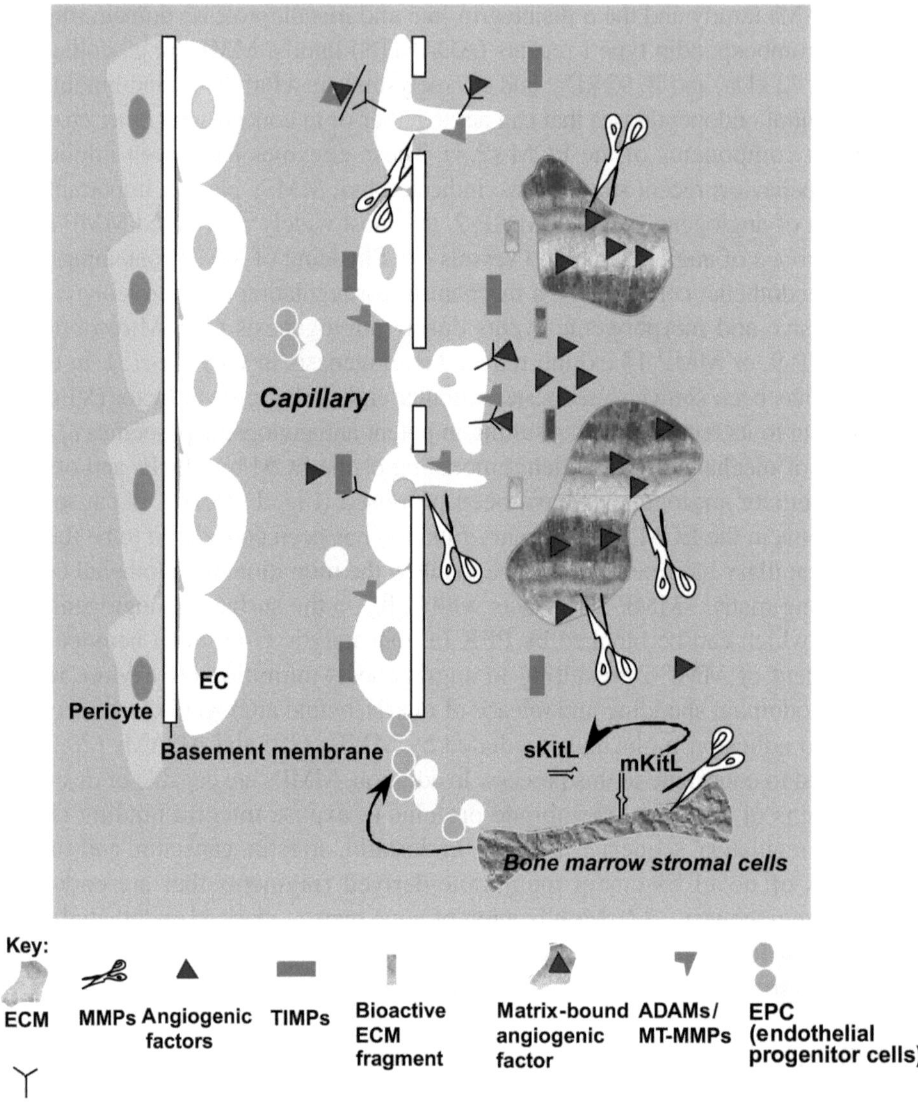

Fig. 1. Role of MMPs in angiogenesis. The matrix metalloproteinases (MMPs) possess both angiogenesis-inducing as well as inhibitory functions. MMPs can break down the capillary basement membrane and allow the migration of endothelial cells into the surrounding extracellular matrix (ECM) when initiated by angiogenic factors such as vascular endothelial growth factor (VEGF). This effect might be a result of removing an inhibitory barrier of basement membrane, inducing a migration stimulatory signal and/or by exposing cryptc binding sites within the matrix molecule to stimulate migration. MMPs can also release matrix-sequestered angiogenic factors such as VEGF and fibroblast growth factor (FGF)-2 and increase their bioavailability. A fragment of cleaved collagen-IV binds to $\alpha_v\beta_3$ integrin and stimulates angiogenesis. MMP-9-mediated Kit ligand processing stimulates the mobilization of endothelial progenitor cells from the bone marrow into the circulation. MMPs play a critical role in the processing of a number of bioactive ECM fragments such as endostatin, arrestin, canstatin, and tumstatin that show potent angio-inhibitory properties. ADAMTS-1 has been shown to sequester VEGF directly and prevent it's binding to KDR. *See* color version on companion CD.

during postnatal mouse retinal development *(42)* suggests that these proteins play an important role in the tightly regulated process of retinal neovascularization.

Retinal Neovascularization

Retinal neovascularization associated with hemorrhage or retinal detachment is a complication of proliferative diabetic retinopathy (PDR), retinopathy of prematurity (ROP), and retinal vascular occlusions. One commonly used model for studying the pathogenesis of retinal neovascularization involves the exposure of newborn mice to hyperoxia. Reduced retinal angiogenesis has been observed in hyperoxic mice deficient in MMP-2, raising the possibility of MMP-2 playing a role in the regulation of pathological retinal neovascularization *(43)*. Furthermore, increased expression as well as increased levels of the active forms of retinal MMP-2 and MMP-9 have been demonstrated during the active phase of angiogenesis in this model *(44,45)*. Reduction in these levels by systemic administration of an MMP inhibitor resulted in reduced retinal neovascularization *(37)*.

Proliferative diabetic retinopathy (PDR) is believed to be the result of a hypoxic stimulus that drives the expression of angiogenic factors such as VEGF, which may stimulate retinal capillary endothelial cells to secrete active MMP-2 *(46)* and initiate neovascularization. Increased expression of MMP-2 and MMP-9 has been observed in the vitreous as well as in the PDR membranes removed from patients' eyes *(26,31, 35,39,47)*. Bone marrow-derived stem cells target retinal astrocytes that serve as a template for developmental and pathological retinal angiogenesis *(48)*. More recently, a role for tissue factor (TF)-VIIa protease complex in the induction of developmental retinal angiogenesis via protease-activated receptor (PAR-2) signaling has been proposed *(49)*.

Choroidal Neovascularization

Age-related macular degeneration (AMD) is the leading cause of legal blindness in the elderly population, with about 35% of people 75 yr or older suffering from some degree of AMD. While the "wet," neovascular form of AMD affects approx 10% of the patients, choroidal neovascularization (CNV) accounts for more than 80% of the severe debilitating vision loss in all AMD patients. It has been proposed that the thickening of Bruch's membrane seen in this disease might be a result of altered matrix turnover or remodeling. Matrix-degrading proteases have been hypothesized to play a role in this as well as in the initiation of the neovascular invasion of the choriocapillaris through Bruch's membrane. Various studies have described the increased expression of MMP-2 and MMP-9 in the Bruch's/choroid complex with age *(29)* as well as in the interphotoreceptor matrix *(27)* and choroidal neovascular membranes *(34)* in AMD eyes. Because the increase in enzyme was mostly the inactive form, the question arises as to whether the increased expression is causative or a consequence of the pathology. MMP-2 is involved in the formation of experimental CNV in mice *(38)* and recently has been shown to synergize with MMP-9 in promoting CNV *(50)*. In addition, an as-yet unanswered question is whether activation of MMPs precedes or is required for neovascularization *(51)*. Localization of MMP-2, MMP-7, and MMP-9 expression to areas of new vessel formation in CNV membranes suggests a possible role in the development of this process

(34,52). In the absence of a good animal model for AMD, this may begin to be addressed by examining a large cohort of well-characterized disease donor eyes at various stages of the disease. Comparisons between the exudative and nonexudative forms of the disease may provide clues to the role of the matrix-degrading proteases in the pathogenesis of the complex phenotype of AMD. The potential efficacy of MMP inhibitors for the prevention of CNV in patients at risk for development or for recurrence following laser photocoagulation or surgical excision remains to be determined.

ENDOGENOUS INHIBITORS OF MMPs: TISSUE INHIBITORS OF METALLOPROTEINASES

MMPs need to be activated before executing their biochemical functions of degrading matrix. MMP activity is tightly regulated in response to the potential consequences of disrupted ECM integrity *(53)*. The complex regulation of these enzymes occurs via numerous mechanisms such as transcriptional regulation, mRNA stability, cell compartmentalization, and activation of secreted proenzymes via proteolysis and via specific endogenous inhibitors. These include the tissue inhibitors of metalloproteinases (TIMPs), which bind to activated MMPs with 1:1 molar stoichiometry *(54,55);* thrombospondins *(56–58);* membrane-anchored glycoprotein **re**version-inducing **c**ysteine-rich protein with **k**azal motifs (RECK); and α2-macroglobulin. Of these inhibitors, TIMPs are considered the key inhibitors in tissue and will be the focus of this review. Four TIMPs (Table 2) have been identified in vertebrates *(54,59);* their expression is regulated during development and tissue remodeling with specific tissues expressing a unique signature of proteinase and inhibitor expression *(60)*.

Mammalian TIMPs show 35 to 40% identity at the amino acid level and are capable of inhibiting the MMP family of enzymes with equal efficacy in in vitro assays *(61)*. Structurally, TIMPs have a two-domain structure (N- and C-terminal domain of 125 and 65 amino acids, respectively), with each domain folded into three loops held together by three disulfide bonds *(62)*. The N-terminal domain contains the highly conserved CXC motif that is responsible for MMP inhibition. TIMP-1, TIMP-2, and TIMP-4 are "soluble" proteins and are present in numerous body fluids *(63)*, whereas TIMP-3 is unique in being tightly bound to the ECM *(64)*. This binding is via the interaction of the C-terminal domain of TIMP-3 with heparan sulfate and chondroitin sulfate chains on the cell surface or with secreted proteoglycans *(65,66)*. Through these interactions, TIMP-3 is localized and this may spatially regulate its activity to specific sites.

Although TIMPs do not show strong selectivity toward active MMPs (except for TIMP-1, which is a poor inhibitor of all the MT-MMPs), they do show specificity in association with the latent MMPs (e.g., TIMP-1 associates preferentially with pro-MMP-9 and TIMP-2 associates with pro-MMP-2). The inhibitory profile of TIMPs toward the ADAMs and ADAMTS molecules appears to be more selective. TIMP-3 is unique in its ability to inhibit ADAM-17 (TACE) *(67)*, ADAM-10 *(68)*, ADAM-12 *(69)*, and the aggrecanases (ADAMTS-4 and ADAMTS-5) *(70)*. It also inhibits the shedding of interleukin-6 (IL-6) *(71)*, L-selectin *(72)*, and syndecans 1 and 4 *(73)* that is thought to be mediated by the ADAM-type proteases. However, more recent evidence suggests that the TIMPs may also show differential inhibition of the MT-MMPs. TIMP-3

Table 2
Biological Properties of Tissue Inhibitors of Metalloproteinases (TIMPs)

Biological property	*TIMP-1*	*TIMP-2*	*TIMP-3*	*TIMP-4*
MMPs inhibited	MMP-1, MMP-2, MMP-3, MMP-7, MMP-8, MMP-9, MMP-10, MMP-11, MMP-12, MMP13, MMP-17, MMP-19, MMP-25, MMP-26	MMP-1, MMP-2, MMP-3, MMP-7, MMP-8, MMP-9, MMP-10, MMP-13, MMP-14, MMP-16, MMP-17, MMP-19, MMP-24, MMP-25, MMP-26	MMP-1, MMP-2, MMP-3, MMP-9, MMP-13, MMP-14, MMP-16, MMP-17, MMP-19, MMP-25, MMP-26	MMP-1, MMP-2, MMP-3, MMP-8, MMP-9, MMP-14, MMP-19
ADAMs inhibited	ADAM-10		ADAM-10, ADAM-12, ADAM-17	
ADAMTSs inhibited	ADAMTS4	ADAMTS1 ADAMTS4	ADAMTS1 ADAMTS4, ADAMTS5	ADAMTS4
MMPs, ADAMs, and ADAMTSs not inhibited	MMP-14, MMP-16, MMP-24, ADAM-12, ADAM-17	ADAM-10, ADAM-12, ADAM-17		ADAM-10, ADAM-17
MMPs activated	None	MMP-2	None	None
Apoptosis	Inhibits	Promotes/inhibits	Promotes/inhibits	Promotes/inhibits

ADAM, a disintegrin and a metalloproteinase; MMP, matrix metalloproteinase.

appears to be a higher-affinity inhibitor of MT3-MMP than MT1-MMP, whereas in contrast, TIMP-2 is a better inhibitor of MT1-MMP *(74)*. The same study showed that TIMP-3 enhances the activation of pro-MMP-2 by MT3-MMP but not by MT1-MMP, in contrast with TIMP-4, which did not support pro-MMP2 activation with either enzyme. Thus the substrate specificity, transcriptional control, as well as tissue localization of the respective TIMPs might be a mechanism to regulate the specific functions associated with each of these molecules.

Biological Activities of TIMPs

In addition to its role in tissue remodeling as a consequence of its metalloprotease-inhibiting functions, TIMPs have been shown to possess other biological activities. TIMP-1 and TIMP-2 have erythroid potentiating *(75,76)* as well as cell growth promoting *(77,78)* activities. Synthetic broad-spectrum MMP inhibitors do not demonstrate similar growth-promoting activities, leading to the speculation that these properties might be independent of the MMP inhibitory functions. In contrast to TIMP-1, TIMP-2, and TIMP-4, which also have antiapoptotic activity *(79–81)*, TIMP-3 induces apoptosis in a number of cell types by stabilization of death receptors *(82,83)*. More recently, TIMP-3 has been shown to initiate cell apoptosis by inhibiting the shedding of TNFα receptor from the cell surface via the Fas-associated death domain-dependent type II pathway *(82,84–87)*. Studies suggest that the induction of apoptosis by TIMP-3 requires MMP inhibition *(67,82)* although synthetic MMP inhibitors do not demonstrate similar properties *(85,88)*. Interestingly, the antiapoptotic activity of TIMP-1 and TIMP-4 *(81)* appears to be MMP-independent *(89)*. Overexpression of TIMPs by cancer cells inhibits tumor growth in mouse models *(90–95)* with one report of stimulation of tumorigenesis by TIMP-4 *(81)*. Adenovirally or retrovirally delivered TIMP-3 has been shown to have potent antitumor activity, as well as a bystander effect in an animal model of human melanoma *(96,97)*. Since mouse genetic models and human diseases are useful tools to dissect the biological functions of proteins, mice engineered to be deficient in TIMPs have been generated and characterized. Absence of the TIMP-2 gene does not lead to developmental defects, which might reflect genetic redundancy. It is interesting to note that in all cases the mice are viable with varied phenotypes (Table 3).

Expression of TIMPs in Retina

Interphotoreceptor matrix, vitreous, and inner and outer nuclear cell layers of the retina express TIMP-1 and TIMP-2 (Table 4) *(27)*. *In situ* hybridization studies demonstrate the presence of TIMP-3 mRNA in retinal pigment epithelium (RPE) cells *(113)*. TIMP-3 protein is present in low levels around blood vessels in human and nonhuman primate choriocapillaris, Bruch's membrane, and drusen *(114,115)*, and more recently, has been shown to bind to sulfated glycosaminoglycans of the ECM *(66)*. Accumulation of TIMP-3 has been observed in ECM deposits in Sorsby's fundus dystrophy (SFD) *(116)*, AMD *(115)*, and malattia leventinese *(117)*. TIMP-3 is the only MMP inhibitor that has been implicated directly in an inherited disease.

Sorsby's Fundus Dystrophy

SFD, a fully penetrant, autosomal dominant, degenerative disease of the macula *(123)*, is manifested by symptoms of night blindness or sudden loss of acuity, usually

Table 3
Phenotype of Mice Deficient in Tissue Inhibitor of Metalloproteinase (TIMP) Genes

Genotype	*Phenotype*
TIMP-1$^{-/-}$	Hyperresistant to corneal infections with *Pseudomonas aeruginosa (98,99)*; decreased atheroslerotic plaque and increased aneurysms *(100)*; alterations in left ventricular geometry *(101)*; increased medial degradation in mouse model of atherosclerosis (apoE–/–) *(102)*; increased postinjury myocardial remodeling *(103)*; impaired nutritionally induced obesity *(104)*; altered reproductive cyclicity and uterine morphology in reproductive-age female mice *(105)* and decreased serum progesterone levels during corpus luteum development *(106)*; decreased retinal neovascularization in transgenic vascular endothelial factor mice *(107)*.
TIMP-2$^{-/-}$	Reduced pro-matrix metalloproteinase (MMP)-2 activation *(108)*; normal development, viability, fertility, and immune responses *(99,108)*.
TIMP-3$^{-/-}$	Spontaneous airspace enlargement in lungs *(87)* and impaired bronchiole branching morphogenesis *(109)*; increased lung compliance defects following septic lung stress *(110)*; accelerated apoptosis in mammary glands *(111)*; dilated cardiomyopathy *(112)*.
TIMP-4$^{-/-}$	nt

Table 4
Expression of Tissue Inhibitors of Metalloproteinases (TIMPs) in Retina

TIMP	*Expression in normal retina*	*Retinal vascular disease*	*Experimental model of ocular neovascularization*
TIMP-1	Interphotoreceptor matrix (IPM) vitreous *(27)*; inner and outer nuclear cell layers *(26)*		
TIMP-2	IPM/vitreous *(27)*; inner and outer nuclear cell layers *(26)*; Bruch's membrane *(118)*		
TIMP-3	Retinal pigment epithelium/ Bruch's membrane *(113–115,118–120)*; IPM/vitreous *(27)*	Age-related macular degeneration *(115)*; Sorsby's fundus dystrophy *(116)*; malattia leventinese *(117)*	Inhibition of choroidal neovascularization *(121)* and angiogenesis in retinopathy of prematurity model *(122)*

in the third to fourth decades of life, due to submacular neovascularization *(124–127)*. Clinically, early, midperipheral drusen and color vision deficits are found *(126,127)*. SFD is a relatively rare disease but has generated significant interest because it closely resembles the exudative or "wet" form of age-related macular degeneration (AMD). SFD is characterized by accumulation of extracellular deposits (drusen) in Bruch's membrane, the five-layered sheet of connective tissue separating the RPE from the choriocapillaris *(128)*. This is distinct from the basal linear deposits seen in AMD,

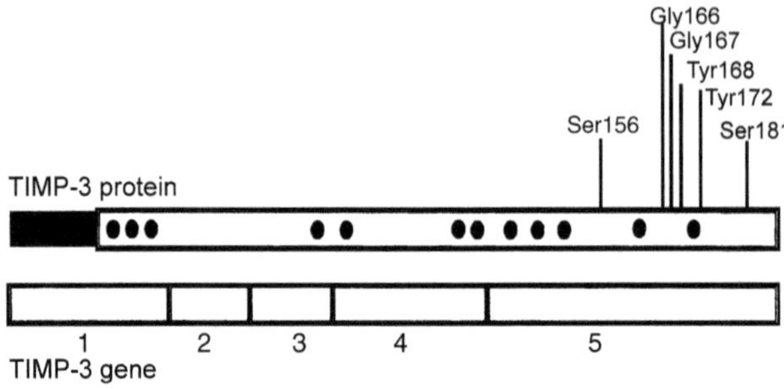

Fig. 2. Cysteine substitutions in exon 5 of the tissue inhibitor of metalloproteinase (TIMP)-3 gene cause Sorsby's fundus dystrophy. *See* color version on companion CD.

which consists of filamentous fine granular material and may represent a thickened basement membrane of the RPE *(128)*. The subretinal deposits in both SFD and AMD have been shown to be rich in TIMP-3 *(115,116,129)*. However, no increase in TIMP-3 RNA was found in the RPE in SFD *(130)*. Possible posttranslational modifications or oxidative processes may contribute to an aggregation of TIMP-3, leading to accumulation of the protein in drusen *(117,129)*. A serious complication of SFD and AMD is the invasion of the thickened Bruch's membrane by newly formed, thin-walled vessels derived from the choriocapillaris. These vessels grow into the subretinal space, causing exudative detachment of the RPE and loss of photoreceptors *(131)*. The symptom of night blindness in SFD can be reversed by large doses of vitamin A, supporting the notion that nutritional deprivation of photoreceptors, owing to the thickened Bruch's membrane, may be a part of the pathophysiology of the disease *(125)*. It is possible that this membrane thickening may also contribute to hypoxic conditions for RPE cells and result in increased secretion of the angiogenic factor, vascular endothelial growth factor (VEGF), which can induce neovascularization. Based on similar clinical and histopathological features, in particular at the level of Bruch's membrane, SFD has been considered to be a genetic model for the more common macular degenerations *(128,132–134)*.

TIMP-3 Mutations Cause Sorsby's Fundus Dystrophy

SFD has been linked with mutations in the TIMP-3 gene *(135–137)*, with eight different missense mutations and a splice site mutation having been identified to date. Interestingly, all mutations identified so far occur in the COOH-terminal portion of the TIMP-3 protein with the introduction of a new cysteine (Fig. 2). These additional thiol groups are located close to the last two conserved cysteine residues, which are believed toparticipate in normal intrachain disulfide bond rearrangements *(138)*. It has been proposed that the C-terminal domains may participate in the modulation of the TIMP/MMP interactions by increasing the low-affinity binding characteristics between the two molecules *(139,140)*. It remains to be determined whether the introduction of a new cysteine in SFD-TIMP-3 affects binding to and/or activation of MMPs. Based on the dominant nature of the disease and its similarity in unrelated families, it is possible that the new cysteine may participate in abnormal interchain bonds with another ECM protein present specifically in the retina. This might explain the presence of an ocular phenotype but sparing of other organs in SFD. It can be hypothesized that SFD mutations in TIMP-3 may lead to an abnormal turnover or localization of TIMP-3

Table 5
Angiogenesis Inhibition by Tissue Inhibitors of Metalloproteinases (TIMPs)

Angiogenesis	*TIMP-1*	*TIMP-2*	*TIMP-3*	*TIMP-4*
Capillary EC proliferation	Stimulates	Inhibits	No effect	nt
In vivo angiogenesis	Inhibits Stimulates None	Inhibits None	Inhibits	nt
Choroidal neovascularization	Stimulates	nt	Inhibits	nt
Retinal neovascularization	nt	nt	Inhibits	nt

together with altered binding to specific ECM molecules present in Bruch's membrane. This might play a role in the thick deposits seen in SFD as well as in changing a biological function attributed to normal TIMP-3. Concomitantly, the increased MMP activity generated by the mutant TIMP-3 may induce CNV *(141)*. SFD is of considerable interest, as it is the only genetic disorder in which hemorrhagic macular degeneration occurs in the majority of affected patients. It is likely that TIMP-3 might be an important physiological angiogenesis inhibitor of the choriocapillaris, and mutations or oxidative modifications might result in the loss of its angioinhibitory activity. Thus, understanding the role of TIMPs in the regulation of angiogenesis may provide clues to deciphering the mysteries of ocular neovascular diseases.

TIMP-3 Expression in the Eye

In situ hybridization studies have demonstrated the presence of TIMP-3 mRNA in RPE cells *(113)*. TIMP-3 protein is present in low levels around blood vessels in human and nonhuman primate choriocapillaris, Bruch's membrane, and drusen *(114,115)*. A progressive increase in expression of TIMP-3 during postnatal mouse retinal development suggests a possible regulatory role during retinal neovascularization *(42)*. Accumulation of TIMP-3 has been observed in ECM deposits in SFD *(116)*, malattia leventinese *(117)*, and AMD *(115)*. Based on previous results of inhibition of angiogenesis by TIMP-3 *(142)*, it can be hypothesized that TIMP-3 may be required to maintain the choriocapillaris in a quiescent state by controlling and localizing the degradation of the matrix around the blood vessels.

DIFFERENTIAL EFFECTS OF TIMPs ON ANGIOGENESIS

TIMPs have been shown to have antiangiogenic properties *(142–147)*. Although structurally similar, members of the TIMP family demonstrate differential effects on the component processes of angiogenesis. Endothelial cell migration is inhibited by TIMP-3 *(142)* and TIMP-2 *(147)* but not by TIMP-1 *(142)*. Microvascular endothelial cell proliferation appears to be inhibited exclusively by TIMP-2, whereas TIMP-1 has been reported to stimulate capillary endothelial cell growth *(77,147)*. TIMP-2, TIMP-3, and TIMP-4 inhibit tube formation induced by basic fibroblast growth factor (bFGF) and VEGF *(142,148)*. VEGF-mediated angiogenesis in an in vivo chicken chorioallantoic membrane assay was inhibited by TIMP-3 but not by TIMP-1 *(149)*. These results suggest that the antiangiogenic activities of TIMP-2 and TIMP-3 are more closely related to each other than to TIMP-1. TIMP-3 inhibits experimental CNV *(121)* and retinal neovascularization in a ROP model *(122)* (Table 5).

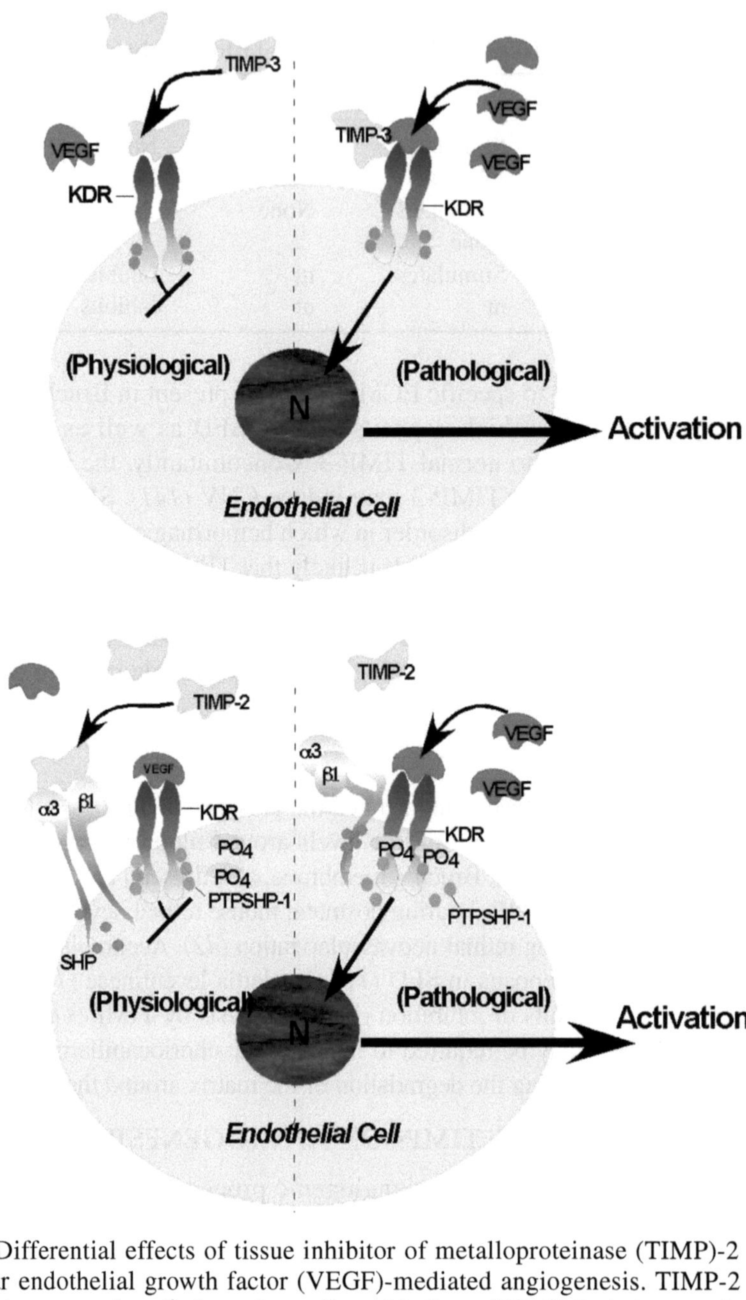

Fig. 3. Differential effects of tissue inhibitor of metalloproteinase (TIMP)-2 and TIMP-3 on vascular endothelial growth factor (VEGF)-mediated angiogenesis. TIMP-2 inhibition of angiogenesis occurs via $\alpha_3\beta_1$ integrin-mediated binding of TIMP-2. A decrease in total protein phosphatase activity associated with β_1 integrin subunits results in an increase in phosphotyrosine phosphatase (PTP) activity associated with fibroblast growth factor receptor (FGFR)-1 and KDR (VEGFR-2), leading to an inhibition of the downstream signaling pathway. TIMP-3 blocks the binding of VEGF to KDR and thereby inhibits VEGF-mediated angiogenesis.

The detailed molecular mechanism by which TIMP-2 and TIMP-3 inhibit angiogenesis have been recently studied and yielded unexpected results (Fig. 3). Both molecules inhibit angiogenesis by MMP-independent mechanisms *(149,150)*. TIMP-2 inhibition of angiogenesis occurs via $\alpha_3\beta_1$ integrin-mediated binding of TIMP-2 to endothelial cells. A concomitant decrease in total protein phosphatase activity associated with β1 integrin subunits along with an increase in phosphotyrosine phosphatase (PTP) activity associated with FGFR-1 and KDR (VEGFR-2) were critical for the inhibitory activity of TIMP-2 *(150)* (Fig. 3). The COOH-terminal loop 6 domain of TIMP-2 was recently found to be critical to inhibiting mitogen-driven angiogenesis *(151)*. In contrast, TIMP-3 blocks the binding of VEGF exclusively to its receptor KDR and inhibits downstream signaling and angiogenesis *(149)* (Fig. 3). This inhibitory activity is also contained in the COOH-terminal end of the protein (Anand-Apte, unpublished observations). TIMP-3 is a secreted protein that distinguishes itself from other members of the TIMP family by its ability to bind to the ECM. In the outer retina, TIMP-3 is synthesized by the RPE and deposited into Bruch's membrane *(113–115,152)*. The specific localization of KDR at the inner choriocapillaris, facing the RPE, supports the notion that VEGF secreted by the RPE is involved in a physiological paracrine association with the choriocapillaris *(153)*. By virtue of its angioinhibitory properties as well as its presence in Bruch's membrane, it could be hypothesized that TIMP-3 plays an important role in the regulation of the angiogenic state of the choriocapillaris. Although the development of the choriocapillaris is being analyzed in detail in mice deficient in TIMP-3 (Anand-Apte, unpublished observations), there appear to be no gross abnormalities on fluorescein angiograms. This suggests the possibility that there may be compensatory mechanisms that come into play or that TIMP-3 might more specifically inhibit pathological neovascularization because of an excess of angiogenic molecules, as seen in AMD. The recent report that TIMP-1 expression increases retinal neovascularization in a mouse model *(107)* reinforces the fact that the control of ocular neovascularization is a complex series of events. It also cautions against a rush to clinical trials prior to gaining knowledge about detailed mechanisms of actions of potential therapeutic molecules.

CONCLUSION

At present, our understanding of the pathogenesis and regulation of ocular neovascularization is at best in its infancy. There are a number of molecules that interplay to regulate this very tightly controlled process. Given that TIMPs have multiple functions, both MMP-dependent and -independent, and that MMPs, ADAMs, ADAMTS, and integrins are all part of a meshwork of molecules that are potent regulators of angiogenesis themselves, further knowledge needs to be gained regarding the role of these proteins in the control of retinal and subretinal neovascularization.

ACKNOWLEDGMENTS

This work was supported by the following grants to B.A-A: NIH (1 R29EY12109-01), Foundation Fighting Blindness (module of center grant), Cleveland Clinic Foundation (seed grant), and American Heart Association (Grant in Aid #455170B).

REFERENCES

1. Pepper MS, Montesano R, Mandriota SJ, Orci L, Vassalli J-D. Angiogenesis: a paradigm for balanced extracellular proteolysis during cell migration and morphogenesis. Enzyme Protein 1996;49:138–162.
2. Matrisian LM. The matrix-degrading metalloproteinases. Bioessays 1992;14:455–463.

3. Somerville RP, Oblander SA, Apte SS. Matrix metalloproteinases: old dogs with new tricks. Genome Biol 2003;4:216.
4. Hiraoka N, Allen E, Apel IJ, Gyetko MR, Weiss SJ. Matrix metalloproteinases regulate neovascularization by acting as pericellular fibrinolysins. Cell 1998;95:365–377.
5. Stetler-Stevenson WG, Yu AE. Proteases in invasion: matrix metalloproteinases. Semin Cancer Biol 2001;11:143–152.
6. Stetler-Stevenson WG. The role of matrix metalloproteinases in tumor invasion, metastasis, and angiogenesis. Surg Oncol Clin N Am 2001;10:383–392, x.
7. Werb Z, Vu TH, Rinkenberger JL, Coussens LM. Matrix-degrading proteases and angiogenesis during development and tumor formation. Apmis 1999;107:11–18.
8. Chang C, Werb Z. The many faces of metalloproteases: cell growth, invasion, angiogenesis and metastasis. Trends Cell Biol 2001;11:S37–S43.
9. Brooks PC. Cell adhesion molecules in angiogenesis. Cancer Metastasis Rev 1996;15: 187–194.
10. Taraboletti G, D'Ascenzo S, Borsotti P, Giavazzi R, Pavan A, Dolo V. Shedding of the matrix metalloproteinases MMP-2, MMP-9, MT1-MMP as membrane vesicle-associated components by endothelial cells. Am J Pathol 2002;160:673–680.
11. Itoh T, Tanioka M, Yoshida H, et al. Reduced angiogenesis and tumor progression in gelatinase A-deficient mice. Cancer Res 1998;58:1048–1051.
12. Vu TH, Shipley JM, Bergers G, et al. MMP-9/gelatinase B is a key regulator of growth plate angiogenesis and apoptosis of hypertrophic chondrocytes. Cell 1998;93: 411–422.
13. Zhou Z, Apte SS, Soininen R, et al. Impaired endochondral ossification and angiogenesis in mice deficient in membrane-type matrix metalloproteinase I. Proc Natl Acad Sci USA 2000;97:4052–4057.
14. Luque A, Carpizo DR, Iruela-Arispe ML. ADAMTS1/METH1 inhibits endothelial cell proliferation by direct binding and sequestration of VEGF165. J Biol Chem 2003;278: 23,656–23,665.
15. Vazquez F, Hastings G, Ortega MA, et al. METH-1, a human ortholog of ADAMTS-1, METH-2 are members of a new family of proteins with angio-inhibitory activity. J Biol Chem 1999;274:23,349–23,357.
16. Lafleur MA, Handsley MM, Edwards DR. Metalloproteinases and their inhibitors in angiogenesis. Expert Rev Mol Med 2003;5:1–39.
17. Brooks PC, Stromblad S, Sanders LC, et al. Localization of matrix metalloproteinase MMP-2 to the surface of invasive cells by interaction with integrin alpha v beta 3. Cell 1996;85:683–693.
18. Brooks PC, Silletti S, von Schalscha TL, Friedlander M, Cheresh DA. Disruption of angiogenesis by PEX, a noncatalytic metalloproteinase fragment with integrin binding activity. Cell 1998;92:391–400.
19. Bergers G, Brekken R, McMahon G, et al. Matrix metalloproteinase-9 triggers the angiogenic switch during carcinogenesis. Nat Cell Biol 2000;2:737–744.
20. Horiuchi K, Weskamp G, Lum L, et al. Potential role for ADAM15 in pathological neovascularization in mice. Mol Cell Biol 2003;23:5614–5624.
21. Garton KJ, Gough PJ, Philalay J, et al. Stimulated shedding of vascular cell adhesion molecule 1 (VCAM-1) is mediated by tumor necrosis factor-alpha-converting enzyme (ADAM 17). J Biol Chem 2003;278:37,459–37,464.
22. Xu J, Rodriguez D, Petitclerc E, Kim JJ, et al. Proteolytic exposure of a cryptic site within collagen type IV is required for angiogenesis and tumor growth in vivo. J Cell Biol 2001;154:1069–1080.
23. Kalluri R. Basement membranes: structure, assembly and role in tumour angiogenesis. Nat Rev Cancer 2003;3:422–433.

24. Heissig B, Hattori K, Dias S, et al. Recruitment of stem and progenitor cells from the bone marrow niche requires MMP-9 mediated release of kit-ligand. Cell 2002;109:625–637.
25. Stupack DG, Cheresh DA. Apoptotic cues from the extracellular matrix: regulators of angiogenesis. Oncogene 2003;22:9022–9029.
26. Salzmann J, Limb GA, Khaw PT, et al. Matrix metalloproteinases and their natural inhibitors in fibrovascular membranes of proliferative diabetic retinopathy. Br J Ophthalmol 2000;84:1091–1096.
27. Plantner JJ, Smine A, Quinn TA. Matrix metalloproteinases and metalloproteinase inhibitors in human interphotoreceptor matrix and vitreous. Curr Eye Res 1998;17:132–140.
28. Yuan L, Neufeld AH. Activated microglia in the human glaucomatous optic nerve head. J Neurosci Res 2001;64:523–532.
29. Guo L, Hussain AA, Limb GA, Marshall J. Age-dependent variation in metalloproteinase activity of isolated human Bruch's membrane and choroid. Invest Ophthalmol Vis Sci 1999;40:2676–2682.
30. Padgett LC, Lui GM, Werb Z, LaVail MM. Matrix metalloproteinase-2 and tissue inhibitor of metalloproteinase-1 in the retinal pigment epithelium and interphotoreceptor matrix: vectorial secretion and regulation. Exp Eye Res 1997;64:927–938.
31. De La Paz MA, Itoh Y, Toth CA, Nagase H. Matrix metalloproteinases and their inhibitors in human vitreous. Invest Ophthalmol Vis Sci 1998;39:1256–1260.
32. Limb GA, Daniels JT, Pleass R, Charteris DG, Luthert PJ, Khaw PT. Differential expression of matrix metalloproteinases 2 and 9 by glial Muller cells: response to soluble and extracellular matrix-bound tumor necrosis factor-alpha. Am J Pathol 2002;160: 1847–1855.
33. Plantner JJ, Jiang C, Smine A. Increase in interphotoreceptor matrix gelatinase A (MMP-2) associated with age-related macular degeneration. Exp Eye Res 1998;67:637–645.
34. Steen B, Sejersen S, Berglin L, Seregard S, Kvanta A. Matrix metalloproteinases and metalloproteinase inhibitors in choroidal neovascular membranes. Invest Ophthalmol Vis Sci 1998;39:2194–2200.
35. Webster L, Chignell AH, Limb GA. Predominance of MMP-1 and MMP-2 in epiretinal and subretinal membranes of proliferative vitreoretinopathy. Exp Eye Res 1999;68:91–98.
36. Kvanta A, Shen WY, Sarman S, Seregard S, Steen B, Rakoczy E. Matrix metalloproteinase (MMP) expression in experimental choroidal neovascularization. Curr Eye Res 2000;21: 684–690.
37. Das A, McLamore A, Song W, McGuire PG. Retinal neovascularization is suppressed with a matrix metalloproteinase inhibitor. Arch Ophthalmol 1999;117:498–503.
38. Berglin L, Sarman S, van der Ploeg I, et al. A Reduced choroidal neovascular membrane formation in matrix metalloproteinase-2-deficient mice. Invest Ophthalmol Vis Sci 2003;44: 403–408.
39. Brown D, Hamdi H, Bahri S, Kenney MC. Characterization of an endogenous metalloproteinase in human vitreous. Curr Eye Res 1994;13:639–647.
40. Lambert V, Munaut C, Jost M, et al. Matrix metalloproteinase-9 contributes to choroidal neovascularization. Am J Pathol 2002;161:1247–1253.
41. Smine A, Plantner JJ. Membrane type-1 matrix metalloproteinase in human ocular tissues. Curr Eye Res 1997;16:925–929.
42. Dorrell MI, Aguilar E, Weber C, Friedlander M. Global gene expression analysis of the developing postnatal mouse retina. Invest Ophthalmol Vis Sci 2004;45:1009–1019.
43. Ohno-Matsui K, Uetama T, Yoshida T, et al. Reduced retinal angiogenesis in MMP-2-deficient mice. Invest Ophthalmol Vis Sci 2003;44:5370–5375.
44. Das A, McGuire PG, Eriqat C, et al. Human diabetic neovascular membranes contain high levels of urokinase and metalloproteinase enzymes. Invest Ophthalmol Vis Sci 1999;40: 809–813.

45. Majka S, McGuire P, Colombo S, Das A. The balance between proteinases and inhibitors in a murine model of proliferative retinopathy. Invest Ophthalmol Vis Sci 2001;42: 210–215.
46. Ben-Yosef Y, Lahat N, Shapiro S, Bitterman H, Miller A. Regulation of endothelial matrix metalloproteinase-2 by hypoxia/reoxygenation. Circ Res 2002;90:784–791.
47. Noda K, Ishida S, Inoue M, et al. Production and activation of matrix metalloproteinase-2 in proliferative diabetic retinopathy. Invest Ophthalmol Vis Sci 2003;44:2163–2170.
48. Otani A, Kinder K, Ewalt K, Otero FJ, Schimmel P, Friedlander M. Bone marrow-derived stem cells target retinal astrocytes and can promote or inhibit retinal angiogenesis. Nat Med 2002;8:1004–1010.
49. Belting M, Dorrell MI, Sandgren S, et al. Regulation of angiogenesis by tissue factor cytoplasmic domain signaling. Nat Med 2004;10:502–509.
50. Lambert V, Wielockx B, Munaut C, et al. MMP-2 and MMP-9 synergize in promoting choroidal neovascularization. FASEB J 2003;17:2290–2292.
51. Sethi CS, Bailey TA, Luthert PJ, Chong NH. Matrix metalloproteinase biology applied to vitreoretinal disorders. Br J Ophthalmol 2000;84:654–666.
52. Kadonosono K, Yazama F, Itoh N, Sawada H, Ohno S. Expression of matrix metalloproteinase-7 in choroidal neovascular membranes in age-related macular degeneration. Am J Ophthalmol 1999;128:382–384.
53. Alexander CM, Werb Z. Targeted disruption of the tissue inhibitor of metalloproteinases gene increases the invasive behavior of primitive mesenchymal cells derived from embryonic stem cells in vitro. J Cell Biol 1992;118:727–739.
54. Visse R, Nagase H. Matrix metalloproteinases and tissue inhibitors of metalloproteinases: structure, function, and biochemistry. Circ Res 2003;92:827–839.
55. Fassina G, Ferrari N, Brigati C, et al. Tissue inhibitors of metalloproteases: regulation and biological activities. Clin Exp Metastasis 2000;18:111–120.
56. Donnini S, Morbidelli L, Taraboletti G, Ziche M. ERK1–2 and p38 MAPK regulate MMP/TIMP balance and function in response to thrombospondin-1 fragments in the microvascular endothelium. Life Sci 2004;74:2975–2985.
57. Bein K, Simons M. Thrombospondin type 1 repeats interact with matrix metalloproteinase 2. Regulation of metalloproteinase activity. J Biol Chem 2000;275:32,167–32,173.
58. Rodriguez-Manzaneque JC, Lane TF, Ortega MA, Hynes RO, Lawler J, Iruela-Arispe ML. Thrombospondin-1 suppresses spontaneous tumor growth and inhibits activation of matrix metalloproteinase-9 and mobilization of vascular endothelial growth factor. Proc Natl Acad Sci USA 2001;98:12,485–12,490.
59. Brew K, Dinakarpandian D, Nagase H. Tissue inhibitors of metalloproteinases: evolution, structure and function. Biochim Biophys Acta 2000;1477:267–283.
60. Nuttall RK, Sampieri CL, Pennington CJ, Gill SE, Schultz GA, Edwards DR. Expression analysis of the entire MMP and TIMP gene families during mouse tissue development. FEBS Lett 2004;563:129–134.
61. Apte SS, Olsen B, Murphy G. The gene structure of tissue inhibitor of metalloproteinases (TIMP)-3 and its inhibitory activities define the distinct TIMP gene family. J Biol Chem 1995;270:14,313–14,318.
62. Woessner JF Jr. That impish TIMP: the tissue inhibitor of metalloproteinases-3. J Clin Invest 2001;108:799–800.
63. Murphy G. The regulation of connective tissue metalloproteinases by natural inhibitors. In: AAS 35: Progress in Inflammation Research and Therapy. Birkhauser, Basel: 1991; 69–76.
64. Blenis J, Hawkes S. Transformation sensitive protein associated with the cell substratum of chicken embryo fibroblasts. Proc Natl Acad Sci USA 1983;80:770–774.

65. Langton K, Barker M, McKie N. Localization of the functional domains of human tissue inhibitor of metalloproteinases-3 and the effects of a Sorsby's fundus dystrophy mutation. J Biol Chem 1998;273:16,778–16,781.
66. Yu WH, Yu S, Meng Q, Brew K, Woessner JF Jr. TIMP-3 binds to sulfated glycosaminoglycans of the extracellular matrix. J Biol Chem 2000;275:31,226–31,232.
67. Amour A, Slocombe P, Webster A, et al. TNF-alpha converting enzyme (TACE) is inhibited by TIMP-3. FEBS Lett 1998;435:39–44.
68. Amour A, Knight CG, Webster A, et al. The in vitro activity of ADAM-10 is inhibited by TIMP-1 and TIMP-3. FEBS Lett 2000;473:275–279.
69. Loechel F, Fox JW, Murphy G, Albrechtsen R, Wewer UM. ADAM 12-S cleaves IGFBP-3 and IGFBP-5 and is inhibited by TIMP-3. Biochem Biophys Res Commun 2000;278: 511–515.
70. Kashiwagi M, Tortorella M, Nagase H, Brew K. TIMP-3 is a potent inhibitor of aggrecanase 1 (ADAM-TS4) and aggrecanase 2 (ADAM-TS5). J Biol Chem 2001;276:12,501–12,504.
71. Hargreaves PG, Wang F, Antcliff J, et al. Human myeloma cells shed the interleukin-6 receptor: inhibition by tissue inhibitor of metalloproteinase-3 and a hydroxamate-based metalloproteinase inhibitor. Br J Haematol 1998;101:694–702.
72. Borland G, Murphy G, Ager A. Tissue inhibitor of metalloproteinases-3 inhibits shedding of L-selectin from leukocytes. J Biol Chem 1999;274:2810–2815.
73. Fitzgerald ML, Wang Z, Park PW, Murphy G, Bernfield M. Shedding of syndecan-1 and -4 ectodomains is regulated by multiple signaling pathways and mediated by a TIMP-3-sensitive metalloproteinase. J Cell Biol 2000;148:811–824.
74. Zhao H, Bernardo MM, Osenkowski P, et al. Differential inhibition of membrane type 3 (MT3)-matrix metalloproteinase (MMP) and MT1-MMP by tissue inhibitor of metalloproteinase (TIMP)-2 and TIMP-3 regulates pro-MMP-2 activation. J Biol Chem 2004; 279:8592–8601.
75. Gasson JC, Golde DW, Kaufman SE, et al. Molecular characterization and expression of the gene encoding human erythroid-potentiating activity. Nature 1985;315:768–771.
76. Stetler-Stevenson WG, Bersch N, Golde DW. Tissue inhibitor of metalloproteinase-2 (TIMP-2) has erythroid-potentiating activity. FEBS Lett 1992;296:231–234.
77. Hayakawa T, Yamashita K, Tanzawa K, Uchijima E, Iwata K. Growth-promoting activity of tissue inhibitor of metalloproteinases-1 (TIMP-1) for a wide range of cells. A possible new growth factor in serum. FEBS Lett 1992;298:29–32.
78. Hayakawa T, Yamashita K, Ohuchi E, Shinagawa A. Cell growth promoting activity of tissue inhibitor of metalloproteinases-2 (TIMP-2). J Cell Science 1994;107:2373–2379.
79. Guedez L, Stetler-Stevenson WG, Wolff L, et al. In vitro suppression of programmed cell death of B cells by tissue inhibitor of metalloproteinases-1. J Clin Invest 1998;102:2002–2010.
80. Valente P, Fassina G, Melchiori A, et al. TIMP-2 over-expression reduces invasion and angiogenesis and protects B16F10 melanoma cells from apoptosis. Int J Cancer 1998;75:246–253.
81. Jiang Y, Wang M, Celiker MY, et al. Stimulation of mammary tumorigenesis by systemic tissue inhibitor of matrix metalloproteinase 4 gene delivery. Cancer Res 2001;61:2365–2370.
82. Bond M, Murphy G, Bennett MR, et al. Localization of the death domain of tissue inhibitor of metalloproteinase-3 to the N terminus. Metalloproteinase inhibition is associated with proapoptotic activity. J Biol Chem 2000;275:41,358–41,363.
83. Ahonen M, Poukkula M, Baker AH, et al. Tissue inhibitor of metalloproteinases-3 induces apoptosis in melanoma cells by stabilization of death receptors. Oncogene 2003; 22: 2121–2134.
84. Ahonen M, Baker AH, Kahari VM. Adenovirus-mediated gene delivery of tissue inhibitor of metalloproteinases-3 inhibits invasion and induces apoptosis in melanoma cells. Cancer Res 1998;58:2310–2315.

85. Baker AH, Zaltsman AB, George SJ, Newby AC. Divergent effects of tissue inhibitor of metalloproteinase-1, -2, or -3 overexpression on rat vascular smooth muscle cell invasion, proliferation, and death in vitro. TIMP-3 promotes apoptosis. J Clin Invest 1998;101: 1478–1487.
86. Smith M, Kung H, Durum S, Colburn N, Sun Y. TIMP-3 induces cell death by stabilizing TNF-alpha receptors on the surface of human colon carcinoma cells. Cytokine 1997; 9:770–780.
87. Leco KJ, Waterhouse P, Sanchez OH, et al. Spontaneous air space enlargement in the lungs of mice lacking tissue inhibitor of metalloproteinases-3 (TIMP-3). J Clin Invest 2001;108:817–829.
88. Bian J, Wang Y, Smith MR, et al. Suppression of in vivo tumor growth and induction of suspension cell death by tissue inhibitor of metalloproteinases (TIMP)-3. Carcinogenesis 1996;17:1805–1811.
89. Guedez L, Courtemanch L, Stetler-Stevenson M. Tissue inhibitor of metalloproteinase (TIMP)-1 induces differentiation and an antiapoptotic phenotype in germinal center B cells. Blood 1998;92:1342–1349.
90. Egeblad M, Werb Z. New functions for the matrix metalloproteinases in cancer progression. Nat Rev Cancer 2002;2:161–174.
91. Gomez DE, Alonso DF, Yoshiji H, Thorgeirsson UP. Tissue inhibitors of metalloproteinases: structure, regulation and biological functions. Eur J Cell Biol 1997;74: 111–122.
92. Anand-Apte B, Bao L, Smith R, et al. A review of tissue inhibitor of metalloproteinases-3 (TIMP-3) and experimental analysis of its effect on primary tumor growth. Biochem Cell Biol 1996;74:853–862.
93. Celiker MY, Wang M, Atsidaftos E, et al. Inhibition of Wilms' tumor growth by intramuscular administration of tissue inhibitor of metalloproteinases-4 plasmid DNA. Oncogene 2001;20:4337–4343.
94. Wang M, Liu YE, Greene J, et al. Inhibition of tumor growth and metastasis of human breast cancer cells transfected with tissue inhibitor of metalloproteinase 4. Oncogene 1997;14:2767–2774.
95. Spurbeck WW, Ng CY, Strom TS, Vanin EF, Davidoff AM. Enforced expression of tissue inhibitor of matrix metalloproteinase-3 affects functional capillary morphogenesis and inhibits tumor growth in a murine tumor model. Blood 2002;100:3361–3368.
96. Ahonen M, Ala-Aho R, Baker AH, et al. Antitumor activity and bystander effect of adenovirally delivered tissue inhibitor of metalloproteinases-3. Mol Ther 2002;5:705–715.
97. Spurbeck WW, Ng CY, Vanin EF, Davidoff AM. Retroviral vector-producer cell-mediated in vivo gene transfer of TIMP-3 restricts angiogenesis and neuroblastoma growth in mice. Cancer Gene Ther 2003;10:161–167.
98. Osiewicz K, McGarry M, Soloway PD. Hyper-resistance to infection in TIMP-1-deficient mice is neutrophil dependent but not immune cell autonomous. Ann NY Acad Sci 1999;878:494–496.
99. Wang Z, Soloway PD. TIMP-1 and TIMP-2 perform different functions in vivo. Ann NY Acad Sci 1999;878:519–521.
100. Silence J, Collen D, Lijnen HR. Reduced atherosclerotic plaque but enhanced aneurysm formation in mice with inactivation of the tissue inhibitor of metalloproteinase-1 (TIMP-1) gene. Circ Res 2002;90:897–903.
101. Roten L, Nemoto S, Simsic J, et al. Effects of gene deletion of the tissue inhibitor of the matrix metalloproteinase-type 1 (TIMP-1) on left ventricular geometry and function in mice. J Mol Cell Cardiol 2000;32:109–120.
102. Lemaitre V, Soloway PD, D'Armiento J. Increased medial degradation with pseudoaneurysm formation in apolipoprotein E-knockout mice deficient in tissue inhibitor of metalloproteinases-1. Circulation 2003;107:333–338.

103. Mukherjee R, Parkhurst AM, Mingoia JT, et al. Myocardial remodeling after discrete radiofrequency injury: effects of tissue inhibitor of matrix metalloproteinase-1 gene deletion. Am J Physiol Heart Circ Physiol 2004;286:H1242–H1247.
104. Lijnen HR, Demeulemeester D, Van Hoef B, Collen D, Maquoi E. Deficiency of tissue inhibitor of matrix metalloproteinase-1 (TIMP-1) impairs nutritionally induced obesity in mice. Thromb Haemost 2003;89:249–255.
105. Nothnick WB. Disruption of the tissue inhibitor of metalloproteinase-1 gene results in altered reproductive cyclicity and uterine morphology in reproductive-age female mice. Biol Reprod 2000;63:905–912.
106. Nothnick WB. Tissue inhibitor of metalloproteinase-1 (TIMP-1) deficient mice display reduced serum progesterone levels during corpus luteum development. Endocrinology 2003;144:5–8.
107. Yamada E, Tobe T, Yamada H, et al. TIMP-1 promotes VEGF-induced neovascularization in the retina. Histol Histopathol 2001;16:87–97.
108. Wang Z, Juttermann R, Soloway PD. TIMP-2 is required for efficient activation of proMMP-2 in vivo. J Biol Chem 2000;275:26,411–26,415.
109. Gill SE, Pape MC, Khokha R, Watson AJ, Leco KJ. A null mutation for tissue inhibitor of metalloproteinases-3 (TIMP-3) impairs murine bronchiole branching morphogenesis. Dev Biol 2003;261:313–323.
110. Martin EL, Moyer BZ, Pape MC, Starcher B, Leco KJ, Veldhuizen RA. Negative impact of tissue inhibitor of metalloproteinase-3 null mutation on lung structure and function in response to sepsis. Am J Physiol Lung Cell Mol Physiol 2003;285:L1222–L1232.
111. Fata JE, Leco KJ, Voura EB, et al. Accelerated apoptosis in the TIMP-3-deficient mammary gland. J Clin Invest 2001;108:831–841.
112. Fedak PW, Smookler DS, Kassiri Z, et al. TIMP-3 deficiency leads to dilated cardiomyopathy. Circulation 2004;19:19.
113. Della NG, Campochiaro PA, Zack DJ. Localization of TIMP-3 mRNA expression to the retinal pigment epithelium. Invest Ophthalmol Vis Sci 1996;37:1921–1924.
114. Fariss RN, Apte SS, Olsen BR, Iwata K, Milam AH. Tissue inhibitor of metalloproteinases-3 is a component of Bruch's membrane of the eye. Am J Pathol 1997;150:323–328.
115. Kamei M, Hollyfield J. TIMP-3 in Bruch's membrane: changes during aging and in age-related macular degeneration. Invest Ophthalmol Vis Sci 1999;40:2367–2375.
116. Fariss RN, Apte SS, Luthert PJ, Bird AC, Milam AH. Accumulation of tissue inhibitor of metalloproteinases-3 in human eyes with Sorsby's fundus dystrophy or retinitis pigmentosa. Br J Ophthalmol 1998;82:1329–1334.
117. Klenotic PA, Munier FL, Marmorstein LY, Anand-Apte B. Tissue inhibitor of metalloproteinases-3 (TIMP-3) is a binding partner of EGF-containing fibulin-like extracellular matrix protein 1 (EFEMP1): Implications for macular degenerations. J Biol Chem 2004;28:28.
118. Vranka JA, Johnson E, Zhu X, et al. Discrete expression and distribution pattern of TIMP-3 in the human retina and choroid. Curr Eye Res 1997;16:102–110.
119. Ruiz A, Brett P, Bok D. TIMP-3 is expressed in the human retinal pigment epithelium. Biochem Biophys Res Commun 1996;226:467–474.
120. Vranka JA, Shepardson A, Johnson EC, Zhu X-H, Alexander JP, Bradley JMB. TIMP3 expression in the human retina and choroid. Invest Ophthalmol Vis Sci 1996;15:S273.
121. Takahashi T, Nakamura T, Hayashi A, et al. Inhibition of experimental choroidal neovascularization by overexpression of tissue inhibitor of metalloproteinases-3 in retinal pigment epithelium cells. Am J Ophthalmol 2000;130:774–781.
122. Auricchio A, Behling KC, Maguire AM, et al. Inhibition of retinal neovascularization by intraocular viral-mediated delivery of anti-angiogenic agents. Mol Ther 2002;6: 490–494.
123. Sorsby A, Mason MEJ, Gardner N. A fundus dystrophy with unusual features. Br J Ophthalmol 1949;33:67–97.

124. Holz FG, Haimovici R, Wagner DG, Bird AC. Recurrent choroidal neovascularization after laser photocoagulation in Sorsby's fundus dystrophy. Retina 1994;14:329–334.
125. Jacobson SG, Cideciyan AV, Regunath G, et al. Night blindness in Sorsby's fundus dystrophy reversed by vitamin A. Nat Genet 1995;11:27–32.
126. Kalmus H, Seedburgh D. Probable common origin of a hereditary fundus dystrophy (Sorsby's familial pseudoinflammatory macular dystrophy) in an English and Australian family. J Med Genet 1976;13:271–276.
127. Polkinghorne PJ, Capon MR, Berninger T, Lyness AL, Sehmi K, Bird AC. Sorsby's fundus dystrophy. A clinical study. Ophthalmology 1989;96:1763–1768.
128. Capon MR, Marshall J, Krafft JI, Alexander RA, Hiscott PS, Bird AC. Sorsby's fundus dystrophy. A light and electron microscopic study. Ophthalmology 1989;96:1769–1777.
129. Crabb JW, Miyagi M, Gu X, et al. Drusen proteome analysis: an approach to the etiology of age-related macular degeneration. Proc Natl Acad Sci USA 2002;99:14,682–14,687.
130. Chong NH, Kvanta A, Seregard S, Bird AC, Luthert PJ, Steen B. TIMP-3 mRNA is not overexpressed in Sorsby fundus dystrophy. Am J Ophthalmol 2003;136:954–955.
131. Polkinghorne PJ, Capon MRC, Berninger T, Lyness AL, Sehmi K, Bird AC. Sorsby's fundus dystrophy. A clinical study. Ophthalmology 1989;96:1763–1768.
132. Wu G, Pruett RC, Baldinger J, Hirose T. Hereditary hemorrhagic macular dystrophy. Am J Ophthalmol 1991;111:294–301.
133. Bird AC. Bruch's membrane change with age. Br J Ophthalmol 1992;76:166–168.
134. Bird AC. Choroidal neovascularisation in age-related macular disease [editorial]. Br J Ophthalmol 1993;77:614–615.
135. Langton KP, McKie N, Curtis A, et al. A novel tissue inhibitor of metalloproteinases-3 mutation reveals a common molecular phenotype in Sorsby's fundus dystrophy. J Biol Chem 2000;275:27,027–27,031.
136. Tabata Y, Isashiki Y, Kamimura K, Nakao K, Ohba N. A novel splice site mutation in the tissue inhibitor of the metalloproteinases-3 gene in Sorsby's fundus dystrophy with unusual clinical features. Hum Genet 1998;103:179–182.
137. Weber BH, Vogt G, Pruett RC, Stohr H, Felbor U. Mutations in the tissue inhibitor of metalloproteinases-3 (TIMP3) in patients with Sorsby's fundus dystrophy. Nat Genet 1994;8: 352–356.
138. Williamson RA, Marston FA, Angal S, et al. Disulphide bond assignment in human tissue inhibitor of metalloproteinases (TIMP). Biochem J 1990;268:267–274.
139. Willenbrock F, Crabbe T, Slocombe PM, et al. The activity of the tissue inhibitors of metalloproteinases is regulated by C-terminal domain interactions: a kinetic analysis of the inhibition of gelatinase A. Biochemistry 1993;32:4330–4337.
140. Nguyen Q, Willenbrock F, Cockett MI, O'Shea M, Docherty AJ, Murphy G. Different domain interactions are involved in the binding of tissue inhibitors of metalloproteinases to stromelysin-1 and gelatinase A. Biochemistry 1994;33:2089–2095.
141. Qi JH, Ebrahem Q, Yeow K, Edwards DR, Fox PL, Anand-Apte B. Expression of Sorsby's fundus dystrophy mutations in human retinal pigment Epithelial cells reduces matrix metalloproteinase inhibition and may promote angiogenesis. J Biol Chem 2002;30:30.
142. Anand-Apte B, Pepper MS, Voest E, et al. Inhibition of angiogenesis by tissue inhibitor of metalloproteinase-3. Invest Ophthalmol Vis Sci 1997;38:817–823.
143. Moses MA. The regulation of neovascularization of matrix metalloproteinases and their inhibitors. Stem Cells 1997;15:180–189.
144. Johnson MD, Kim HR, Chesler L, Tsao-Wu G, Bouck N, Polverini PJ. Inhibition of angiogenesis by tissue inhibitor of metalloproteinase. J Cell Physiol 1994;160:194–202.
145. Moses MA, Langer R. A metalloproteinase inhibitor as an inhibitor of neovascularization. J Cell Biochem 1991;47:230–235.

146. Takigawa M, Nishida Y, Suzuki F, Kishi J, Yamashita K, Hayakawa T. Induction of angiogenesis in chick yolk-sac membrane by polyamines and its inhibition by tissue inhibitors of metalloproteinases (TIMP and TIMP-2). Biochem Biophys Res Commun 1990; 171:1264–1271.
147. Murphy AN, Unsworth EJ, Stetler-Stevenson WG. Tissue inhibitor of metalloproteinases-2 inhibits bFGF-induced human microvascular endothelial cell proliferation. J Cell Physiol 1993;157:351–358.
148. Lafleur MA, Handsley MM, Knauper V, Murphy G, Edwards DR. Endothelial tubulogenesis within fibrin gels specifically requires the activity of membrane-type-matrix metalloproteinases (MT-MMPs). J Cell Sci 2002;115:3427–3438.
149. Qi JH, Ebrahem Q, Moore N, et al. A novel function for tissue inhibitor of metalloproteinases-3 (TIMP3): inhibition of angiogenesis by blockage of VEGF binding to VEGF receptor-2. Nat Med 2003;9:407–415.
150. Seo DW, Li H, Guedez L, et al. TIMP-2 mediated inhibition of angiogenesis: an MMP-independent mechanism. Cell 2003;114:171–180.
151. Fernandez CA, Butterfield C, Jackson G, Moses MA. Structural and functional uncoupling of the enzymatic and angiogenic inhibitory activities of tissue inhibitor of metalloproteinase-2 (TIMP-2): loop 6 is a novel angiogenesis inhibitor. J Biol Chem 2003;278: 40,989–40,995.
152. Ruiz A, Peterson B, Bok D. Localization and quantification of TIMP-3 mRNA in the human retina. Invest Ophthalmol Vis Sci 1996;37:S1143.
153. Blaauwgeers HG, Holtkamp GM, Rutten H, et al. Polarized vascular endothelial growth factor secretion by human retinal pigment epithelium and localization of vascular endothelial growth factor receptors on the inner choriocapillaris. Evidence for a trophic paracrine relation. Am J Pathol 1999;155:421–428.

16
Integrins in Ocular Angiogenesis

Matthew R. Ritter, PhD and Martin Friedlander, MD, PhD

CONTENTS

INTEGRINS

The integrin family of membrane proteins are ubiquitously expressed cell surface receptors that not only mediate cell anchorage to the surrounding extracellular matrix, but are also critically important in transducing environmental cues to subcellular signaling pathways. Integrins play important roles in cell differentiation and survival and have generated interest in diverse fields ranging from structural biology and immunology to tumor biology and ophthalmology. Much of the interest has centered on the roles of integrins during cell–cell adhesion, such as that which occurs between endothelial cells and leukocytes during arrest and extravasation from blood vessels during inflammation. Another major area of interest has been the function of integrins and their interaction with the extracellular matrix (ECM). Integrins specifically bind components of the ECM such as fibronectin and vitronectin, but also non-ECM molecules such as von Willebrand factor and thrombospondin. The specificity of interaction with various ligands is a result of the noncovalently linked α/β chains that form the functional integrin heterodimer. The α-subunit is comprised of approx 1000 amino acids and contains calcium-binding motifs that are critical to integrin function *(1)*. Integrin β-subunits are made up of approx 750 amino acids and introduce additional variability through alternative splicing of the cytoplasmic regions. Different pairings of α- and β-subunits produce at least 20 different integrin heterodimers with distinct but overlapping binding specificities *(2)*. In turn, each ECM component may be recognized by several integrins. In general, integrins recognize amino acid sequences that contain a key acidic residue that is critical for binding *(3)*. A common example of an integrin

From: *Ophthalmology: Ocular Angiogenesis: Diseases, Mechanisms, and Therapeutics*
Edited by: J. Tombran-Tink and C. J. Barnstable © Humana Press Inc., Totowa, NJ

ligand sequence is the RGD (Arg-Gly-Asp) sequence, which is found in a number of integrin-binding proteins *(4)*. Integrin-binding sequences that are unrelated to the RGD motif show structural and topological similarities to the RGD sequence, suggesting that specific spatial elements are required for recognition *(5)*. Some integrins are known to require activation in order to bind their corresponding ligands, a mechanism referred to as "inside-out" signaling. For example, the $\alpha_{IIb}\beta_3$ integrin is a constitutively expressed receptor on platelets but is able to bind its primary ligand, fibrinogen, only after a conformational change induced by platelet activation *(6)*.

In addition to their roles as adhesion molecules, integrins have been described in a large body of work as signal-transducing molecules that regulate important cellular functions such as proliferation, gene expression, migration, and apoptosis *(7)*. Integrins possess no intrinsic biochemical activity. Thus, in order to serve as signal transducers, they must recruit other molecules to perform these functions. Integrin cytoplasmic domains associate with a large number of adapter proteins and tyrosine kinases that carry out the signaling functions of these receptors *(8)*. The integrins are named for this function as *integrators* of the ECM and cytoplasmic complexes. Through various adapter proteins, the integrins are indirectly linked to the cytoskeleton and exert control over its functions. The small GTPase, Rho, has been shown to mediate effects of integrins on the cytoskeleton, although the events downstream of Rho are complex and still being elucidated *(9)*. A reciprocal relationship exists in this system in which integrins regulate the cytoskeleton and, in turn, the cytoskeleton can influence integrin function, for example, integrin clustering and focal adhesion formation *(10)*. Integrin ligation results in increased levels of tyrosine phosphorylation, events that are carried out by protein tyrosine kinases that propagate extracellular signals initiated by integrin receptors *(11)*. Phosphorylated tyrosines can be recognized by proteins that contain the modular adapter domain known as the Src homology 2 (SH2) domain, named after a central player in integrin signaling, Src *(12)*. This domain, along with a number of other modular domains, including SH3 and protein tyrosine binding (PTB) domains, are present in different combinations in proteins that lack catalytic activity but serve important functions as adapter proteins. Thus, extremely complex signaling networks exist that use tyrosine kinases and their corresponding recognition domains as "switches" to turn particular pathways "on" or "off." Also included in these networks are phosphatases, which play important roles in the regulation of pathways involving tyrosine phosphorylation events *(13,14)*. The endpoints of these integrin-regulated pathways include control of cell migration, gene expression, and cell survival. These cellular functions are also regulated by the receptor tyrosine kinase family, which includes many of the growth factor receptors. In contrast with integrins, these transmembrane proteins possess intrinsic kinase activity and therefore do not depend on other enzymes to initiate signals *(15)*. Integrins and receptor tyrosine kinases have been shown to cooperate, as integrin input is necessary for optimal activation of receptors for insulin, epidermal growth factor (EGF), and vascular endothelial growth factor (VEGF) *(16–18)*. The mitogen-activated protein (MAP) kinases are regulated by both receptor types and appear to reside at a major point of intersection of integrin- and growth factor receptor-mediated signaling pathways *(19,20)*.

INTEGRINS IN NEOVASCULAR DISEASES OF THE EYE

Neovascularization is a major finding in the majority of eye diseases that result in catastrophic loss of vision. The leading cause of vision loss in individuals over age 55 is age-related macular degeneration (AMD), whereas proliferative diabetic retinopathy (PDR) is the leading cause of blindness in those under 55 *(21)*. These two diseases differ in the site of new vessel growth. AMD is characterized by neovascularization in the choriocapillaries, whereas in PDR, retinal blood vessels proliferate.

Blood vessels are formed by two major processes: vasculogenesis or angiogenesis. Vasculogenesis occurs as a result of differentiation of precursor cells, which are already present in the tissue, into the endothelial cells that contribute to the formation of blood vessels. It is this process that is prevalent during early development. Angiogenesis differs in that new blood vessels are generated by sprouting from the preexisting vasculature. Although both vasculogenesis and angiogenesis occur during development, the adult vasculature is normally quite stable, with little turnover of vessels. New blood vessel formation occurs in the normal adult during menstruation and wound healing and under pathological circumstances such as arthritis and tumor growth.

Neovascular eye diseases are the result of angiogenesis, which is a complex series of events coordinated at the cellular and molecular levels. Endothelial cells, which comprise the lining of blood vessels, are the major cellular component of angiogenesis, which can be broken into three major initial steps: (1) endothelial cell activation and breakdown of the basement membrane; (2) adhesion to the intact and proteolytically modified extracellular matrix; and (3) endothelial cell migration through the extracellular milieu. Integrins have roles in all three of these steps. Integrins interact with growth factor receptors to transmit signals from outside the cell to the interior, where cellular activities are altered. For example, integrin $\alpha_v\beta_3$ has been shown to be involved in the activation of vascular endothelial growth factor receptor-2 (VEGFR-2) *(22)*. VEGF is a well-characterized initiator of angiogenesis that has been shown to be important in the growth of new vessels in many contexts by stimulating the growth and migration of endothelial cells and inhibiting their apoptosis. In order for endothelial cells to sprout off their parent vessel and migrate toward the source of the angiogenic signal, the basement membrane that underlies them in the normal vessel must be degraded. The basement membrane is rich in collagen type IV and is degraded by a number of enzymes including MMP-2 and MMP-9, both of which have been shown to be regulated by integrins in their activation and/or localization *(23,24)*. The third step in the described sequence involves the migration of endothelial cells through the surrounding matrix. This involves highly coordinated cellular events that translate cell adhesion and tension generated on the cytoskeleton into directional movement of the cell. Integrins have a central role in cell motility, as they are important adhesion molecules and they transmit and integrate signals to the cytoskeleton. By interfering with any of these three steps, angiogenesis can be inhibited, and as central players in all steps, integrins are reasonable targets for therapeutic intervention in pathological neovascular disease.

Work from our laboratory and others has shown that blocking integrin function effectively inhibits angiogenesis in the eye *(25–28)*. In a model of cytokine-induced corneal angiogenesis, anti-integrin antibodies were shown to be effective inhibitors of vessel growth *(25)*. This model uses cytokine-containing pellets that are implanted into rabbit corneas, establishing a gradient toward which limbal vessels are stimulated to grow into the normally avascular cornea. Pellets containing an antibody against $\alpha_v\beta_5$ integrin were shown to inhibit VEGF-induced angiogenesis, whereas those containing anti-$\alpha_v\beta_3$ antibody inhibited blood vessel growth stimulated by basic fibroblast growth factor (bFGF). Only minimal inhibition was seen with reverse combinations of antibody and cytokine. These findings were extended by employing these same anti-integrin antibodies with a panel of angiogenic cytokines and measuring blood vessel growth in the chick chorioallantoic membrane (CAM) assay *(29)*. Here, cytokine-saturated filter disks are placed on the CAM of 10-d-old chick embryos. Blood vessels are stimulated to grow toward the disks and the degree of angiogenesis can be quantified by analyzing the number and extent of branching blood vessels within the area of the disk. Under these conditions, a single dose of antibody against $\alpha_v\beta_5$ inhibited angiogenesis induced by VEGF, transforming growth factor (TGF)-α, and phorbol 12-myristate 13-acetate (PMA), but had minimal effects on that induced by bFGF and tumor necrosis factor (TNF)-α. Antibody against $\alpha_v\beta_3$ proved effective at inhibiting angiogenesis stimulated by bFGF and TNF-α but not the other growth factors tested. Preliminary investigations into downstream signaling pathways involved in integrin-mediated angiogenesis revealed that blocking protein kinase C (PKC) inhibited vessel growth induced by PMA, VEGF, and TGF-α, but had little effect on bFGF- or TNF-α-mediated angiogenesis. Thus two pathways of angiogenesis were identified: one that involves $\alpha_v\beta_3$ and is largely independent of PKC, and a second that relies on $\alpha_v\beta_5$ but also requires PKC activity.

Angiogenesis-related integrins have been shown to be expressed in tissue from patients with proliferative vascular diseases such as PDR, AMD, and presumed ocular histoplasmosis syndrome *(26,28,30,31)*. These findings prompted studies to investigate whether systemically administered antagonists of these integrins could inhibit retinal angiogenesis in mouse models. Two models of retinal blood vessel growth were used to investigate this concept. The hypoxia-induced retinopathy model described by Smith et al. *(32)* was used to test the efficacy of α_v integrin antagonists in inhibiting retinal neovascularization. Mice are exposed to 75% oxygen from postnatal days 7 to 12 and then are returned to normoxia. This period of hyperoxia causes obliteration of retinal vessels. After return to normoxia, the areas of obliteration then become ischemic and pathological preretinal neovascularization ensues. In two studies using this model, it was demonstrated that administration of antagonists of α_v integrins reduced the formation of preretinal neovascular tufts up to 75% *(27,28)*. Different routes of administration were used in these studies, including subcutaneous, intraperitoneal, and periorbital injection, with all routes showing efficacy.

The second model of retinal angiogenesis used to explore the potential of integrin antagonists for the treatment of ocular vascular disease was the neonatal mouse retinal angiogenesis model. At birth, the mouse retina is avascular but becomes vascularized over about the first month of life through radial growth of vessels from the central retinal artery, which enters the eye through the optic nerve. Vessels are guided to the peripheral retina by astrocytes that precede the advancing vasculature and establish a template on which these vessesls are patterned *(33)*. Twice-daily subcutaneous treatment of newborn mice with cyclic RGDfV peptide, which blocks both $\alpha_v\beta_3$ and $\alpha_v\beta_5$ integrins, significantly inhibited the growth of retinal vessels in this developmental model,

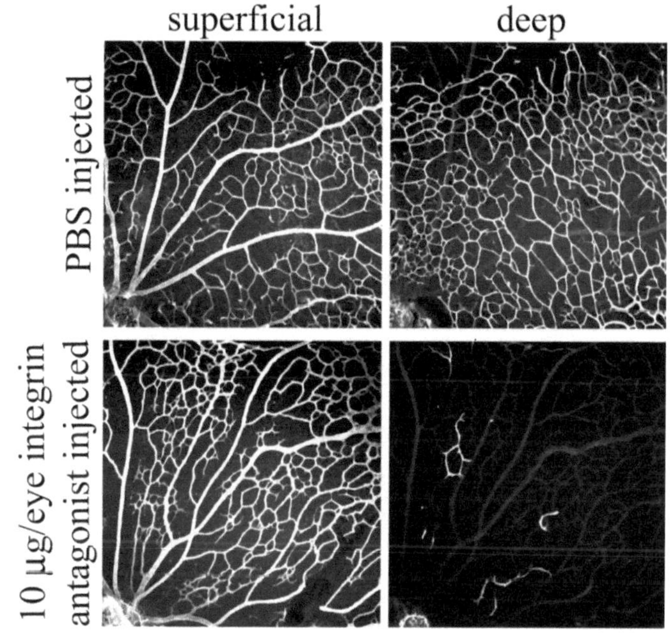

Fig. 1. Inhibition of retinal angiogenesis by integrin antagonism. Injection of a small-molecule antagonist of $\alpha_v\beta_3$ and $\alpha_v\beta_5$ at postnatal day 8 (P8) inhibits the growth of the deep retinal vasculature when visualized at P12, while having no effect on the previously established superficial vessels.

whereas control RADfV peptide-treated retinas appeared identical to untreated controls. Using confocal microscopy and a computerized method of estimating blood vessel volume, treatment with RGDfV peptide antagonist resulted in a 78% reduction of vascularization relative to control peptide treatment. More recent studies using highly potent small-molecule antagonists of both $\alpha_v\beta_3$ and $\alpha_v\beta_5$ also inhibit retinal angiogenesis in a neonatal mouse model after intravitreal injection (Fig. 1). In this model, small-molecule antagonists of $\alpha_v\beta_3$ and $\alpha_v\beta_5$ integrins will completely inhibit retinal angiogenesis in approx 35 to 50% of animal eyes. Thus, integrin antagonism is an effective approach to inhibition of corneal and retinal angiogenesis in a number of mouse models.

DOWNSTREAM EFFECTS OF INTEGRIN ANTAGONISM

Deeper investigations into integrin antagonism and the effects on cell signaling in the context of angiogenesis have been conducted. One study examined the role of p53, a well known regulator of the cell cycle, in α_v integrin signaling during retinal angiogenesis *(34)*. Starting with the observation that p53 activity is induced upon blockage of α_v integrins during angiogenesis, these investigators were interested in determining whether loss of p53 could compensate for α_v integrin function in retinal neovascularization. It was first confirmed that systemic treatment of wild-type mice with an α_v antagonist inhibited developmental retinal angiogenesis, as previously reported *(26)*. By showing that mice lacking p53 had normal retinal vascularization with anti-α_v

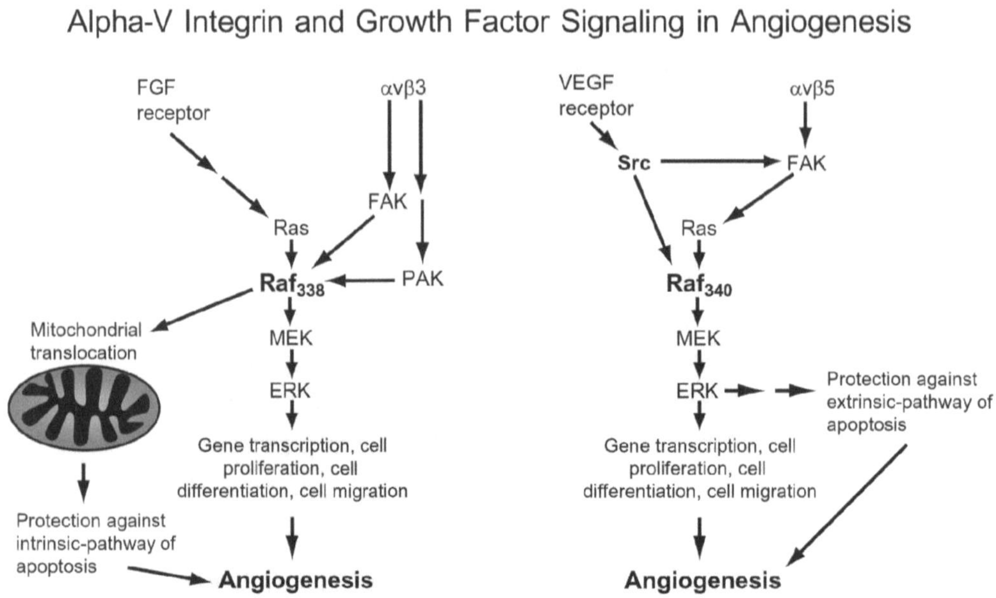

Fig. 2. bFGF/$\alpha_v\beta_3$ and VEGF/$\alpha_v\beta_5$ signaling pathways. Proposed model whereby each of these signaling pathways accounts for protection of endothelial cells from distinct mediators of apoptosis. The $\alpha_v\beta_3$ pathway promotes an ERK-independent survival mechanism preventing stress-mediated death based on Raf coupling to the mitochondria, whereas the $\alpha_v\beta_5$ pathway prevents receptor-mediated death in an ERK-dependent manner. In addition, ERK is likely playing a general role in both pathways of angiogenesis because it regulates gene transcription, cell cycle progression, and cell migration, which are critical to the growth and differentiation of new blood vessels. (Reproduced from ref. *35* with permission of The Rockefeller University Press.)

treatment, a role for p53 was indicated during integrin-mediated angiogenesis in the retina. It was concluded from this work that loss of p53 compensates for the function of α_v integrins in retinal neovascularization, possibly by interfering with α_v integrin regulation of vascular cell apoptosis.

Further elucidation of the two pathways of integrin-mediated angiogenesis *(25)* were provided by studies aimed at understanding the different ways $\alpha_v\beta_3$ and $\alpha_v\beta_5$ integrins regulate the Ras-extracellular signal regulated kinase (Ras-ERK) signaling pathway *(35)*. This pathway is influenced by both growth-factor stimulation and integrin-mediated adhesion and is involved in the control of cellular functions critical to angiogenesis. The conclusions from this work indicate that during angiogenesis in the chick CAM, VEGF and $\alpha_v\beta_5$ or bFGF and $\alpha_v\beta_3$ lead to activation of the Ras-ERK pathway in distinct ways. Integrin $\alpha_v\beta_5$ and focal adhesion kinase (FAK) cooperate with VEGF to activate Ras and Src, which causes phosphorylation of Raf and the propagation of signals important in angiogenesis. bFGF uses $\alpha_v\beta_3$, FAK, and p21-activated kinase (PAK) downstream of Ras to activate Raf. Both pathways result in sustained activity of the Ras-ERK pathway and promote angiogenesis, but the different players involved may partially explain the divergent responses of the vasculature to bFGF and VEGF (Fig. 2). Although complex, a better understanding of the function of integrins and their roles in regulating intracellular signaling pathways during angiogenesis is beginning to emerge.

INVESTIGATING INTEGRIN FUNCTION THROUGH GENETICS

The studies discussed thus far have depended on probing integrin function by blocking their adhesion, and likely their signaling function, with various compounds. Another approach is to genetically manipulate animals so that they lack expression of the particular integrin subunits of interest. This approach has been implemented in a number of studies and, interestingly, it has been shown that in mice lacking α_v, β_3, or β_5 extensive developmental angiogenesis is observed *(36–38)*. All α_v-null mice show normal development up to embryonic day 9.5 with approx 20% of them surviving until birth *(36)*. β_3 knockout mice are viable and fertile with apparently normal developmental angiogenesis, including postnatal development of the retinal vasculature *(37)*. Also viable and fertile, β_5-null mice display normal wound healing responses, suggesting that not only is developmental angiogenesis not disrupted, but adult neovascularization proceeds normally as well *(38)*. These findings show clearly that α_v integrins are not required for angiogenesis in all contexts and brings into question the importance of $\alpha_v\beta_3$ and $\alpha_v\beta_5$ integrins in adult pathological angiogenesis. To address this question specifically, studies using various models of pathological angiogenesis were carried out in β_3- and/or β_5-deficient mice *(39)*. In tumor models, β_3- and β_3/β_5-deficient mice showed enhanced tumor growth and angiogenesis. Angiogenesis was measured by vessel density in histological sections and was shown to be elevated only in tumors and not in normal skin when compared to wild-type mice. β_3-null mice were used in a model of oxygen-induced retinopathy that demonstrated that these mice had increased preretinal neovascularization compared with wild-type mice. Based on other reports of VEGF involvement in this model, it was concluded in this study that β_3 deficiency enhances VEGF-induced blood vessel growth. This contention was bolstered by experiments showing that vessel growth into VEGF-containing Matrigel implants was increased in the β_3 knockouts. It was also shown that, although the absence of β_3 does not affect the expression of other integrins, β_3-null endothelial cells showed higher levels of VEGF receptor-2 (VEGFR-2), indicating a possible mechanism by which $\alpha_v\beta_3$ could act as a negative regulator of angiogenesis. In this scenario, $\alpha_v\beta_3$ would normally suppress VEGFR-2 expression and function, and knockout of this integrin would relieve this suppression. Antagonists of $\alpha_v\beta_3$ could then be viewed to cause dysregulation of VEGFR-2, possibly explaining the observed effects of these compounds.

The apparent discrepancies between the large body of work using integrin antagonists in angiogenesis studies and the more recent genetic findings have generated considerable controversy. The discovery that β_3/β_5 knockout mice not only support pathological angiogenesis, but show enhanced vessel growth, would likely come as a surprise to most in this field. Although these data appear to erode the idea of $\alpha_v\beta_3$ and $\alpha_v\beta_5$ integrins as positive regulators of angiogenesis, consideration of other work may provide a mechanistic interpretation of the genetic findings. A major point used as evidence to support the idea of integrins as negative regulators of angiogenesis is that some integrin antagonists have been found to activate integrin signaling functions *(40)*. Although this may be true for some integrin-blocking agents, it is not true for all. Using a dimeric RGD-containing disintegrin derived from Southern copperhead snake venom, it was shown that this homodimer activated $\alpha_v\beta_3$-mediated signaling whereas monomeric RGD-containing disintegrins with similar sequences flanking the RGD did not, and in fact when used simultaneously, the monomeric molecules inhibited the signaling initiated by the dimer.

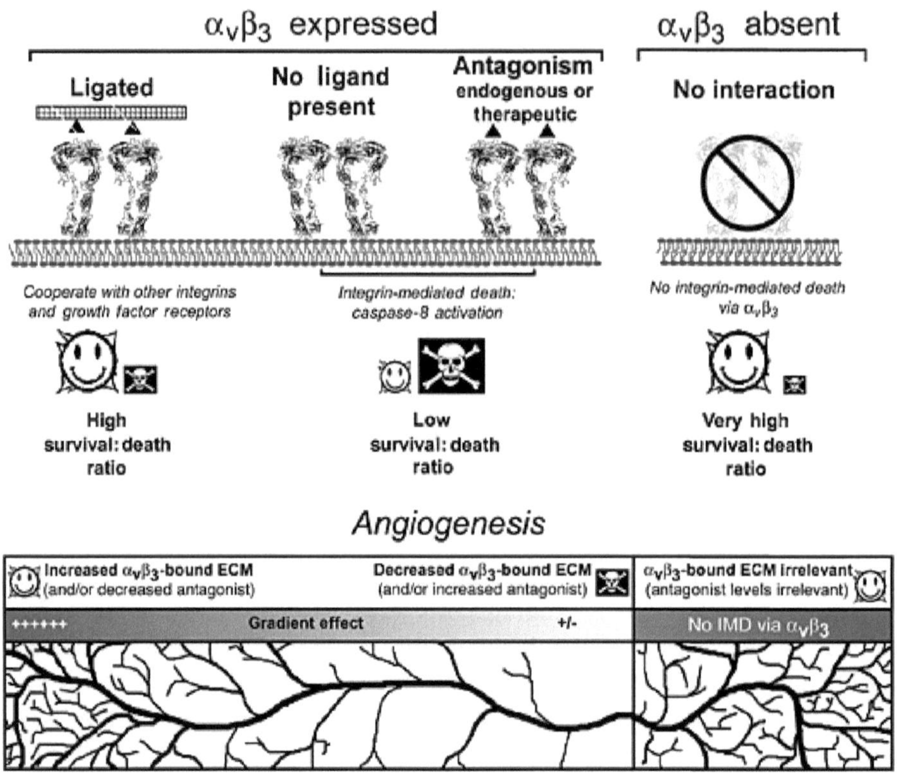

Fig. 3. A role for integrin $\alpha_v\beta_3$ in governing survival of angiogenic endothelial cells. Data from inhibitor studies and genetic investigations suggest that integrin $\alpha_v\beta_3$ (and likely other integrins) can function as a biosensor. When ligated by an immobilized matrix, they provide mechanical anchorage to the extracellular matrix (ECM), and trigger survival signals (left). When ligands are absent, or in the presence of (soluble) endogenous or therapeutic antagonists, the integrin activates a death pathway, leading to cell death (center) and suppressing angiogenesis (lower panels). However, when $\alpha_v\beta_3$ is absent, the ability to sense ECM and to trigger endothelial cell apoptosis through this integrin is lost (right), contributing to increased pathological angiogenesis (lower right). (Reproduced from ref. *46*, with permission.)

Furthermore, antibodies directed against $\alpha_v\beta_3$ similarly blocked the signals initiated by this dimeric integrin-binding molecule when used simultaneously *(41,42)*. This illustrates the point that ligation by an antagonist does not ensure the transmission of integrin signals to the cell interior and highlights the idea that the signaling properties of each integrin-blocking agent need to be investigated on an individual basis.

Other recent studies have shown that integrins can act as negative regulators of cell survival by promoting apoptosis mediated by caspase-8 *(43)*. This “integrin-mediated death” is initiated by unligated $\alpha_v\beta_3$ integrin in endothelial cells when they are seeded into 3D collagen matrices, which supports adhesion but does not ligate $\alpha_v\beta_3$. Furthermore, when $\alpha_v\beta_3$ expression on endothelial cells is reduced, survival is prolonged in this environment (Fig. 3). Resolution of this controversy requires additional studies, but at this point most of available data support the concept of α_v integrins as important pro—angiogenic molecules with complex biofeedback mechanisms that can prevent inappropriate blood vessel growth.

INTEGRIN ANTAGONISTS IN THE CLINICS

Based on extensive preclinical studies, clinical trials using integrin antagonists have been initiated, primarily in oncology. Merck KGaA (Darmstadt) and the National Cancer Institute have initiated a clinical trial with a cyclic peptide antagonist of $\alpha_v\beta_3$ and $\alpha_v\beta_5$ *(44)*. As no dose-limiting toxicities were observed in earlier phase I trials, the potential application of these molecules to therapeutic utility are significant *(45)*. Small-molecule antagonists of these integrins are currently being considered for clinical trials in ophthalmology. Another integrin, $\alpha_5\beta_1$, has also been targeted for therapeutic inhibition and clinical trials in ophthalmology are being planned with an antibody antagonist of this integrin. Although several integrins are clearly associated with neovascularization, it may be necessary to combine antagonists that target multiple integrins and/or other angiogenic mechanisms. Such combination angiostatic therapy may be the key to clinical success in suppressing the growth of abnormal, new blood vessels in a variety of neovascular eye diseases and such studies are currently under way.

ACKNOWLEDGMENTS

The authors would like to thank the members of the Friedlander laboratory for valuable discussions and critical insights into the work discussed in this review. We also thank Dave Cheresh, John Hood, and Dwayne Stupack for critical discussions of the field and permission to use figures from their published work. We apologize, in advance, to our colleagues whose work we may have unintentionally overlooked or "over-interpreted." The work discussed from our own laboratory was supported by grants from the National Eye Institute (EY11254) and The Robert Mealy Program for the Study of Macular Degenerations to M.F. M.R. was supported by a Ruth L. Kirschstein National Research Service Award from the National Eye Institute (F32 EY13916).

REFERENCES

1. Tuckwell DS, Brass A, Humphries MJ, Homology modelling of integrin EF-hands. Evidence for widespread use of a conserved cation-binding site. Biochem J 1992;285:325–331.
2. Hynes RO. Integrins: versatility, modulation, and signaling in cell adhesion. Cell 1992;69:11–25.
3. Pierschbacher MD, Ruoslahti E. Influence of stereochemistry of the sequence Arg-Gly-Asp-Xaa on binding specificity in cell adhesion New perspectives in cell adhesion: RGD and integrins. J Biol Chem 1987;262:17,294–17,298.
4. Ruoslahti E, Pierschbacher MD. New perspectives in cell adhesion: RGD and integrins. Science 1987;238:491–497.
5. Main AL, Harvey TS, Baron M, Boyd J, Campbell ID. The three-dimensional structure of the tenth type III module of fibronectin: an insight into RGD-mediated interactions. Cell 1992;71:671–678.
6. Plow EF, Ginsberg MH. Cellular adhesion: GPIIb-IIIa as a prototypic adhesion receptor. Prog Hemost Thromb 1989;9:117–156.
7. Giancotti FG, Ruoslahti E. Integrin signaling. Science 1999;285:1028–1032.
8. Sastry SK, Horwitz AF. Integrin cytoplasmic domains: mediators of cytoskeletal linkages and extra- and intracellular initiated transmembrane signaling. Curr Opin Cell Biol 1993;5:819–831.
9. Barry ST, Flinn HM, Humphries MJ, Critchley DR, Ridley AJ. Requirement for Rho in integrin signalling. Cell Adhes Commun 1997;4:387–398.
10. Ridley AJ, Hall A. The small GTP-binding protein rho regulates the assembly of focal adhesions and actin stress fibers in response to growth factors. Cell 1992;70:389–399.

11. Kornberg LJ, Earp HS, Turner CE, Prockop C, Juliano RL. Signal transduction by integrins: Increased protein tyrosine phosphorylation caused by clustering of β1 integrins. Proc Natl Acad Sci USA 1991;88:8392–8396.
12. Schaller MD, Hildebrand JD, Shannon JD, Fox JW, Vines RR, Parsons JT. Autophosphorylation of the focal adhesion kinase, $pp125^{FAK}$, directs SH2-dependent binding of $pp60^{src}$. Mol Cell Biol 1994;14:1680–1688.
13. Harder KW, Moller NP, Peacock JW, Jirik FR. Protein-tyrosine phosphatase alpha regulates Src family kinases and alters cell-substratum adhesion. J Biol Chem 1998;273:31,890–31,900.
14. Garton AJ, Tonks NK. Regulation of fibroblast motility by the protein tyrosine phosphatase PTP-PEST. J Biol Chem 1999;274:3811–3818.
15. Egan SE, Giddings BW, Brooks MW, Buday L, Sizeland AM, Weinberg RA. Association of Sos Ras exchange protein with Grb2 is implicated in tyrosine kinase signal transduction and transformation. Nature 1993;363:45–51.
16. Vuori K, Ruoslahti E. Association of insulin receptor substrate-1 with integrins. Science 1994;266:1576–1578.
17. Cybulsky AV, McTavish AJ, Cyr MD. Extracellular matrix modulates epidermal growth factor receptor activation in rat glomerular epithelial cells. J Clin Invest 1994;94:68–78.
18. Jones PL, Crack J, Rabinovitch M. Regulation of tenascin-C, a vascular smooth muscle cell survival factor that interacts with the alpha v beta 3 integrin to promote epidermal growth factor receptor phosphorylation and growth. J Cell Biol 1997;139:279–293.
19. Chen Q, Kinch MS, Lin TH, Burridge K, Juliano RL. Integrin-mediated cell adhesion activates mitogen-activated protein kinases. J Biol Chem 1994;269:26,602–26,605.
20. Canagarajah BJ, Khokhlatchev A, Cobb MH, Goldsmith EJ. Activation mechanism of the MAP kinase ERK2 by dual phosphorylation. Cell 1997;90:859–869.
21. Klein R, Klein BE, Moss SE, Cruickshanks KJ. The Wisconsin Epidemiologic Study of diabetic retinopathy. XIV. Ten-year incidence and progression of diabetic retinopathy. Arch Ophthalmol 1994;112:1217–1228.
22. Soldi R, Mitola S, Strasly M, Defilippi P, Tarone G, Bussolino F. Role of alphavbeta3 integrin in the activation of vascular endothelial growth factor receptor-2. EMBO J 1999;18:882–892.
23. Brooks PC, Stromblad S, Sanders LC, et al. Localization of matrix metalloproteinase MMP-2 to the surface of invasive cells by interaction with integrin αvβ3. Cell 1996;85:683–693.
24. Seftor RE, Seftor EA, Gehlsen KR, et al. Role of the alpha v beta 3 integrin in human melanoma cell invasion. Proc Natl Acad Sci USA 1992;89:1557–1561.
25. Friedlander M, Brooks PC, Shaffer RW, Kincaid CM, Varner JA, Cheresh DA. Definition of two angiogenic pathways by distinct alpha v integrins. Science 1995;270:1500–1502.
26. Friedlander M, Theesfeld CL, Sugita M, et al. Involvement of integrins alpha v beta 3 and alpha v beta 5 in ocular neovascular diseases. Proc Natl Acad Sci USA 1996;93:9764–9769.
27. Hammes HP, Brownlee M, Jonczyk A, Sutter A, Preissner KT. Subcutaneous injection of a cyclic peptide antagonist of vitronectin receptor-type integrins inhibits retinal neovascularization. Nat Med 1996;2:529–533.
28. Luna J, Tobe T, Mousa SA, Reilly TM, Campochiaro PA. Antagonists of integrin alpha v beta 3 inhibit retinal neovascularization in a murine model. Lab Invest 1996;75:563–573.
29. Brooks PC, Clark RA, Cheresh DA. Requirement of vascular integrin alpha v beta 3 for angiogenesis. Science 1994;264:569–571.
30. Casaroli Marano RP, Vilaro S. The role of fibronectin, laminin, vitronectin and their receptors on cellular adhesion in proliferative vitreoretinopathy. Invest Ophthalmol Vis Sci 1994;35:2791–2803.
31. Casaroli Marano RP, Preissner KT, Vilaro S. Fibronectin, laminin, vitronectin and their receptors at newly-formed capillaries in proliferative diabetic retinopathy. Exp Eye Res 1995;60:5–17.

32. Smith LE, Wesolowski E, McLellan A, et al. Oxygen-induced retinopathy in the mouse. Invest Ophthalmol Vis Sci 1994;35:101–111.
33. Dorrell MI, Aguilar E, Friedlander M. Retinal vascular development is mediated by endothelial filopodia, a preexisting astrocytic template and specific R-cadherin adhesion. Invest Ophthalmol Vis Sci 2002;43:3500–3510.
34. Stromblad S, Fotedar A, Brickner H, et al. Loss of p53 compensates for alpha v-integrin function in retinal neovascularization. J Biol Chem 2002;277:13,371–13,374.
35. Hood JD, Frausto R, Kiosses WB, Schwartz MA, Cheresh DA. Differential alphav integrin-mediated Ras-ERK signaling during two pathways of angiogenesis. J Cell Biol 2003; 162:933–943.
36. Bader BL, Rayburn H, Crowley D, Hynes RO. Extensive vasculogenesis, angiogenesis, and organogenesis precede lethality in mice lacking all alpha v integrins. Cell 1998;95:507–519.
37. Hodivala-Dilke KM, McHugh KP, Tsakiris DA, et al. Beta3-integrin-deficient mice are a model for Glanzmann thrombasthenia showing placental defects and reduced survival. J Clin Invest 1999;103:229–238.
38. Huang X, Griffiths M, Wu J, Farese RV Jr, Sheppard D. Normal development, wound healing, and adenovirus susceptibility in beta5-deficient mice. Mol Cell Biol 2000;20: 755–759.
39. Reynolds LE, Wyder L, Lively JC, et al. Enhanced pathological angiogenesis in mice lacking beta3 integrin or beta3 and beta5 integrins. Nat Med 2002;8:27–34.
40. Hynes RO. A reevaluation of integrins as regulators of angiogenesis. Nat Med 2002;8: 918–921.
41. Ritter MR, Zhou Q, Markland FS Jr. Contortrostatin, a snake venom disintegrin, induces alphavbeta3-mediated tyrosine phosphorylation of CAS and FAK in tumor cells. J Cell Biochem 2000;79:28–37.
42. Ritter MR, Zhou Q, Markland FS Jr. Contortrostatin, a homodimeric disintegrin, actively disrupts focal adhesion and cytoskeletal structure and inhibits cell motility through a novel mechanism. Cell Commun Adhes 2001;8:71–86.
43. Stupack DG, Puente XS, Boutsaboualoy S, Storgard CM, Cheresh DA. Apoptosis of adherent cells by recruitment of caspase-8 to unligated integrins. J Cell Biol 2001;155:459–470.
44. Smith JW. Cilengitide Merck. Curr Opin Investig Drugs 2003;4:741–745.
45. Eskens FA, Dumez H, Hoekstra R, et al. Phase I and pharmacokinetic study of continuous twice weekly intravenous administration of Cilengitide (EMD 121974), a novel inhibitor of the integrins alphavbeta3 and alphavbeta5 in patients with advanced solid tumours. Eur J Cancer 2003;39:917–926.
46. Cheresh DA, Stupack DG. Integrin–Mediated death: an explanation of the integrin—knockout phenotype? Nat Med 2002;8:193–194.

17

Ocular Inflammation and Neovascularization

Chi-Chao Chan, MD and Robert B. Nussenblatt, MD

CONTENTS

INTRODUCTION

Neovascularization, also termed "angiogenesis," is the process of generating new capillary blood vessels as an extension of existing vasculature *(1)*. Neovascularization is an integral part of normal developmental processes and numerous pathologies, ranging from tumor growth and metastasis to inflammation and ocular disease. This process is driven by a cocktail of proangiogenic growth factors and cytokines and is tempered by an equally diverse group of inhibitors of neovascularization.

Ocular neovascularization is an uncommon but well-recognized complication of uveitis *(2)*. Although the exact pathogenesis is still not clear, uveitic neovascularization is definitely related to inflammation. New vessel growth often appears in the retina, optic nerve head, and choroid rather than in the iris and ciliary body. Immunosuppressive therapy is the first choice for treatment of uveitic neovascularization.

CLINICAL MANIFESTATION

Uveitic neovascularization affects both uveal and retinal tissues. It more commonly involves the retina—either through neovascularization of the disk (NVD) or neovascularization elsewhere (NVE)—and the choroid (choroidal neovascularization, CNV). Both NVD and NVE can be detected by fundoscopy and angiography. The new vessels tend to grow on the retinal surface. Later these vessels will penetrate the internal limiting membrane and posterior vitreous hyaloid face, and proliferate into the vitreous (Fig. 1A). They are fragile and tend to bleed, resulting in vitreous hemorrhage. Due to the lack of tight junctions on these neovascular endothelial cells, early and progressive

From: *Ophthalmology: Ocular Angiogenesis: Diseases, Mechanisms, and Therapeutics*
Edited by: J. Tombran-Tink and C. J. Barnstable © Humana Press Inc., Totowa, NJ

leakage is the classic finding on fluorescein angiography (Fig. 1B). CNV can be detected by fundoscopy, angiography, and indocyanine green angiography.

Retinal Neovascularization

Retinal neovascularization often occurs in uveitides that are associated with occlusive retinal vasculitis, such as Behçet's and Eales' diseases *(3–6)*. Eales' disease, first described by Henry Eales in 1880, is notable for its presentation of retinal periphlebitis, ischemia, and neovascularization. In contrast, Behçet's disease, first described by Dr. T. Shigeta in 1924 and Dr. B. Adamantiades in 1931 but popularized and named by Hulûsi Behçet in 1937, presents with intraocular inflammation consisting of retinal vasculitis, oral and mucosal ulcerations, and skin lesions. In a large study, Atmaca and colleagues reported that 47 of 912 eyes with Behçet's disease developed retinal neovascularization: 25 with NVD and 22 with NVE *(7)*. Although retinal neovascularization rarely occurs in pars planitis *(8)*, both NVE and NVD leading to vitreous hemorrhage have been reported *(9–11)*. Other uveitides reported to develop NVD and NVE include systemic lupus erythematosus *(12,13)*, sarcoidosis *(14)*, birdshot retinochoroidopathy *(15)*, and retinal vasculitis (Fig. 1). Infectious uveitis such as AIDS *(16)* and others can also be associated with retinal neovascularization *(2)*.

Choroidal Neovascularization

CNV includes choroidal and subchoroidal neovascularization. CNV occurs in both infectious and noninfectious choroiditis. Although CNV has been considered less common than NVD and NVE in older literature, we have now detected more uveitic CNV with advanced clinical equipment and skills. Usually CNV presents with subretinal or intraretinal hemorrhage, pigment epithelial detachment and a grayish-green subretinal membrane (Fig. 2A). It is often associated with chorioretinal scar. Either classic or occult CNV has been described in uveitic CNV. It can be detected by fluorescent angiogram (Fig. 2B,C). Indocyanine green angiography is helpful for identifying feeder vessels (Fig. 3).

CNV is an important feature of ocular histoplasmosis *(17,18)*, which manifests as the classic triad of discrete atrophic choroidal scars in the macula or midperiphery (histo spots), peripapillary atrophy, and choroidal neovascularization *(19)*. CNV has also been associated with serpiginous choroidopathy *(20,21)*. Blumenkranz and associates reported CNV in 56% (14 of 53) of patients with serpiginous choroidopathy *(22)*. CNV is associated with a poor prognosis in Vogt-Koyanagi-Harada syndrome (VKH) *(23,24)*. We reported the development of CNV in 14.7% (11 of 75) of patients with VKH who had a poor visual outcome *(25)*. Several infections are known to be complicated by CNV, including toxoplasmosis and *Candida* choroidoretinitis *(26–28)*.

All CNV, including that which is developed in age-related macular degeneration, involves some degree of inflammation. This inflammatory component varies in intensity depending on the underlying disease and dynamic stage of CNV development *(29)*. The growth pattern of CNV varies from individual to individual and disease to disease. As a result, no two CNV presentations are exactly alike. In addition, the varying clinical manifestations are due to the dynamic evolution of CNV, which involves initiation, inflammatory activity, and evolutional (fibrotic) stages *(30)*.

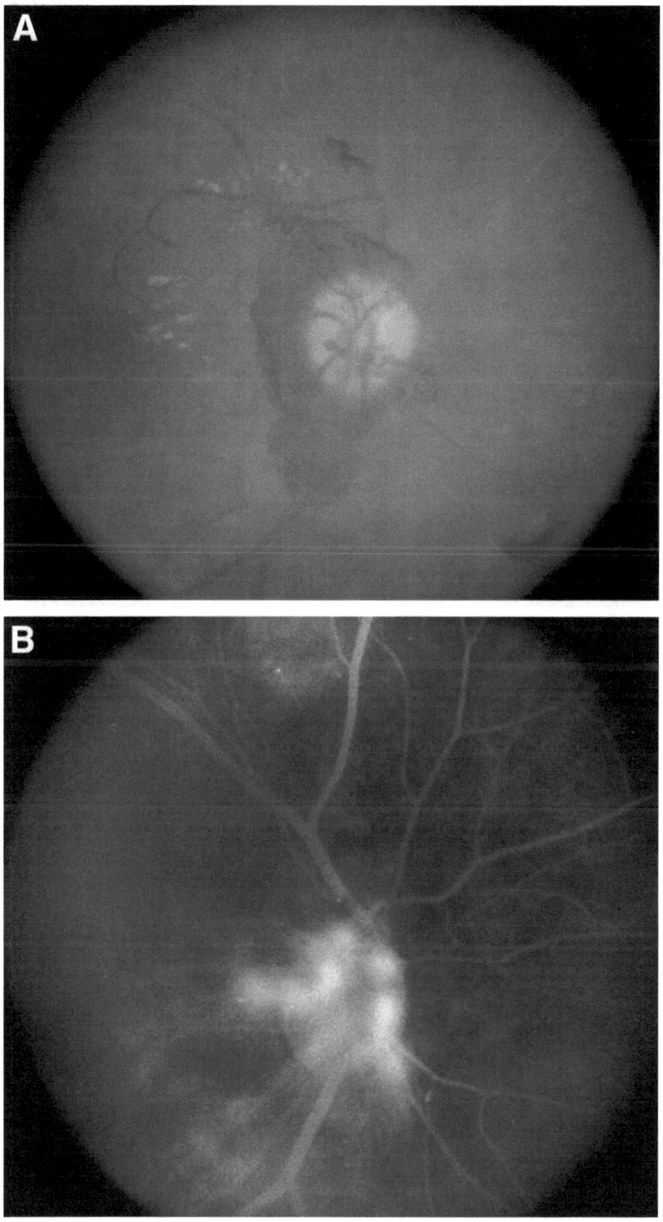

Fig. 1. (**A**) Fundoscopy shows neovascularization of the disk (NVD) at the optic disk in a patient with retinal vasculitis. (**B**) Late phase of fluorescent angiography shows vascular leakage from NVD in a patient with Vogt-Koyanagi-Harada syndrome. *See* color version on companion CD.

Iris and Ciliary Neovascularization

Neovascularization in the iris and ciliary body is a rare and ominous complication of uveitis. An Iris neovascularization, or rubeosis irides, is new vessel growth on the surface of the iris, which can result in hyphema and/or rubeotic glaucoma (Fig. 3). Ciliary

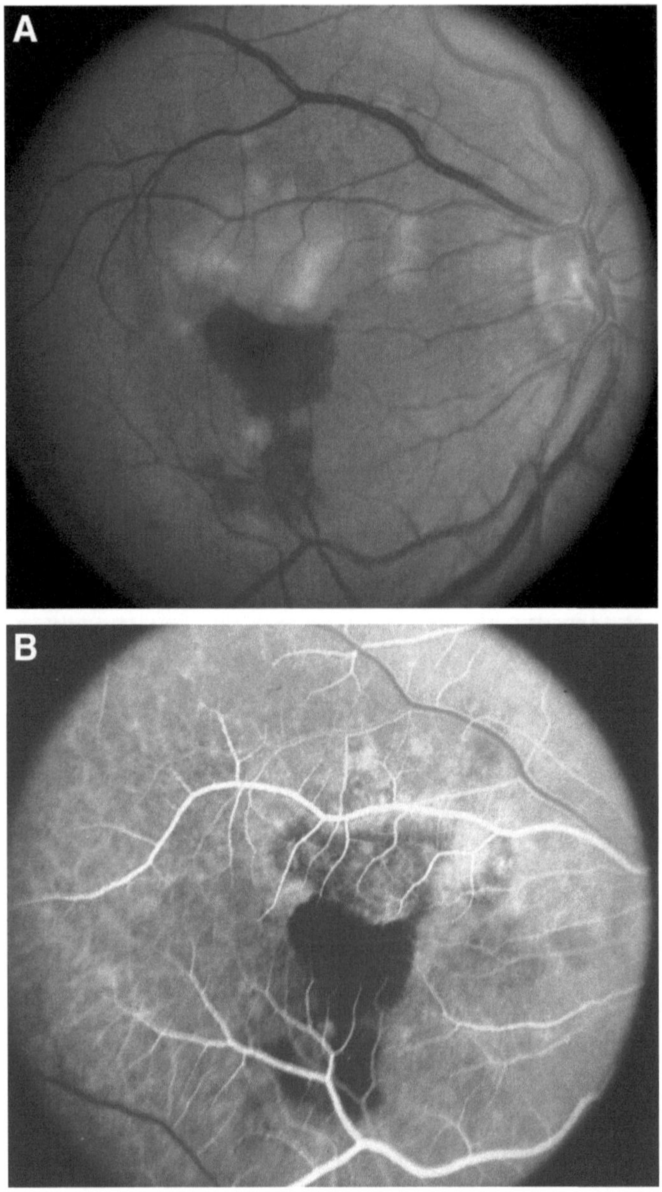

Fig. 2. Clinical illustrations of choroidal neovascularization (CNV) in a patient with Vogt-Koyanagi-Harada syndrome show (**A**) grayish membrane and blood at the central macula, (**B**) early phase of fluorescent angiogram with blockage, and (**C**) late phase of fluorescent angiogram with leakage. (**D**) Indocyanine green angiogram of a patient with ocular toxoplasmosis shows choroidal feeder vessel from CNV. *See* color version on companion CD.

neovascularization arises from a fibrovascular cyclitic membrane, which is formed from long-standing chronic uveitis with ciliary body involvement *(31)*.

PATHOGENESIS

Ocular neovascularization, like neovascularization elsewhere in the body, is driven by various proangiogenic growth factors and cytokines, which include a potentially

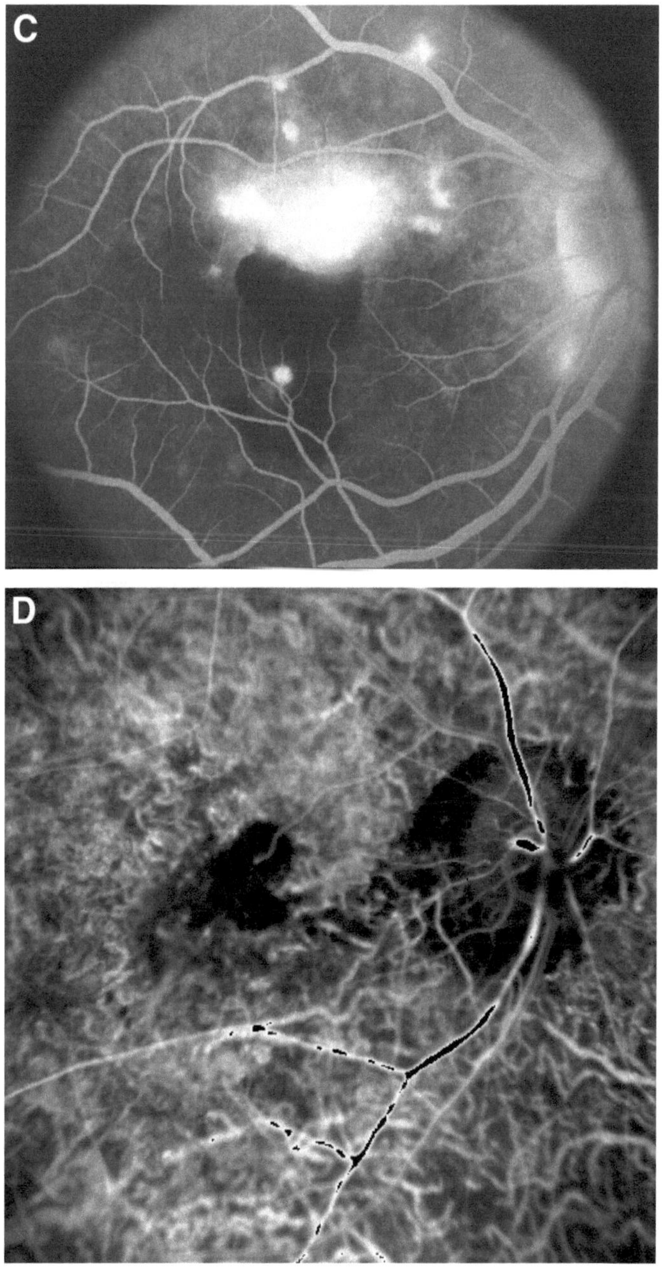

Fig. 2. (*Continued*)

large group of participating proteins involved in a complex interaction. Despite the participation of multiple stimulatory factors for ocular neovascularization, vascular endothelial growth factor (VEGF) is a key regulator *(32–34)*. Cytokines, growth factors, and gonadotropins that do not stimulate angiogenesis directly can modulate angiogenesis by adjusting VEGF expression in specific cells, thus exerting an indirect angiogenic or antiangiogenic effect.

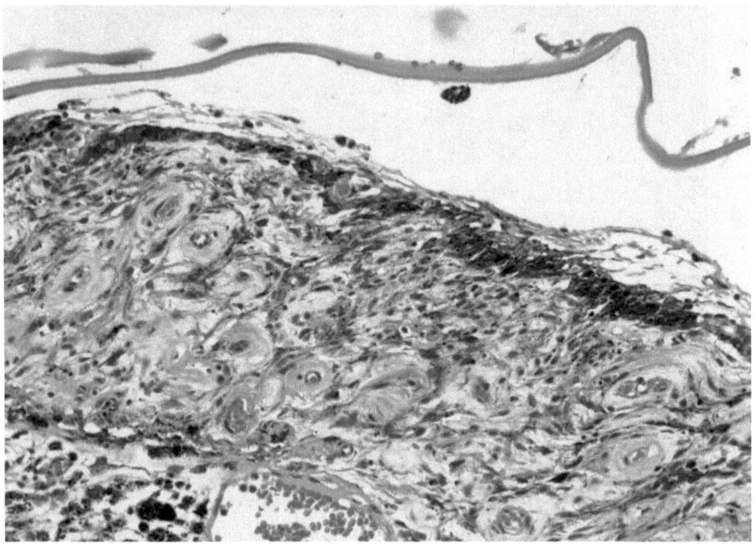

Fig. 3. Photomicrograph shows small vessels on the iris surface (rubeosis iridis) of a patient with Vogt-Koyanagi-Harada syndrome (hematoxylin and eosin, original magnification ×200). *See* color version on companion CD.

Inflammation and immune-derived angiogenesis is observed in numerous disorders, in part because most leukocyte subtypes affect many angiogenic processes by producing myriad angiogenic growth factors such as VEGF, placenta growth factor (PIGF), platelet-derived growth factor (PDGF), hypoxia-induced factor (HIF), transforming growth factor (TGF)-β, various chemokines and cytokines, as well as proteinases including tryptase, chymase, matrix metalloprotein kinases (MMPs), and heparanase *(35)*. These angiogenic factors amplify the inflammatory process by recruiting leukocytes and affecting their function *(36)*. Leukocytes and vascular endothelial cells can influence each other in many ways. In addition, neutrophils, nature killer (NK) cells, macrophages, and mast cells have been associated with stimulation of angiogenesis in tumors and allergic conditions. Recently, bone marrow-derived endothelial progenitor cells are reported to incorporate into sites of physiological and pathological neovascularization.

VEGF

VEGF is a highly specific mitogen for vascular endothelial cells *(37,38)*. Vascular permeability factor has been characterized as a protein that promotes extravasation of protein from tumor-associated blood vessels *(39)*. Vascular permeability factor and VEGF are encoded by a single VEGF gene *(40,41)*, which produces several VEGF isoforms such as $VEGF_{120}$, $VEGF_{145}$, $VEGF_{165}$, and $VEGF_{206}$. The VEGF family, including VEGF-A to -E and PIGF, shares the common receptors VEGFR-1 to VEGFR-3, heparan-sulfate proteoglycan, and neurophilin-1 and neurophilin-2 *(34)*. VEGF is a survival factor for vascular endothelial cells, both in vitro and in vivo *(42,43)*. VEGF prevents apoptosis and induces expression of the antiapoptotic protein Bcl-2 in endothelial cells. VEGF also induces vascular leakage.

VEGF has been implicated in various inflammatory disorders *(44)*. Transgenic overexpression of VEGF results in increased density of torturous cutaneous blood capillaries and enhanced leukocyte rolling and adhesion in skin venules, suggesting that overexpression of VEGF in the skin is sufficient to induce a chronic dermatitis similar to human psoriasis *(45,46)*. In a rat model of CNV induced by subretinal injection of adenoviral vector encoding the $VEGF_{165}$ gene, we have also observed a considerable infiltration of macrophages and lymphocytes in the lesion *(47)*. In differential leukocyte and endothelial responses, $VEGF_{165}$ was found to be the pathological isoform working through VEGFR-1 and VEGFR-2 *(48)*. In vivo blockade of VEGFR-1 significantly suppresses $VEGF_{165}$-induced corneal inflammation and monocyte chemotaxis. In vitro, $VEGF_{165}$ more potently stimulates intracellular adhesion molecule-1 expression on endothelial cells in a process mediated by VEGFR-2. More details about VEGF are discussed in Chapters 11 and 18.

VEGF may be a mediator of angiogenesis and permeability in inflammatory disorders, including uveitis *(34)*. Factors that can potentiate VEGF production include growth factors such as PDGF, TGF-α and -β, fibroblast growth factor (FGF)-4, keratinocyte growth factor (KGF), insulin-like growth factor (IGF)-I, and cytokines/chemokines, such as tumor necrosis factor (TNF)-α, interleukin (IL)-1β, IL-6, IL-8, CCL-2, CCL5, and all four CXC chemokines *(49)*. Some cytokines, such as IL-10 and IL-13, can inhibit the release of VEGF. Inflammatory cytokines such as IL-1 and IL-6 induce expression of VEGF in several cell types; therefore, inflammation can trigger VEGF release that results in neovascularization.

Hypoxia-Inducible Factor

Hypoxia-inducible factor (HIF) is another potent mediator of angiogenesis. The regulation of angiogenesis by hypoxia is an important component of homeostatic mechanisms that link the vascular oxygen supply to metabolic demand. HIF, an αβ-heterodimer, is a DNA-binding factor that mediates hypoxia-inducible activity of the erythropoietin and VEGF genes *(50)*. HIF-1β subunits are constitutive nuclear proteins, whereas HIF-α subunits are regulatory and induced by hypoxia. HIF is activated in hypoxic cells; HIF not only modulates production of several angiogenic growth factors, but also regulates expression of their receptors and has important effects on matrix metabolism *(51)*.

Several inflammatory mediators and cytokines, including nitric oxide *(52)*, IL-1 *(53)*, and TNF-α *(54)*, can regulate HIF-α. A decrease in HIF-α is reported to be correlated with a marked reduction of IL-8 production by a potent angiogenic agent, carboxyaminotriazole *(55)*. *CXCR4*, the gene for the receptor of chemokine CXCL12 (stromal cell-derived factor-1α, SDF-1α), is recognized as a novel target gene of the DNA-binding transcriptional activator HIF *(56)*. *CXCR4* is now considered a hypoxia-inducible gene.

Chemokines and Cytokines

Chemokines are a group of small (8–14 kDa), mostly basic, structurally related molecules that regulate cell trafficking of leukocytes through interactions with a subset of seven-transmembrane, G protein-coupled receptors. Chemokines are defined by structure and classified and named according to patterns of conserved cysteines. They are divided into four subfamilies: CXC (an amino acid between the two N-terminal cysteine residues), CC (two cysteines adjacent to each other), C (only one cysteine), or CX3C (three amino acids between the two cysteines). Chemokines have been shown to play a critical role in the regulation of angiogenesis during pathophysiological processes, such as tumor growth, wound healing, and ischemia. Chemokines may exert their regulatory activity on angiogenesis directly or as a consequence of leukocyte infiltration, induction of growth factor expression, and direct stimulation of vascular endothelial cells *(57)*.

CXC chemokines represent a large family of homologous peptides exhibiting positive (angiogenesis) or negative (angiostasis) activity on the control of angiogenesis *(49)*. Among the angiogenic CXC chemokines are CXCL1, CXCL2, CXCL3, CXCL5, CXCL6, CXCL7, CXCL8 (IL-8), and CXCL12; among the angiostatic CXC chemokines are CXCL4, CXCL9, CXCL10, CXCL11, and CXCL13. Thus, CXC chemokines not only influence the sequential participation of inflammatory cells but also regulate, in a coordinated fashion, the inflammatory reaction leading to angiogenesis, tissue repair, and new tissue generation. The coordination of angiogenesis and inflammation is a result of the shared ability of vascular endothelial cells and leukocytes to respond to chemokines. Indeed, dysregulation of CXCL chemokines could lead to chronic inflammation and neovascularization.

Among the CXCL chemokines, IL-8 (CXCL8) is a notorious angiogenic molecule. This chemokine functions in the direct enhancement of endothelial cell proliferation, survival, MMP expression in CXCR1- and CXCR2-expressing endothelial cells, and the direct regulation of angiogenesis *(58)*. IL-8 also mediates vascular endothelial cell migration and promotes neovascularization.

Proangiogenic cytokines can directly drive neovascularization. The angiogenic activity of TNF-α has been elicited by the synthesis of direct angiogenic inducers or of proteases *(43)*. TNF-α upregulates the expression and the function of VEGFR-2 and neurophilin-1 in human endothelium in a dose- and time-dependent manner. In a recent study of cyclooxygenase 2 (COX-2, an important enzyme in arachidonic acid metabolism) and neovascularization, prostanoids (products of the COX-2 pathway) are found to be independently involved in the VEGF/VEGFR pathway for inflammatory cytokine-induced angiogenesis. IL-1β markedly induces angiogenesis in vitro and in vivo. This process can be significantly inhibited by COX-2 selective inhibitors but not by a VEGF receptor tyrosine kinase inhibitor *(59)*.

Other inflammatory mediators such as nitric oxide and prostanoids also play active roles in angiogenesis during inflammatory processes. Indeed, there are reports of uveitic patients who develop neovascularization without evidence of retinal ischemia *(60–63)*. The curious finding of marked capillary dropout but no neovascularization in some uveitic cases may result from the complex interaction among various angiogenic and angiostatic growth factors, ischemic factors, cytokines, chemokines, and inflammatory mediators.

EXPERIMENTAL OCULAR INFLAMMATION AND NEOVASCULARIZATION

A spectrum of chronic noninfectious uveitides has been simulated by the pathological changes seen in the animal model of experimental autoimmune uveitis (EAU). EAU in animals is induced by immunization with retinal antigens or their fragments. Examples of the retinal antigens are arrestin (retinal-soluble antigen, S-Ag), interphotoreceptor retinoid-binding protein (IRBP), rhodopsin and its illuminated form opsin, recoverin, and phosducin *(64)*. The pathogenesis of EAU, and likely of human endogenous uveitis, involves cell-mediated destruction of retinal tissues that is dependent on retinal antigen-specific T cells *(65)*. EAU can include vitritis, chorioretinal inflammatory infiltration, retinal vasculitis, edema, and atrophy, in addition to inflammation in the uvea. Neovascularization is one of the recognizable complications of EAU.

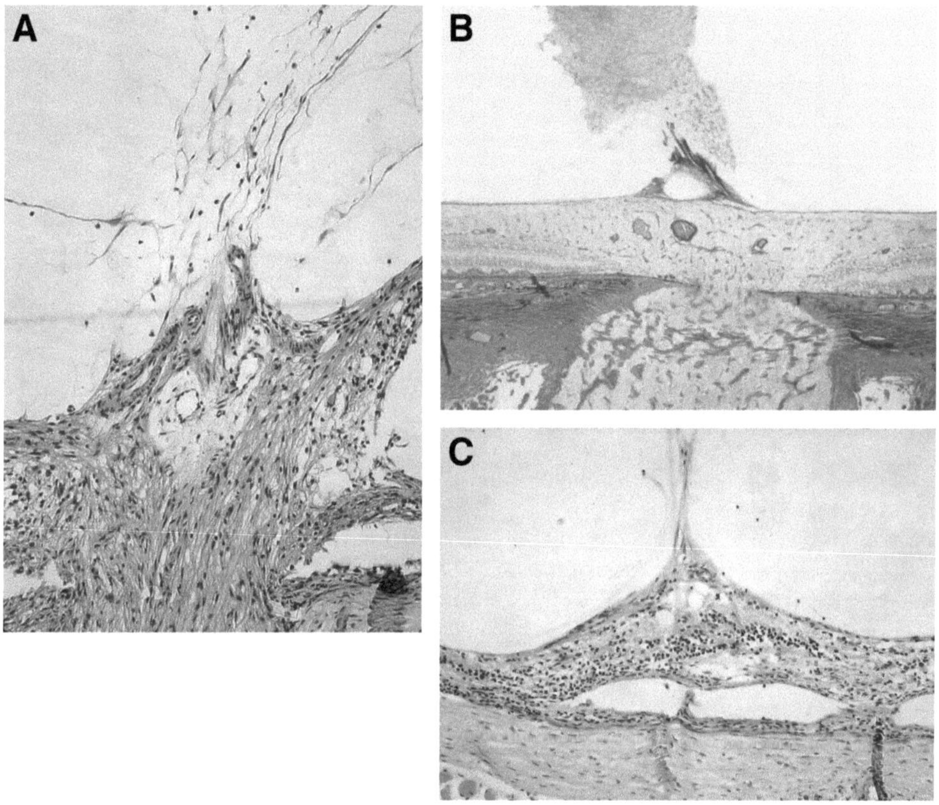

Fig. 4. Photomicrographs show neovascularization of the disk (NVD) arising from the optic disc vessels in **(A)** a rat with experimental autoimmune uveitis (EAU) and **(B)** a patient with Behçet disease. **(C)** neovascularization elsewhere (NVE) is shown in an EAU rat (hematoxylin and eosin; original magnification: A, ×400; B, ×100; C, ×200). *See* color version on companion CD.

EAU and Neovascularization

In mouse EAU, CNV occurs in 10% of eyes *(66)*. In rat EAU, NVE, and NVD, but rarely CNV, may develop in those animals with a total loss of photoreceptors *(67)*. In monkey EAU, different forms of ocular neovascularization including CNV, NVE, and NVD may develop *(68)*. Although the exact pathogenesis remains elusive, cytokines/chemokines and inflammatory mediators certainly play an important role in the angiogenic process *(69)*. Increased VEGF has also been reported in EAU even in cases without neovascularization in the eye *(70)*.

Pathology of Neovascularization

Histopathologically, neovascularization in EAU closely resembles that observed in human uveitis. In both NVD and NVE, the new vessels arise from the capillaries in the nerve fiber layer and proliferate as naked channels in the early stage. Later fibrosis and gliosis occur around these small vessels, which are noted more frequently in rat EAU eyes with loss of photoreceptors. Because these vessels often lack tight junctions and bleed easily, vitreous hemorrhage is common (Fig. 4A,B). Scarring and shrinkage tend to occur around these proliferating channels and may lead to wrinkling of the retina and even to the development of a retinal traction detachment (Fig. 4C). In humans,

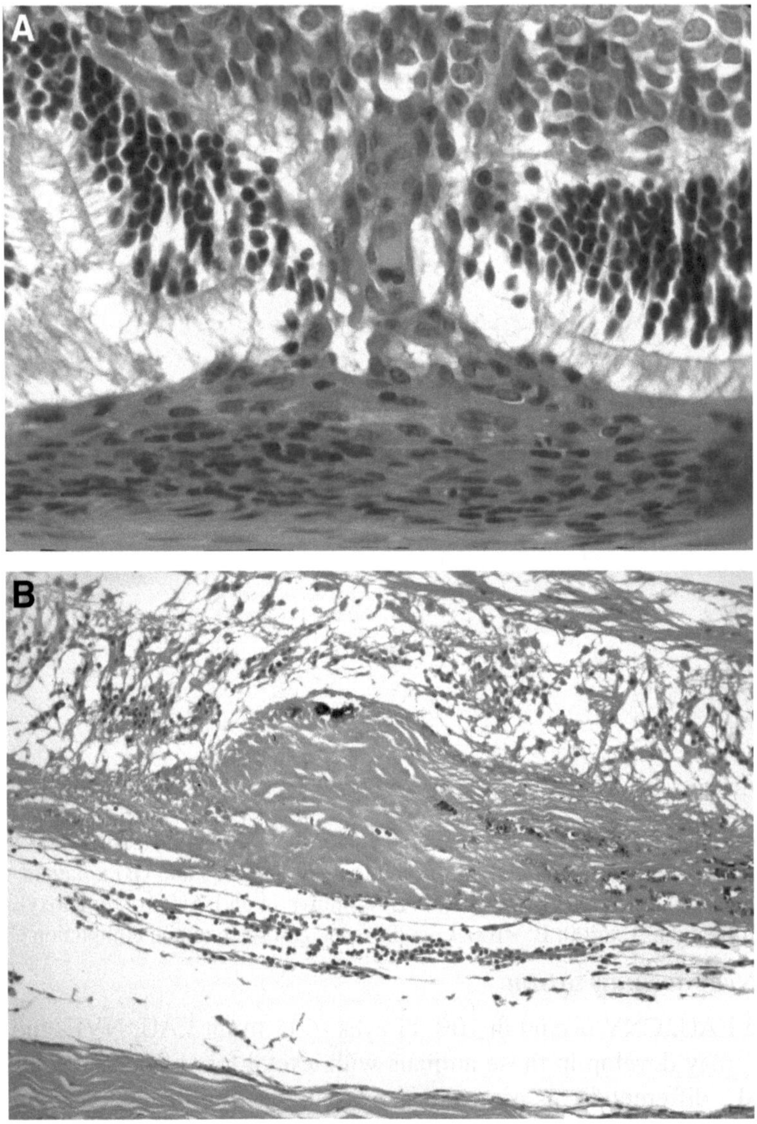

Fig. 5. Photomicrographs show choroidal neovascularization arising from the choroid in **(A)** a mouse with experimental autoimmune uveitis and **(B)** a patient with Vogt-Koyanagi-Harada syndrome. Inflammatory cells are present in the choroid (hematoxylin and eosin; original magnification: A, ×400; B, ×200). *See* color version on companion CD.

retinal neovascularization associated with massive VEGF expression is reported in Eales' disease that is frequently complicated by extensive retinal neovascularization and vitreous hemorrhages *(71)*.

CNV occurs through associated breaks in Bruch's membrane. In general, CNV presents as a sub-retinal pigment epithelium (RPE) neovascular membrane with capillary and/or small vessel-like lumens arising from the choroidal vasculature. Frequently, the sub-RPE neovascularization leads to serous and hemorrhagic detachment of the RPE or the retina, and this, in turn, may lead to disciform scarring (Fig.5A,B).

Usually there is an inflammatory cellular component in CNV lesions associated with uveitis. A typical example is ocular histoplasmosis or the presumed histoplasmosis syndrome, in which macrophages and lymphocytes are mediators of angiogenesis or modifiers of CNV *(72,73)*.

THERAPY

Currently available treatments for uveitic neovascularization include immunotherapy, photocoagulation, photodynamic therapy (PDT), and surgical excision of the CNV neovascular membrane. Therapeutic approaches for ocular neovascularization will be discussed in greater detail in later chapters.

In uveitic neovascularization, there is always an inflammatory component. Therefore, antiinflammatory and/or immunosuppressive therapies should be prescribed. Corticosteroids are antiinflammatory and antiangiogenic. Local (including periocular) injections and vitreal implants, as well as systemic corticosteroids, have been reported to treat NVD effectively in sarcoidosis, multiple sclerosis, juvenile rheumatoid arthritis, cyclitis, and idiopathic uveitis *(2,61)*. Although corticosteroids alone may be less favorable for CNV, additional immunosuppressive agents such as cyclosporine and azathioprine have been used successfully to regress neovascularization in sympathetic ophthalmia, multifocal choroiditis, ocular histoplasmosis syndrome, serpiginous choroiditis, and endogenous posterior uveits *(74,75)*.

With the recent advance in understanding of angiogenesis, antiangiogenic factors such as anti-VEGF agents are being introduced as treatments for neovascularization, including ocular neovascularization *(76,77)*. These novel agents, in combination with immunotherapy, may have promising effects for better control of uveitic neovascularization.

Laser photocoagulation and PDT for uveitic neovascularization have been reported in a few small case series *(2,78)*. PDT appeared to stabilize or improve vision in a few patients with subfoveal CNV secondary to multifocal choroiditis and panuveitis. However, these encouraging results need further investigation and longer follow-up.

The surgical removal of uveitic CNV in the subfoveal area was described in 1991 as yielding significant therapeutic success *(79)*. Since then it has been recognized that the mechanical excision of CNV associated with ocular histoplasmosis and multifocal choroiditis produces less damage to the photoreceptor cells than laser photocoagulation *(80,81)*. However, this surgical procedure is rather difficult and requires skillful surgeons. Surgical complications are frequent. Therefore, surgery should be reserved for selected patients who fail to respond to medical therapy, because the neovascular membrane often grows back. In addition, it is technically difficult to remove a recurrent CNV if there is scarring.

In summary, ocular neovascularization associated with uveitis is a serious complication. Uveitic neovascularization is a consequence of a complex interaction between genetic and environmental factors such as neovascular growth factors, cytokines, chemokines, and inflammatory mediators. The pathology of NVD, NVE, and CNV in EAU closely mimics that seen in human uveitides. Uveitic neovascularization occurs more often in eyes with both severe inflammation and ischemia. Immunotherapy is the first choice for uveitic neovascularization.

REFERENCES

1. Polverini PJ. The pathophysiology of angiogenesis. Crit Rev Oral Biol Med 1995;6:230–247.
2. Kuo IC, Cunningham ET Jr. Ocular neovascularization in patients with uveitis. Int Ophthalmol Clin 2000;40:111–126.
3. Graham EM, Stanford MR, Shilling JS, Sanders MD. Neovascularisation associated with posterior uveitis. Br J Ophthalmol 1987;71:826–833.
4. Nussenblatt RB. Uveitis in Behcet's disease. Int Rev Immunol 1997;14:67–79.
5. Atmaca LS, Batioglu F, Atmaca Sonmez P. A long-term follow-up of Eales' disease. Ocul Immunol Inflamm 2002;10:213–221.
6. Biswas J, Sharma T, Gopal L, Madhavan HN, Sulochana KN, Ramakrishnan S. Eales disease—an update. Surv Ophthalmol 2002;47:197–214.
7. Atmaca LS, Batioglu F, Idil A. Retinal and disc neovascularization in Behcet's disease and efficacy of laser photocoagulation. Graefes Arch Clin Exp Ophthalmol 1996;234:94–99.
8. Green WR, Kincaid MC, Michels RG, Pederson JE, Kenyon KR, Maumenee AE. Pars planitis. Trans Ophthalmol Soc UK 1981;101:361–367.
9. Phillips WB 2nd, Bergren RL, McNamara JA. Pars planitis presenting with vitreous hemorrhage. Ophthalmic Surg 1993;24:630–631.
10. Park SE, Mieler WF, Pulido JS. 2 peripheral scatter photocoagulation for neovascularization associated with pars planitis. Arch Ophthalmol 1995;113:1277–1280.
11. Pulido JS, Mieler WF, Walton D, et al. Results of peripheral laser photocoagulation in pars planitis. Trans Am Ophthalmol Soc 1998;96:127–137; discussion 137–141.
12. Vine AK, Barr CC. Proliferative lupus retinopathy. Arch Ophthalmol 1984;102:852–854.
13. Read RW, Chong LP, Rao NA. Occlusive retinal vasculitis associated with systemic lupus erythematosus. Arch Ophthalmol 2000;118:588–589.
14. Duker JS, Brown GC, McNamara JA. Proliferative sarcoid retinopathy. Ophthalmology 1988;95:1680–1686.
15. Barondes MJ, Fastenberg DM, Schwartz PL, Rosen DA. Peripheral retinal neovascularization in birdshot retinochoroidopathy. Ann Ophthalmol 1989;21:306–308.
16. Wright ME, Suzman DL, Csaky KG, Masur H, Polis MA, Robinson MR. Extensive retinal neovascularization as a late finding in human immunodeficiency virus-infected patients with immune recovery uveitis. Clin Infect Dis 2003;36:1063–1066.
17. Ciulla TA, Piper HC, Xiao M, Wheat LJ. Presumed ocular histoplasmosis syndrome: update on epidemiology, pathogenesis, and photodynamic, antiangiogenic, and surgical therapies. Curr Opin Ophthalmol 2001;12:442–449.
18. Callanan D, Jost BF. New findings in ocular histoplasmosis. Curr Opin Ophthalmol 1995;6:8–12.
19. Smith RE. Studies of the presumed ocular histoplasmosis syndrome. Trans Ophthalmol Soc UK 1981;101:328–334.
20. Jampol LM, Orth D, Daily MJ, Rabb MF. Subretinal neovascularization with geographic (serpiginous) choroiditis. Am J Ophthalmol 1979;88:683–689.
21. Lee DK, Suhler EB, Augustin W, Buggage RR. Serpiginous choroidopathy presenting as choroidal neovascularisation. Br J Ophthalmol 2003;87:1184–1185.
22. Blumenkranz MS, Gass JD, Clarkson JG. Atypical serpiginous choroiditis. Arch Ophthalmol 1982;100:1773–1775.
23. Read RW, Rao NA, Cunningham ET. Vogt-Koyanagi-Harada disease. Curr Opin Ophthalmol 2000;11:437–442.
24. Moorthy RS, Chong LP, Smith RE, Rao NA. Subretinal neovascular membranes in Vogt-Koyanagi-Harada syndrome. Am J Ophthalmol 1993;116:164–170.
25. Lertsumitkul S, Whitcup SM, Nussenblatt RB, Chan CC. Subretinal fibrosis and choroidal neovascularization in Vogt-Koyanagi-Harada syndrome. Graefes Arch Clin Exp Ophthalmol 1999;237:1039–1045.

26. Brezin AP, Kasner L, Thulliez P, et al. Ocular toxoplasmosis in the fetus. Immunohistochemistry analysis and DNA amplification. Retina 1994;14:19–26.
27. Fine SL, Owens SL, Haller JA, Knox DL, Patz A. Choroidal neovascularization as a late complication of ocular toxoplasmosis. Am J Ophthalmol 1981;91:318–322.
28. Jampol LM, Sung J, Walker JD, et al. Choroidal neovascularization secondary to Candida albicans chorioretinitis. Am J Ophthalmol 1996;121:643–649.
29. Grossniklaus HE, Ling JX, Wallace TM, et al. Macrophage and retinal pigment epithelium expression of angiogenic cytokines in choroidal neovascularization. Mol Vis 2002;8:119–126.
30. Grossniklaus HE, Green WR. Choroidal neovascularization. Am J Ophthalmol 2004;137: 496–503.
31. Chan CC, Fujikawa LS, Rodrigues MM, Stevens G Jr, Nussenblatt RB. Immunohistochemistry and electron microscopy of cyclitic membrane. Report of a case. Arch Ophthalmol 1986;104:1040–1045.
32. Campochiaro PA, Hackett SF. Ocular neovascularization: a valuable model system. Oncogene 2003;22:6537–6548.
33. Ferrara N. Role of vascular endothelial growth factor in regulation of physiological angiogenesis. Am J Physiol Cell Physiol 2001;280:C1358–C1366.
34. Neufeld G, Cohen T, Gengrinovitch S, Poltorak Z. Vascular endothelial growth factor (VEGF) and its receptors. FASEB J 1999;13:9–22.
35. Carmeliet P. Angiogenesis in health and disease. Nat Med 2003;9:653–660.
36. Luttun A, Tjwa M, Moons L, et al. Revascularization of ischemic tissues by PlGF treatment, and inhibition of tumor angiogenesis, arthritis and atherosclerosis by anti-Flt1. Nat Med 2002;8:831–840.
37. Tischer E, Gospodarowicz D, Mitchell R, et al. Vascular endothelial growth factor: a new member of the platelet-derived growth factor gene family. Biochem Biophys Res Commun 1989;165:1198–1206.
38. Ferrara N, Henzel WJ. Pituitary follicular cells secrete a novel heparin-binding growth factor specific for vascular endothelial cells. Biochem Biophys Res Commun 1989;161:851–858.
39. Senger DR, Galli SJ, Dvorak AM, Perruzzi CA, Harvey VS, Dvorak HF. Tumor cells secrete a vascular permeability factor that promotes accumulation of ascites fluid. Science 1983;219:983–985.
40. Leung DW, Cachianes G, Kuang WJ, Goeddel DV, Ferrara N. Vascular endothelial growth factor is a secreted angiogenic mitogen. Science 1989;246:1306–1309.
41. Keck PJ, Hauser SD, Krivi G, et al. Vascular permeability factor, an endothelial cell mitogen related to PDGF. Science 1989;246:1309–1312.
42. Gerber HP, McMurtrey A, Kowalski J, et al. Vascular endothelial growth factor regulates endothelial cell survival through the phosphatidylinositol 3′-kinase/Akt signal transduction pathway. Requirement for Flk-1/KDR activation. J Biol Chem 1998;273:30,336–30,343.
43. Giraudo E, Primo L, Audero E, et al. Tumor necrosis factor-alpha regulates expression of vascular endothelial growth factor receptor-2 and of its co-receptor neuropilin-1 in human vascular endothelial cells. J Biol Chem 1998;273:22,128–22,135.
44. Ferrara N, Gerber HP, LeCouter J. The biology of VEGF and its receptors. Nat Med 2003;9:669–676.
45. Detmar M, Yeo KT, Nagy JA, et al. Keratinocyte-derived vascular permeability factor (vascular endothelial growth factor) is a potent mitogen for dermal microvascular endothelial cells. J Invest Dermatol 1995;105:44–50.
46. Xia YP, Li B, Hylton D, Detmar M, Yancopoulos GD, Rudge JS. Transgenic delivery of VEGF to mouse skin leads to an inflammatory condition resembling human psoriasis. Blood 2003;102:161–168.
47. Baffi J, Byrnes G, Chan CC, Csaky KG. Choroidal neovascularization in the rat induced by adenovirus mediated expression of vascular endothelial growth factor. Invest Ophthalmol Vis Sci 2000;41:3582–3589.

48. Usui T, Ishida S, Yamashiro K, et al. VEGF164(165) as the pathological isoform: differential leukocyte and endothelial responses through VEGFR1 and VEGFR2. Invest Ophthalmol Vis Sci 2004;45:368–374.
49. Romagnani P, Lasagni L, Annunziato F, Serio M, Romagnani S. CXC chemokines: the regulatory link between inflammation and angiogenesis. Trends Immunol 2004;25:201–209.
50. Pugh CW, Ratcliffe PJ. Regulation of angiogenesis by hypoxia: role of the HIF system. Nat Med 2003;9:677–684.
51. Maxwell PH, Ratcliffe PJ. Oxygen sensors and angiogenesis. Semin Cell Dev Biol 2002;13: 29–37.
52. Sandau KB, Faus HG, Brune B. Induction of hypoxia-inducible-factor 1 by nitric oxide is mediated via the PI 3K pathway. Biochem Biophys Res Commun 2000;278:263–267.
53. Thornton RD, Lane P, Borghaei RC, Pease EA, Caro J, Mochan E. Interleukin 1 induces hypoxia-inducible factor 1 in human gingival and synovial fibroblasts. Biochem J 2000;350:307–312.
54. Hellwig-Burgel T, Rutkowski K, Metzen E, Fandrey J, Jelkmann W. Interleukin-1beta and tumor necrosis factor-alpha stimulate DNA binding of hypoxia-inducible factor-1. Blood 1999;94:1561–1567.
55. Oliver VK, Patton AM, Desai S, Lorang D, Libutti SK, Kohn EC. Regulation of the proangiogenic microenvironment by carboxyamido-triazole. J Cell Physiol 2003;197:139–148.
56. Staller P, Sulitkova J, Lisztwan J, Moch H, Oakeley EJ, Krek W. Chemokine receptor CXCR4 downregulated by von Hippel-Lindau tumour suppressor pVHL. Nature 2003; 425:307–311.
57. Bernardini G, Ribatti D, Spinetti G, et al. Analysis of the role of chemokines in angiogenesis. J Immunol Methods 2003;273:83–101.
58. Li A, Dubey S, Varney ML, Dave BJ, Singh RK. IL-8 directly enhanced endothelial cell survival, proliferation, and matrix metalloproteinases production and regulated angiogenesis. J Immunol 2003;170:3369–3376.
59. Kuwano T, Nakao S, Yamamoto H, et al. Cyclooxygenase 2 is a key enzyme for inflammatory cytokine-induced angiogenesis. FASEB J 2004;18:300–310.
60. Shorb SR, Irvine AR, Kimura SJ. Optic disk neovascularization associated with chronic uveitis. Am J Ophthalmol 1976;82:175–178.
61. Sanislo SR, Lowder CY, Kaiser PK, et al. Corticosteroid therapy for optic disc neovascularization secondary to chronic uveitis. Am J Ophthalmol 2000;130:724–731.
62. Kelly PJ, Weiter JJ. Resolution of optic disk neovascularization associated with intraocular inflammation. Am J Ophthalmol 1980;90:545–548.
63. Gray T, Kanski J, Lightman S. Steroid responsive disc neovascularisation in uveitis associated with juvenile chronic arthritis. Br J Ophthalmol 1998;82:327–328.
64. Gery I, Streilein JW. Autoimmunity in the eye and its regulation. Curr Opin Immunol 1994;6:938–945.
65. Caspi RR. Th1 and Th2 responses in pathogenesis and regulation of experimental autoimmune uveoretinitis. Int Rev Immunol 2002;21:197–208.
66. Chan CC, Caspi RR, Ni M, et al. Pathology of experimental autoimmune uveoretinitis in mice. J Autoimmun 1990;3:247–255.
67. al-Mahdawi S, McGettrick PM, Lee WR, Graham DI, Shallal A, Converse CA. Experimental autoimmune uveoretinitis and pinealitis induced by interphotoreceptor retinoid-binding protein and S-antigen: induction of intraretinal and subretinal neovascularization. J Clin Lab Immunol 1990;32:21–28.
68. Singh VK, Usukura J, Shinohara T. Molecular mimicry: uveitis induced in Macaca fascicularis by microbial protein having sequence homology with retinal S-antigen. Jpn J Ophthalmol 1992;36:108–116.

69. Wakefield D, Lloyd A. The role of cytokines in the pathogenesis of inflammatory eye disease. Cytokine 1992;4:1–5.
70. Vinores SA, Chan CC, Vinores MA, et al. Increased vascular endothelial growth factor (VEGF) and transforming growth factor beta (TGFbeta) in experimental autoimmune uveoretinitis: upregulation of VEGF without neovascularization. J Neuroimmunol 1998;89:43–50.
71. Perentes Y, Chan CC, Bovey E, Uffer S, Herbort CP. Massive vascular endothelium growth factor (VEGF) expression in Eales' disease. Klin Monatsbl Augenheilkd 2002;219:311–314.
72. Mann ES, Fogarty SJ, Kincaid MC. Choroidal neovascularization with granulomatous inflammation in ocular histoplasmosis syndrome. Am J Ophthalmol 2000;130:247–250.
73. Spencer WH, Chan CC, Shen D, Rao NA. Detection of histoplasma capsulatum DNA in lesions of chronic ocular histoplasmosis syndrome. Arch Ophthalmol 2003;121:1551–1555.
74. Dees C, Arnold JJ, Forrester JV, Dick AD. Immunosuppressive treatment of choroidal neovascularization associated with endogenous posterior uveitis. Arch Ophthalmol 1998;116:1456–1461.
75. Kilmartin DJ, Forrester JV, Dick AD. Cyclosporine-induced resolution of choroidal neovascularization associated with sympathetic ophthalmia. Arch Ophthalmol 1998;116:249–250.
76. Eyetech Study Group. Preclinical and phase 1A clinical evaluation of an anti-VEGF pegylated aptamer (EYE001) for the treatment of exudative age-related macular degeneration. Retina 2002;22:143–152.
77. Eyetech Study Group. Anti-vascular endothelial growth factor therapy for subfoveal choroidal neovascularization secondary to age-related macular degeneration: phase II study results. Ophthalmology 2003;110:979–986.
78. Spaide RF, Freund KB, Slakter J, Sorenson J, Yannuzzi LA, Fisher Y. Treatment of subfoveal choroidal neovascularization associated with multifocal choroiditis and panuveitis with photodynamic therapy. Retina 2002;22:545–549.
79. Thomas MA, Kaplan HJ. Surgical removal of subfoveal neovascularization in the presumed ocular histoplasmosis syndrome. Am J Ophthalmol 1991;111:1–7.
80. Eckstein M, Wells JA, Aylward B, Gregor Z. Surgical removal of non-age-related subfoveal choroidal neovascular membranes. Eye 1998;12:775–780.
81. Atebara NH, Thomas MA, Holekamp NM, Mandell BA, Del Priore LV. Surgical removal of extensive peripapillary choroidal neovascularization associated with presumed ocular histoplasmosis syndrome. Ophthalmology 1998;105:1598–1605.

III

Therapeutics and Delivery for Angiogenic Eye Diseases

18
Anti-VEGF Therapies for Diseases of the Retina and Choroid

Ming Lu, MD, PhD and Donald J. D'Amico, MD

CONTENTS

INTRODUCTION

Angiogenesis, and the closely related problems of ischemia and vascular leakage, play an important role in a spectrum of ocular diseases. A variety of angiogenic and angiostatic factors have been identified in the pathological neovascularization of the retina and choroid. This chapter reviews the major retinal and choroidal neovascular diseases, and focuses on the rationale and current therapeutic attempts with anti-vascular endothelial growth factor (VEGF) strategies, as well as the drug delivery modalities to the loci of pathological neovascularization. The term "neovascularization" has been used to describe the development of pathological new vessels and is considered synonymous with angiogenesis in this chapter.

Diabetic retinopathy, branch and central retinal vein occlusions (BRVO and CRVO), retinopathy of prematurity (ROP), and age-related macular degeneration (AMD) are distinct disorders with many individually characteristic features. Nevertheless, common angiogenic and angiostatic factors have been found pivotal in the pathogenesis of each

From: *Ophthalmology: Ocular Angiogenesis: Diseases, Mechanisms, and Therapeutics*
Edited by: J. Tombran-Tink and C. J. Barnstable © Humana Press Inc., Totowa, NJ

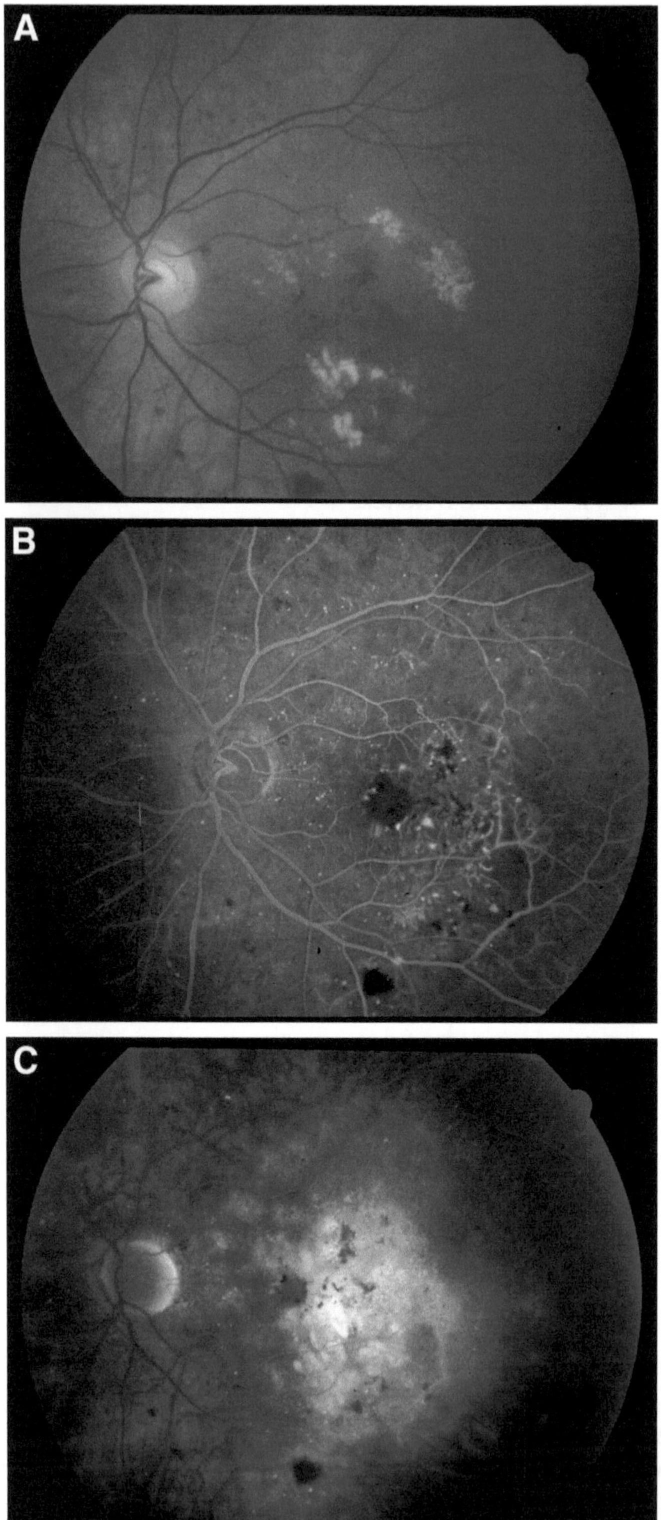
A
B
C

of these diseases. The discovery of these factors, such as VEGF, as well as their mechanisms of action, has led to the development of drugs specifically targeting the molecules or their signal transduction pathways.

Although neovascularization is the most dramatic outcome in these conditions, the understanding of each clinical entity and therapy is aided by considering a more inclusive central triad consisting of ischemia, vascular leakage, and neovascularization. Indeed, ischemia and vascular leakage frequently dominate the clinical presentation in these diseases, and are often responsible for significant visual loss. Ischemia is seen as a precursor to neovascularization that is mediated through biochemical signals that have been steadily elucidated *(1–3)*. Vascular leakage with exudation and/or transudation can occur as a consequence of vascular damage to previously normal vessels. This vascular damage may be a result of endothelial injury induced by abnormal leukocyte adhesion and enzymatic activity *(4)*, ischemia, metabolic derangements, and many other causes. Profound vascular leakage is also a hallmark of new vessels in the retina and choroid, and contributes greatly to the dysfunction of adjacent structures and tissues by diverse fluid accumulations such as edema, hemorrhage, and serous retinal and retinal pigment epithelium (RPE) detachment.

As a precursor to retinal neovascularization in diabetes or retinal vascular occlusions, ischemia of the retinal circulation is easily visible with fluorescein angiography in many eyes. In macular degeneration, the stimulus for choroidal neovascularization is not demonstrable on available tests such as fluorescein angiography, but ischemia is still presumed to play a central role. In all of these conditions, this triad of ischemia, vascular leakage, and neovascularization is evident and interrelated, and produces visual loss in diverse but predictable ways.

DIABETIC RETINOPATHY

Diabetic retinopathy is discussed first as a prototypical neovascular retinal disease because of the extensive basic science research into the role of VEGF in its causation. Diabetic retinopathy is an extremely complicated disease and is one of the leading causes of visual loss in the world *(5)*. It is typically bilateral and progressive, although there are wide variations in progression and severity across affected individuals, ranging from asymptomatic manifestations to profound visual loss. The vasculopathic model suggests that the initial damage begins in the diabetic blood vessel and is characterized by leakage and ischemia. These two processes result in an increasing failure of the retinal circulation to deliver oxygen and support the metabolism of the retina.

The sequence of anatomical changes in the retina leading to blindness in diabetes is fairly well defined. There is general agreement that diabetic retinopathy can be classified into nonproliferative and proliferative stages *(6)*. Multiple progressive microvascular changes characterize the two stages. The hallmark of the mild and moderate nonproliferative stages is leakage of the retinal vessels. The clinical findings are dot and blot hemorrhages, microaneurysms, venous dilation, hard exudates, and edema (Fig. 1). The

Fig. 1. Nonproliferative diabetic retinopathy. **(A)** Fundus photo shows hemorrhages and exudates in the macula. **(B)** Fluorescein angiogram of same eye discloses bright leakage from numerous microaneurysms; an additional finding of retinal capillary nonperfusion is visible as the dark area in the lower right of the photo, and in the increased avascular zone near the fovea. **(C)** Later phase of angiogram depicts extensive bright fluorescein leakage with macular edema. *See* color version on companion CD.

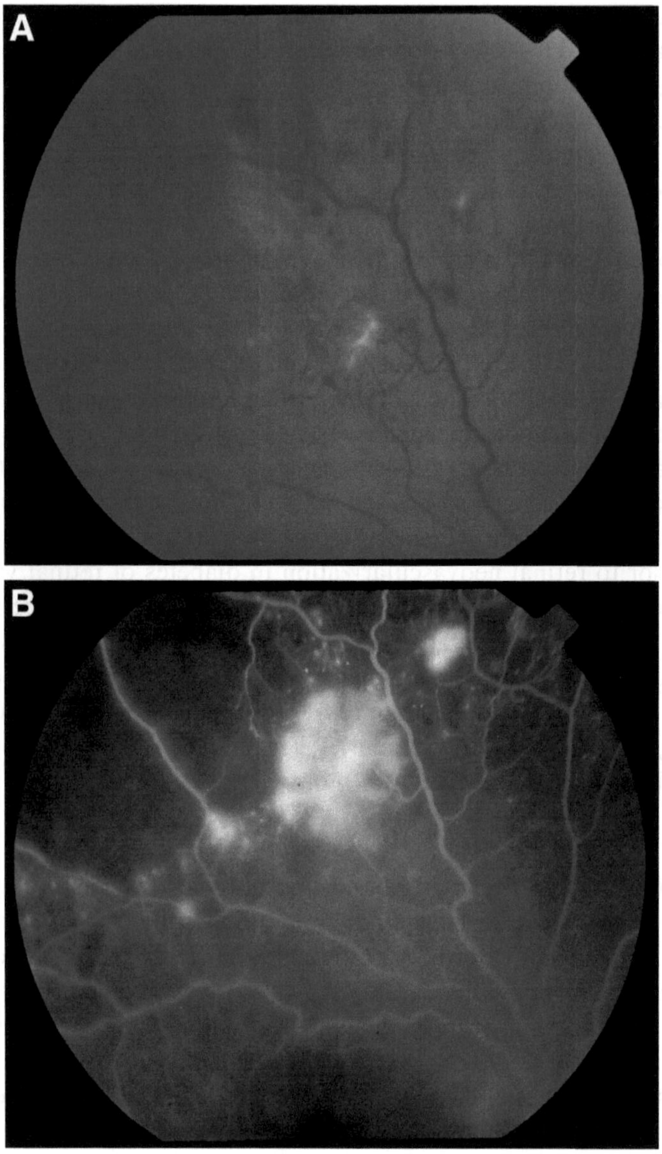

Fig. 2. Proliferative diabetic retinopathy. (**A**) Fundus photograph shows an area of retinal neovascularization with some associated fibrosis in the center of the photograph; intraretinal hemorrhages are also present. (**B**) Fluorescein angiogram of the same eye reveals the neovascularization in detail, and also clearly defines the broad extent of associated ischemic retina, visible as the dark area at the upper left, which borders the neovascular complex. *See* color version on companion CD.

hallmark of the severe nonproliferative stage is ischemia of the retina. The clinical findings are cotton-wool spots, which are caused by microinfarction of the retina, intraretinal microvascular abnormalities, venous beading, arteriolar narrowing, and large blot hemorrhage. The hallmark of the proliferative stage is angiogenesis. The clinical findings are retinal neovascularization, vitreous hemorrhage, and retinal detachment (Figs. 2 and 3).

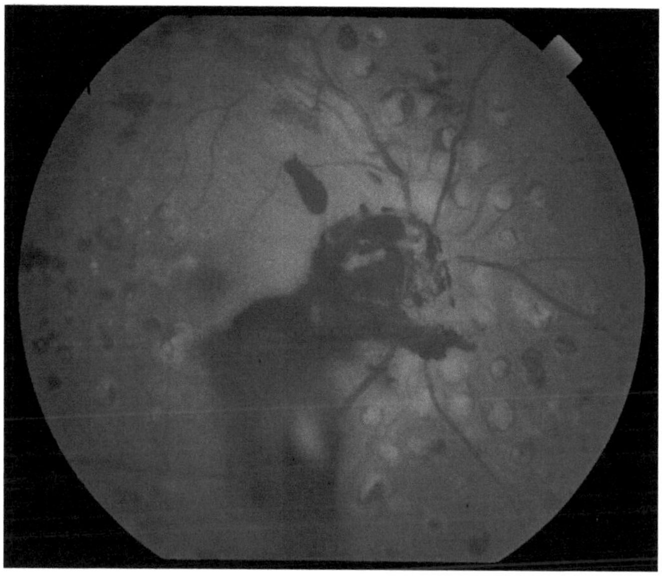

Fig. 3. Vitreous hemorrhage from disk neovascularization in proliferative diabetic retinopathy. Fundus photo shows fresh hemorrhage obscuring the disk and posterior retina. Previous panretinal laser photocoagulation treatment is visible in the numerous variably pigmented spots throughout the nonmacular retina. *See* color version on companion CD.

Proliferative diabetic retinopathy is primarily an ischemic disease. Neovascularization of the retina, optic nerve, and iris is preceded temporally and associated spatially by retinal capillary nonperfusion *(7,8)*, which is demonstrable on fluorescein angiography. Ablation of ischemic retina by laser photocoagulation, which has been the mainstay of treatment for diabetic retinopathy in the past 30 yr, leads to stabilization and regression of neovascularization *(6)*. These observations support the hypothesis that an angiogenic factor(s) released from the ischemic retina stimulates angiogenesis both locally and at a distance *(9)*. The candidate factor must meet at least three criteria: mitogenic for endothelial cells, secreted and freely diffusible, and induced by ischemia. Only VEGF fits all three criteria.

In the nonproliferative form of the disease, visual loss usually results from leakage of the macular vessels and consequent macular edema. Current treatment for macular edema is not satisfactory. A laser photocoagulation treatment in the nonfoveal macula has been demonstrated to be beneficial in reducing retinal thickness and stabilizing vision, but usually does not restore visual acuity to predisease levels (Fig. 4). Surgery, including vitrectomy, with removal of the vitreous gel, posterior hyaloid, or even the internal limiting membrane has also shown success (Fig. 5), but visual recovery is usually incomplete and capricious. Most recently, intravitreal injection of triamcinolone acetonide has become popular (Fig. 6), and has shown the ability to reduce edema and restore visual acuity in many cases, but with the problems of relapse in a few months and the development of glaucoma and cataract in a substantial subgroup *(10)*. Regardless, the efficacy of triamcinolone acetonide has supported the search for other pharmacological approaches, including intraocular steroid implants and intravitreal injections

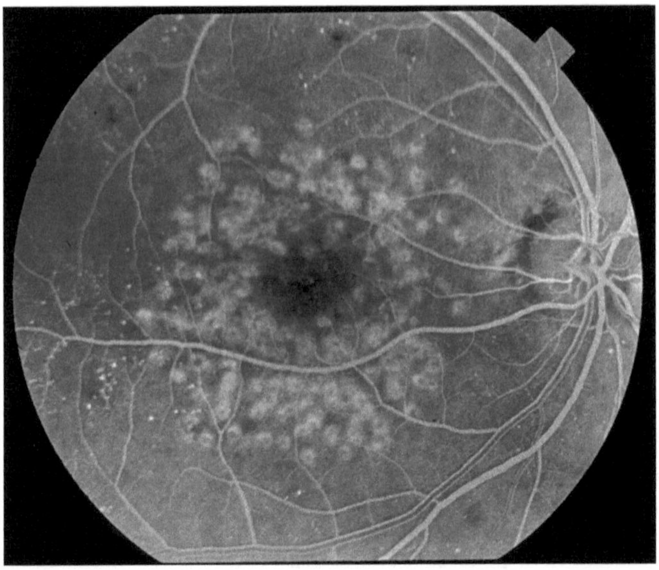

Fig. 4. Grid laser photocoagulation for diabetic macular edema. A midphase fluorescein angiogram shows a pattern of photocoagulation spots surrounding the fovea. Numerous bright, smaller microaneurysms are also visible.

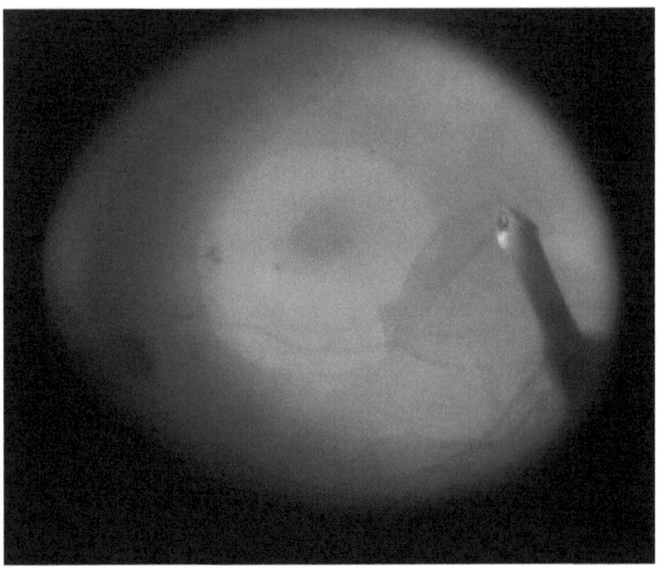

Fig. 5. Surgical peeling of the internal limiting membrane for diabetic macular edema. Intraoperative photo during vitrectomy of indocyanine green-stained internal limiting membrane being removed from the surface of the macular retina. *See* color version on companion CD.

of anti-VEGF agents. Indeed, the use of these anti-VEGF agents in an attempt to control the abnormal vascular leakage in macular edema is most attractive. In addition, it is likely that combination approaches, such as surgery combined with drug treatment, will be increasingly explored.

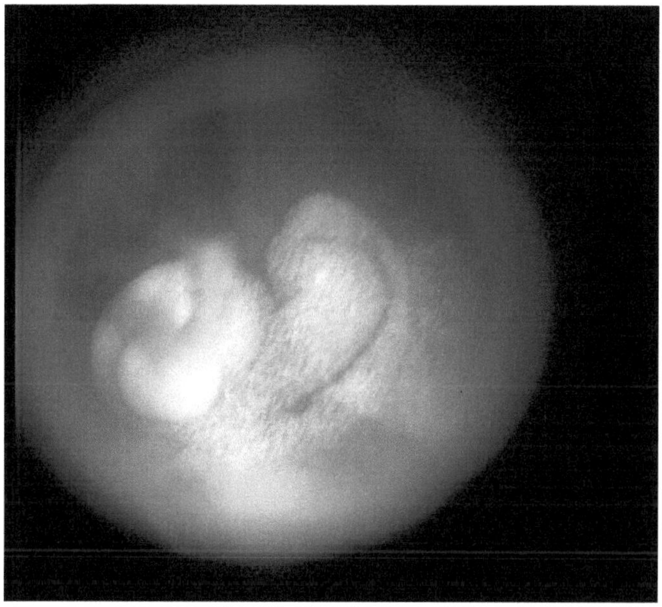

Fig. 6. Intravitreal triamcinolone acetonide for diabetic macular edema. Fundus photo demonstrates that the whitish drug is visible immediately after injection into the vitreous. *See* color version on companion CD.

Proliferative retinopathy is typically treated by panretinal photocoagulation, which results in regression of retinal neovascularization in most cases (Fig. 7). However, this treatment is destructive to the peripheral retina and visual field, and does not reverse the intrinsic retinal ischemia, which is often severe and visually damaging. In addition, many patients with proliferative diabetic retinopathy require complicated vitreoretinal surgery for vitreous hemorrhage or retinal detachment *(11)* (Fig. 8).

OVERVIEW OF VEGF BASIC SCIENCE

The VEGF family includes placenta growth factor (PlGF), VEGF-A, VEGF-B, VEGF-C, VEGF-D, and VEGF-E (for review, *see* refs. *3* and *12*). Briefly, VEGF-A plays a pivotal role in the development of pathological angiogenesis in ischemic and inflammatory diseases. VEGF-B is currently being investigated for its role in nonangiogenic tumor progression. VEGF-C and VEGF-D are being investigated for their role in tumor angiogenesis and lymphangiogenesis. PlGF acts synergistically with VEGF-A in angiogenesis and plasma extravasation in pathological conditions *(13)*. VEGF-E is the viral VEGF homolog and an angiogenic factor *(14)*. The abbreviation VEGF in this chapter represents VEGF-A.

VEGF is a 35- to 45-kDa homodimeric protein that was originally isolated as a vasopermeability factor (VPF) *(15)* and later as an angiogenesis factor *(16–19)*. The structure and function of VEGF protein and its gene regulation have been reviewed extensively *(3,12)*. Briefly, up to six different VEGF isoforms are derived through alternative splicing of mRNA *(12,20)*. The smaller isoforms ($VEGF_{110}$, $VEGF_{121}$, $VEGF_{144}$, and $VEGF_{165}$) are secreted and freely diffusible, whereas the larger isoforms ($VEGF_{189}$

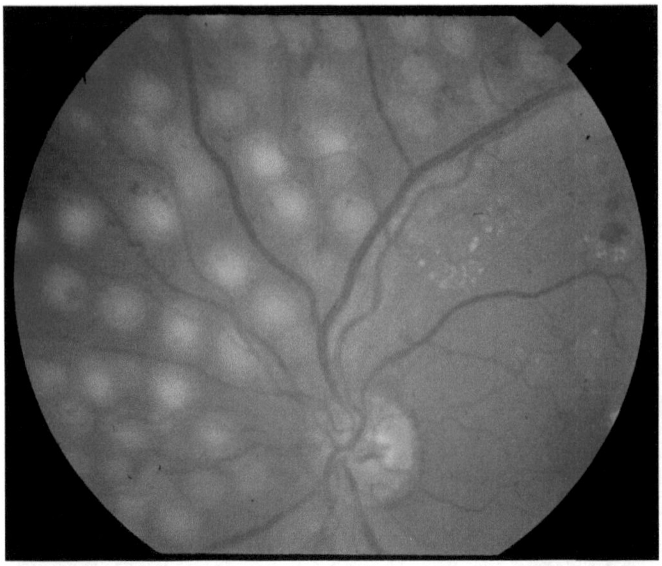

Fig. 7. Panretinal laser photocoagulation for proliferative diabetic retinopathy. A pattern of whitish recent laser spots is seen outside the macula area. *See* color version on companion CD.

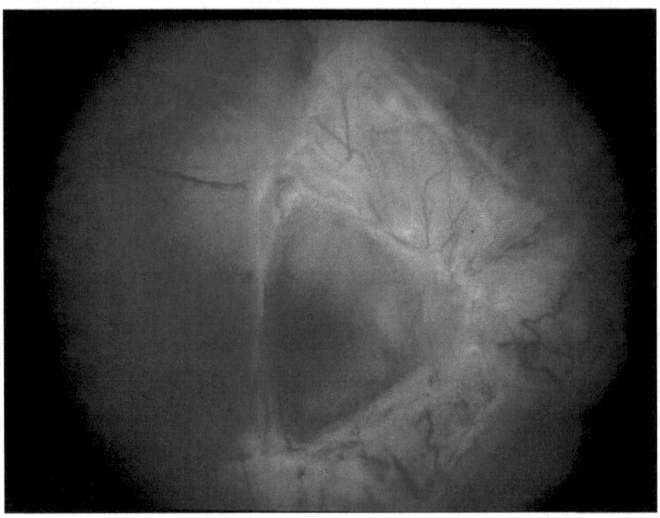

Fig. 8. Severe proliferative diabetic retinopathy with fibrovascular overgrowth and distortion of the retina. Fundus photo demonstrates that the underlying retinal anatomy is completely obscured, and extensive traction detachment of the retina, due to progressive growth and contracture of the neovascular tissue, is seen. *See* color version on companion CD.

and $VEGF_{206}$) are bound to heparin-containing proteoglycans on the cell surface or basement membrane *(21)*. In terms of permeability, VEGF is 50,000 times more potent at increasing dermal microvascular permeability than histamine *(22)*. VEGF induces expression of urokinase-type and tissue-type plasminogen activators, as well as that of metalloproteinase interstitial collagenase. This coinduction promotes degradation of the local extracellular matrix and facilitates endothelial cell migration *(23)*. VEGF is an endothelial cell-specific mitogen *(24,25)*. It has been shown that VEGF is involved in normal vascular development, ovulation, and tumor angiogenesis *(12)*. Hypoxia is a major regulator of VEGF expression *(12)*, which distinguishes VEGF from other growth factors that have been postulated to have a role in ocular neovascular diseases, including insulin-like growth factor (IGF)-1, fibroblast growth factors (FGFs), epidermal growth factor (EGF), PlGF, and VEGF-B *(26)*. VEGF expression is upregulated by hypoxia *(24–28)*.

Three members of the VEGF receptor (VEGFR) family have been identified so far. VEGFR-1 (fms-like tyrosine kinase-1, Flt-1) is predominantly expressed in pericytes and has been implicated in vessel survival *(3)*. VEGFR-2 (kinase insert domain-containing receptor or KDR) is considered to be the receptor that mediates functional VEGF signaling in endothelial cells *(29,30)*. VEGFR-3 is implicated in lymphangiogenesis *(31)*. The critical role of VEGF in developmental angiogenesis and vasculogenesis is demonstrated by the fact that deletion of the genes for VEGF, or its receptors, results in abnormal blood vessel development and death in utero *(3,12,32–35)*.

EVIDENCE FOR ROLE OF VEGF IN DIABETIC RETINOPATHY

Many cells in the eye produce VEGF. Within the retina, these include RPE cells, pericytes, endothelial cells, glial cells, Müller cells, and ganglion cells *(9)*. VEGF is causally linked to retinal ischemia-associated neovascularization *(10,36–41)*. The levels of VEGF in the retina and vitreous of patients with proliferative diabetic retinopathy are elevated, and they decrease when treatment with laser photocoagulation induces remission of these diseases *(42,43)*. It is expressed at high levels in response to hypoxia *(25,44)*. Increased levels of VEGF are present in ischemic retinal cells in vivo *(38–40)* and in vitro *(41)*.

VEGF preferentially binds to high-affinity receptors on retinal endothelial cells *(45)*. VEGF receptors on endothelial cells appear to be tyrosine kinases capable of phosphorylating other proteins involved in cellular signal transduction *(46)*. Furthermore, in vitro inhibition experiments have identified VEGF as the sole endothelial cell mitogen synthesized and secreted by hypoxic retinal cells *(37,41)*. VEGF levels were shown to correlate both spatially and temporally with iris neovascularization in a monkey model *(38)*. The correlation of VEGF with neovascularization of the retina was found in a neonatal mouse model of hypoxia-induced neovascularization *(40)*. These studies demonstrated that VEGF expression was increased in the retina prior to the development of neovascularization in this mouse model of proliferative retinopathy. In addition, VEGF levels declined as the neovascularization regressed in these animals. Injection of VEGF into normal primate eyes is sufficient to produce retinal edema, hemorrhage, venous beading, capillary occlusion with ischemia, microaneurysms, and retinal and iris neovascularization and neovascular glaucoma, characteristic findings of all stages of diabetic retinopathy *(47,48)*. Moreover, the inhibition of intraocular VEGF suppresses retinal ischemia-associated iris *(36)* and retinal neovascularization *(37)*. Blockade of VEGF receptor signaling is sufficient to completely prevent retinal neovascularization *(49)*. Therefore, VEGF appears to be the mediator of ischemia-induced intraocular angiogenesis. Retinal VEGF levels are also increased at the nonproliferative stage in diabetic animal models *(50–52)*.

In the human eye, elevated vitreous and aqueous VEGF levels correlate strongly with retinal ischemia-associated neovascularization in diabetic retinopathy, retinal vein occlusion, and retinopathy of prematurity *(42,43,52,53)*. The vitreous concentrations of VEGF were higher than aqueous levels, suggesting the existence of an intraocular VEGF concentration gradient between the vitreous and aqueous. After successful laser panretinal photocoagulation for retinal neovascularization, the intraocular concentration of VEGF was reduced by an average of 75% *(43)*. Furthermore, the VEGF present in the vitreous of individuals with active intraocular neovascularization was capable of binding VEGF receptors, as well as stimulating retinal endothelial cell growth in vitro *(43)*. In a study evaluating the presence of angiogenic growth factors expressed in neovascular membranes obtained from diabetic patients, VEGF was consistently detected *(54)*. High VEGF mRNA levels were detected in the retinas of enucleated eyes from patients with neovascularization secondary to diabetes, central retinal vein occlusion, retinal detachment, and intraocular tumors *(39)*. Increased VEGF expression was also demonstrated in the retinal and choroidal vessels of subjects with diabetes using immunohistochemical localization of postmortem tissue *(55)*. These data demonstrate a close correlation between elevated intraocular VEGF concentration and active intraocular neovascularization in humans.

Both glucose *(56,57)* and advanced glycation endproducts (AGEs) *(58)* stimulate VEGF expression. The increase in VEGF by hyperglycemia and AGEs may cause the leakage of the retinal vasculature at the mild nonproliferative stage of diabetic retinopathy. VEGF induces leukostasis via the induction of endothelial cell expression of intercellelular adhesion molecule (ICAM)-1 *(4,59–61)*. In both streptozotocin-induced diabetes in rats and VEGF-induced retinopathy in rats, the adhesion molecule ICAM-1 to which leukocytes adhere, is upregulated on retinal endothelium *(60)*. The adhered leukocytes obstruct blood flow and cause capillary nonperfusion. Hypertrophy and hyperplasia of the retinal capillary endothelial cells in VEGF-induced retinopathy may also contribute to the narrowing of capillary lumina *(62,63)*. Ischemia further increases VEGF gene expression by increasing VEGF mRNA stability and enhancing VEGF gene transcription *(64,65)*. Thus there is a positive feedback loop that increases VEGF production in an accelerated manner. The positive feedback loop of VEGF and ischemia contributes to the accelerated accumulation of VEGF seen at the advanced stages of diabetic retinopathy. Once the VEGF concentration in the retina and vitreous exceeds the threshold of angiogenesis, new vessels grow and the proliferative stage ensues.

OTHER MOLECULES—PIGMENT EPITHELIUM-DERIVED FACTOR, INSULIN-LIKE GROWTH FACTOR-1, ANGIOPOIETIN-1 AND -2

The ancient Chinese yin-yang theory also applies to ocular angiogenic and angiostatic homeostasis. Neovascularization not only is a response to a rise in the local concentration of angiogenic molecules but also requires a fall in the levels of endogenous angiostatic molecules *(66)*. Numerous inhibitors of angiogenesis have been reported to counteract the effects of VEGF. Pigment epithelium-derived factor (PEDF) is one such putative inhibitor that is found in the normal eye responsible for the avascularity of cornea and vitreous *(67)*. PEDF has been reported to be increased by hyperoxia and decreased by hypoxia *(67)*, unlike many other angiostatic factors discovered so far, such as angiostatin *(68)* and endostatin *(69)*. Expression of PEDF causes the regression of ocular neovascularization by promoting apoptosis of cells within neovascular lesions *(70,71)*. Lower levels of PEDF were found in the vitreous of patients with diabetic retinopathy where VEGF level was increased *(72,73)*. These data suggest that the induction of angiogenesis in the eye requires not only an elevation of VEGF but also a decrease in PEDF—the loss of balance between angiogenic and angiostatic factors. Overexpression of PEDF inhibits retinal neovascularization *(70,74–76)*. Therapeutically, antagonists of VEGF and agonists of PEDF could have synergistic effects in inhibiting neovascularization in diabetic retinopathy and other ocular diseases. However, the role of PEDF in diabetic retinopathy remains to be elucidated, as genetic deletion of PEDF does not significantly alter the development of ocular vasculature *(77)*, and high levels of immunoreactive PEDF were found in the vitreous of individuals with or without ocular neovascularization *(78)*, contradictory to some previous reports *(72,73)*.

Growth hormone and IGF-1 are also involved in the pathogenesis of diabetc retinopathy *(79)*. Ablation of the pituitary gland has been associated with regression of retinal neovascularization *(80)*. The incidence and severity of diabetic retinopathy in growth hormone-deficient dwarfs are much lower than in other diabetic patients *(81)*. Furthermore, the concentrations of IGF-1 in the vitreous correlate positively with serum concentrations in patients with diabetes but not in normal subjects *(82,83)*. Thus, leakage into the vitreous from systemic circulation is probably the primary source of this factor, although local production in the eye cannot be ruled out. IGF-1 is an endothelial cell mitogen and it stimulates VEGF gene expression by enhancing VEGF gene transcription *(84)*. An IGF-1 receptor antagonist suppresses retinal neovascularization in vivo *(85)*. Inhibition of growth hormone and/or IGF-1 resulted in decreased retinal neovascularization *(85–87)*. IGF-1 has been hypothesized as a permissive agent for VEGF to stimulate new vessel growth *(88)*.

A number of additional angiogenesis modulators were discovered in the last decade. Angiopoietins are regulators of vascular integrity and are involved in pathological neovascularization *(89)*. Angiopoietin (Ang)-1 protects the adult's vasculature against plasma leakage *(90)*. Ang-2 enhances VEGF effect in ischemia-induced angiogenesis. Both hypoxia and VEGF upregulate the expression of Ang2 but not Ang1 in endothelial cells *(91)*. The opposite effects of the angiopoietins owe to their respective agonist and antagonist signaling action through the endothelial Tie2 receptor. The combined inhibition of Ang2 and VEGF signaling may be more effective in treating ischemic retinal disorders *(92)*. Vessels in Ang1-overexpressing mice were resistant to leaks caused by inflammatory agents. Coexpression of Ang1 and VEGF had an additive effect on angiogenesis but resulted in leakage-resistant vessels typical of Ang1 *(93)*. Therefore, Ang1 may be useful for reducing microvascular leakage and, in combination with VEGF, for promoting growth of competent vessels.

BRANCH AND CENTRAL RETINAL VENOUS OCCLUSIONS

Occlusion of a branch retinal vein causes regional retinal hemorrhages and edema, with some patients experiencing retinal ischemia and secondary neovascularization and vitreous hemorrhage *(94)*. The typical mechanism of visual loss is retinal edema (Fig. 9),

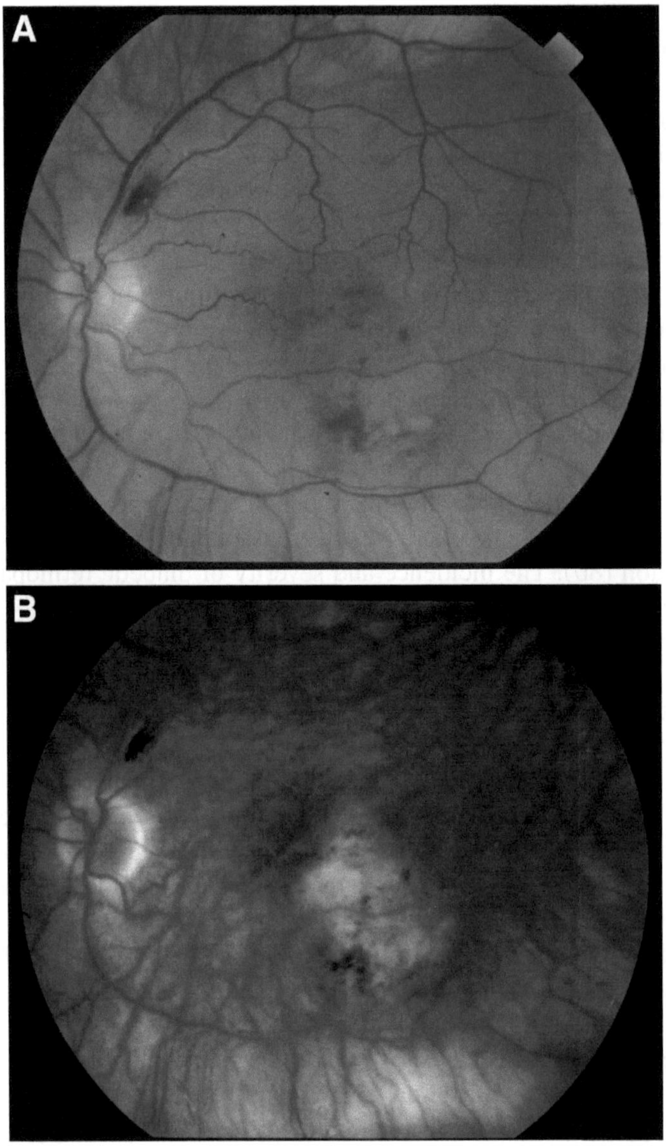

Fig. 9. Branch retinal vein occlusion (BRVO) with macular edema. (**A**) Fundus photo shows sectoral pattern of hemorrhage and a cotton-wool spot (nerve-fiber layer infarct) at and inferior to the fovea; the hemorrhage above the disk is related to the underlying hypertension, and is not part of the BRVO. (**B**) Fluorescein angiogram reveals corresponding macular edema in the late phases of the study. *See* color version on companion CD.

more commonly without the accumulation of the hard exudates seen in diabetic retinopathy, although loss of perfusion in the macula may also develop and severely reduce vision (Fig. 10). Neovascularization, if it develops, may reduce vision due to vitreous hemorrhage, or rarely, retinal detachment. Central retinal vein occlusion is usually caused by a thrombus in the region of the lamina cribrosa, and causes a profound engorgement of the retinal circulation with widespread retinal venous tortuousity,

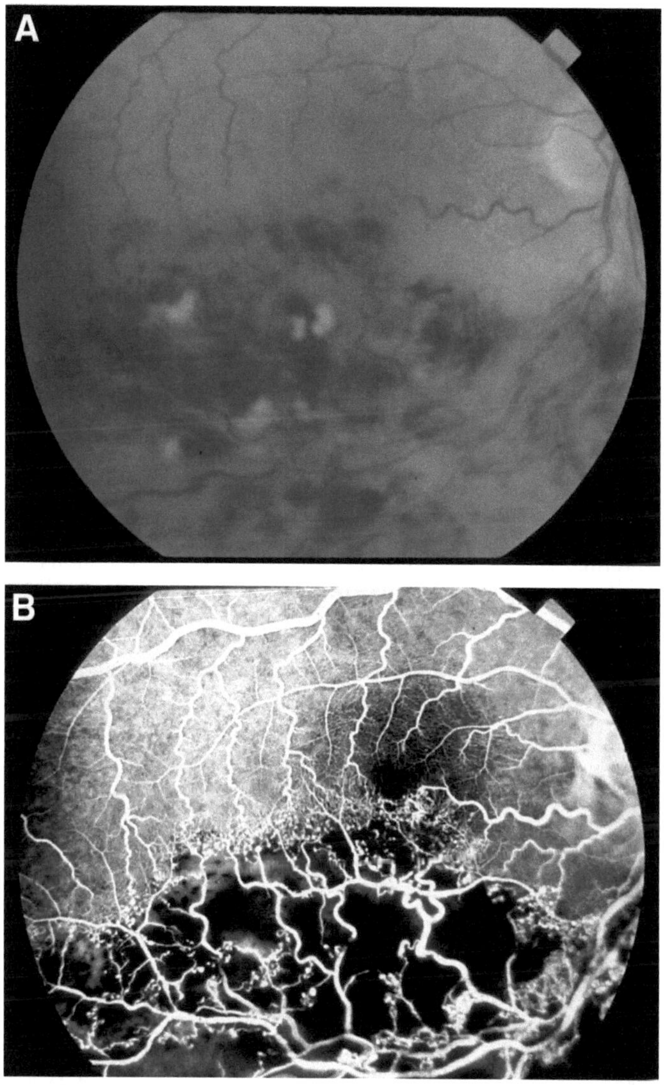

Fig. 10. Branch retinal vein occlusion with severe retinal ischemia. **(A)** Fundus photograph reveals extensive hemorrhage in a sectoral pattern inferiorly, consistent with involvement of a branch retinal vein. **(B)** Fluorescein angiogram discloses profound retinal capillary ischemia in the affected territory, visible as extensive nonperfused dark areas between the remaining large vascular trunks. *See* color version on companion CD.

hemorrhages, and macular edema *(95)* (Fig. 11). Although a substantial number of younger patients with the disease may show spontaneous improvement, in patients older than 65 yr of age the prognosis is poor. Visual acuity is reduced by either persistent macular edema or by the development of retinal ischemia (Fig. 12) frequently followed by neovascularization of the iris and severe painful glaucoma that may require enucleation to control.

VEGF was temporally and spatially correlated with ocular angiogenesis in a primate model of BRVO *(38)*. In human eyes surgically removed from patients with CRVO

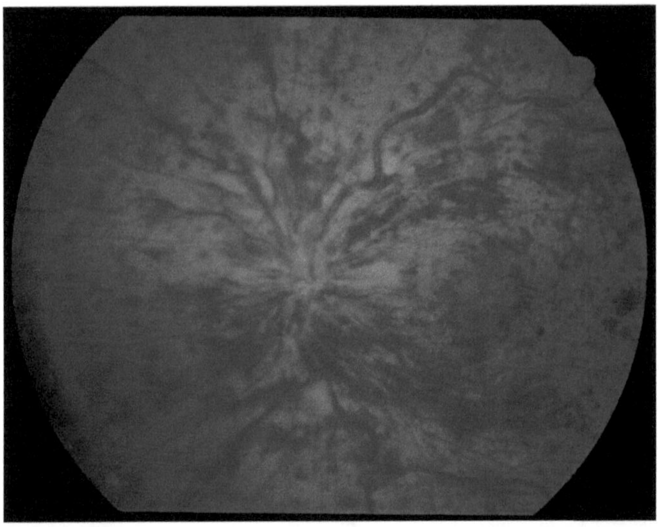

Fig. 11. Central retinal vein occlusion (CRVO) with recent onset. Fundus photograph reveals extensive retinal hemorrhages and vascular tortuousity due to CRVO. *See* color version on companion CD.

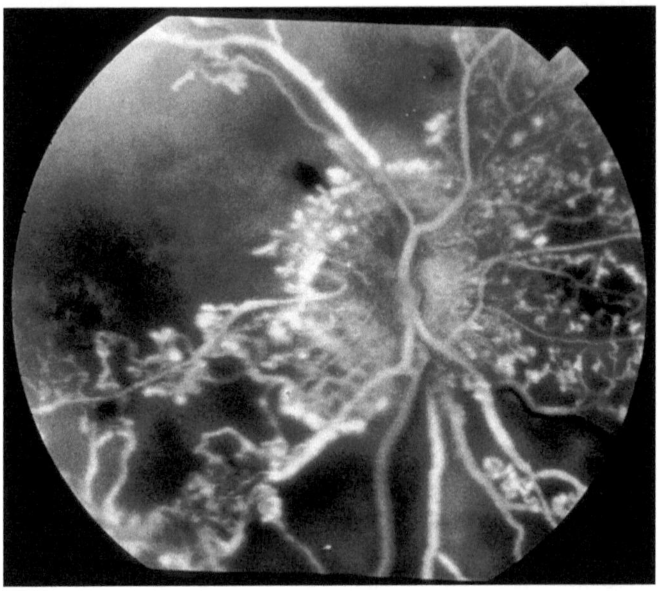

Fig. 12. Central retinal vein occlusion with severe retinal ischemia. Fluorescein angiogram shows extensive loss of retinal circulation, visible as dark, nonperfused areas in much of the photo.

and neovascular glaucoma, the VEGF-producing retinal cells resided in the ischemic regions of the retina *(53)*. There was a correlation of increased VEGF levels in the aqueous with neovascularization and permeability in patients with ischemic CRVO *(96)*. The role of VEGF in retinal arteriolar occlusive diseases, including central retinal artery occlusion and branch retinal artery occlusion, seems similar to that in diabetic retinopathy, in that retinal ischemia/hypoxia increases VEGF expression.

The use of anti-VEGF agents for BRVO and CRVO might be envisioned for both control of neovascularization (particularly rubeosis in CRVO) as well as the more common problem of macular edema in both conditions. Trials of intravitreal anti-VEGF agents to control the macular edema are in progress, but results are not yet available.

RETINOPATHY OF PREMATURITY

ROP is a major cause of blindness in children in developed countries *(88)*. It is a condition in which the immature peripheral retinal vessels proliferate abnormally with neovascularization and associated fibrous tissue contracture, often resulting in profound visual loss due to opacified fibrovascular membrane overgrowth across the anterior vitreous with secondary traction retinal detachment due to contraction of this anterior fibrovascular tissue. The process appears to consist of two phases: (1) ischemia in the incompletely vascularized peripheral retina in the premature infant, followed by (2) neovascularization. It has been well modeled in neonatal experimental animals that are first exposed to hyperoxemia (with suppression of normal peripheral retinal vascularization) followed by return to room air with relative ischemia in the incompletely vascularized retinal periphery *(40)*.

Retinal vascular growth is delayed after premature birth, due to the low level of IGF-1 normally provided by the placenta and the amniotic fluid. IGF-1 is required for VEGF signaling for vascular endothelial cell growth and survival *(88)*. Hyperoxia (supplemental oxygen) inhibits vessel formation by suppressing endogenous VEGF production *(97)*. Insufficient vascularization of the developing retina creates hypoxia, which stimulates VEGF production. Once the VEGF expression supercedes the threshold level, retinal neovascularization ensues. In the mouse and rat models of ROP, hyperoxia causes cessation of normal vessel growth through suppression of VEGF expression, causing loss of the physiological wave of VEGF anterior to the growing vascular front *(40,98)*. Non-oxygen-regulated factors such as IGF-1 also play a role. IGF-1 levels, low at premature birth, rise with ROP progression, permitting VEGF-induced retinopathy *(85,88)*. Furthermore, IGF-1 stimulates VEGF expression in retinal cells *(84)*, and its effect on retinal neovascularization is mediated, at least in part, through VEGF expression.

The animal model of ROP appears to mirror the human situation quite closely, and has provided specifics into the role of VEGF and other factors in the development of the condition. Although it is clear that VEGF is critically involved in this disease, a direct therapeutic trial with anti-VEGF agents is not ongoing at present, because of the advanced stage at which the disease presents, as well as many other difficulties in the management of ROP. Nevertheless, it is likely that a successful angiostatic agent, with an acceptable route of administration, would be of great benefit in this condition in the control of fibrovascular proliferation and retinal detachment. Such a drug therapy would reduce the need for retinal ablative therapies with laser and cryo-therapy that are currently used to control neovascularization in these infants.

CHOROIDAL NEOVASCULARIZATION AND ROLE OF VEGF IN PATHOGENESIS OF AGE-RELATED MACULAR DEGENERATION

AMD is a complex, multistage, bilateral, and frequently progressive disease that is a substantial cause of visual impairment and suffering in older patients. Although there are marked racial, regional, and other differences in occurrence, no group is spared, and it is worldwide in its distribution. AMD accounts for over 50% of blindness in Caucasian patients in the United States who are over 40 yr of age; this will increase substantially over the next decades as the aging of industrialized populations continues *(99)*.

The earliest ophthalmoscopically visible manifestations of the disease include drusen and areas of hypo- or hyperpigmentary change in the macular RPE. These findings may be minor, asymptomatic, and nonprogressive for a given individual, or they may produce progressive visual loss due to increasing atrophic or hyperplastic changes in the macular retina and RPE. Most important, studies have shown that patients with larger and more extensive drusen and pigmentary abnormalities have a relatively higher chance of developing neovascular AMD, with the development of choroidal new vessels that break through the Bruch's membrane into the subretinal pigment epithelial space and/or subretinal space, frequently affecting the fovea and producing substantial visual loss (Figs. 13 and 14). Although the pathogenesis of CNV in AMD is not fully understood, VEGF plays an important role (reviewed in refs. *1–3,23*). The increased thickness and hydrophobicity of Bruch's membrane with lipophilic material may decrease the diffusion of oxygen from the choroid to retina *(100)*. Hypoxia is a potent stimulus of VEGF expression. Other factors implicated in AMD, such as AGE and reactive-oxygen intermediates, are potent stimuli of VEGF expression in RPE cells *(58,101)*. VEGF is overexpressed in the RPE of autopsy eyes with AMD and in transdifferentiated RPE cells of surgically excised CNV membranes *(102–104)*. Vitreous VEGF levels were found to be significantly higher in patients with AMD and CNV as compared with healthy controls *(105–106)*. Studies on transgenic mice and other animal models indicate that overexpressing VEGF in retinal RPE cells leads to CNV formation *(107–109)*.

It is helpful to view the neovascular AMD lesion in two important contexts. First, it is clearly and advanced stage of a complex disease, and it would certainly be better to prevent it than to treat it. Second, each lesion is capable of including a great diversity of anatomic derangements (e.g., blood, exudation, atrophy, fibrosis, etc.) which, given the micron-by-micron importance of the macular retina, can have a profound influence on visual function. These anatomic/clinical elements encountered in AMD lesions are listed in Table 1. As a result of this variability, one lesion with subretinal hemorrhage that avoids the foveal area will produce very different symptoms from one in which the hemorrhage involves the fovea. Similarly, a lesion with an extrafoveal eruption of choroidal new vessels without a broad overlying serous elevation of the sensory retina will have a much different prognosis from one in which the new vessels involve the fovea. These differences are frequently obliterated in the need to study patients and treatments with "neovascular AMD" but are critical to understanding the pathophysiology of AMD and the potential for treatment. Table 2 revisits the basic lesion elements and suggests the potential reversibility of each with current or future therapies.

The attractiveness of VEGF as a therapeutic target derives from its roles in two of the most basic processes within a typical lesion of advanced AMD, namely neovascularization and vascular leakage. The role of VEGF as a critical factor in the control of the growth of abnormal blood vessels from the choroid directly attacks a central problem in this disease. However, the profound vascular permeability induced by VEGF is potentially of even greater importance in the treatment of established neovascular AMD

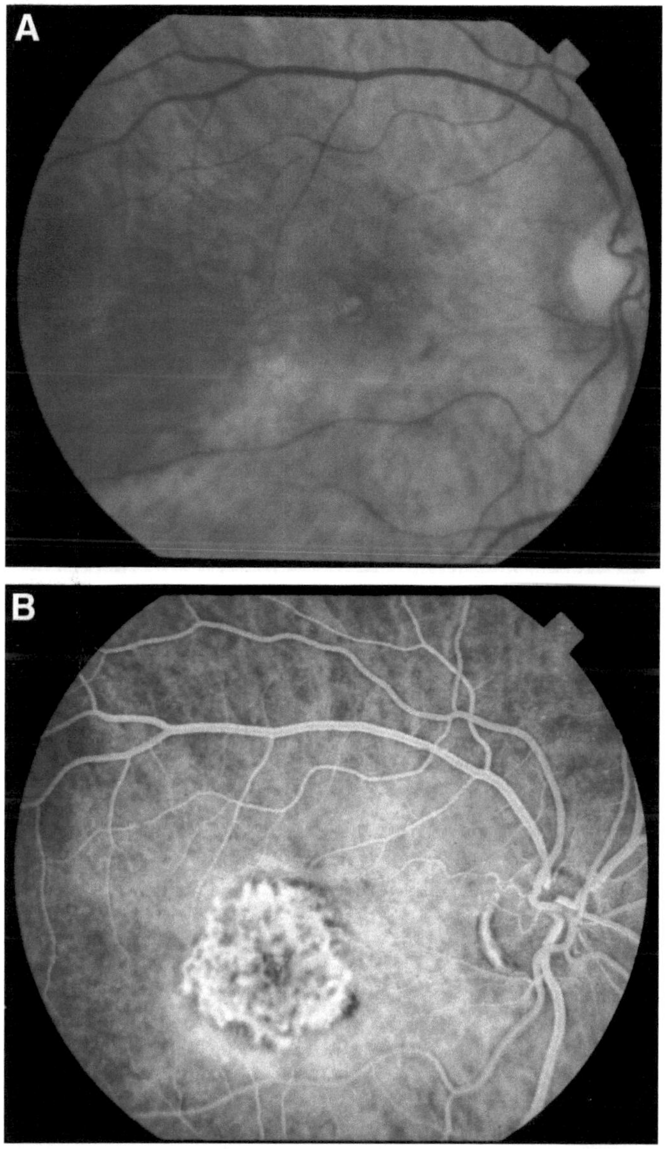

Fig. 13. Age-related macular degeneration with choroidal neovascularization. (**A**) Fundus photograph shows an area of hypopigmentation near the fovea, with a smaller subretinal hemorrhage visible at the four o'clock direction from the fovea. (**B**) Fluorescein angiogram of the same eye reveals a large cartwheel pattern typical of classic choroidal neovascularization, which in this eye involves the entire central macula. *See* color version on companion CD.

lesions, in which leakage of fluid from new vessels causes visual loss through retinal edema and exudation, subretinal fluid, and hemorrhage. Furthermore, these permeability-related derangements appear to be reversible, offering the prospect of restoring function to retinal elements encumbered by edema.

Laboratory evidence suggesting the efficacy of the anti-VEGF approach in treating AMD is emerging. Repetitive intravitreous injection of rhuFabV2, an active fragment

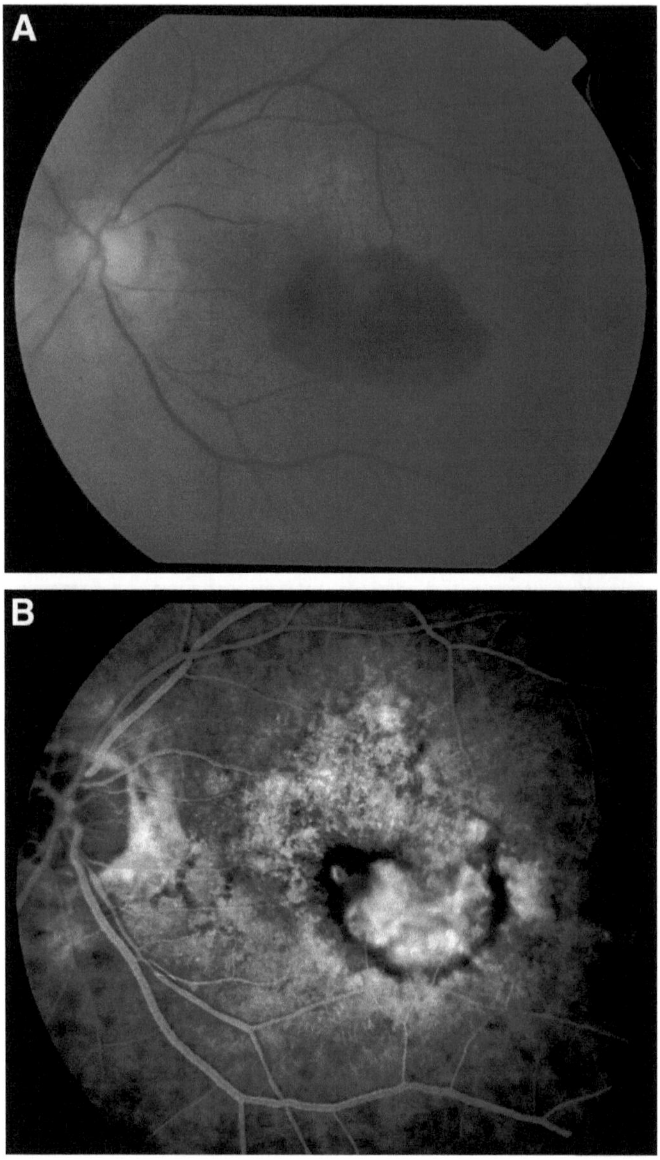

Fig. 14. Age-related macular degeneration with choroidal neovascularization. **(A)** Fundus photo at initial patient presentation demonstrates subretinal hemorrhage in the macula. **(B)** Fluorescein angiogram of the same eye several months later shows the choroidal neovascular membrane visible in the lower left center of the photo; there are extensive other pigmentary changes due to chronic exudation and retinal pigment epithelium alterations. **(C)** Fundus photograph of the same eye at a later date reveals subretinal fibrosis has developed, indicated by whitish scar tissue with pigmented borders. *See* color version on companion CD.

of a recombinant humanized monoclonal VEGF antibody, inhibits the development of laser-induced CNV in a primate model *(110)*. Adenoviral transfection of a soluble VEGF receptor into the RPE of rats inhibited the development of laser-induced CNV *(111)*. Clinical trials with anti-VEGF agents are ongoing, and are discussed below.

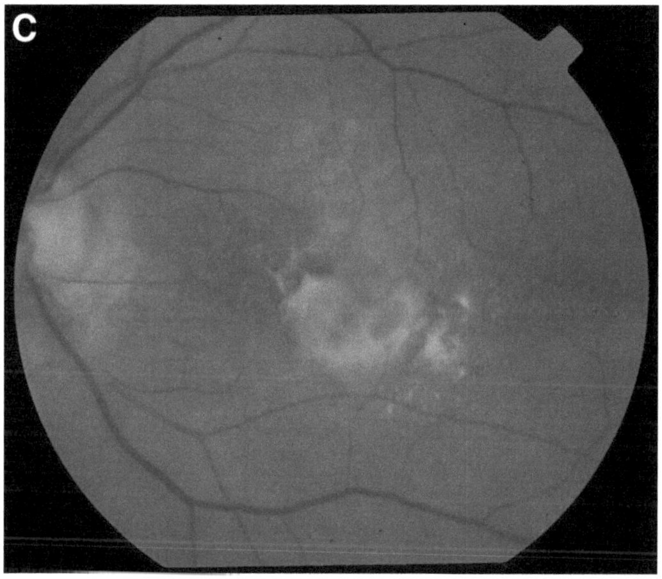

Fig. 14. *(Continued)*

Table 1
Anatomic/Clinical Elements of Age-Related Macular Degeneration Lesions

Leakage from choroidal neovascularization membrane	Neovascularization
Retinal edema	SubRPE
Hemorrhage	Subretinal
Sub-retinal pigment epithelium (RPE)	Intraretinal
Subretinal	Fibrosis
Retinal	Intraretinal
Vitreous	Preretinal
Detachment	Subretinal
Drusen	Sub-RPE
RPE ± tear	Photoreceptor/retinal cell atrophy
Retinal	Choriocapillaris atrophy
RPE hyperplasia	Chorioretinal anastomosis
RPE atrophy	

As in diabetic retinopathy, imbalance of angiogenic and angiostatic factors occurs in AMD. Expression of PEDF was decreased in cells within choroidal neovascular tissues, where VEGF level was increased *(112–113)*. An inverse correlation of the expression of PEDF and the formation of CNV has been found in an experimental animal model *(114)*, suggesting that PEDF alone or in combination with anti-VEGF agents may be used as alternative strategies for the treatment of CNV. CNV was significantly decreased after intraocular injection of adenoviral vectors expressing PEDF *(74)*. A phase I study of gene therapy with adenovirus vector containing the PEDF gene is under way for advanced CNV in patients with AMD *(115)*.

Angiopoietins also play a role in CNV formation. Histological examination of CNV in AMD and other diseases disclosed that Ang1 and Ang2 were present *(116)*. The Tie2

Table 2
Treatment Possibilities for Age-Related Macular Degeneration Lesion Elements

Element	*Potential reversability with therapy*
Neovascularization	Reversible (controllable) with Laser if extrafoveal Photodynamic therapy Surgery and numerous experimental therapies Antiangiogenic drugs
Leakage (and bleeding) from choroidal neovascularization membrane	Reversible with Closure, reduction, or elimination of vessels as above Drugs to control permeability Surgery or observation for hemorrhage in many sites
Fibrosis	Irreversible
Retinal pigment epithelium (RPE) atrophy	Irreversible (possible RPE transplantation in future)
RPE hyperplasia	Irreversible (possible RPE transplantation in future)
Photoreceptor/retinal cell atrophy	Irreversible (neuroregenerative growth factors, neural retinal transplants, or chip implants in distant future)
Choriocapillaris atrophy	Irreversible
Chorioretinal anastomosis	Irreversible

receptor is expressed in the vascular structures as well as the RPE and in fibroblast-like cells. VEGF upregulates Ang1 synthesis and secretion by RPE cells *(117)*. Systemically expressed soluble Tie2 receptor via adenoviral-mediated gene delivery markedly inhibits the development of laser-induced CNV in mice *(118)*. Ang1 may have a potential therapeutic use as it suppresses VEGF-induced leukostasis and inflammation by inhibiting expression of ICAM-1, vascular cell adhesion molecule-1 (VCAM-1), and E-selectin *(119)*.

CLINICAL INVESTIGATION OF PHARMACOLOGICAL THERAPIES

Anti-VEGF Approaches

Because VEGF is both a permeability factor and an angiogenic factor, anti-VEGF agents may be used to treat both leakage and neovascularization of the retina and choroid. The strategies used in the development of antiangiogenic agents involve the inhibition of angiogenic factors as well as therapy with endogenous inhibitors of angiogenesis, such as PEDF, endostatin, and angiostatin. VEGF antagonists have been developed by many research laboratories and pharmaceutical companies, including, among others, an aptamer (Macugen®, Eyetech Pharmaceuticals) which neutralizes VEGF in the extracellular milieu; neutralizing antibody fragment rhufab (Lucentis®, Genentech); signal transduction inhibitors, LY333531 (ruboxistaurin, Eli Lilly); ribozymes (Ribozyme Pharmaceuticals).

Macugen

Macugen is a pegylated anti-VEGF aptamer that binds to, and inhibits the function of, VEGF. It competitively binds to the major isoform of VEGF, $VEGF_{165}$, like an antibody.

Aptamers are chemically synthesized short strands of RNA (oligonucleotides) that adopt highly specific three-dimensional conformations. There are two Phase II/III clinical trials for the use of Macugen in the treatment of exudative AMD and one Phase II/III clinical trial of Macugen for its use in the treatment of diabetic macular edema. Macugen is also being tested for the treatment of retinal vein occlusions. The drug is given by intravitreal injection, and initial treatment plans call for reinjection every 6 wk.

Results from two large, prospective, randomized, multicenter pivotal trials of patients with neovascular AMD have recently been released *(120)*. Patients with vision of 20/40 to 20/320 and evidence of subfoveal involvement were assigned to one of three doses (0.3, 1, or 3.0 mg) of Macugen or sham injections. The trial achieved statistical significance in its primary endpoint, namely, the ability to limit further visual loss of 15 or more letters in a treated patient. In August 2004, data presented to the FDA demonstrated that intravitreous 0.3 mg Macugen treatment, given at 6-wk intervals and measured at an endpoint of 1 yr, stabilized or improved vision in 33% of the patients compared with 23% of controls. Seventy percent of the patients given 0.3 mg Macugen lost less than three lines of vision during the year, compared with 55% in the control group. In addition to visual results, the treatment decreased the leakage and lesion size over time, but other measures of leakage, such as optical coherence tomography (OCT), were not included in the trial. The 1.0-mg dose was also significant, but the 3.0-mg dose did not achieve statistical significance—a finding that is currently unexplained. There were no drug-related systemic or ocular toxicities noted, but complications of the injection procedure were seen. Twelve of the 1190 patients developed endophthalmitis as a result of the injections, but the majority were treatable and remained in the trial; only one patient experienced severe visual loss from endophthalmitis. Given the fact that more than 7500 injections were administered, the safety profile appeared quite comparable to other intravitreal injection procedures. From the patient's perspective, the multiple injections were well tolerated, with most other adverse events being mild and transient.

Also recently, results have been released on a pilot trial of 169 patients given 0.3 mg Macugen every 6 wk by intravitreous injection for the treatment of diabetic macular edema *(121)*. Seventy-three percent of treated patients had stable or improved vision at 36 wk, compared with 51% of controls ($p = 0.02$). Additional data are forthcoming.

Lucentis (Rhufab V2)

Lucentis is a recombinantly produced, humanized, antibody Fab fragment to VEGF. It was designed to bind to and inhibit all isoforms of VEGF. Lucentis penetrates through all retinal layers, whereas IgG penetrates only superficially *(122)*. Phase I/II study indicated that Lucentis was well tolerated and inflammation was not significant. Lucentis inhibits the development of laser-induced CNV in a primate model *(110)*. A pilot trial of 53 patients with subfoveal neovascular AMD treated with intravitreal injection with one of two doses every 4 wk showed that 94% had stable or improved vision *(123)*. Compared with 11 untreated controls, who lost an average 4.9 letters of acuity at day 98, treated patients gained an average of 9.0 letters. These highly favorable results, notable for a substantial number of patients with visual gain, encouraged Genentech to conduct the ongoing pivotal Phase III randomized trials for patients with predominantly occult and predominately classic CNV due to AMD.

Ruboxistaurin

Ruboxistaurin (PKC B inhibitor, LY333531) mesylate was designed to block the signal transduction pathway of VEGF. VEGF binds to its receptor Flk-1 (KDR), activates specific PKC isoforms including β-2, and causes edema and neovascularization. LY333531 inhibited more than 95% of the edema formation in the retina of diabetic animal models *(124)*. Treatment with LY333531 attenuated the increase of leukocyte entrapment in the retinal microcirculation during the period of early diabetes *(125)*. Clinical trials by Eli Lilly and Company showed that ruboxistaurin delays the occurrence of moderate visual loss in patients with moderately severe to very severe nonproliferative diabetic retinopathy, according to the results of a multicenter trial presented during the 63rd Scientific Session of the American Diabetes Association (ADA). Ruboxistaurin is also being studied by Eli Lilly as a possible treatment for diabetic peripheral neuropathy and diabetic nephropathy, the other two major diabetic microvascular complications.

VEGF-TRAP

VEGF-TRAP(R1R2) is a fusion protein, which combines ligand binding elements taken from the extracellular domains of VEGFR-1 and VEGFR-2 fused to the Fc portion of IgG *(126)*. This potent high-affinity VEGF blocker effectively suppresses tumor growth and vascularization in vivo, resulting in almost completely avascular tumors *(126)*. Subcutaneous injections or a single intravitreous injection of VEGF-TRAP(R1R2) strongly suppressed choroidal neovascularization in mice with laser-induced rupture of Bruch's membrane, as well as subretinal neovascularization in transgenic mice expressing VEGF in photoreceptor cells *(127)*. VEGF-TRAP(R1R2) significantly reduced the vascular leakage in two models of VEGF-induced breakdown of the blood–retinal barrier. These data confirm that VEGF is a critical stimulus for the development of choroidal neovascularization and indicate that VEGF-TRAP(R1R2) may provide a new agent for the treatment of choroidal neovascularization and diabetic macular edema *(127)*. The compound is not yet in clinical trials.

Other Approaches

Retaane

Anecortave acetate (Retaane®, Alcon Laboratories) is a modified steroid derivative without glucocorticoid activity. It inhibits extracellular matrix protease activity induced by angiogenic stimuli and thus blocks cell migration. Retaane significantly reduced retinal neovascularization in a rat model of retinopathy of prematurity *(128)* as well as in numerous other experimental neovascularization models. For patient use, it is delivered using posterior juxtascleral injection. Clinical trials on patients with subfoveal neovascular AMD are ongoing, and 24-mo data on the Retaane phase II/III were recently released *(129)*. Retaane was significantly better than placebo for preserving vision, preventing severe vision loss, and inhibiting the growth of all lesion types in patients with wet AMD. At 2 yr, 73% of patients treated with Retaane showed stable or improved vision, whereas only 47% of placebo-treated patients showed a similar vision outcome ($p = 0.035$). In addition, 94% of patients experienced no severe vision loss after 2 yr of treatment with Retaane. At 12 mo, 79% of patients treated with Retaane had stable or improved vision, whereas only 53% of placebo-treated patients showed a similar vision outcome. Treated patients also showed no increase in choroidal neovascularization. To date, there have been no clinically relevant safety issues. Alcon has recently completed enrollment in a large randomized, prospective, multicenter Phase III clinical trial comparing the effectiveness of Retaane with photodynamic therapy (PDT).

Other Drugs

Other angiostatic agents in development include angiostatic steroids, cyclooxygenase inhibitors, integrin antagonists, thalidomide, prolactin, octreotide, matrix metalloproteinase inhibitors, thrombospondin-2, curcumin, angiostatin, endostatin, plasminogen kringle 5 (K5), and TNP-470 *(3,12,130)*. K5 exerts its angiostatic activity by decreasing VEGF and increasing PEDF *(131)*. Steroids' antiinflammatory effect translates into antiangiogenic activity. Intravitreal triamcinolone acetonide effectively inhibited preretinal and optic nerve head neovascularization in the pig retinal vein occlusion model *(132)*. In human studies, intravitreal triamcinolone has been shown to be effective in treating macular edema in diabetic retinopathy that is refractory to laser photocoagulation *(10,133,134)*. Inflammatory mechanisms influence neovascularization of the retina and choroids and cyclooxygenase-2 (COX-2) is induced in retinal astrocytes in human diabetic retinopathy, in the murine and rat model of ischemic proliferative retinopathy in vivo, and in hypoxic astrocytes in vitro. Specific COX-2 but not COX-1 inhibitors prevented intravitreal neovascularization *(135)*. Intravitreal administration of indomethacin, a cyclooxygenase inhibitor, inhibits the formation of laser-induced subretinal neovascularization in monkey eyes *(136)*. Integrin antagonists inhibited retinal neovascularization and CNV in animal models and may provide additional targeting sites for the treatment of ocular angiogenic diseases *(137–139)*. The integrin family of adhesion receptors mediate endothelial cell proliferation *(140)*.

DRUG DELIVERY MODALITIES FOR ANTI-VEGF AND OTHER AGENTS

The pharmacological approaches discussed above offer a new hope for the successful treatment of ocular disorders associated with neovascularization. However, there are a number of potential problems that warrant caution in clinical trials. For the eye, the method of drug delivery is important. Local delivery presumably has fewer side effects than systemic administration. Local delivery may be done by using extraocular depot injections, intravitreal injections, delivery through gene therapy, or administration through intraocular or extraocular slow-release implant devices. Compounds delivered by eyedrops usually do not reach the posterior segment of the eye with therapeutic concentrations, where pathological neovascularization most often occurs. Gene therapy is promising for delivery of antiangiogenic proteins, as the RPE is an easy target for viral transfection and strategically located, but problems remain in developing safe viral vectors. Multiple intravitreal injections, as are used in some of the current clinical trials, involve the risks of endophthalmitis and retinal detachment. Slow-release implants involve intraocular surgery, whereas discontinuation of drug delivery, if needed in case of side effects, can be problematic. Intravitreal polymer implants have been used to release drugs with first-order kinetics over an extended duration. Anti-VEGF receptor (KDR) antibody delivered by slow-release pellets inhibited the formation of retinal vessels in oxygen-induced retinopathy in dogs, an animal model of ROP *(141)*.

Transscleral delivery is an innovative modality of delivering drugs to the posterior segment *(142)*. Sustained transscleral delivery of medications may be achieved by a controlled-release device. The loading of aptamer EYE001-containing poly (lactic-co-glycolic) acid microspheres into a device and placing it on the orbital surface of the sclera was shown to be feasible *(143)*. Additional investigational drug delivery modalities are iontophoresis and sonophoresis, the application of an electrical current or ultrasound to facilitate diffusion of a drug across tissue barriers. For systemic therapy, inhibition of VEGF may lead to suppression of the normal neovascular response, at times when it is needed, such as for the cardiac circulation and reproductive system. Suppression of normal wound healing is not desired as well. It is still unknown whether excessive inhibition of VEGF in the eye will lead to side effects due to unknown functions of VEGF, e.g., physiological level for endothelial survival. VEGF is constitutively expressed in retina of humans and primates *(144)*. In knockout mice in which the hypoxia-responsive gene of VEGF was inactivated, a neurodegenerative disorder developed, suggesting that a neurotrophic function of hypoxia-induced VEGF is essential under physiological conditions *(145)*.

CONCLUSIONS

VEGF is an exciting point of attack in the treatment of neovascular diseases of the retina and choroid. The underlying biochemistry is complex, however, and combination approaches, utilizing drugs, surgery, laser, and other modalities, will be explored to treat neovascularization, vascular leakage, and ischemia, and thereby secure the maximum visual benefit for affected patients. The exciting clinical results seen in early trials of AMD and diabetic macular edema represent the beginning, and not the limit, of the pharmacotherapy for the retina.

REFERENCES

1. Adamis AP, Aiello LP, D'Amato RA. Angiogenesis and ophthalmic disease. Angiogenesis 1999;3:9–14.
2. Campochiaro PA. Retinal and choroidal neovascularization. J Cell Physiol 2000;184: 301–310.
3. Witmer AN, Vrensen GF, Van Noorden CJ, et al. Vascular endothelial growth factors and angiogenesis in eye disease. Prog Retin Eye Res 2003;22:1–29.
4. Miyamoto K, et al. In vivo demonstration of increased leukocyte entrapment in retinal microciculation of diabetic rats. Invest Ophthalmol Vis Sci 1998;39:2190–2194.
5. Frank RN. Diabetic retinopathy. N Engl J Med 2004;350:48–58.
6. Aiello LP, Gardner TW, King GL, et al. Diabetic retinopathy. Diabetes Care 1998;21: 143–156.
7. Michaelson I. The mode of development of the vascular system of the retina with some observations on its significance for certain retinal diseases. Trans Ophthalmol Soc UK 1948;68:137–180.
8. Ashton N. Neovascularization in ocular disease. Transfusion (Paris) 1961;81:145–161.
9. Miller JW, Adamis AP, Aiello LP. Vascular endothelial growth factor in ocular neovascularization and proliferative diabetic retinopathy. Diabetes/Metabolism Rev 1997;13:37–50.
10. Massin P, Audren F, Haouchine B, et al. Intravitreal triamcinolone acetonide for diabetic diffuse macular edema: preliminary results of a prospective controlled trial. Ophthalmology 2004;111:218–224.

11. Gotzaridis EV, Lit ES, D'Amico DJ. Progress in vitreoretinal surgery for proliferative diabetic retinopathy. Sem Ophthalmol 2001;16:31–40.
12. Ferrara N. VEGF and the quest for tumour angiogenesis factors. Nat Rev Cancer 2002;2:795–803.
13. Carmeliet P, Moons L, Luttun A, et al. Synergism between vascular endothelial growth factor and placental growth factor contributes to angiogenesis and plasma extravasation in pathological conditions. Nat Med 2001;7:575–583.
14. Meyer M, Clauss M, Lepple-Wienhues A, et al. A novel vascular endothelial growth factor encoded by Orf virus, VEGF-E, mediates angiogenesis via signalling through VEGFR-2 (KDR) but not VEGFR-1 (Flt-1) receptor tyrosine kinases. EMBO J 1999;18:363–374.
15. Senger DR, Galli SJ, Dvorak AM, Perruzzi CA, Harvey VS, Dvorak HF. Tumor cells secrete a vascular permeability factor that promotes accumulation of ascites fluid. Science 1983;219:983–985.
16. Ferrara N, Henzel WJ. Pituitary follicular cells secrete a novel heparin-binding growth factor for vascular endothelial cells. Biochem Biophys Res Commun 1989;161:851–858.
17. Keck PJ, Hauser SD, Krivi G, et al. Vascular permeability factor, an endothelial cell mitogen related to PDGF. Science 1989;246:1309–1312.
18. Leung DW, Cachianes G, Kuang WJ, Goeddel DV, Ferrara N. Vascular endothelial growth factor is a secreted angiogenic mitogen. Science 1989;246:1306–1309.
19. Clauss M, Gerlach M, Gerlach B, et al. Vascular permeability factor: a tumor-derived polypeptide that induces endothelial cell and monocyte procoagulant activity, and promotes monocyte migration. J Exp Med 1990;172:1535–1545.
20. Burchardt M, Burchardt T, Chen MW, et al. Expression of mRNA splice variants for VEGF in the penis of adult rats and humans. Biol Reprod 1999;60:398–404.
21. Houck KA, Leung DW, Rowland AM, et al. Dual regulation of vascular endothelial growth factor. J Biol Chem 1992;267:26,031–26,037.
22. Senger D, Connolly D, Van De Water L, et al. Purification and NH2-terminal amino acid sequence of guinea pig tumor secreted VPF. Cancer Res 1990;50:1774–1778.
23. Ambati J, Ambati BK, Yoo SH, et al. Age-related macular degeneration: etiology, pathogenesis, and therapeutic strategies. Surv Ophthalmol 2003;48:257–293.
24. Plate KH, Brier G, Weich HA, Risau W. Vascular endothelial growth factor is a potential tumor angiogenesis factor in human gliomas in vivo. Nature 1992;359:845–848.
25. Shweiki D, Itin A, Soffer D, Keshet E. Vascular endothelial growth factor induced by hypoxia may mediate hypoxia-initiated angiogenesis. Nature 1992;359:843–845.
26. Cao Y, Linden P, Shima D, Browne F, Folkman J. In vivo angiogenic activity and hypoxia induction of heterodimers of placenta growth factor/vascular endothelial growth factor. J Clin Invest 1996;98:2507–2511.
27. Blaauwgeers HG, Holtkamp GM, Rutten H, et al. Polarized vascular endothelial growth factor secretion by human retinal pigment epithelium and localization of vascular endothelial growth factor receptors on the inner choriocapillaris. Evidence for a trophic paracrine relation. Am J Pathol 1999;155:421–428.
28. Marti HH, Risau W. Systemic hypoxia changes the organ-specific distribution of vascular endothelial growth factor and its receptors. Proc Nat Acad Sci USA 1998;95;15,809–15,814.
29. Millauer B, Wizigmann-Voos S, Schnurch H, et al. High affinity VEGF binding and developmental expression suggest Flk-1 as a major regulator of vasculogenesis and angiogenesis. Cell 1993;72:835–846.
30. De Vries C, Escobedo JA, Ueno H, et al. The fms-like tyrosine kinase, a receptor for VEGF. Science 1992;255:989–991.
31. Kukk E, Lymboussaki A, Taira S, et al. VEGF-C receptor binding and pattern of expression with VEGFR-3 suggests a role in lymphatic vascular development. Development 1996;122;3829–3837.

32. Carmeliet P, Ferreira V, Breir G, et al. Abnormal blood vessel development and lethality in embryos lacking a single VEGF allele. Nature 1996;380:435–439.
33. Dumont DJ, Jussila L, Taipale J, et al. Cardiovascular failure in mouse embryos deficient in VEGF receptor-3. Science 1998;282:946–949.
34. Fong G-H, Rossant J, Gertssenstein M, Breitman ML. Role of the flt-1 receptor tyrosine kinase in regulating the assembly of vascular endothelium. Nature 1995;376:66–70.
35. Shalaby F, Rossand J, Yamaguchi TP, et al. Failure of blood-island formation and vasculogenesis in Flk-1 deficient mice. Nature 1995;376:62–66.
36. Adamis AP, Shima DT, Tolentino M, et al. Inhibition of VEGF prevents retinal ischemia-associated iris neovascularization in a primate. Arch Ophthalmol 1996;114:66–71.
37. Aiello LP, Pierce EA, Foley ED, et al. Suppression of retinal neovascularization in vivo by inhibition of vascular endothelial growth factor (VEGF) using soluble VEGF-receptor chimeric proteins. Proc Nat Acad Sci USA 1995;92:10,457–10,461.
38. Miller J, Adamis AP, Shima DT, et al. Vascular endothelial growth factor/vascular permeability factor is temporally and spatially correlated with ocular angiogenesis in a primate model. Am J Pathol 1994;145:574–584.
39. Pe'er J, Shweiki D, Itin A, Hemo I, Gnessin H, Keshet E. Hypoxia-induced expression of vascular endothelial growth factor by retinal cells is a common factor in neovascularizing ocular diseases. Lab Invest 1995;72:638–645.
40. Pierce EA, Avery RL, Foley ED, Aiello LP, Smith LEH. Vascular endothelial growth factor/vascular permeability factor expression in a mouse model of retinal neovascularization. Proc Natl Acad Sci USA 1995;2:905–909.
41. Shima DT, Deutsch U, D'Amore PA. Hypoxic induction of vascular endothelial growth factor (VEGF) in human epithelial cells is mediated by increases in mRNA stability. FEBS Lett 1995;370:203–208.
42. Adamis AP, Miller J, Bernal M, et al. Increased vascular endothelial growth factor levels in the vitreous of eyes with proliferative diabetic retinopathy. Am J Ophthalmol 1994;118:445–450.
43. Aiello LP, Avery RL, Arrigg PG, et al. Vascular endothelial growth factor in ocular fluid of patients with diabetic retinopathy and other retinal disorders. N Eng J Med 1994;331: 1480–1487.
44. Adamis AP, Shima DT, Yeo KT, et al. Synthesis and secretion of vascular permeability factor/vascular endothelial growth factor by human retinal pigment epithelial cells. Biochem Biophys Res Commun 1993;193:631–638.
45. Thieme H, Aiello LP, Takagi H, Ferrara N, King GL. Comparative analysis of vascular endothelial growth factor receptors on retinal and aortic vascular endothelial cells. Diabetes 1995;44:98–103.
46. Xia P, Aiello LP, Ishii H, et al. Characterization of vascular endothelial growth factor's effect on the activation of protein kinase C, its isoforms, and endothelial cell growth. J Clin Invest 1996;98:2018–2026.
47. Tolentino MJ, Miller JW, Gragoudas ES, et al. Intravitreal injections of vascular endothelial growth factor produce retinal ischemia and microangiopathy in an adult primate. Ophthalmology 1996;103:1820–1828.
48. Tolentino MT, Miller JW, Gragoudas ES, Chatzistefanou K, Ferrara N, Adamis AP. Vascular endothelial growth factor is sufficient to produce iris neovascularization and neovascular glaucoma in a non-human primate. Arch Ophthalmol 1996;114:964–970.
49. Ozaki H, Seo MS, Ozaki K, et al. Blockade of VEGF receptor signaling is sufficient to completely prevent retinal neovascularization. Am J Pathol 2000;156:697–707.
50. Murata T, Nakagawa K, Khalil A, Ishibashi T, Inomata H, Sueishi K. The relation between expression of vascular endothelial growth factor and breakdown of the blood retinal barrier in diabetic rat retinas. Lab Invest 1996;74:819–825.

51. Sone H, Kawakami Y, Okuda Y, et al. Ocular vascular endothelial growth factor levels in diabetic rats are elevated before observable retinal proliferative changes. Diabetologia 1997;40:726–730.
52. Amin RH, Frank RN, Kennedy A, Eliott D, Puklin JE, Abrams GW. Vascular endothelial growth factor is present in glial cells of the retina and optic nerve of human subjects with nonproliferative diabetic retinopathy. Invest Ophthalmol Vis Sci 1997;38:36–47.
53. Pe'er J, Folberg R, Itin A, Gnessin H, Hemo I, Keshet E. Vascular endothelial growth factor upregulation in human central retinal vein occlusion. Ophthalmology 1998;105:412–416.
54. Malecaze F, Clamens S, Simorre-Pinatel V, et al. Detection of vascular endothelial growth factor messanger RNA and vascular endothelial growth factor-like activity in proliferative diabetic retinopathy. Arch Ophthalmol 1994;112:1476–1482.
55. Lutty GA, McLeod S, Merges C, et al. Localization of VEGF in human retina and choroid. Arch Ophthalmol 1996;114:971–977.
56. Williams B, Gallacher B, Patel H, Orme C. Glucose-induced protein kinase C activation regulates VPF mRNA expression and peptide production by human smooth muscle cells in vitro. Diabetes 1997;46:1497–1503.
57. Tilton RG, Kawamura T, Chang KC, et al. Vascular dysfunction induced by elevated glucose levels in rats is mediated by vascular endothelial growth factor. J Clin Invest 1997;99:2192–2202.
58. Lu M, Kuroki M, Amano S, et al. Advanced glycation end products increase retinal vascular endothelial growth factor expression. J Clin Invest 1998;101:1219–1224.
59. Lu M, Perez VL, Ma N, et al. VEGF increases retinal vascular ICAM-1 expression in vivo. Invest Ophthalmol Vis Sci 1999;40:1808–1812.
60. Miyamoto K, Khosrof S, Bursell SE, et al. Vascular endothelial growth factor (VEGF)-induced retinal vascular permeability is mediated by intercellular adhesion molecule-1 (ICAM-1). Am J Pathol 2000;156:1733–1739.
61. Paques M, Boval B, Richard S, et al. Evaluation of fluorescein-labeled autologous leukocytes for examination of retinal circulation in humans. Curr Eye Res 2000;21:560–565.
62. Hofman P, Van Blijswijk BC, Gaillard PJ, Vrensen GF, Schlingemann RO. Endothelial cell hypertrophy induced by vascular endothelial growth factor in the retina: new insights into the pathogenesis of capillary nonperfusion. Arch Ophthalmol 2001;119:861–866.
63. Tolentino MJ, McLeod DS, Taomoto M, Otsuji T, Adamis AP, Lutty GA. Pathologic features of vascular endothelial growth factor-induced retinopathy in the nonhuman primate. Am J Ophthalmol 2002;133:373–385.
64. Levy AP, Levy NS, Wegner S, Goldberg MA. Transcriptional regulation of vascular endothelial growth factor gene by hypoxia. J Biol Chem 1995;270:13,333–13,340.
65. Levy AP, Levy NS, Goldberg MA. Post-transcriptional regulation of vascular endothelial growth factor by hypoxia. J Biol Chem 1996;34:19,761–19,766.
66. Bouck N. PEDF: anti-angiogenic guardian of ocular function. Trends Mol Med 2002;8: 330–334.
67. Dawson DW, Volpert OV, Gillis P, et al. Pigment epithelium-derived factor: a potent inhibitor of angiogenesis. Science 1999;285:245–248.
68. O'Reilly MS, Holmgren L, Shing Y, et al. Angiostatin: a circulating endothelial cell inhibitor that suppresses angiogenesis and tumor growth. Cold Spring Harb Symp Quant Biol 1994;59:471–482.
69. O'Reilly MS, Boehm T, Shing Y, et al. Endostatin: an endogenous inhibitor of angiogenesis and tumor growth. Cell 1997;88:277–285.
70. Duh EJ, Yang HS, Suzuma I, et al. Pigment epithelium-derived factor suppresses ischemia-induced retinal neovascularization and VEGF-induced migration and growth. Invest Ophthalmol Vis Sci 2002;43:821–829.

71. Mori K, Gehlbach P, Ando A, et al. Regression of ocular neovascularization in response to increased expression of pigment epithelium-derived factor. Invest Ophthalmol Vis Sci 2002;43:2428–2434.
72. Gao Y, Li D, Zhang S, Gee C, Crosson, J Ma. Unbalanced expression of VEGF and PEDF in ischemia-induced retinal neovascularization. FEBS Lett 2001;489:270–276.
73. Spranger J, Osterhoff M, Reimann M, et al. Loss of the antiangiogenic pigment epithelium-derived factor in patients with angiogenic eye disease. Diabetes 2110;50: 2641–2645.
74. Mori K, Gehlbach P, Yamamoto S, et al. AAV-mediated gene transfer of pigment epithelium-derived factor inhibits choroidal neovascularization. Invest Ophthalmol Vis Sci 2000;43:1994–2000.
75. Raisler BJ, Berns KI, Grant MB, et al. Adeno-associated virus type-2 expression of pigmented epithelium-derived factor or Kringles 1-3 of angiostatin reduce retinal neovascularization. Proc Natl Acad Sci USA 2002;99:8909–8914.
76. Stellmach V, Crawford SE, Zhou W, et al. Prevention of ischemia-induced retinopathy by the natural ocular antiangiogenic agent pigment epithelium-derived factor. Proc Natl Acad Sci USA 2001;98:2593–2597.
77. Wiegand SJ. Angiogenesis 2004, presentation at Bascom Palmer Eye Institute, Miami, FL, 2004.
78. Duh EJ, Yang HS, Haller JA, et al. Vitreous levels of pigment epithelium-derived factor and vascular endothelial growth factor: implications for ocular angiogenesis. Am J Ophthalmol 2004;137:668–674.
79. Merimee TJ. Diabetic retinopathy. N Eng J Med 1990;322:978–983.
80. Poulsen JE. Recovery from retinopathy in a case of diabetes with Simmonds' disease. Diabetes 1953;2:7–12.
81. Alzaid AA, Dinneen SF, Melton III LJ, Rizza RA. The role of growth hormone in the development of diabetic retinopathy. Diabetes Care 1994;17:531–534.
82. Grant MB, Russel B, Fitzgerald C, Merimee TJ. Insulin-like growth factors in vitreous: studies in controls and diabetics with neovascularization. Diabetes 1986;35:416–420.
83. Meyer-Schwickerath R, Pfeiffer A, Blum WF, et al. Vitreous levels of the insulin-like growth factors I and II, and the insulin-like growth factor binding proteins 2 and 3, increase in neovascular eye disease. J Clin Invest 1993;92:2620–2625.
84. Punglia RS, Lu M, Hsu J, et al. Regulation of vascular endothelial growth factor expression by insulin-like growth factor I. Diabetes 1997;46:1619–1626.
85. Smith LEH, Shen W, Perruzzi C, et al. Regulation of vascular endothelial growth factor-dependent receptor neovascularization by IGF-1 receptor. Nat Med 1999;5:1390–1395.
86. Grant MB, Mames RN, Fitzgerald C, et al. The efficacy of octreotide in the therapy of severe nonproliferative and early proliferative diabetic retinopathy: a randomized controlled study. Diabetes Care 2000;23:504–509.
87. Smith LEH, Kopchick JJ, Chen W, et al. Essential role of growth hormone in ischemia-induced retinal neovascularization. Science 1997;276:1706–1709.
88. Smith LEH. Pathogenesis of retinopathy of prematurity. Semin Neonatol 2003;8:469–473.
89. Yancopoulos GD, Davis S, Gale NW, Rudge JS, Wiegand SJ, Holash J. Vascular-specific growth factors and blood vessel formation. Nature 2000;407:242–248.
90. Thurston G, Rudge JS, Ioffe E, et al. Angiopoietin-1 protects the adult vasculature against plasma leakage. Nat Med 2000;6:460–463.
91. Oh H, Takagi H, Suzuma K, et al. Hypoxia and vascular endothelial growth factor selectively up-regulate angiopoietin-2 in bovine microvascular endothelial cells. J Biol Chem 1999;274:15,732–15,739.
92. Takagi H, Koyama S, Seike H, et al. Potential role of the angiopoietin/tie2 system in ischemia-induced retinal neovascularization. Invest Ophthalmol Vis Sci 2003;44:393–402.

93. Thurston G, Suri C, Smith K, et al. Leakage-resistant blood vessels in mice transgenically overexpressing angiopoietin-1. Science 1999;286:2511–2514.
94. Hayreh SS, Zimmerman MB, Podhajsky P. Incidence of various types of retinal vein occlusion and their recurrence and demographic characteristics. Am J Ophthalmol 1994; 117:429–441.
95. Green WR, Chan CC, Hutchins GM, Terry JM. Central retinal vein occlusion: a prospective histopathologic study of 29 eyes in 28 cases. Trans Am Ophthalmol Soc 1981;79:371–422.
96. Boyd SR, Zachary I, Chakravarthy U, et al. Correlation of increased vascular endothelial growth factor with neovascularization and permeability in ischemic central vein occlusion. Arch Ophthalmol 2002;120:1644–1650.
97. Stone J, Chan-Ling T, Pe'er J, Itin A, Gnessin H, Keshet E. Roles of vascular endothelial growth factor and astrocyte degeneration in the genesis of retinopathy of prematurity. Invest Ophthalmol Vis Sci 1996;37:290–299.
98. Alon T, Hemo I, Itin A, et al. Vascular endothelial growth factor as a survival factor for newly formed retinal vessels and has implications for retinopathy of prematurity. Nat Med 1995;1:1024–1028.
99. The Eye Diseases Prevalence Research Group. Causes and prevalence of visual impairment among adults in the United States. Arch Ophthalmol 2004;122:477–485.
100. Holz FG, Sheraidah G, Pauleikhoff D, Bird AC. Analysis of lipid deposits extracted from human macular and peripheral Bruch's membrane. Arch ophthalmol 1994;112: 402–406.
101. Kuroki M, Voest EE, Amano S, et al. Reactive oxygen intermediates increase vascular endothelial growth factor expression in vitro and in vivo. J Clin Invest 1996;98:495–504.
102. Frank RN, Amin HR, Eliott D, et al. Basic fibroblast growth factor and vascular endothelial growth factor are present in epiretinal and choroidal neovascular membranes. Am J Ophthalmol 1996;122:393–403.
103. Kvanta A, Algvere VP, Berglin L, Seregard S. Subfoveal fibrovascular membranes in age-related macular degeneration express vascular endothelial growth factor. 1996;37: 1929–1934.
104. Lopez PF, Sippy DB, Lambert MH, Thach AB, Hinton DR. Transdifferentiated retinal pigment epithelial cells are immunoreactive for vascular endothelial growth factor in surgically excised age-related macular degeneration-related choroidal neovascular membranes. Invest Ophthalmol Vis 1996;37:855–868.
105. Wells JA, Murthy R, Chibber R, et al. Levels of vascular endothelial growth factor are elevated in the vitreous of patients with subretinal neovascularisation. Br J ophthalmol 1996;80:363–366.
106. Holekamp NM, Bouck N, Volpert O. Pigment epithelium-derived factor is deficient in the vitreous of patients with choroidal neovascularization due to age-related macular degeneration. Am J Ophthalmol 2002;134:220–227.
107. Baffi J, Byrnes G, Chan CC, Csaky KG. Choroidal neovascularization in the rat induced by adenovirus mediated expression of vascular endothelial growth factor. Invest Ophthalmol Vis Sci 2000;41:3582–3589.
108. Schwesinger C, Yee C, Rohan RM, et al. Intrachoroidal neovascularization in transgenic mice overexpressing vascular endothelial growth factor in the retinal pigment epithelium. Am J Pathol 2001;158:1161–1172.
109. Spilsbury K, Garrett LK, Shen WY, et al. Overexpression of vascular endothelial growth factor (VEGF) in the retinal pigment epithelium leads to the development of choroidal neovascularization. Am J Pathol 2000;157:135–144.
110. Krzystolik MG, Afshari AM, Adamis AP, et al. Prevention of experimental choroidal neovascularization with intravitreal anti-vascular endothelial growth factor antibody fragment. Arch Ophthalmol 2002;120:338–346.

111. Honda M, Sakamoto T, Ishibashi T, et al. Experimental subretinal neovascularization is inhibited by adenovirus-mediated soluble VEGF/flt-1 receptor gene transfection: a role of VEGF and possible treatment for SRN in age-related macular degeneration. Gene Ther 2000;7:978–985.
112. Ogata N, Nishikawa M, Nishimura T, et al. Inverse levels of pigment epithelium-derived factor and vascular endothelial growth factor in the vitreous of eyes with rhegmatogenous retinal detachment and proliferative vitreoretinopathy. Am J Ophthalmol 2002;133:851–852.
113. Ohno-Matsui K, Morita I, Tombran-Tink J, et al. Novel mechanism for age-related macular degeneration: an equilibrium shift between the angiogenesis factors VEGF and PEDF. J Cell Physiol 2001;189:323–333.
114. Renno RZ, Youssri IA, Michaud N, Gragoudas ES, Miller JW. Expression of pigment epithelium-derived factor in experimental choroidal neovascularization. Invest Ophthalmol Vis Sci 2002;43:1574–1580.
115. Rasmussen HS, Rasmussen CS, Curham RG, King CR, Wei L. Looking into anti-angiogenic gene therapies for disorders of the eye. Drug Discov Today 2001;6:1171–1175.
116. Otani A, Takagi H, Oh H, et al. Expressions of angiopoietins and Tie2 in human choroidal neovascular membranes. Invest Ophthalmol Vis Sci 1999;40:1912–1920.
117. Hangai M, Moon SY, Kitaya N, et al. Systemically expressed soluble tie2 inhibits intraocular neovascularization. Hum Gene Ther 2001;12:1311–1321.
118. Hangai M, Murata T, Miyawaki N, et al. Angiopoietin-1 upregulation by vascular endothelial growth factor in human retinal pigment epithelial cells. Invest Ophthalmol Vis Sci 2001;42:1617–1625.
119. Kim I, Moon OS, Park SK, et al. Angiopoietin-1 reduces VEGF-stimulated leukocyte adhesion to endothelial cells by reducing ICAM-1, VCAM-1, and E-selectin expression. Circ Res 2001;89:477–479.
120. Gragondes ES, Adamis AP, Cunningham ET Jr, et al. Pegaptanib for neovascular age-related muscular degeneration. New Engl J Med 2004;351:2805–2816.
121. Eyetech Pharmaceuticals, Inc., NY. (2004) Press release May 3, 2004.
122. Mordenti J, Cuthbertson RA, Ferrara N, et al. Comparisons of the intraocular tissue distribution, pharmacokinetics, and safety of 125I-labeled full-length and Fab antibodies in rhesus monkeys following intravitreal administration. Toxicol Pathol 1999;27:536–544.
123. Genentech CA. Press release Oct 1, 2002.
124. Aiello LP, Bursell SE, Clermont A, et al. Vascular endothelial growth factor-induced retinal permeability is mediated by protein kinase C in vivo and suppressed by an orally effective beta-isoform-selective inhibitor. Diabetes 1997;46:1473–1480.
125. Nonaka A, Kiryu J, Tsujikawa A, et al. PKC-beta inhibitor (LY333531) attenuates leukocyte entrapment in retinal microcirculation of diabetic rats. Invest Ophthalmol Vis Sci 2000;41:2702–2706.
126. Holash J, Davis S, Papadopoulos N, et al. VEGF-Trap: a VEGF blocker with potent antitumor effects. Proc Natl Acad Sci USA 2002;99:11,393–11,398.
127. Saishin Y, Saishin Y, Takahashi K, et al. VEGF-TRAP(R1R2) suppresses choroidal neovascularization and VEGF-induced breakdown of the blood-retinal barrier. J Cell Physiol 2003;195:241–248.
128. Penn JS, Rajaratnam VS, Collier RJ, Clark AF. The effect of an angiostatic steroid on neovascularization in a rat model of retinopathy of prematurity. Invest Ophthalmol Vis Sci 2001;42:283–290.
129. The Anecortave Acetate Clinical Study Group. (in press) Anecortave acetate monotherapy for treatment of subfoveal neovascularization in age-related macular degeneration (AMD): clinical outcomes at month 24. Ophthalmology, in press.
130. Folkman J. Role of antiogenesis in tumor growth and metastasis. Semin Oncol 2002;29:15–18.

131. Gao G, Li Y, Gee S, et al. Down-regulation of vascular endothelial growth factor and up-regulation of pigment epithelium-derived factor: a possible mechanism for the anti-angiogenic activity of plasminogen kringle 5. J Biol Chem 2002;277:9492–9497.
132. Danis RP, Bingaman DP, Yang Y, et al. Inhibition of preretinal and optic nerve head neovascularization in pigs by intravitreal triamcinolone acetonide. Ophthalmology 1996;103: 2099–2104.
133. Jonas JB, Kreissig I, Sofker A, et al. Intravitreal injection of triamcinolone for diffuse diabetic macular edema. Arch Ophthalmol 2003;121:57–61.
134. Martidis A, Duker JS, Greenberg PB, et al. Intravitreal triamcinolone for refractory diabetic macular edema. Ophthalmology 2002;109:920–927.
135. Sennlaub F, Valamanesh F, Vazquez-Tello A, et al. Cyclooxygenase-2 in human and experimental ischemic proliferative retinopathy. Circulation 2003;108:198–204.
136. Sakamoto T, Soriano D, Nassaralla J, et al. Effect of intravitreal administration of indomethacin on experimental subretinal neovascularization in the subhuman primate. Arch Ophthalmol 1995;113:222–226.
137. Hammes HP, Brownlee M, Jonczyk A, Sutter A, Preissner KT. Subcutaneous injection of a cyclic peptide antagonist of vitronectin receptor-type integrins inhibits retinal neovascularization. Nat Med 1996;2:529–533.
138. Kamizuru H, Kimura H, Yasukawa T, Tabata Y, Honda Y, Ogura Y. Monoclonal antibody-mediated drug targeting to choroidal neovascularization in the rat. Invest Ophthalmol Vis Sci 2001;42:2664–2672.
139. Luna J, Tobe T, Mousa SA, Reilly TM, Campochiaro PA. Antagonists of integrin alpha v beta 3 inhibit retinal neovascularization in a murine model. Lab Invest 1996;75:563–573.
140. Mousa SA. Anti-integrin as novel drug-discovery targets: potential therapeutic and diagnostic implications. Curr Opin Chem Biol 2002;6:534–541.
141. McLeod DS, Taomoto M, Cao J, et al. Localization of VEGF receptor-2 (KDR/Flk-1) and effects of blocking it in oxygen-induced retinopathy. Invest Ophthalmol Vis Sci 2002;43: 474–482.
142. Ambati J, Adamis AP. Transscleral drug delivery to the retina and choroid. Prog Retin Eye Res 2002;21:145–151.
143. Carrasquillo KG, Ricker JA, Rigas IK, et al. Controlled delivery of the anti-VEGF aptamer EYE001 with poly(lactic-co-glycolic)acid microspheres. Invest Ophthalmol Vis Sci 2003;44: 290–299.
144. Kim I, Ryan AM, Rohan R, et al. Constitutive expression of VEGF, VEGFR-1, and VEGFR-2 in normal eyes. Invest Ophthalmol Vis Sci 1999;40:2115–2121
145. Oosthuyse B, Moons L, Storkebaum E, et al. Deletion of the hypoxia-response element in the vascular endothelial growth factor promoter causes motor neuron degeneration. Nat Genet 2001;28:131–138.

19

Anecortave Acetate

A Novel Ocular Angiostatic Agent

Stella M. Robertson, PhD, Alberta A. Davis, PhD, David C. Dahlin, PhD, and Abbot F. Clark, PhD

CONTENTS

RELEVANCE OF ANECORTAVE ACETATE TO CNV ASSOCIATED WITH AMD

A variety of angiogenic factors have been identified in choroidal neovascularization (CNV) membranes of patients with exudative age-related macular degeneration (AMD) *(1)*, and several different angiogenic factors can cause experimental CNV *(2,3)*. One of the rate-limiting steps for neovascularization is the angiogenic factor-induced activation of vascular endothelial cells and induction of the angiogenic proteolytic cascade, which allows the endothelial cells to break through the vessel wall and migrate through interstitial tissue to form new blood vessels. An ideal therapeutic agent for the treatment of exudative AMD should be able to inhibit CNV independent of the factor(s) inducing neovascularization and should attack the rate-limiting step of neovascularization. In addition, this agent should be locally administered via a mechanism that does not pierce the eye, deliver the therapeutic agent to the macula, and not require frequent administration. Due to the chronic nature of AMD, the therapeutic agent should have superior ocular and systemic safety.

RETAANE® 15 mg (anecortave acetate suspension) meets all these criteria. Anecortave acetate is an angiostatic cortisene that is being evaluated clinically for the treatment of CNV. Unlike other therapies being tested, it is administered by transscleral delivery outside the eye as a posterior juxtascleral depot once every 6 mo. Anecortave acetate has been extensively tested and shown to have angiostatic activity in 12 preclinical models of neovascularization and has been shown to work independently of the inciting cause of neovascularization.

From: *Ophthalmology: Ocular Angiogenesis: Diseases, Mechanisms, and Therapeutics*
Edited by: J. Tombran-Tink and C. J. Barnstable © Humana Press Inc., Totowa, NJ

PRECLINICAL EVALUATION OF ANECORTAVE ACETATE

Design of Anecortave Acetate

Anecortave acetate is a derivative of cortisol that was designed to enhance angiostatic activity but eliminate glucocorticoid activity. Although glucocorticoids are well known for their antiinflammatory and angiostatic activities, they have serious side effects, including the development of ocular hypertension and glaucoma in susceptible individuals *(4)* and the development of posterior subcapsular cataracts *(5)*. Three modifications were made to cortisol to generate anecortave acetate (Fig. 1). The 11β-hydroxyl group, which is essential for glucocorticoid activity, was removed from cortisol. A double bond between C9 and C11 was added to prevent in vivo enzymatic rehydroxylation at C11. And finally, an acetate group was added at C21 to enhance ocular penetration and provide ideal physical–chemical properties for the administration of a slow-release depot.

The first two modifications have generated a new class of compounds known as angiostatic cortisenes. This name is derived from replacement of the 11β-hydroxyl ("ol") in cortis*ol* with a C9-11 double bond ("ene") to form a cortis*ene*. Anecortave acetate is one of several compounds in this new cortisene class of pregnanes with a C9-11 double bond, which have significant angiostatic activity but are devoid of glucocorticoid activity.

Preclinical Angiostatic Efficacy of Anecortave Acetate

Anecortave acetate and/or its deacetylated active metabolite derivative, anecortave desacetate, have significant angiostatic activity in 12 different preclinical models of neovascularization (Table 1). Unlike many other angiostatic agents, anecortave acetate inhibits neovascularization regardless of the inciting cause of neovascularization, and is active in seven different species.

More than 100 compounds were assayed for angiostatic activity in a chick embryo chorioallantoic membrane (CAM) model of neovascularization *(6)*. An agarose dosing pellet containing the test agent was placed on the CAMs of shell-less 6 d embryos, and the ability to inhibit new blood vessel formation was assessed 48 h later. Unlike previous studies *(14)*, no heparin cofactor was needed to see the angiostatic activity of anecortave acetate and many of these compounds. Anecortave acetate and anecortave desacetate, in addition to several other cortisenes, were much more active than the angiostatic steroids tetrahydrocorticol (THF) and tetrahydrocortexolone (THS) *(6)*.

Fourteen of these compounds were further tested for angiostatic activity in a rabbit corneal neovascularization model. A florid corneal neovascularization was induced by implantation of Elvax pellets containing LPS, a potent angiogenic stimulus, in the midstroma of rabbit corneas. The compounds were placed in another pellet adjacent to the LPS implant. Again, the cortisene, including anecortave acetate and anecortave desacetate, were the most active compounds, almost totally inhibiting this neovascular response *(6)*. There was a statistically significant correlation of angiostatic activity for the compounds tested in the CAM and corneal neovascularization models. Topical application of anecortave acetate dose-dependently inhibited LPS-induced corneal neovascularization, with the 1% suspension almost totally shutting down angiogenesis (Fig. 2) *(7)*. Efficacy was even greater with basic fibroblast growth factor (bFGF)-induced corneal neovascularization.

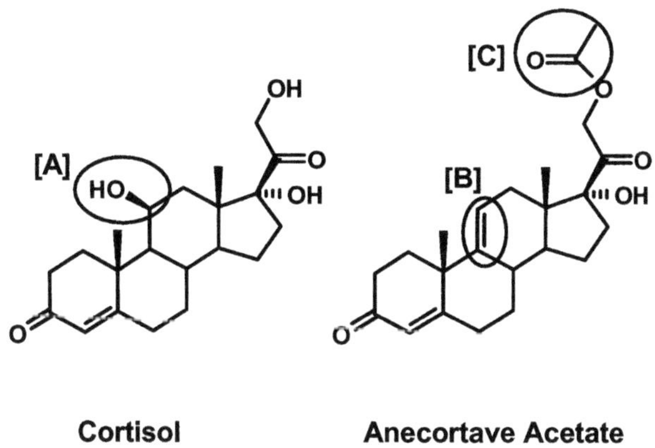

Fig. 1. Design and structure of anecortave acetate. Three structural modifications made to cortisol to derive anecortave acetate. The 11β-hydroxyl group of cortisol **(A)** was removed and a C9-11 double bond was added **(B)** to eliminate glucocorticoid activity. The 21-acetate group **(C)** enhanced the pharmacokinetic properties of anecortave acetate for ocular delivery.

Table 1
Angiostatic Efficacy of Anecortave Acetate in a Variety of Preclinical Models of Neovascularization

Model	*Reference*
Chicken embryo chorioallantoic membrane (CAM)	*6*
Rabbit corneal pocket (LPS- and bFGF-induced)	*7*
Kitten retinopathy of prematurity (ROP)	*8*
Rat pup model of ROP	*9*
Rabbit model of choroidal neovascularization (CNV) (bFGF-induced)	**
Mouse model of CNV (laser-induced)	*10*
Rat RCS retinal neovascularization	*8*
Mouse retinal angiogenesis	**
Mouse intraocular melanoma	*11*
Mouse retinoblastoma	*12,13*
Bovine RVEC proliferation (VEGF-induced)	**
Human RVEC proliferation and tube formation (VEGF-induced)	Manuscript in preparation

** = unpublished data (Alcon Research, Ltd.).

Anecortave acetate and anecortave desacetate were evaluated for angiostatic activity against oxygen-induced retinopathy in experimental models of retinopathy of prematurity (ROP). Newborn rat pups reared in an environment of cyclic 10 to 50% oxygen for 14 d develop a well-characterized oxygen-induced retinopathy that mimics many features of ROP *(15,16)*. In this model system, a single intravitreal injection of anecortave acetate at the time of return to room air (day 14) or 2 d later (day 16) resulted in a highly significant 66% and 50% inhibition of retinopathy, respectively *(9)* (Fig. 3). An additional study also showed that a single intravitreal administration of anecortave desacetate inhibited aberrant retinal vessel growth by 50% in a kitten model of ROP *(8)*.

The effect of anecortave acetate on subretinal neovascularization was examined in two different models of CNV. In the first model, subretinal implantation of a slow-release

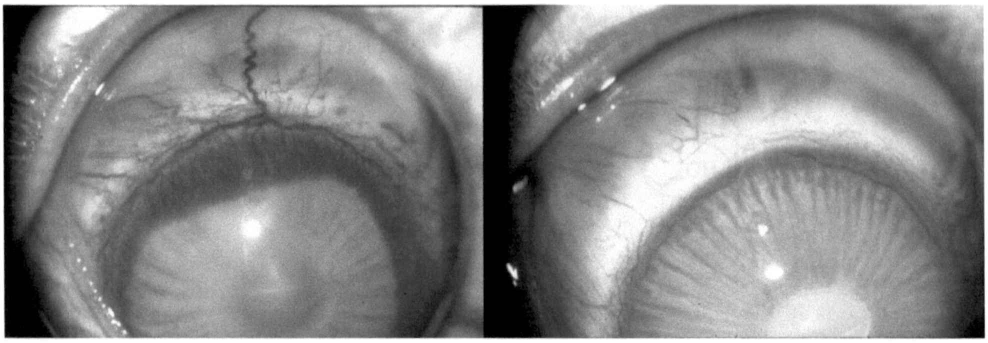

Fig. 2. Anecortave acetate inhibition of LPS-induced corneal neovascularization in rabbits. Midstromal implants of LPS-impregnated pellets were placed in rabbit corneas to induce neovascularization. The eyes were treated topically bid with either vehicle or 1% suspensions of anecortave acetate for 14 d. Corneal neovascularization and edema were almost totally inhibited by anecortave acetate treatment *(7)*. *See* color version on companion CD.

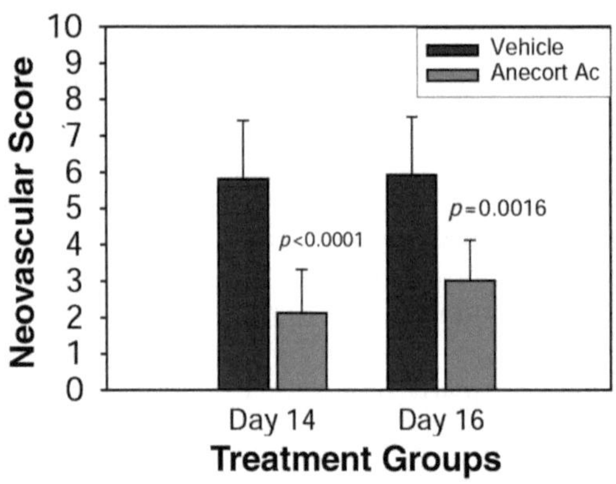

Fig. 3. Inhibition of retinopathy in rat pup model of retinopathy of prematurity (ROP) by anecortave acetate. A single intravitreal injection of anecortave acetate immediately after return to room air (d 14) or 2 d subsequent to return to room air (d 16) significantly inhibited retinal neovascularization by 66% and 50%, respectively *(9)*. *See* color version on companion CD.

formulation of bFGF in rabbits caused marked choroidal neovascularization as assessed histologically and by fluorescein angiography *(3)*. A single posterior juxtascleral administration of two different concentrations of anecortave acetate inhibited any sign of CNV by 50 to 60% over the 8 wk of study (Fig. 4). A second study of laser-induced CNV in mice confirmed the angiostatic activity of anecortave acetate against subretinal neovascularization *(10)*.

The growth of solid tumors is associated with the development of their own blood supply, and angiostatic agents have been an attractive anticancer therapeutic target *(17)*. Anecortave acetate was tested for activity in two different ocular tumor models. A mouse model of a highly angiogenic melanoma was generated in which 99E1 tumor cells were injected into the anterior chamber of nude mice. The topical ocular administration of anecortave acetate significantly inhibited tumor growth by 70% and prevented the tumor from perforating the eye *(11)*. Subconjunctival administration of

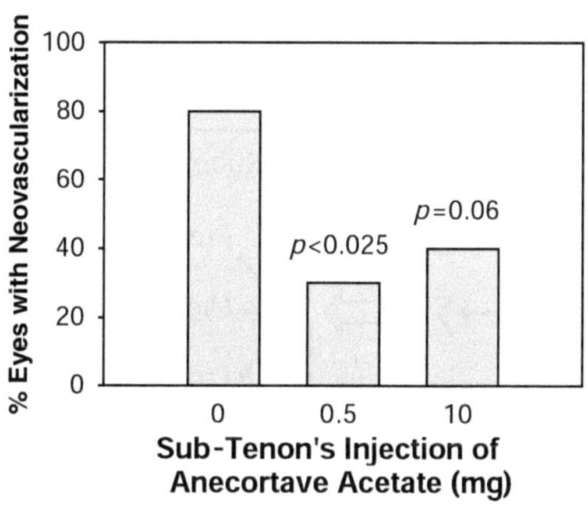

Fig. 4. Anecortave acetate mediated inhibition of bFGF-induced choroidal neovascularization in rabbits. A slow-release subretinal implant of bFGF induced significant choroidal neovascularization (CNV) in the majority of rabbits. A single posterior juxtascleral administration of 0.5 or 10 mg anecortave acetate inhibited CNV by 50 to 60% during the 8-wk duration of the study ($n = 8$ per group; $p < 0.025$ for the 0.5-mg group and $p = 0.06$ for the 10-mg group; CNV was not statistically different between the 0.5-mg and the 10-mg groups). *See* color version on companion CD.

Table 2
Preclinical Summary of Anecortave Acetate

- Extensively studied ocular angiostatic agent
- Active in a wide variety of neovascular models
  - In 7 different species
  - In various ocular and nonocular tissues
  - Independent of inciting cause of neovascularization
  - Inhibits rate-limiting steps in neovascular process
- No safety-related issues identified
- Posterior juxtascleral administration provides prolonged delivery of anecortave acetate to the macular choroid and retina for up to 6 mo after single administration

anecortave acetate dose dependently inhibited tumor growth and tumor vascularity in a murine retinoblastoma model *(12,13)*.

Anecortave acetate and anecortave desacetate were also inhibitory in several in vitro models of angiogenesis. Both compounds partially inhibited the proliferation of human vascular endothelial cells *(18)*. Anecortave acetate dose-dependently inhibited VEGF-induced proliferation of both bovine and human retinal vascular endothelial cells as well as inhibited VEGF-induced tube formation in cultured human retinal vascular endothelial cells (Penn et al., manuscript in preparation). *See* Table 2 for a preclinical summary of anecortave acetate.

Mechanism of Action

Although neovascularization is a continuous process, it can be broken down into a series of stages. The first stage consists of activation of vascular endothelial cells

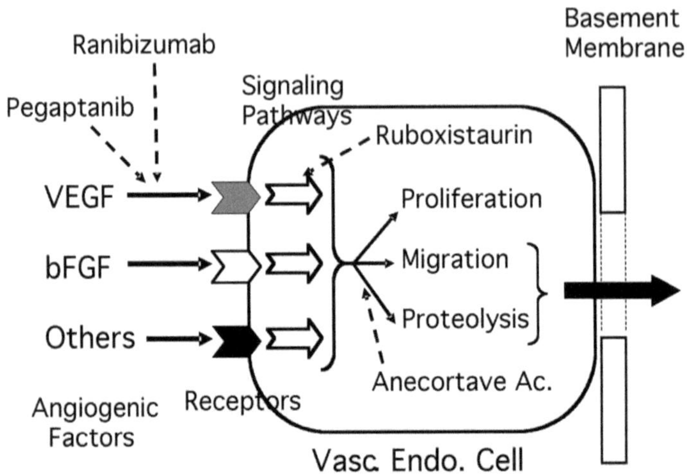

Fig. 5. Comparison of angiostatic mechanism of action among the angiostatic agents being tested clinically. Three different anti-vascular endothelial growth factor (VEGF) therapies target either VEGF directly (pegaptanib sodium *[26,27]* and ranibizumab *[28]*), or the VEGF signaling pathway (ruboxistaurin *[29]*). In contrast, anecortave acetate inhibits neovascularization downstream of the initial signaling event, independent of the inciting cause, by suppressing the angiogenic proteolytic cascade and by inhibiting vascular endothelial cell proliferation.

(VECs) by an angiogenic factor(s). A wide variety of angiogenic factors have been identified, including vascular endothelial growth factor (VEGF), FGF2, platelet-derived growth factor (PDGF), and lipopolysaccharide (LPS) *(19,20)*. Activated endothelial cells produce a set of extracellular proteinases (urokinase plasminogen activator [uPA] and matrix metalloproteinases [MMPs]), which degrade the basement membrane, allowing the cells to break through their vessel wall and migrate through the surrounding interstitial tissues. The VECs proliferate and associate with parenchymal cells (pericytes) to form capillaries that allow blood flow. A number of different classes of therapeutic agents have been explored to inhibit each one of these steps.

Anecortave acetate is unique among the classes of angiostatic agents in several ways (Fig. 5). It inhibits neovascularization independent of the inciting cause of angiogenesis. Many other angiostatic agents are directed at inhibiting only one specific angiogenic factor (such as VEGF). Anecortave acetate inhibits several steps of the neovascular process, downstream of the initial signaling event. It inhibits the angiogenic proteolytic cascade by inhibiting the expression of uPA and MMPs *(18)* as well as upregulating the expression of the uPA inhibitor PAI-1 *(9)*. In addition, anecortave acetate inhibits VEC proliferation.

Preclinical Safety Studies

Anecortave acetate was extensively tested in a wide variety of preclinical ocular and systemic safety models as well as toxicology studies. No safety-related issues have been identified. Both anecortave acetate and anecortave desacetate lack glucocorticoid activity. Neither exhibited glucocorticoid-mediated anti-inflammatory activity in four inflammation models, including an in vitro model of LPS-induced inflammation *(6)*, LPS-induced uveitis in rats and rabbits, and carrageenan-induced footpad edema in rats. In addition, these agents did not have the propensity to raise IOP, and did not cause the development of cataracts, which are typical glucocorticoid activities. These last two preclinical observations have been confirmed by the safety results from clinical studies in exudative AMD patients.

Posterior Juxtascleral Administration of Anecortave Acetate

The development of a safe and clinically practical method for delivery of the active metabolite of anecortave acetate, anecortave desacetate, to the retina and choroid was based initially on the assessment of various routes of administration in animals. The oral route was found to be impractical due to rapid systemic metabolism in rats (and later confirmed in humans). Topical ocular drops and subconjunctival injections provided effective concentrations in anterior tissues of the rabbit (iris-ciliary body C_{max} of approx 0.3 μM), but concentrations in the posterior retina and choroid were subtherapeutic. Intravitreal injections in rabbits and monkeys were found to provide substantial and prolonged levels in the vitreous, retina, and choroid. However, delivery by intravitreal administration was not pursued in the development of RETAANE® 15 mg suspension due to concerns about potential serious complications associated with intravitreal injections, such as endophthalmitis and retinal detachment.

Effective concentrations of anecortave desacetate were generally attained in rabbit retina and choroid using sub-Tenon's injections with a narrow-gauge needle, similar to the technique described by Smith and Nozik for periocular corticosteroid injections *(21)*. Because of the low solubility of anecortave acetate, this slow-release depot delivered drug for months. However, subsequent studies demonstrated that in order to provide appropriate concentrations at the target tissues the suspension depot must be in direct contact with the sclera (juxtascleral) and positioned over the macula, and that needle injections were unreliable in this placement. The literature indicates that periocular needle injections are similarly inaccurate in the clinic *(22)*.

Therefore, to maximize delivery to the retina and choroid, a method for delivery of the drug to the outer surface of the sclera, over the macula, was devised. This included a new proprietary curved cannula (Fig. 6), which was designed for administration of a slow-release posterior juxtascleral depot of anecortave acetate. The curvature of this cannula matched the radius of the human globe. A 56-degree bend was incorporated 16 mm from the tip to ease insertion through a small incision through conjunctiva and Tenon's capsule. When the incision is positioned 8 mm posterior to the limbus, the bend also provided control of depth of insertion, thereby properly positioning the rounded tip relative to the macula and optic nerve. Studies in rabbits and monkeys have demonstrated consistent distribution of anecortave desacetate to the retina and choroid when administered by the posterior juxtascleral cannula technique. In addition, data from monkeys have shown that a single posterior juxtascleral administration delivers concentrations of the active anecortave desacetate above the therapeutic target (approx 0.1 μM) to the retina under the dose site for about 6 mo and that the levels in the choroid were about 10-fold higher.

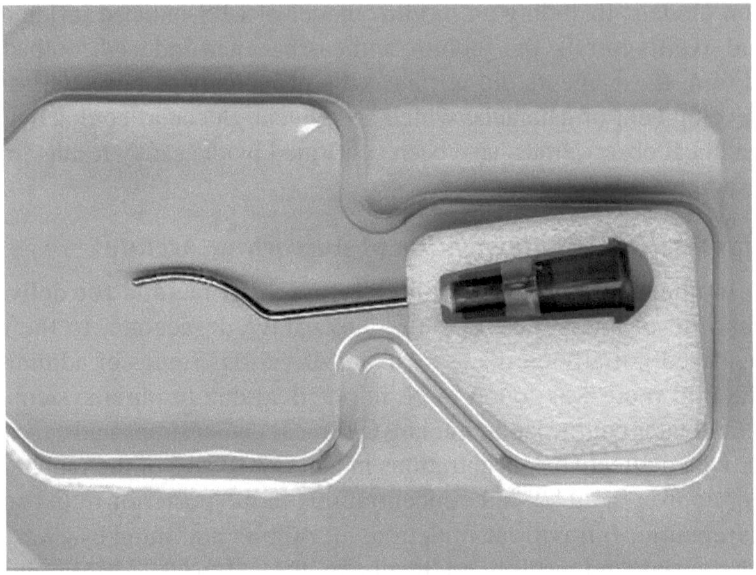

Fig. 6. Specially designed cannula for posterior juxtascleral administration. The proprietary cannula was designed so that the curvature matched the radius of the human globe. A 56-degree bend was incorporated 16 mm from the tip to facilitate insertion through a small incision 8 mm from the limbus through the conjunctiva and Tenon's capsule. *See* color version on companion CD.

THERAPEUTICS

Clinical Trials of Anecortave Acetate for Exudative AMD

Three double-masked randomized clinical studies (Clinical Study C-98-03, C-00-07, and C-01-99) to assess the safety and efficacy of anecortave acetate have been completed. Transscleral drug delivery with a posterior juxtascleral depot (PJD) administration of anecortave acetate was used to place a depot of drug onto the bare sclera in the region of the macula, for treatment of patients with subfoveal exudative (wet) AMD, once every 6 mo (Fig. 7).

In Clinical Study C-98-03, treatments were administered as single-agent therapy, while in Clinical Study C-00-07 the treatments were administered approx 7 d postphotodynamic therapy with Visudyne® PDT. Both masked, randomized studies employed a placebo control, were conducted as dose-response studies, and are comparable in patient demographics, baseline logarithm of the minimum angle of resolution (logMAR) visual acuity, and lesion location.

The small 6-mo Phase II study (C-00-07) evaluating the safety and efficacy of anecortave acetate 15 or 30 mg vs placebo following initial treatment with Visudyne® PDT was completed in 2002. Data from this study show that anecortave acetate can be safely administered with photodynamic therapy. Results from this study suggest a trend (not statistically significant) at month 6 favoring both anecortave acetate concentrations tested (15 mg and 30 mg) combined with Visudyne PDT over Visudyne® PDT alone (plus placebo) for both preservation of vision and inhibition of lesion growth.

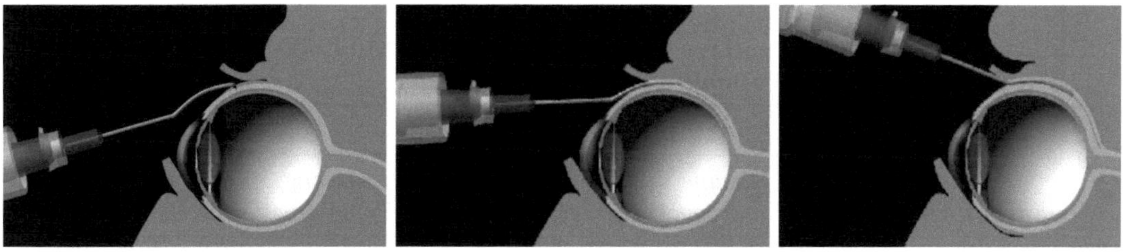

- **1 drop local anesthesia**
- **Small incision (1–1.5 mm) from limbus through Tenon's**
- **Smooth insertion, maintaining contact scleral surface**
- **Slow delivery (0.5 mL)**
- **Touch insertion site with counter pressure device and gently withdraw cannula**

Fig. 7. Posterior juxtascleral administration of 15 mg Retaane depot. The new cannula, designed for administration of a slow-release posterior juxtascleral depot of anecortave acetate, is used to deliver the drug in therapeutic concentrations to the choroid and retina once every 6 mo. *See* color version on companion CD.

Phase II/III 24-Mo Clinical Study (C-98-03)

One hundred twenty-eight patients with minimally classic or predominantly classic subfoveal CNV lesions secondary to AMD were enrolled and randomized 1:1:1:1 to anecortave acetate (3, 15, or 30 mg) versus placebo. Mean change from baseline for best-corrected logMAR visual acuity was the primary efficacy variable. Patients received a posterior juxtascleral depot of study medication or placebo every 6 mo if the masked investigator thought the CNV lesion would benefit from treatment. Follow-up examinations included detailed ophthalmic examinations (best-corrected logMAR visual acuity evaluation, query of patient as to double vision, external examination of the eye(s), routine screening for changes in extraocular motility and/or restriction of gaze, pupil responsiveness, slit-lamp examination of anterior segment lens, dilated fundus examination, and IOP measurement).

Results from this safety and efficacy trial, Clinical Study C-98-03, demonstrate that 15 mg anecortave acetate for depot suspension administered as a posterior juxtascleral depot is effective as primary therapy for the treatment of wet AMD in patients with subfoveal CNV *(23,24)*. This efficacy was demonstrated by measures of both visual function and lesion growth. The analyses of the month 24 results support the month 12 clinical outcomes. The collective results from these evaluations support the overall efficacy conclusion that 15 mg anecortave acetate is superior to placebo for preservation of visual acuity. At both months 12 and 24, anecortave acetate 15 mg suspension was statistically superior ($p < 0.05$) to placebo treatment for stabilization of vision (<3 logMAR line change in visual acuity from baseline) in the overall analysis of all eyes treated in the study. Patients in the placebo group showed a mean decrease from baseline logMAR vision of more than 3 lines at months 12 and 24, whereas patients in the anecortave acetate 15 mg group showed a mean decrease of about 1.5 logMAR lines, a difference that is statistically significant ($p < 0.05$).

The timepoint for primary inference in this study was month 12. The percentage of patients who maintained vision (loss of <3 logMAR lines) at month 12 was statistically significantly greater in the anecortave acetate 15 mg group than in the placebo group

Table 3
Clinical Outcomes in Anecortave Acetate Monotherapy Study (C-98-03) 12 Mo and 24 Mo for All Patients

	12-mo Results			*24-mo Results*		
Clinical outcomes	*Retaane 15 mg depot*	*placebo*	p *value*	*Retaane 15 mg depot*	*placebo*	p *value*
Mean change in VA (lines of vision lost)	1.5	3.0	0.013	1.5	3.0	0.033
% of patients with stable or improved VA	79	53	0.032	73	47	0.035
% of patients with severe vision loss	3	23	0.022	6	23	0.073
% Change in total lesion size	172	242	0.432	178	440	0.004

VA, logMAR visual acuity. Stable vision: <3 logMAR line change in VA from baseline. Severe vision loss: 6 or more logMAR line change in VA from baseline.

(79 vs 53%, $p = 0.032$). Month 24 results confirm the longer-term benefit of the anecortave acetate 15 mg group relative to placebo where the percentage of patients who maintained vision at month 24 is greater in the 15 mg group (73 vs. 47%, $p < 0.05$) relative to placebo (Table 3).

The mechanism of action for anecortave acetate has been shown to be independent of the angiogenic stimulus and to inhibit proliferation, migration, and thus formation of new blood vessels in the eye (*see* Preclinical section). Therefore, it is reasonable to expect that this inhibition will occur whether the lesion is minimally classic or predominantly classic. Indeed, when a subgroup analysis was done for predominantly classic lesions, the most aggressive type of lesions, and the ones frequently responsible for sudden, severe vision loss, anecortave acetate was also effective in this patient population. In this patient group, the 15-mg dose continued to demonstrate superiority over placebo at 24 mo, for both the percentage of patients who maintain vision (80 vs 42%, $p < 0.05$) and for mean change from baseline in logMAR visual acuity. Patients in the placebo group showed a mean decrease from baseline logMAR vision of about 3.5 lines at month 24, whereas patients in the anecortave acetate 15 mg group showed a mean decrease of about 1.0 logMAR line, a difference of 2.5 logMAR lines which is also statistically significant ($p \leq 0.05$).

In this study, anecortave acetate 15 mg inhibited all aspects of lesion growth, including growth of the total lesion, total CNV, and the classic neovascular component of the lesion compared to placebo. By month 24, the advantage of the anecortave acetate 15 mg group over the placebo group was statistically significant ($p \leq 0.05$) for minimally classic and predominantly classic lesions (Fig. 8).

Phase III Clinical Study C-01-99

The third study, C-01-99, was designed to demonstrate the statistical noninferiority of anecortave acetate 15 mg to PDT with verteporfin in patients eligible for treatment with PDT. Although a brief summary of the results will be reported here, the results from this study are being published elsewhere (Slakter et al., in press).

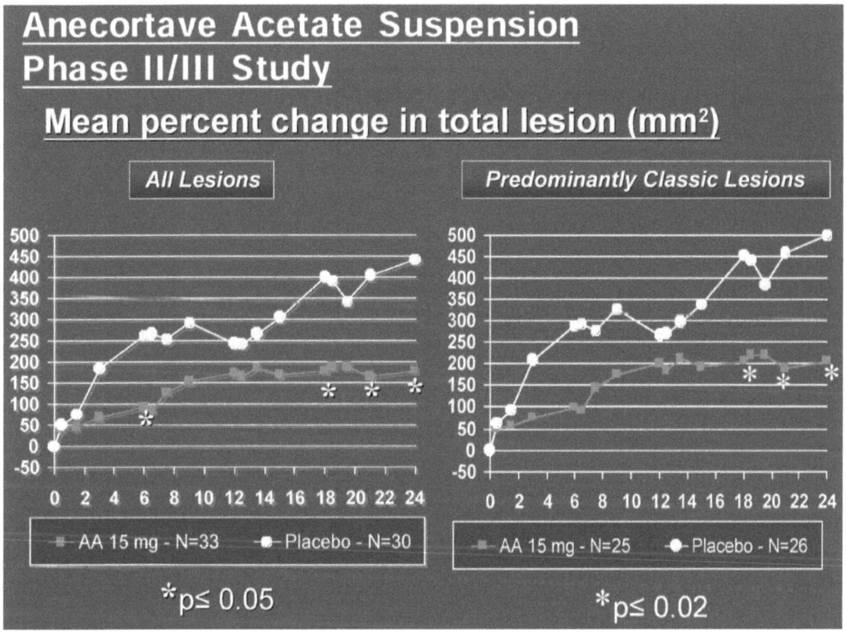

Fig. 8. Inhibition of choroidal neovascularization lesion growth by Retaane® 15 mg suspension. The advantage of the anecortave acetate 15 mg group over the placebo group for inhibition of total lesion growth was statistically significant ($p \geq 0.05$) in the overall analysis, as well as for patients with a predominantly classic lesion. *See* color version on companion CD.

Five hundred thirty AMD patients with predominantly classic subfoveal CNV were enrolled in this prospective, double-masked, active controlled, randomized study designed to evaluate the efficacy and safety of anecortave acetate 15 mg vs PDT.

The 12-mo results from this study show that the percentages of patients with less than a three-line loss of VA were 44.9% and 48.6%, for the anecortave acetate 15 mg and PDT treatment groups ($p = 0.4305$), respectively, and the difference was not statistically significant.

Reflux of study drug during or immediately after depot administration and the dosing interval between depot administrations were identified as two controllable factors that made a difference in the efficacy observed among patients treated with anecortave acetate 15 mg. Differences in maintenance of visual acuity were evident for patients that had no reflux of study drug (50% vs 45%) and for patients who were treated within the 6-mo treatment window (50% vs 33%). When reflux was controlled and the dosing window was within 6 mo, the responder rate for anecortave acetate 15 mg was 57% vs 49% for PDT ($p = 0.1932$).

A counter pressure device (CPD) was developed to eliminate reflux, and is presently being used in all ongoing and future studies. All physicians administering the drug in clinical trials with anecortave acetate have been trained in the proper method for performing the posterior juxtascleral depot procedure using the CPD. The importance of eliminating reflux and retreatment at or shortly before 6 mo is being re-emphasized in the ongoing clinical trials. *See* Table 4 for a clinical summary of anecortave acetate.

Table 4
Clinical Summary of Anecortave Acetate

- Efficacious in all forms of wet age-related macular degeneration
  - Minimally classic
  - Predominantly classic
- Superior to placebo for
  - Reducing loss of vision from baseline
  - Avoiding severe vision loss (≥6 lines)
  - Inhibiting growth of choroidal neovascularization lesions (2 mm^2)
- Transscleral delivery in a posterior juxtascleral depot is safe and provides prolonged delivery of anecortave acetate to the choroid and retina for up to 6 mo after single administration
- No treatment-related serious adverse events

Safety

To date, the collective safety results from these completed studies as well as ongoing studies indicate that anecortave acetate administered as a posterior juxtascleral depot is safe and well-tolerated. There have been no serious treatment-related adverse events reported in these studies. The majority of adverse events reported have not been related to therapy and occurred in incidences similar to placebo. The events assessed as treatment related are commonly reported following conjunctival and/or periocular/ sub-Tenon's injections; and the safety data continue to support the safety of the posterior juxtascleral depot administration procedure *(23,24)*.

Ongoing Studies

Exudative (Wet) AMD

Currently there are four ongoing clinical efficacy and safety studies to evaluate anecortave acetate 15 mg suspension for treatment of subfoveal CNV in patients with wet AMD.

Two additional Phase III studies that compare anecortave acetate 15 mg to placebo, following juxtascleral administration at 6-mo intervals, in patients with all lesion types have completed enrollment.

Interval Dose Evaluation of Anecortave Acetate Study

The Interval Dose Evaluation of Anecortave Acetate (IDEAA) study (C-04-59) is currently enrolling patients. This 2 yr study will evaluate the dose concentration and administration frequency of anecortave acetate when administered by posterior juxtascleral depot every 3 mo (anecortave acetate 15 mg) or 6 mo (anecortave acetate 15 mg, anecortave acetate 30 mg). Patients eligible for this study will be 50 yr of age or older and have a clinical diagnosis of exudative AMD and a primary or recurrent (after laser photocoagulation) subfoveal CNV lesion (predominantly classic, minimally classic, or occult with evidence of progression).

An open-label rollover phase II study, designed to allow continued treatment of patients exited from Clinical Study C-98-03 (at its conclusion) with anecortave acetate 15 mg, is ongoing. Patients rolled from that study into this 24-mo study will receive posterior juxtascleral depot administrations of anecortave acetate 15 mg at 6-mo intervals.

As of July 2005 more than 2400 depot administrations of anecortave acetate (30, 15, or 3 mg) or placebo have been given at 6-mo intervals as part of ongoing or completed clinical trials. There have been no perforations of the globe, no evidence of optic nerve damage, and no evidence of damage to the posterior ciliary arteries.

Non-Exudative (Dry) AMD

Anecortave Acetate Risk Reduction Trial (AART)

Anecortave acetate shows clinical efficacy in the treatment of subfoveal CNV in patients with wet AMD. In view of the positive safety profile and demonstrated clinical efficacy of anecortave acetate administered as a posterior juxtascleral depot every 6 mo, Alcon Research, Ltd. is conducting a 2500 patient clinical trial for an unmet medical need, a new indication with no approved treatment options. This indication is for the treatment of eyes with dry AMD (i.e., intermediate or large soft/confluent drusen and focal hyperpigmentation and no CNV or geographic atrophy) that are at risk for progression to CNV.

Transscleral Drug Delivery Device (Implant)

Alcon Research, Ltd. is developing a method for the long-term delivery of drugs to the retina. The device that is in development is a curved silicone holder with a cavity that holds the drug at the proximal end. It can be implanted juxtasclerally, in the sub-Tenon's space for the treatment of retinal diseases such as age-related macular degeneration *(25)*.

REFERENCES

1. Rakic JM, Lambert V, Devy L, et al. Placental growth factor, a member of the VEGF family, contributes to the development of choroidal neovascularization. Invest Ophthalmol Vis Sci 2003;44:3186–3193.
2. Cui JZ, Kimura H, Spee C, et al. Natural history of choroidal neovascularization induced by vascular endothelial growth factor in the primate. Graefes Arch Clin Exp Ophthalmol 2000;238:326–333.
3. Kimura H, Sakamoto T, Hinton DR, et al. A new model of subretinal neovascularization in the rabbit. Invest Ophthalmol Vis Sci 1995;36:2110–2119.
4. Clark AF, Morrison JC. Corticosteroid glaucoma. In: Glaucoma: Science and Practice. Morrison JC, Pollack IP, eds. Thieme Medical Publishers, New York: 2002.
5. Carnahan MC, Goldstein DA. Ocular complications of topical, peri-ocular, and systemic corticosteroids. Curr Opin Ophthalmol 2000;11:478–483.
6. McNatt LG, Weimer L, Yanni J, Clark AF. Angiostatic activity of steroids in the chick embryo CAM and rabbit cornea models of neovascularization. J Ocul Pharmacol Ther 1999;15:413–423.
7. BenEzra D, Griffin BW, Maftzir G, et al. Topical formulations of novel angiostatic steroids inhibit rabbit corneal neovascularization. Invest Ophthalmol Vis Sci 1997;38:1954–1962.
8. Clark AF. AL-3789: a novel ophthalmic angiostatic steroid. Exp Opin Invest Drugs 1997;6: 1867–1877.
9. Penn JS, Rajaratnam VS, Collier RJ, Clark AF. The effect of an angiostatic steroid on neovascularization in a rat model of retinopathy of prematurity. Invest Ophthalmol Vis Sci 2001;42:283–290.
10. Bingaman DP, Liu C, Landers RA, Gu X. Local delivery of anecortave acetate inhibits laser-induced choroidal neovascularization (CNV) in the mouse. ARVO Annual Meeting. Fort Lauderdale, FL, 2004.

11. Clark AF, Mellon J, Li XY, et al. Inhibition of intraocular tumor growth by topical application of the angiostatic steroid anecortave acetate. Invest Ophthalmol Vis Sci 1999;40:2158–2162.
12. Murray TG, Escalona-Benz E, Hayden BC, et al. Subconjunctival anecortave acetate, an angiostatic steroid, in the treatment of a murine model of retinoblastoma. ARVO Annual Meeting. Fort Lauderdale, FL, 2003.
13. Murray TG. Combined anti-angiogenic and peri-ocular chemotherapy using anecortave acetate and carboplatin in the treatment of retinal tumors in the LHbetaTag murine transgenic model of retinoblastoma. ARVO Annual Meeting. Fort Lauderdale, FL, 2004.
14. Crum R, Szabo S, Folkman J. A new class of steroids inhibits angiogenesis in the presence of heparin or a heparin fragment. Science 1985;230:1375–1378.
15. Madan A, Penn JS. Animal models of oxygen-induced retinopathy. Front Biosci 2003;8: d1030–d1033.
16. Penn JS, Henry MM, Tolman BL. Exposure to alternating hypoxia and hyperoxia causes severe proliferative retinopathy in the newborn rat. Pediatr Res 1994;36:724–731.
17. Folkman J. Angiogenesis inhibitors: a new class of drugs. Cancer Biol Ther 2003;2(4 Suppl 1): S127–S133.
18. DeFaller JM, Clark AF. A new pharmacological treatment for angiogenesis. In: Pterygium. Taylor HR, ed. Kugler Publications, The Hague: 2000.
19. Das A, McGuire PG. Retinal and choroidal angiogenesis: pathophysiology and strategies for inhibition. Prog Retin Eye Res 2003;22:721–748.
20. Casey R, Li WW. Factors controlling ocular angiogenesis. Am J Ophthalmol 1997;124: 521–529.
21. Smith RE, Nozik RA. In Uveitis: A Clinical Approach to Diagnosis and Management, 2nd Edition. Williams and Wilkins Publishers, Baltimore: 1989;51–76.
22. Freeman WR, Green RL, Smith RE. Echographic localization of corticosteroids after periocular injection. Am J Ophthalmol 1987;103(3 Pt 1):281–288.
23. D'Amico DJ, Goldberg MF, Hudson H, et al. Anecortave acetate as monotherapy for treatment of subfoveal neovascularization in age-related macular degeneration: twelve-month clinical outcomes. Ophthalmology 2003;110:2372–2383; discussion 2384, 2385.
24. D'Amico DJ, Goldberg MF, Hudson H, et al. Anecortave acetate as monotherapy for the treatment of subfoveal lesions in patients with exudative age-related macular degeneration (AMD): interim (month 6) analysis of clinical safety and efficacy. Retina 2003;23:14–23.
25. Yaacobi Y, Chastain J, Lowseth L, et al. In-vivo studies with trans-scleral anecortave acetate delivery device designed to treat choroidal neovascularization in AMD. ARVO Annual Meeting. Fort Lauderdale, FL, 2003.
26. Anti-vascular endothelial growth factor therapy for subfoveal choroidal neovascularization secondary to age-related macular degeneration: phase II study results. Ophthalmology 2003;110:979–986.
27. Preclinical and phase 1A clinical evaluation of an anti-VEGF pegylated aptamer (EYE001) for the treatment of exudative age-related macular degeneration. Retina 2002;22:143–152.
28. Krzystolik MG, Afshari MA, Adamis AP, et al. Prevention of experimental choroidal neovascularization with intravitreal anti-vascular endothelial growth factor antibody fragment. Arch Ophthalmol 2002;120:338–346.
29. Wheeler GD. Ruboxistaurin (Eli Lilly). IDrugs 2003;6:159–163.

20
Gene Therapy for Neovascular Retinopathies

Brian J. Raisler, PhD, Kenneth I. Berns, MD, PhD, and William W. Hauswirth, PhD

CONTENTS

INTRODUCTION

Normal control of retinal angiogenesis, the formation of new blood vessels in either the retinal or choroidal beds from preexisting vasculature, is essential for vision. Conversely, pathological neovascularization (NV) of retinal and choroidal vessels is a key process leading to vision loss in several prevalent ocular diseases, including retinopathy of prematurity (ROP), proliferative diabetic retinopathy (PDR), and age-related macular degeneration (AMD). PDR and AMD are the leading causes of blindness in developed countries, and ROP is the leading cause of infant blindness. Proper regulation of retinal vascularization is thought to depend on an equilibrium between ocular vascular growth factors, primarily vascular endothelial growth factor (VEGF) *(1)*, and natural inhibitors of angiogenesis, primarily pigment epithelium-derived factor (PEDF) *(2)*. When this balance becomes disturbed—as may happen, for example, during and after the hyperoxic treatment of premature infants—pathological angiogenesis often occurs that ultimately leads to vision loss.

NEOVASCULAR RETINAL DISEASES AS TARGETS FOR GENE THERAPY

AMD, Associated Choroidal Neovascularization, and Need for New Therapies

The late forms of AMD are the primary cause of irreversible legal blindness on the three developed continents *(3,4)*. Late clinical hallmarks include choroidal neovascularization (CNV) accompanied by progressive retinal degeneration. This is typically preceded by abnormalities of the underlying retinal pigment epithelium (RPE) and

From: *Ophthalmology: Ocular Angiogenesis: Diseases, Mechanisms, and Therapeutics*
Edited by: J. Tombran-Tink and C. J. Barnstable © Humana Press Inc., Totowa, NJ

choroidal vasculature. An early clinical sign is the accumulation of lipoproteinaceous deposits (drusen) in the RPE/choroid extracellular matrix. Although a relatively common age-related phenomenon, drusen deposition is a significant risk factor in exudative AMD due to CNV. An impediment to developing effective AMD therapies has been the lack of good animal models for AMD. Although many individual clinical facets of AMD are mimicked in one or more experimental rodent models, including high-fat diets and phototoxicity *(5,6)*, aging studies *(7,8)*, and candidate AMD gene manipulations *(9–12)*, none fully replicates drusen or spontaneous CNV, both key vascular and RPE features of human AMD *(13,14)*. The use of moderate energy laser burns in Bruch's membranes to stimulate CNV in various species *(15)* has become the model of choice for validating CNV therapies. Recently several genetic models in mice have been reported to exhibit accumulation of drusen-like deposits followed by late retinal/choroidal NV *(13)*. These models appear to be the first to recapitulate the key age-related hallmarks of AMD, and they involve eliminating either functional gene for the macrophage chemotactic receptor/ligand pair CCR2 or CCL2. These mice may provide a second animal target for validating gene therapy approaches to AMD.

Because prevention of CNV is one central focus of retinal gene therapy, an understanding of its anatomy and natural history in AMD are important. A typical CNV vascular membrane typically has a plexus of incompletely formed blood vessels that leak serum components. Such local vascular defects allow angiographic detection of CNV foci after intravenous fluorescein. Based primarily on the timing and appearance of the fluorescence angiography, CNV is divided into two types, classic or occult. In the classic form, regions around CNV membranes hyperfluoresce quickly and continue to leak over larger areas with time, often with increased intensity. In occult CNV, hyperfluorescence is usually slower to appear and more punctuate, owing to leakage into regions of irregularly detached RPE. The progression of initially diagnosed CNV to measurable vision loss is disappointingly common. Laser photocoagulation, the most common current option for extrafoveal and juxtafoveal CNV, is of some value; however, because most CNV is occult, nearly 90% of patients with newly diagnosed AMD are not suitable for laser treatment *(16,17)*. Photodynamic therapy (PDT) is also partially effective and is gaining in acceptance. However, PDT is intended primarily for classic CNV and its effects are transient, with most patients requiring repeated sessions over the long term *(18)*. Importantly, many patients do not experience visual improvement after PDT. It is now becoming clear that effective AMD treatment will require long-term management of classic and occult CNV and that no current therapy satisfies this criterion very well. The central aim of gene therapy approaches, therefore, is to develop a safe, minimally invasive, and long-term therapy for CNV.

Diabetic Retinopathy and Need for New Therapies

In developed countries diabetic retinopathy is the primary reason for severe visual loss in patients under the age of 60 *(19)*. Retinal NV, the hallmark of PDR, can progress to retinal detachment and eventually to blindness. Accompanying retinal vascular permeability is also common in these patients, and, if in or near the macula, leads to diabetic macular edema (DME), the most prevalent cause of moderate vision loss in diabetics. PDR and DME are the two major ocular complications in diabetics that require treatment.

Panretinal laser photocoagulation can significantly decrease severe vision loss due to PDR; however, in addition to injuring peripheral retina, this treatment often also exacerbates DME and occasionally causes constriction of visual fields *(16,17,20,21)*. Because a clear view of the retina is needed to effectively deliver laser photocoagulation and diabetic patients often present with vitreous hemorrhage or cataract obscuring a clear view, laser treatment is often delayed and/or coupled with additional surgery. For patients with DME, focal laser photocoagulation slows the rate of vision loss but, as with focal laser treatment for AMD, multiple treatments are required and substantial visual loss may still occur. Therefore, for both PDR and DME, new, more permanent treatments are clearly needed.

Retinopathy of Prematurity

Retinopathy of prematurity is the leading cause of blindness in children in developed countries *(22,23)*. ROP is a proliferative ischemia-induced retinopathy that occurs primarily in low-birth-weight preterm infants owing to the required high oxygen support. Many mechanistic aspects of ROP are also found in the more prevalent NV ocular diseases, including AMD and diabetic retinopathy. The initial phase of ROP is induced by oxygen therapy after premature birth and leads to retarded growth of the retinal vasculature (phase I). The resulting insufficient perfusion of the developing retina creates a hypoxic environment, leading to induction of proangiogenic factors that stimulate subsequent abnormal retinal vessel proliferation (phase II). The process of retinal neovascularization in ROP and in animal models of oxygen-induced retinopathy (OIR) is complex, and involves proangiogenic factors, such as VEGF, as well as basement membrane components. Potential medical therapies for ROP, including modulators of angiogenic factors, inhibitors of basement membrane changes, endogenous inhibitors of VEGF such as PEDF, and antiinflammatory drugs, have shown efficacy against neovascularization in several animal models but are not yet in general clinical practice. The OIR mouse model (*see* below) most closely mimics the pathology, and very likely the mechanism, of ROP.

Candidate Antineovascular Factors

Although several proangiogenic agents have been suggested to play key roles in the induction and maintenance of retinal NV, multiple lines of evidence indicate that VEGF plays the central role *(24)*. In fact, despite the likely participation by other proangiogenic factors, expression of VEGF is both necessary *(25)* and sufficient for retinal NV to occur *(26,27)*. Increased expression of VEGF occurs early in diabetic retinopathy *(28,29)* and has been implicated in increased retinal vascular permeability *(30,31)*. In fact, sustained intravitreous release of VEGF in monkeys has been shown to cause macular edema *(31)*. Thus, VEGF is an important, and perhaps key, stimulatory factor for both PDR and DME, and its therapeutic inhibition is central to most anti-NV gene therapies. It has been postulated that the proangiogenic effects of VEGF are modulated by endogenous inhibitors of angiogenesis *(29,32)*. With regard to ocular NV, this hypothesis has been supported by studies in which increased ocular levels of PEDF *(33–36)*, endostatin *(37)*, or angiostatin *(38,39)* have been demonstrated to inhibit various types of ocular neovascularization. As PEDF and endostatin are normally present in the eye and both angiostatin and endostatin can induce ocular PEDF expression

(Hauswirth and Raisler, unpublished), it is reasonable to expect that increasing their concentration in the eye may be a nontoxic way to treat AMD and PDR.

ADENO-ASSOCIATED VIRUS VECTORS

General Properties

In large part because it is nonpathogenic and causes persistent infections, adeno-associated virus (AAV) has been developed as a vector for gene therapy *(40)*. The generic AAV-based vector has had its two normal genes removed; in their place the passenger gene and regulatory sequences are inserted, bounded on both ends by AAV inverted terminal repeats (ITRs). Since all the AAV coding sequences are missing, there is minimal response by the host except to the virion itself. As a consequence there has been little evidence of immune-modulated inflammatory responses to AAV vectors, albeit the transgene-encoded product itself may engender an immune reaction. Vector production requires the vector construct, the AAV coding sequences for the Rep and structural capsid proteins in a separate construct lacking the ITRs, and the adenovirus genes required for AAV replication (E1, 2, and 4). Administered AAV vectors exist primarily in an extrachromosomal state. After prolonged periods of time (months in mice) there is evidence of rare integration into the host genome *(41)*, but the integration is at random sites *(41,42)*. Expression with constitutive promoters has been long-lived, over 1 yr in many cases, with remarkably little evidence of toxicity. One advantage of AAV vectors is that they can transduce nondividing cells, making them particularly well suited for the retina. A limitation of AAV vectors is that the upper limit of inserted transgene size is only 4.7 kb; however, Duan and collaborators *(43)* have demonstrated that coadministration of several AAV vectors encoding different parts of a large protein can lead to synthesis of the intact protein by homologous recombination.

Treatment of Nonneovascular Retinal Diseases Using AAV Vectors

Progress toward safe and effective retinal gene therapies has focused largely on AAV vectors, although more limited data have been reported for adenovirus *(44,45)*, lentivirus *(46)*, or "gutted" adenovirus *(47)* vectors as well. In the longest-term rodent study to date, AAV-delivered ribozymes designed against P23H rod opsin gene *(48)*, a common cause of human autosomal dominant RP, preserved photoreceptors for at least 8 mo in a transgenic rat model of P23H opsin RP *(49,50)*.

There have also been promising results using virally vectored gene replacement for recessive retinal disease in animals. A 4-bp deletion in the RPE65 gene leads to a stop codon in a strain of homozygous Swedish Briard dogs (RPE65–/–) and results in the absence of a functional RPE65 protein. This effectively disrupts the visual cycle and causes an autosomal recessive retinal degeneration very similar to Leber congenital amaurosis (LCA) in humans. Before treatment, all RPE65–/– dogs had severe visual deficits, including very-low-amplitude electroretinography (ERG) responses to light stimuli and large lipid-like inclusions in their RPE. Subretinally injected AAV2 vector carrying wild-type canine RPE65 (AAV2-CBA-cRPE65) stably restored visual function in this large-animal model of childhood blindness, as assessed by ERG analysis, immunohistochemistry, and behavioral testing *(51)*. Function was preserved for at least 3 yr after a single treatment *(52)*. An AAV-delivered rds-peripherin gene regulated by a rod opsin promoter was found to partially rescue photoreceptor structure in the rds mouse for up to 6 wk *(53)*, although ERG function was not proportionately restored and rescue depended on early treatment *(54)*. Recessive mutations in the MERTK gene cause an RP-like phenotype in the RCS rat that responded well to Ad-MERTK gene replacement *(55)*.

Several neurotrophin gene therapies have also shown promise in rodent RP models. Human CNTF (ciliary neurotrophic factor) cDNA in AAV vectors rescues rods in the P23H opsin transgenic rat *(56)*; opsin knockout mouse *(57)*, and the P216L rds/peripherin transgenic mouse *(58)*, however, distinct rod toxicity was reported in all cases. In contrast, results with AAV-GDNF (glial cell line-derived neurotrophic factor) demonstrated rod preservation and no apparent toxicity in the S334ter opsin transgenic rat *(59)*. In summary, AAV is presently the best-documented retinal vector in terms of efficiency of cell-specific gene delivery, level of passenger gene expression, persistence of expression, and lack of toxicity. It also has the best current record at delaying retinal degenerations and/or restoring retinal function in animal models of dominant and recessive RP. These vector properties bode well for developing gene-based therapies for AMD, PDR, and ROP.

GENE THERAPY STRATEGIES FOR TREATING NEOVASCULAR OCULAR DISEASE

Animal Models of Neovascular Retinopathies

In order to effectively study the potential of any antiangiogenic treatment, it is necessary to have appropriate animal models. In the case of diabetic retinopathy, the neovascular insult arises from the inner retinal vascular bed, sometimes also referred to as preretinal neovascularization. The most commonly used animal model for this condition is the oxygen-induced retinopathy (OIR) mouse model as described by Smith et al. *(60)*. This model can also serve as a surrogate for ROP, as it encompasses many of the stimuli and pathophysiological hallmarks of neonatal ischemic retinopathy. For the CNV seen in exudative AMD, the most prevalent animal model employs laser burns in Bruch's membrane to induce CNV in an adult mouse *(61)*.

The OIR mouse model involves exposing neonatal mice to elevated levels of oxygen (~75%) for a period of 5 d. This leads to a pattern of central retinal vasoobliteration. Upon the return to room air, the neonatal mouse pups experience a relative retinal hypoxia, resulting in an ischemia-driven retinal neovascularization that is maximal at postnatal day 17. This neovascular response can be visualized by fluorescein angiography and is quantified by enumerating the endothelial cell nuclei internal to the inner limiting membrane of the retina in histological thin sections. The neovascular response in this model is relatively short-lived, however, and the new vessels that form in response to retinal ischemia cease to proliferate and then regress spontaneously by postnatal day 21 *(60)*.

Although a fully accurate model of exudative AMD has yet to be developed, the current model of choice for studying CNV consists of laser-induced ruptures of Bruch's membrane in the mouse *(62)*. Three or four 100-μm burns are introduced into Bruch's membrane at one to two disk diameters from the optic nerve. The subsequent focal rupture of membrane integrity at each burn allows local proliferation choroidal vessels into the subretinal space within 2 to 4 wk. The extent of the CNV response can be quantified through fluorescein angiographic imaging of choroidal whole mounts *(34)*. Recently a mouse model of AMD has been developed that implicates macrophage dysfunction in AMD pathogenesis *(13)*. These knockout mice are deficient in either monocyte chemoattractant protein-1 (Ccl-2; also known as MCP-1) or its cognate receptor (Ccr-2). At senescence, these mice spontaneously form lipoproteinaceous drusen and share other pathophysiological markers with AMD, including the eventual development of CNV. This is a potentially significant development, as it heralds the first animal model exhibiting drusen deposition followed by development of CNV, very similar to that observed in AMD. A direct connection between human AMD and macrophage disfunction, however, has yet to be made.

VEGF and Hypoxia Signaling Pathway as Targets for Gene Therapy

VEGF appears to be the major proangiogenic factor in the retina and is induced through a hypoxia-signaling pathway. VEGF is a 46-kDa glycopeptide that is active in a homodimeric state and is expressed in several cell types within the eye, including vascular endothelial cells, pericytes, ganglion cells, and pigmented epithelium *(25,42,63–65)*. Expression of VEGF is upregulated in low oxygen conditions and its levels are increased in animal models of retinal neovascularization *(42,65)* and in human patients with ROP *(66)*, PDR *(67–69)*, and CNV *(70)*.

There is evidence to suggest that VEGF may be involved in the development and maintenance of CNV. VEGF is present at elevated levels in fibroblastic cells and RPE cells of surgically removed choroidal neovascular membranes *(70–73)*. Also, in both rat and monkey models of laser-induced CNV, increases in VEGF mRNA are seen in RPE-like cells, choroidal vascular endothelial cells, and fibroblast-like cells in the lesions *(74,75)*. Intravitreal injection of an antibody fragment against VEGF reduced CNV in a primate model *(76)*, indicating some role for VEGF in the development or persistence of CNV. However, increased expression of VEGF in photoreceptors of mice did not result in frank CNV in initial studies *(27,77)*. More recent work, though, has documented proliferation of retinal vessels in the deep capillary bed when VEGF expression was under the control of the strong rhodopsin promoter *(26)*, suggesting that high levels of VEGF and/or the prior breakdown of Bruch's membrane may be required for CNV.

The process by which VEGF expression is increased in response to hypoxia has been more completely elucidated in recent years. A cytosolic heme protein appears to act as a sensor to detect decreased oxygen tension and to generate free radicals. This process, in turn, activates various transcription factors, including hypoxia-inducible factor (HIF-1) *(78)*, which stimulate transcription of multiple proangiogenic genes, including VEGF *(79,80)*. This action of HIF-1 requires binding to hypoxia response element (HRE) promoter regions *(81)* in VEGF and other proangiogenic factor genes, suggesting that HIF-1 signaling plays a role in VEGF-mediated neovascularization in response to local retinal ischemia. Thus VEGF acts as a major angiogenic stimulator relatively early in the signaling cascade, is clearly involved in retinal NV, and may also have a role in choroidal NV. Most new approaches to controlling retinal NV involve attempts to modulate these VEGF induction pathways (*see* next section).

Another potential mechanism for interfering with VEGF-mediated NV is to block VEGF from binding to its cognate receptors, VEGFR-1, a fms-like tyrosine kinase receptor (Flt-1), and VEGFR-2, kinase insert domain-containing receptor (KDR). Expression of a soluble fragment of the Flt-1 receptor (sFlt-1) might be a particularly attractive approach to ameliorating VEGF-based NV because it is likely to inhibit VEGF signaling at two levels. sFlt-1 binds to and sequesters VEGF and also binds endogenous membrane spanning isoforms of Flt-1 and KDR, thus creating inactive heterodimers *(82,83)*. Other factors have also been used to inhibit VEGF in animal models, including soluble chimeric proteins that bind to VEGFR-1 *(25)*, inhibition of the VEGFR-2 (KDR) receptor by novel synthetic amines and indoles *(84–86)*, anti-VEGF monoclonal antibodies *(87,88)*, and VEGF antisense oligonucleotides *(89,90)*.

Current Non-Gene-Based Treatment Options for Neovascular Retinal Disease

Current treatment options for patients with ocular neovascularization do not include antiangiogenic treatments. However, two approaches to inhibiting VEGF are being currently evaluated in clinical trials. EYE001 (Macugen), an anti-VEGF pegylated aptamer for the treatment of CNV in wet AMD *(91)*, operates by acting like an anti-VEGF antibody to sequester VEGF from binding to its receptor. RhuFab (Lucentis) is an engineered antibody fragment directed against VEGF that was initially shown to be safe and efficacious in a monkey model of CNV *(76)*. Recent studies in mice have examined orally active drugs that inhibit the VEGF receptor kinase pathway and demonstrate significant reduction in ocular neovascularization *(92,93)*. However, such systemic inhibition of VEGF-mediated angiogenesis raises safety concerns that must be addressed before this could be applied clinically. To avoid such concerns, local delivery of several agents is being investigated. Intravitreal injection of soluble VEGF receptors and antisense oligonucleotides for VEGF both reduce retinal NV in the OIR mouse model *(25,94)*. Work in nonhuman primates has shown a reduction in iris NV following intravitreal injection of anti-VEGF antibody *(88)*. Recently, intraocular injections of an anti-VEGF antibody or an aptamer that binds VEGF have been tested for safety in phase II clinical trials for treatment of cancer, and phase III trials both for cancer and control of angiogenesis in AMD are under way *(95)*. Preliminary reports suggest that injection of the anti-VEGF antibody may induce a local inflammatory response, but it is not considered a severe enough problem to discontinue these approaches *(96)*. Alternative proteins with antiangiogenic activity such as PEDF have been identified *(42,97)*, and intraocular injection alone or in combination with other factors could also be considered. All these treatments, however, share the potentially limiting disadvantage of requiring repeated intraocular injection.

GENE-BASED THERAPIES FOR NEOVASCULAR RETINAL DISEASE

Vector and Vector Administration Properties

Gene-based therapy for the treatment of ocular neovascular disease offers advantages over conventional methods. By using a vector with a strong selective promoter to express the antiangiogenic protein or factor locally, expression can be limited to a specific cell type or subset of cell types within the retina. This reduces the safety concerns compared with systemic administration of antiangiogenic agents. Delivery of the vector to discreet compartments within the eye by subretinal or intravitreal injection may also allow additional topological control of expression by limiting vector access to only those local vessels affected. Choice of the appropriate vector for delivery of the therapeutic gene might also allow modulation of the duration of expression. For example, adenoviral vectors support expression in the eye that is rapid in onset but lasts for periods of only days to weeks *(98)*. This short period of expression would, in theory, limit its effectiveness for long-term treatment of recurring NV. However, a finite expression window also limits exposure of the retina to factors that might be damaging in the long term. An alternative is to use a drug-regulated promoter in a vector such as AAV that otherwise would lead to persistent expression. The idea would be to express the therapeutic gene only when needed by systemic administration of the nontoxic inducer. Two such systems have been tested in the retina using AAV vectors *(99,100)*. In one the tetracycline-inducible expression system demonstrated tight regulation of reporter gene expression in photoreceptors and RPE cells in response to doxycycline levels in the drinking water *(100)*. The second, employing a rapamycin induction system, found high levels of the passenger gene product, a secreted erythropoietin, after the drug consumption that, upon withdrawal, decayed rapidly *(99)*. The use of either in a neovascular disease setting remains to be tested.

For optimizing the safety of ocular gene therapy for NV diseases it may be important to limit expression of a therapeutic protein even more specifically, to just a single retinal cell type and/or to a more defined retinotopographic area. By altering the promoter used to drive expression of an antiangiogenic factor it may be possible to fine-tune therapeutic gene expression to a pharmacologically significant but highly localized cellular pattern. The commonly used cytomegalovirus enhancer-promoter (CMV) and the chimeric CMV enhancer-chicken beta-actin (CBA) promoters both drive vector passenger gene expression in multiple retinal cell types. A more cell-specific promoter could be employed to target expression selectively. Alternatively, delivering the vector specifically to the intravitreal or subretinal space in a larger human eye may also serve to define the localization of expression. Advanced stages of AMD are characterized by a neovascularization of the chorocapillaris within or adjacent to the macula where treatment might be most effective if the vector were administered subretinally near potentially active CNV regions. This type of subretinal administration effectively limits the lateral spread of vector-mediated expression *(51)*, whereas vitreal administration may allow less constrained vector diffusion leading to a wider, less controlled retinal area of transduction. Full testing of these ideas will require more detailed studies in larger, more human-sized animal models of NV such as the laser-induced CNV monkey.

Several improvements in current AAV vectors are possible, and could be evaluated in the context of ocular NV. Incorporation of vascular targeting signal into the viral capsid at sites that still allow efficient vector assembly may increase the transduction efficiency of endothelial cells *(101)*. An alternative is to screen random peptide insertions into the viral capsid for those that lead to enhanced vascular endothelial cell transduction *(102)*. Combined with the compartmentalization of the eye, this approach offers the distinct advantage of being able to target viral vector delivery directly to the cell type undergoing pathology. Clearly, such vector capsid modifications depend on our knowledge of the appropriate epitopes to target. In this regard there is growing evidence that vessels involved in NV can be distinguished from normal preexisting vessels. Endothelial precursor cell levels are increased by proangiogenic factors that promote new capillary formation in the adult *(103)*. This process can be differentiated from normal prenatal vasculogenesis, in which cells known as hemangioblasts act as pluripotent progenitors capable of forming both blood and blood vessels *(104,105)*. While both angiogenesis and vasculogenesis have a role in the formation and maintenance of the vasculature, there are important differences. Vasculogenesis, primarily involved in developmental vessel formation, takes place by the *de novo* assembly of vasculature from hemangioblasts. In contrast, angiogenesis, involved both in developmental vessel formation and later processes such as wound healing, forms new microvessels by migration and proliferation of endothelial cells from larger, extant vessels. Although the two processes are distinct, evidence suggests that they may share certain regulatory mechanisms. Lineage-specific markers might be used to distinguish existing vasculature from pathologically forming angiogenic vessels, although a recent study suggests that a subpopulation of adult bone marrow stem cells may function as hemangioblasts *(106)*, potentially making such a distinction more difficult. Other candidate cell markers are integrins $\alpha_v\beta_3$ and $\alpha_v\beta_5$, present on endothelial cells participating in angiogenesis but absent on normal retinal endothelial cells *(107,108)*. For a more complete review of angiogenesis and vasculogenesis, including the cell types and markers involved and the key regulatory players, interested readers should consult the review by Beck and D'Amore *(109)*. In summary, the possibility of distinguishing normal vessels from those participating in pathological NV opens the door to reengineering vectors to specifically target such hyperproliferative endothelial cells involved in NV while sparing the normal vasculature.

AAV-Vectored Gene Therapy for Neovascular Retinal Disease

Two of the most potent general inhibitors of neovascularization are kringle domains 1 through 3 of angiostatin (K1K3) and PEDF. K1K3 is a proteolytic fragment of plasminogen *(32)* that retains potent angiostatic properties. It is an endogenous regulator of vasculogenesis and, as a naturally occurring peptide, it is not likely to stimulate an immunogenic response *(110,111)*. Neither plasminogen nor plasmin inhibits endothelial cell proliferation, nor does angiostatin affect coagulation. Although angiostatin is known to inhibit tumor growth in vivo by increasing endothelial apoptosis and inhibiting tumor-associated angiogenesis, its precise mechanism of action is unclear. Apoptosis in vitro is induced in endothelial cells by multiple forms of angiostatin *(112)*, and cells have been shown to be arrested at the G2/M transition interface *(113)*. Administration of angiostatin to tumor-bearing mice has not resulted in detectable systemic cytotoxicity; only angiogenic proliferation is inhibited *(32,114,115)*. In the OIR mouse model, AAV mediated-K1K3 treated eyes had 78% fewer endothelial cells above the inner limiting membrane (ILM) compared with paired controls, indicating that K1K3 gene therapy can effectively control retinal NV *(38)*. Angiostatin therefore appears to be an effective and nontoxic inhibitor of NV that is worth evaluating for potential clinical use in the treatment of retinal NV. A recent study has indicated that kringle 5 of angiostatin induces PEDF and inhibits VEGF both in cell culture and a rat model of ischemic retinopathy *(116)*, thus suggesting a potential mechanism for the potency of angiostatin.

PEDF, first purified from human retinal pigment epithelial cultures as a factor that induces neuronal differentiation of cultured retinoblastoma cells *(97,117)*, has been recently shown to regulate normal angiogenesis in the eye *(2)*. PEDF is found both intracellularly and extracellularly in the fetal and early adult eye but is lost at the onset of senescence *(118,119)*. It is downregulated by hypoxia and induced in the retina as a result of hyperoxia; it is a very potent inhibitor of corneal NV and prevents endothelial cell migration toward a wide variety of angiogenic inducers *(2)*. PEDF therefore appears to be a major natural antiangiogenic regulator of the retinal vasculature and is an excellent candidate gene for therapy against ocular NV. As an intraocularly injected protein, PEDF delays the loss of photoreceptors in the rd mouse *(120)*, implying that it may also possess neurotrophic activity in the retina and that the extracellular protein can effectively disperse throughout the retina. In the OIR mouse model, AAV-mediated PEDF-treated eyes had 74% fewer NV endothelial cells compared to paired control eyes, indicating that vectored PEDF can effectively control retinal NV *(38)*. Expression of PEDF from either AAV *(34)* or adenovirus *(33)* vectors was also effective in reducing CNV in rodent models. This anti-CNV strategy is currently in phase I clinical testing using an adenovirus vector to deliver PEDF as a potential treatment for exudative AMD *(121)*. Interestingly, the effectiveness of the AAV–PEDF vector was independent of whether it was administered to the vitreous or subretinal space *(34)*, suggesting that expression of naturally secreted angiostatic factors such as PEDF may be relatively independent of the retinal cell type supporting expression.

Endostatin, a proteolytic fragment of collagen XVIII, is an endogenous inhibitor of tumor angiogenesis *(77)*. It has been suggested that vectored expression of this agent could be used to regulate pathological angiogenesis in human diseases such as cancer and various retinopathies *(77,122,123)*. Because it is a naturally occurring inhibitor of angiogenesis, like PEDF, vectored expression should have minimal side effects. Recently endostatin has been demonstrated to inhibit VEGF-induced retinal vascular permeability, neovascularization, and retinal detachment when delivered intraocularly *(124)*. Endostatin has also been effective in reducing CNV when expressed from a systemically administered adenoviral vector *(37)*. Another recent study examined the correlation of VEGF and endostatin levels with the severity of diabetic retinopathy in human patients. Concentrations of VEGF and endostatin in aqueous humor and vitreous fluid were significantly correlated with the severity of disease. Specifically, the levels of VEGF and endostatin were inversely correlated significantly between active and quiescent NV disease *(125)*, suggesting that increased ocular endostatin might be effective in controlling retinal as well as CNV. Consistent with this idea, AAV vectors carrying cDNAs for either PEDF or endostatin reduced NV endothelial cell levels in the OIR mouse *(126)*.

AAV vectors encoding the soluble VEGFR-1, sFlt-1, have also shown promise for long-term inhibition of three types of ocular neovascularization *(127,128)*. When injected into the anterior chamber, these vectors resulted in expression in both the corneal endothelium and iris pigment epithelium and reduced corneal NV by 36% *(128)*. Subretinal injection of similar vectors reduced choroidal NV subsequent to laser lesions around the optic nerve *(128)* and in the OIR mouse *(127)*, suggesting that a secretable factor expressed in one or more transduced cell populations can be effective in the control of ocular NV occurring in distant retinal tissue. Similarly, secreted exon 6 and 7 peptides of VEGF as cDNAs in AAV2 vectors reduced angiogenesis in the OIR mouse *(129,130)*.

CONCLUSIONS

Effective, long-lasting treatment of retinal neovascular disorders, including proliferative diabetic retinopathy, exudative AMD, and ROP, remain one of the greatest challenges in ophthalmology today. Advances in gene delivery to the posterior ocular segment, particularly with AAV-based vectors, provide new approaches toward the treatment of such debilitating retinal diseases. As these neovascular conditions all share the pathophysiology of an overproliferating vasculature, a variety of antiangiogenic factors are candidates for treatment by gene therapy.

REFERENCES

1. Shweiki D, Itin A, Soffer D, Keshet E. Vascular endothelial growth factor induced by hypoxia may mediate hypoxia-initiated angiogenesis. Nature 1992;359:843–845.
2. Dawson DW, Volpert OV, Gillis P, et al. Pigment epithelium-derived factor: a potent inhibitor of angiogenesis. Science 1999;285:245–248.
3. Ambati J, Ambati BK, Yoo SH, Ianchulev S, Adamis AP. Age-related macular degeneration: Etiology, pathogenesis, and therapeutic strategies. Surv Ophthalmol 2003;48:257–293.
4. Smith W, Assink J, Klein R, et al. Risk factors for age related macular degeneration - Pooled findings from three continents. Ophthalmology 2001;108:697–704.
5. Cousins SW, Espinosa-Heidmann DG, Alexandriou A, Sall J, Dubovy S, Csaky K. The role of aging, high fat diet and blue light exposure in an experimental mouse model for basal laminar deposit formation. Exp Eye Res 2002;75:543–553.
6. Dithmar S, Sharara NA, Curcio CA, et al. Murine high-fat diet and laser photochemical model of basal deposits in Bruch membrane. Arch Ophthalmol 2001;119:1643–1649.
7. Majji AB, Cao JT, Chang KY, et al. Age-related retinal pigment epithelium and Bruch's membrane degeneration in senescence-accelerated mouse. Invest Ophthalmol Vis Sci 2000;41:3936–3942.
8. Cao J, Majji AB, Chang KY, et al. Retinal pigment epithelium and Bruch's membrane degeneration in senescence accelerated mouse (SAM). Invest Ophthalmol Vis Sci 2000;41:S23.
9. Dithmar S, Curcio CA, Le NA, Brown S, Grossniklaus HE. Ultrastructural changes in Bruch's membrane of apolipoprotein E-deficient mice. Invest Ophthalmol Vis Sci 2000;41: 2035–2042.
10. Lu B, Rutledge BJ, Gu L, et al. Abnormalities in monocyte recruitment and cytokine expression in monocyte chemoattractant protein 1-deficient mice. J Exp Med 1998;187: 601–608.
11. Rakoczy PE, Zhang D, Robertson T, et al. Progressive age-related changes similar to age-related macular degeneration in a transgenic mouse model. Am J Pathol 2002;161:1515–1524.
12. Weng J, Mata NL, Azarian SM, Tzekov RT, Birch D, Travis GH. Insights into the function of Rim protein in photoreceptors of Statgardt's disease from the phenotype of the abcr knockout mouse. Cell 1999;98:13–23.
13. Ambati J, Anand A, Fernandez S, et al. An animal model of age-related macular degeneration in senescent Ccl-2- or Ccr-2-deficient mice. Nat Med 2003;9:1390–1397.
14. Zarbin MA. Current concepts in the pathogenesis of age-related macular degeneration. Arch Ophthalmol 2004;122:598–614.

15. Ohkuma H, Ryan SJ. Experimental subretinal neovascularization in the monkey—permeability of new vessels. Arch Ophthalmol 1983;101:1102–1110.
16. Bressler NM, Bressler SB, Gragoudas ES. Clinical characteristics of choroidal neovascular membranes. Arch Ophthalmol 1987;105:209–213.
17. Folk JC. Aging macular degeneration—Clinical features of treatable disease. Ophthalmology 1985;92:594–602.
18. Blumenkranz MS, Bressler NM, Potter MJ, et al. Photodynamic therapy of subfoveal choroidal neovascularization in age-related macular degeneration with verteporfin—two-year results of 2 randomized clinical trials—TAP report 2. Arch Ophthalmol 2001;119:198–207.
19. Klein R, Klein BEK, Moss SE, Davis MD, Demets DL. The Wisconsin Epidemiologic Study of Diabetic Retinopathy 3. Prevalence and risk of diabetic retinopathy when age at diagnosis is 30 or more years. Arch Ophthalmol 1984;102:527–532.
20. Chew EY, Ferris FL, Csaky KG, et al. The long-term effects of laser photocoagulation treatment in patients with diabetic retinopathy—The Early Treatment Diabetic Retinopathy Follow-Up Study. Ophthalmology 2003;110:1683–1689.
21. Mcdonald HR, Schatz H. Macular edema following panretinal photocoagulation. Retina 1985;5:5–10.
22. Simons BD, Flynn JT. Retinopathy of prematurity and associated factors. Internat Ophthalmol Clin 1999;39:29–48.
23. Smith LEH. Pathogenesis of retinopathy of prematurity. Sem Neonatol 2003;8:469–473.
24. Campochiaro PA. Retinal and choroidal neovascularization. J Cell Physiol 2000;184: 301–310.
25. Aiello LP, Pierce EA, Foley ED, et al. Suppression of retinal neovascularization in vivo by inhibition of vascular endothelial growth factor (VEGF) using soluble VEGF-receptor chimeric proteins. Proc Natl Acad Sci USA 1995;92:10,457–10,461.
26. Ohno-Matsui K, Hirose A, et al. Inducible expression of vascular endothelial growth factor in adult mice causes severe proliferative retinopathy and retinal detachment. Am J Pathol 2002;160:711–719.
27. Okamoto N, Tobe T, Hackett SF, et al. Transgenic mice with increased expression of vascular endothelial growth factor in the retina: a new model of intraretinal and subretinal neovascularization [see comments]. Am J Pathol 1997;151:281–291.
28. Lutty GA, McLeod DS, Merges C, Diggs A, Plouet J. Localization of vascular endothelial growth factor in human retina and choroid. Arch Ophthalmol 1996;114:971–977.
29. Vinores SA, Youssri AI, Luna JD, et al. Upregulation of vascular endothelial growth factor in ischemic and non-ischemic human and experimental retinal disease. Histol Histopathol 1997;12:99–109.
30. Derevjanik NL, Vinores SA, Xiao WH, et al. Quantitative assessment of the integrity of the blood-retinal barrier in mice. Invest Ophthalmol Vis Sci 2002;43:2462–2467.
31. Ozaki H, Hayashi H, Vinores SA, Moromizato Y, Campochiaro PA, Oshima K. Intravitreal sustained release of VEGF causes retinal neovascularization in rabbits and breakdown of the blood–retinal barrier in rabbits and primates. Exp Eye Res 1997;64:505–517.
32. O'Reilly MS, Holmgren L, Shing Y, et al. Angiostatin: a novel angiogenesis inhibitor that mediates the suppression of metastases by a Lewis lung carcinoma. Cell 1994;79:315–328.
33. Mori K, Duh E, Gehlbach P, et al. Pigment epithelium-derived factor inhibits retinal and choroidal neovascularization. J Cell Physiol 2001;188:253–263.
34. Mori K, Gehlbach P, Yamamoto S, et al. AAV-mediated gene transfer of pigment epithelium-derived factor inhibits choroidal neovascularization. Invest Ophthalmol Vis Sci 2002;43: 1994–2000.
35. Duh EJ, Yang HS, Suzuma I, et al. Pigment epithelium-derived factor suppresses ischemia-induced retinal neovascularization and VEGF-induced migration and growth. Invest Ophthalmol Vis Sci 2002;43:821–829.

36. Mori K, Gehlbach P, Ando A, McVey D, Wei L, Campochiaro PA. Regression of ocular neovascularization in response to increased expression of pigment epithelium-derived factor. Invest Ophthalmol Vis Sci 2002;43:2428–2434.
37. Mori K, Ando A, Gehlbach P, et al. Inhibition of choroidal neovascularization by intravenous injection of adenoviral vectors expressing secretable endostatin. Am J Pathol 2001;159:313–320.
38. Raisler BJ, Berns KI, Grant MB, Beliaev D, Hauswirth WW. Adeno-associated virus type-2 expression of pigmented epithelium-derived factor or kringles 1–3 of angiostatin reduce retinal neovascularization. Proc Natl Acad Sci USA 2002;99:8909–8914.
39. Lai CC, Wu WC, Chen SL, et al. Suppression of choroidal neovascularization by adeno-associated virus vector expressing angiostatin. Invest Ophthalmol Vis Sci 2001;42: 2401–2407.
40. Muzyczka N. Use of AAV as a general transducetion vector for mammalian cells. In: Current Topics in Microbiology and Immunology, V. 158. Muzyczka N, ed. Springer Verlag, Berlin: 1992:97–129.
41. Song S, Laipis PJ, Berns KI, Flotte TR. Effect of DNA-dependent protein kinase on the molecular fate of the rAAV2 genome in skeletal muscle. Proc Natl Acad Sci USA 2001;98:4084–4088.
42. Miller JW, Adamis AP, Shima DT, et al. Vascular endothelial growth factor/vascular permeability factor is temporally and spatially correlated with ocular angiogenesis in a primate model. Am J Pathol 1994;145:574–584.
43. Duan D, Yue Y, Engelhardt JF. Dual vector expansion for the recombinant AAV packaging capacity. Methods Mol Biol 2003;219:29–51.
44. Cayouette M, Gravel C. Adenovirus-mediated gene transfer of ciliary neurotrophic factor can prevent photoreceptor degeneration in the retinal degeneration (rd) mouse. Hum Gene Ther 1997;8:423–430.
45. Bennett J, Tanabe T, Sun D, et al. Photoreceptor cell rescue in retinal degeneration (rd) mice by in vivo gene therapy. Nat Med 1996;2:649–654.
46. Takahashi M, Miyoshi H, Verma IM, Gage FH. Rescue from photoreceptor degeneration in the rd mouse by human immunodeficiency virus vector-mediated gene transfer. J Virol 1999;73:7812–7816.
47. Kumar-Singh R, Farber DB. Encapsidated adenovirus mini-chromosome-mediated delivery of genes to the retina: application to the rescue of photoreceptor degeneration. Hum Mol Genet 1998;7:1893–1900.
48. Drenser KA, Timmers AM, Hauswirth WW, Lewin AS. Ribozyme-targeted destruction of RNA associated with autosomal-dominant retinitis pigmentosa. Invest Ophthalmol Vis Sci 1998;39:681–689.
49. LaVail MM, Yasumura D, Matthes MT, et al. Ribozyme rescue of photoreceptor cells in P23H transgenic rats: long- term survival and late-stage therapy. Proc Natl Acad Sci USA 2000;97:11,488–11,493.
50. Lewin AS, Drenser KA, Hauswirth WW, et al. Ribozyme rescue of photoreceptor cells in a transgenic rat model of autosomal dominant retinitis pigmentosa. Nat Med 1998;4:967–971.
51. Acland GM, Aguirre GD, Ray J, et al. Gene therapy restores vision in a canine model of childhood blindness. Nat Genet 2001;28:92–95.
52. Acland GM, Aguirre GD, Aleman TS, et al. Continuing evaluation of gene therapy in the Rpe65 mutant dog. Invest Ophthalmol Vis Sci 2002;43:U1306.
53. Ali RR, Sarra GM, Stephens C, et al. Restoration of photoreceptor ultrastructure and function in retinal degeneration slow mice by gene therapy. Nat Genet 2000;25:306–310.
54. Sarra GM, Stephens C, De Alwis M, et al. Gene replacement therapy in the retinal degeneration slow (rds) mouse: the effect on retinal degeneration following partial transduction of the retina. Hum Mol Genet 2001;10:2353–2361.

55. Vollrath D, Feng W, Duncan JL, et al. Correction of the retinal dystrophy phenotype of the RCS rat by viral gene transfer of Mertk. Proc Natl Acad Sci USA 2001;98:12,584–12,589.
56. Peterson WA, Flannery JG, Hauswirth WW, et al. Enhanced survival of photoreceptors in P23H mutant rhodopsin transgenic rats by adeno-associated virus(AAV)-mediated delivery of neurotrophic genes. Inv Ophthalmol Vis Sci 1999;39:S1117 (Abstr.)
57. Liang FQ, Dejneka NS, Cohen DR, et al. AAV-mediated delivery of ciliary neurotrophic factor prolongs photoreceptor survival in the rhodopsin knockout mouse. Mol Ther 2001; 3:241–248.
58. Bok D, Yasumura D, Matthes MT, et al. Effects of adeno-associated virus-vectored ciliary neurotrophic factor on retinal structure and function in mice with a P216L rds/peripherin mutation. Exp Eye Res 2002;74:719–735.
59. Sanftner LH, Abel H, Hauswirth WW, Flannery JG. Glial Cell Line Derived Neurotrophic Factor Delays Photoreceptor Degeneration in a Transgenic Rat Model of Retinitis Pigmentosa. Mol Ther 2001;4:622–629.
60. Smith LE, Wesolowski E, McLellan A, et al. Oxygen-induced retinopathy in the mouse. Invest Ophthalmol Vis Sci 1994;35:101–111.
61. D'Amore PA. Mechanisms of retinal and choroidal neovascularization. Invest Ophthalmol Vis Sci 1994;35:3974–3979.
62. Ryan SJ. The development of an experimental model of subretinal neovascularization in disciform macular degeneration. Trans Am Ophthalmol Soc 1979;77:707–745.
63. Mousa SA, Lorelli W, Campochiaro PA. Role of hypoxia and extracellular matrix-integrin binding in the modulation of angiogenic growth factors secretion by retinal pigmented epithelial cells. J Cell Biochem 1999;74:135–143.
64. Shima DT, Gougos A, Miller JW, et al. Cloning and mRNA expression of vascular endothelial growth factor in ischemic retinas of *Macaca fascicularis*. Invest Ophthalmol Vis Sci 1996;37:1334–1340.
65. Pierce EA, Avery RL, Foley ED, Aiello LP, Smith LE. Vascular endothelial growth factor/vascular permeability factor expression in a mouse model of retinal neovascularization. Proc Natl Acad Sci USA 1995;92:905–909.
66. Stone J, Chan-Ling T, Pe'er J, Itin A, Gnessin H, Keshet E. Roles of vascular endothelial growth factor and astrocyte degeneration in the genesis of retinopathy of prematurity. Invest Ophthalmol Vis Sci 1996;37:290–299.
67. Adamis AP, Miller JW, Bernal MT, et al. Increased vascular endothelial growth factor levels in the vitreous of eyes with proliferative diabetic retinopathy. Am J Ophthalmol 1994; 118:445–450.
68. Aiello LP, Avery RL, Arrigg PG, et al. Vascular endothelial growth factor in ocular fluid of patients with diabetic retinopathy and other retinal disorders. N Engl J Med 1994; 331:1480–1487.
69. Boulton M, Gregor Z, McLeod D, et al. Intravitreal growth factors in proliferative diabetic retinopathy: correlation with neovascular activity and glycaemic management. Br J Ophthalmol 1997;81:228–233.
70. Kvanta A, Algvere PV, Berglin L, Seregard S. Subfoveal fibrovascular membranes in age-related macular degeneration express vascular endothelial growth factor. Invest Ophthalmol Vis Sci 1996;37:1929–1934.
71. Amin R, Puklin JE, Frank RN. Growth factor localization in choroidal neovascular membranes of age-related macular degeneration. Invest Ophthalmol Vis Sci 1994;35:3178–3188.
72. Frank RN, Amin RH, Eliott D, Puklin JE, Abrams GW. Basic fibroblast growth factor and vascular endothelial growth factor are present in epiretinal and choroidal neovascular membranes. Am J Ophthalmol 1996;122:393–403.
73. Lopez PF, Sippy BD, Lambert HM, Thach AB, Hinton DR. Transdifferentiated retinal pigment epithelial cells are immunoreactive for vascular endothelial growth factor in surgically

excised age-related macular degeneration-related choroidal neovascular membranes. Invest Ophthalmol Vis Sci 1996;37:855–868.
74. Yi X, Ogata N, Komada M, et al. Vascular endothelial growth factor expression in choroidal neovascularization in rats. Graefes Arch Clin Exp Ophthalmol 1997;235:313–319.
75. Ishibashi T, Hata Y, Yoshikawa H, Nakagawa K, Sueishi K, Inomata H. Expression of vascular endothelial growth factor in experimental choroidal neovascularization. Graefes Arch Clin Exp Ophthalmol 1997;235:159–167.
76. Krzystolik MG, Afshari MA, Adamis AP, et al. Prevention of experimental choroidal neovascularization with intravitreal anti-vascular endothelial growth factor antibody fragment. Arch Ophthalmol 2002;120:338–346.
77. O'Reilly MS, Boehm T, Shing Y, et al. Endostatin: an endogenous inhibitor of angiogenesis and tumor growth. Cell 1997:277–285.
78. Bunn HF, Poyton RO. Oxygen sensing and molecular adaptation to hypoxia. Physiol Rev 1996;76:839–885.
79. Forsythe JA, Jiang BH, Iyer NV, et al. Activation of vascular endothelial growth factor gene transcription by hypoxia-inducible factor 1. Mol Cell Biol 1996;16:4604–4613.
80. Gerber HP, Condorelli F, Park J, Ferrara N. Differential transcriptional regulation of the two vascular endothelial growth factor receptor genes. Flt-1, but not Flk-1/KDR, is up-regulated by hypoxia. J Biol Chem 1997;272:23,659–23,667.
81. Iyer NV, Kotch LE, Agani F, et al. Cellular and developmental control of O2 homeostasis by hypoxia-inducible factor 1 alpha. Genes Dev 1998;12:149–162.
82. Kendall RL, Thomas KA. Inhibition of vascular endothelial cell growth factor activity by an endogenously encoded soluble receptor. Proc Natl Acad Sci USA 1993;90:10,705–10,709.
83. Kendall RL, Wang G, Thomas KA. Identification of a natural soluble form of the vascular endothelial growth factor receptor, FLT-1, and its heterodimerization with KDR Biochem Biophys Res Commun 1996;226:324–328.
84. Bilodeau MT, Cunningham AM, Koester TJ, et al. Design and synthesis of 1,5-diarylbenzimidazoles as inhibitors of the VEGF-receptor KDR Bioorg Med Chem Lett 2003;13: 2485–2488.
85. Bilodeau MT, Rodman LD, McGaughey GB, et al. The discovery of N-(1,3-thiazol-2-yl) pyridin-2-amines as potent inhibitors of KDR kinase. Bioorg Med Chem Lett 2004;14: 2941–2945.
86. Fraley ME, Arrington KL, Hambaugh SR, et al. Discovery and evaluation of 3-(5-thien-3-ylpyridin-3-yl)-1H-indoles as a novel class of KDR kinase inhibitors. Bioorg Med Chem Lett 2003;13:2973–2976.
87. Sone H, Kawakami Y, Segawa T, et al. Effects of intraocular or systemic administration of neutralizing antibody against vascular endothelial growth factor on the murine experimental model of retinopathy. Life Sci 1999;65:2573–2580.
88. Adamis AP, Shima DT, Tolentino MJ, et al. Inhibition of vascular endothelial growth factor prevents retinal ischemia-associated iris neovascularization in a nonhuman primate. Arch Ophthalmol 1996;114:66–71.
89. Berdugo M, Valamanesh F, Andrieu C, et al. Delivery of antisense oligonucleotide to the cornea by iontophoresis. Antisense Nucleic Acid Drug Dev 2003;13:107–114.
90. Lai CM, Spilsbury K, Brankov M, Zaknich T, Rakoczy PE. Inhibition of corneal neovascularization by recombinant adenovirus mediated antisense VEGF RNA Exp Eye Res 75:625–634.
91. The Eyetech Study Group. Preclinical and phase 1A clinical evaluation of an anti-VEGF pegylated aptamer (EYE001) for the treatment of exudative age-related macular degeneration. Retina 2002;22:143–152.
92. Bold G, Altmann KH, Frei J, et al. New anilinophthalazines as potent and orally well absorbed inhibitors of the VEGF receptor tyrosine kinases useful as antagonists of tumor-driven angiogenesis. J Med Chem 2000;43:2310–2323.

93. Aiello LP, Bursell SE, Clermont A, et al. Vascular endothelial growth factor-induced retinal permeability is mediated by protein kinase C in vivo and suppressed by an orally effective beta-isoform-selective inhibitor. Diabetes 1997;46:1473–1480.
94. Robinson GS, Pierce EA, Rook SL, Foley E, Webb R, Smith LE. Oligodeoxynucleotides inhibit retinal neovascularization in a murine model of proliferative retinopathy. Proc Natl Acad Sci USA 1996;93:4851–4856.
95. Ferrara N. Role of vascular endothelial growth factor in physiologic and pathologic angiogenesis: therapeutic implications. Semin Oncol 2002;29:10–14.
96. Ferrara N, Gerber HP. The role of vascular endothelial growth factor in angiogenesis. Acta Haematol 2001;106:148–156.
97. Tombran-Tink J, Chader GG, Johnson LV. PEDF: a pigment epithelium-derived factor with potent neuronal differentiative activity [letter]. Exp Eye Res 1991;53:411–414.
98. Reichel MB, Ali RR, Thrasher AJ, Hunt DM, Bhattacharya SS, Baker D. Immune responses limit adenovirally mediated gene expression in the adult mouse eye. Gene Ther 1998;5:1038–1046.
99. Auricchio A, Rivera VM, Clackson T, et al. Pharmacological regulation of protein expression from adeno-associated viral vectors in the eye. Mol Ther 2002;6:238–242.
100. McGee Sanftner LH, Rendahl KG, Quiroz D, et al. Recombinant AAV-mediated delivery of a tet-inducible reporter gene to the rat retina. Mol Ther 2001;3:688–696.
101. Nicklin SA, Buening H, Dishart KL, et al. Efficient and selective AAV2-mediated gene transfer directed to human vascular endothelial cells. Mol Ther 2001;4:174–181.
102. Muller OJ, Kaul F, Weitzman MD, et al. Random peptide libraries displayed on adeno-associated virus to select for targeted gene therapy vectors. Nat Biotechnol 2003;21: 1040–1046.
103. Asahara T, Masuda H, Takahashi T, et al. Bone marrow origin of endothelial progenitor cells responsible for postnatal vasculogenesis in physiological and pathological neovascularization. Circ Res 1999;85:221–228.
104. Noden DM. Embryonic origins and assembly of blood vessels. Am Rev Respir Dis 1989;140:1097–1103.
105. Choi K. Hemangioblast development and regulation. Biochem Cell Biol 1998;76:947–956.
106. Grant MB, May WS, Caballero S, et al. Adult hematopoietic stem cells provide functional hemangioblast activity during retinal neovascularization. Nat Med 2002;8:607–612.
107. Friedlander M, Theesfeld CL, Sugita M, et al. Involvement of integrins alpha v beta 3 and alpha v beta 5 in ocular neovascular diseases. Proc Natl Acad Sci USA 1996;93:9764–9769.
108. Luna J, Tobe T, Mousa SA, Reilly TM, Campochiaro PA. Antagonists of integrin alpha v beta 3 inhibit retinal neovascularization in a murine model. Lab Invest 1996;75:563–573.
109. Beck L Jr, D'Amore PA. Vascular development: cellular and molecular regulation. FASEB J 1997;11:365–373.
110. Kirsch M, Schackert G, Black PM. Angiogenesis, metastasis, and endogenous inhibition. J Neurooncol 2000;50:173–180.
111. Cao Y. Endogenous angiogenesis inhibitors and their therapeutic implications. Int J Biochem Cell Biol 2001;33:357–369.
112. Lucas R, Holmgren L, Garcia I, et al. Multiple forms of angiostatin induce apoptosis in endothelial cells. Blood 1998;92:4730–4741.
113. Griscelli F, Li H, Bennaceur-Griscelli A, Soria J, et al. Angiostatin gene transfer: inhibition of tumor growth in vivo by blockage of endothelial cell proliferation associated with a mitosis arrest. Proc Natl Acad Sci USA 1998;95:6367–6372.
114. OReilly MS, Holmgren L, Chen C, Folkman J. Angiostatin induces and sustains dormancy of human primary tumors in mice. Nat Med 1996;2:689–692.
115. Wu ZG, OReilly MS, Folkman J, Shing Y. Suppression of tumor growth with recombinant murine angiostatin. BBRC 1997;236:651–654.

116. Gao G, Li Y, Gee S, et al. Down-regulation of vascular endothelial growth factor and up-regulation of pigment epithelium-derived factor: a possible mechanism for the anti-angiogenic activity of plasminogen kringle 5. J Biol Chem 2002;277:9492–9497.
117. Steele FR, Chader GJ, Johnson LV, Tombran-Tink J. Pigment epithelium-derived factor: neurotrophic activity and identification as a member of the serine protease inhibitor gene family. Proc Natl Acad Sci USA 1993;90:1526–1530.
118. Becerra SP. Structure-function studies on PEDF A noninhibitory serpin with neurotrophic activity. Adv Exp Med Biol 1997;425:223–237.
119. Araki T, Taniwaki T, Becerra SP, Chader GJ, Schwartz JP. Pigment epithelium-derived factor (PEDF) differentially protects immature but not mature cerebellar granule cells against apoptotic cell death. J Neurosci Res 1998;53:7–15.
120. Cayouette M, Smith SB, Becerra SP, Gravel C. Pigment epithelium-derived factor delays the death of photoreceptors in mouse models of inherited retinal degenerations. Neurobiol Dis 1999;6:523–532.
121. Rasmussen H, Chu KW, Campochiaro P, et al. Clinical protocol. An open-label, phase I, single administration, dose- escalation study of ADGVPEDF11D (ADPEDF) in neovascular age-related macular degeneration (AMD). Hum Gene Ther 2001;12:2029–2032.
122. Zatterstrom UK, Felbor U, Fukai N, Olsen BR. Collagen XVIII/endostatin structure and functional role in angiogenesis. Cell Struct Funct 2000;25:97–101.
123. Nguyen JT. Adeno-associated virus and other potential vectors for angiostatin and endostatin gene therapy. Adv Exp Med Biol 2000;465:457–466.
124. Takahashi K, Saishin Y, Saishin Y, et al. Intraocular expression of endostatin reduces VEGF-induced retinal vascular permeability, neovascularization, and retinal detachment. FASEB J 2003;17:896–898.
125. Noma H, Funatsu H, Yamashita H, Kitano S, Mishima HK, Hori S. Regulation of angiogenesis in diabetic retinopathy: possible balance between vascular endothelial growth factor and endostatin. Arch Ophthalmol 2002;120:1075–1080.
126. Auricchio A, Behling KC, Maguire AM, et al. Inhibition of retinal neovascularization by intraocular viral-mediated delivery of anti-angiogenic agents. Mol Ther 2002;6:490–494.
127. Bainbridge JW, Mistry A, De Alwis M, et al. Inhibition of retinal neovascularisation by gene transfer of soluble VEGF receptor sFlt-1. Gene Ther 2002;9:320–326.
128. Lai CM, Brankov M, Zaknich T, et al. Inhibition of angiogenesis by adenovirus-mediated sFlt-1 expression in a rat model of corneal neovascularization. Hum Gene Ther 2001;12: 1299–1310.
129. Bainbridge JW, Jia H, Bagherzadeh A, Selwood D, Ali RR, Zachary I. A peptide encoded by exon 6 of VEGF (EG3306) inhibits VEGF-induced angiogenesis in vitro and ischaemic retinal neovascularisation in vivo. Biochem Biophys Res Commun 2003;302:793–799.
130. Jia HY, Jezequel S, Lohr M, et al. Peptides encoded by exon 6 of VEGF inhibit endothelial cell biological responses and angiogenesis induced by VEGF. Biochem Biophys Res Commun 2001;283:164–173.

21
Noninvasive Delivery of DNA Into the Eye

John M. Nickerson, PhD, R. Keith Shuler, Jr., MD,
John B. Davies, MD, Phyllis K. Dioguardi, MD,
Steven M. Wolchok, MD, Vincent T. Ciavatta, PhD,
Jeffrey H. Boatright, PhD, and Henry F. Edelhauser, PhD

CONTENTS

INTRODUCTION

This article reviews and summarizes recent promising findings *(1–3)* from our laboratories showing that DNA, despite its large size and mass, can be transported through pores in the sclera and delivered into the interior of the eye. We speculate that these approaches may be modified to deliver large amounts of therapeutic DNAs into retinal pigment epithelium (RPE) cells, neurosensory retinal cells, and many other cells in the eye.

We hypothesized that a continuum of connected pores exists in the sclera through which naked DNA or submicroscopic particles can pass. This hypothesis was based on the delivery of charged drugs into the cornea and skin by iontophoresis, and the delivery of lipophilic drugs into the anterior chamber by passive diffusion. We tested this hypothesis by (1) electrophoretically but noninvasively forcing various forms of DNA through preparations of human sclera from which Tenon's capsule and the choroid-RPE-retina had been removed, (2) passive diffusion of oligonucleotides across the same preparation, (3) electrophoresis of dyes into an isolated intact mouse globe, forcing dyes into the interior of the eye, and (4) electrophoresis of a plasmid, which expressed a fluorescent protein in an eye of a living mouse.

Delivery Strategies to Posterior Segment

An important consideration in ocular gene therapy is the delivery of therapeutic agents to specific tissues within the eye. We review here tests of whether the sclera is a

From: *Ophthalmology: Ocular Angiogenesis: Diseases, Mechanisms, and Therapeutics*
Edited by: J. Tombran-Tink and C. J. Barnstable © Humana Press Inc., Totowa, NJ

barrier to efficient delivery of DNA to the posterior segment. Several approaches are being considered, including ocular injection, systemic injection, surface applicants, and electric fields to deliver genes to the eye. The DNA being delivered may be "naked," conjugated to transfection agents such as liposomal agents, or packaged in hobbled viruses (for reviews, *see* refs. *4–6*). Achieving adequate levels of therapeutic agents in the posterior segment has been difficult by topical application *(7–9)*. Intraocular administration via intravitreal injections or surgical implantation of intraocular sustained-release devices are effective in achieving therapeutic drug levels, but due to their invasive nature, these methods carry risk for significant complications. Ocular injections are routinely performed in the clinic in order to deliver a drug to a target tissue. Such an injection may cause direct tissue damage by the needle and may result in infection or inflammatory responses. Repeated intravitreal injections are required for chronic diseases and have the potential complications of retinal detachment, endophthalmitis, vitreous hemorrhage, and cataract formation *(10)*. Surgical implantation of intraocular sustained-release devices, such as the Vitrasert ganciclovir implant used in the treatment of cytomegalovirus, avoids repeated injections *(11,12)*. However, periodic intraocular surgery is required to insert and replace these implants. Surgical placement and removal carries the risk of complications similar to those associated with intravitreal injection *(11,12)*. Systemic administration can deliver drugs to the posterior eye, but the systemic levels necessary to penetrate the blood–retinal barrier are often associated with dose-limiting side effects and toxicity *(13)*. The dilution of the preparation through systemic administration remains problematic. Systemic administration may require viral *(14,15)* or pegylated liposomal *(16)* packaging of therapeutic DNA constructs for ocular targeting and treatment. Delivering bioactive agents to the posterior segment either across the sclera or via intrascleral injection may prevent many complications associated with intraocular delivery as well as limit systemic toxicity.

DNA Delivery Strategies

Many techniques to deliver large DNA fragments (entire genes or cDNAs) have been developed: DNA compaction, liposomes, viruses, hydrodynamic pressure, biolistic delivery, and many other inventive delivery approaches have been successful to some degree. Each approach has benefits and drawbacks. Various forms of viral packaging are thought to have resulted in adverse reactions in humans, including immune responses in the eye *(17,18)*, leukemia-like symptoms *(19,20)*, or death *(21,22)*. Adeno-associated virus (AAV)-mediated DNA delivery appears to have fewer side effects *(17)* and has been used to rescue vision in some animal models of blindness *(23–27)*. However, AAV delivery may require direct ocular injection to achieve efficacy *(4)*. Further, the randomness of integration of the therapeutic DNA inserts in the genome following recombinant AAV infection is of concern *(28)*. Topical application (eyedrops) of therapeutic DNA is noninvasive and can be given repeatedly. It has been used to deliver virally packaged DNA in treatment of excimer laser-induced corneal haze *(29)*, but seems unlikely to be able to deliver DNA to posterior segment targets. Retrobulbar or periocular injections may be a viable option *(30)*. Stechschulte and coworkers *(31)* injected a plasmid containing the flt-1 cDNA into the stroma of the cornea, which expressed flt-1, a soluble VEGF receptor, and achieved inhibition of VEGF-induced neovascularization. They concluded that

(1) the cornea was a readily accessible target for gene therapy, and (2) naked DNA injected into the corneal stroma was an effective method to deliver, transfect, and express a gene in therapeutic doses.

Oligonucleotide-Based Therapies

Experimental strategies that use oligonucleotides are under active investigation as potential treatments for human eye diseases. Some of these strategies include antisense *(32)*, genoplasty *(33)*, RNAi *(34)*, and ribozyme technologies *(35)*.

Electric Fields Induce Electrotransfer

A completely different delivery modality is available for ocular gene therapy. This approach takes advantage of the fact that DNA is highly charged at neutral pH and can be driven through sieves such as agarose or even high concentrations of tightly crosslinked polyacrylamide in electric fields. Tough but pliable tissues often possess an architecture of spongy material having numerous pores throughout a matrix. These pores may interconnect, forming sieve-like channels extending through the tissue. Aqueous channels supported by such a structural framework are thought to explain transcorneal and transdermal delivery of small charged compounds in several animal models *(36–45)*. These successes in cornea and skin suggest that electric fields should drive DNA across the sclera, as the latter exhibits a similar porous morphology.

It is useful to distinguish among the terms electroporation, iontophoresis, and electrophoresis as applied to DNA delivery. Electroporation employs a high field-strength, short-duration pulse of electricity to reversibly create holes in the plasma membrane of a cell. Once a pore is opened, by diffusion, nearby molecules may cross into the cell through the transient pore. This technique is commonly used in the laboratory to introduce DNAs into cultured eukaryotic cells, bacteria, tissue explants, and living animals. It has been highly successful in the rat eye following subretinal injection of a plasmid DNA *(46)*. Electroporation is not electrotransfer and does not cause significant bulk or net movement of DNA, and the DNA must be positioned immediately adjacent to a cell that is to be transfected.

Electroporation should be contrasted with two electrotransfer approaches that do cause a substantial net and directional movement of DNA. These two methods are iontophoresis and electrophoresis. Iontophoresis is the introduction into and replacement of ions in tissues mediated by an electric field. Usually the bulk of the current is carried by a charged drug itself as other ions such as those of buffers or physiological salts such as NaCl would reduce the number of drug ions delivered. This is in contrast to electrophoresis, in which several buffer constituents are used to maintain a discrete band of one analyte (CF, a short DNA) migrating at a velocity different from another analyte (CF, a longer DNA). A low-voltage, constant-current electric field (iontophoresis) is commonly used clinically to drive charged molecules across tissue layers (notably the skin) *(47)*. Previously, it was common practice in ophthalmology *(48)*, and now is being reintroduced into the clinic *(49,50)*. Electrophoresis is defined as the movement of charged molecules under the influence of an electric field through a liquid medium in a porous support (which can take on many forms, including agarose, polyacrylamide, paper, and others). This approach is most often used in the laboratory as an analytical or preparative bench science technique rather than a clinical delivery approach.

Pores Through the Sclera

The corneal stroma and the sclera are similar in that their main constituents are intermingled layers of bundled collagen fibers, with an occasional fibroblast. The water content of the sclera in adults is 65 to 75%, apparently providing ample aqueous volume for transscleral drug delivery and depot *(51,52)*. These similarities suggest that intra- or transscleral transit would be just as effective as intracorneal transit. The scleral permeability of drugs is well-established (reviewed in refs. *53–57)*. A continuum of pores is thought to be the most likely route *(49,58,59)*. The pores may be quite large, as molecules such as IgGs and serum albumin can diffuse across the sclera *(60)*. Charge properties may affect the permeability *(61)*. These studies establish that many classes and sizes of agents can diffuse through sclera pores. Our experiments test the hypothesis that (1) nucleic acids under the influence of an electric field should migrate though these scleral pores, (2) the pores are large enough for plasmid-sized DNAs, (3) the fibers making up the matrix do not irreversibly bind the nucleic acids or interfere with flow of the DNA through the pores, and (4) nucleic acids may pass through the same pores by passive diffusion.

Modeling DNA Mass Transfer Across the Sclera

Here we review the testing of two ocular DNA delivery schemes for potential use in humans. We investigated whether nucleic acids in any of several forms and sizes can be delivered across human sclera by a constant-voltage electric field (i.e., by electrophoresis). Also, we report here new findings that show the migration of dyes and oligonucleotides into an intact globe in vitro and *in situ*. These same dyes are frequently used in DNA gel electrophoreses as indicators of DNA migration through a given sieving medium.

EXPERIMENTS REVIEWED

In experiment 1, we began by asking whether we could transfer bulk amounts of DNA across only the sclera, and we continued by asking whether the DNA was intact. Experiments 1 and 2 were conducted with cadaveric human sclera to assure that the same thickness and pore characteristics of sclera would be tested as those that might be found in human patients. Conventional molecular biological equipment and methods for analyzing DNA were adapted to test whether dyes or DNAs of various sizes could be driven across human sclera. Experiment 3 employed an intact excised mouse eye, and experiment 4 tested the delivery of a fluorescently tagged oligonucleotide into the eye of a living mouse. Our results raise the prospect of treating the interior of the eye with potentially therapeutic DNAs encoding proteins that could cure genetically inherited diseases or treat other eye diseases for which no alternative treatments exist, including glaucoma, macular degeneration, diabetic retinopathy, and cataracts. The central hypothesis of these studies is that the sclera, despite its durability and strength, has many microscopic to molecular-scale water-filled pores throughout it. The pores allow the sclera to behave as a hydrophilic network of fibers like a regular meshwork. The hypothesized scleral pores appear large enough for nucleic acids up to plasmid sizes to pass through under the influence of an electric field. We expect a continuum of small scleral pores reaching from the outside surface to the choroid. Experiment 1 investigated electrotransfer of dyes and DNAs through the hypothesized channels in the sclera.

Experimental Systems and Methods

In experiment 2 we model the behavior of the sclera in a modified Ussing chamber that allows passive diffusion of drugs or DNA from an upper chamber into a lower chamber. From the lower chamber, the contents are periodically collected and the concentration of the drug or DNA is measured. The permeability of the agent is calculated according to a simple mass transfer equation *(2)* by calculating the permeability constant, K_{trans} (cm/s), using the following equation:

$$K_{trans} = (R_{total}/(A \times t)) \times (1/D)$$

where R_{total} is the total moles transferred through the sclera in time t (s), A represents the surface area of the sclera (cm^2), and D is the initial concentration of the solution in the donor chamber (mol/mL).

The cadaveric sclera is a valid and important model, as (1) human tissue is the ultimate long-term treatment target; (2) in many ways, except for the density and thickness contributed by collagen fibers, there are relatively few fundamental differences in scleral tissues ranging in age from embryonic to adult *(62)*; (3) from a practical standpoint, experiments 1 and 2 enable us to simply, easily, and rapidly test many experimental variants and parameters with human tissue that might otherwise go to waste. The size of the human scleral rectangles makes them easy to manipulate, speeding up the prototyping process. The more prototyping we do in experiments 1 and 2, the more impact is obtained in developing electric fields as an effective therapeutic treatment.

In experiment 4, we modeled the live *in situ* eye with a simpler model (an intact but excised eye), having several obvious stipulated differences: (1) In the apparatus, current flow may pass only through the removed globe or along surface moisture and cannot pass through the normally attached tissues such as the extraorbital muscles, optic nerve, or capsular connecting tissues (which are removed during dissection). (2) The current can no longer "short-circuit" through extraocular muscles, extraocular tissues, optic nerve, and other tissues to the grounding electrode. (3) There is no perfusion through the blood supply, and the cells of the eye are dying because of hypoxia in the experimental apparatus. Despite these caveats, this experimental system provides a simple, fast, and robust experimental apparatus to determine how to best drive DNA across an experimentally manageable number of eye-specific discrete barriers in a simple approach to DNA delivery to the RPE—in other words, as we become successful in passing DNA through a single barrier, we subsequently add additional layers, one at a time.

RESULTS

Experiment 1: Electrophoresis of DNA Through Sclera

Figure 1 (from ref. *1*) illustrates the experimental apparatus. Conventional molecular biological equipment and methods for analyzing DNA were adapted to test whether DNAs of various sizes could be driven across the sclera. Figures 2 and 3 show typical results from the electrophoresis of dyes and DNAs of differing sizes through human sclera. (The movie version of Fig. 2 can be viewed at http://www.molvis.org/molvis/v9/a69/davies-fig2.html.)

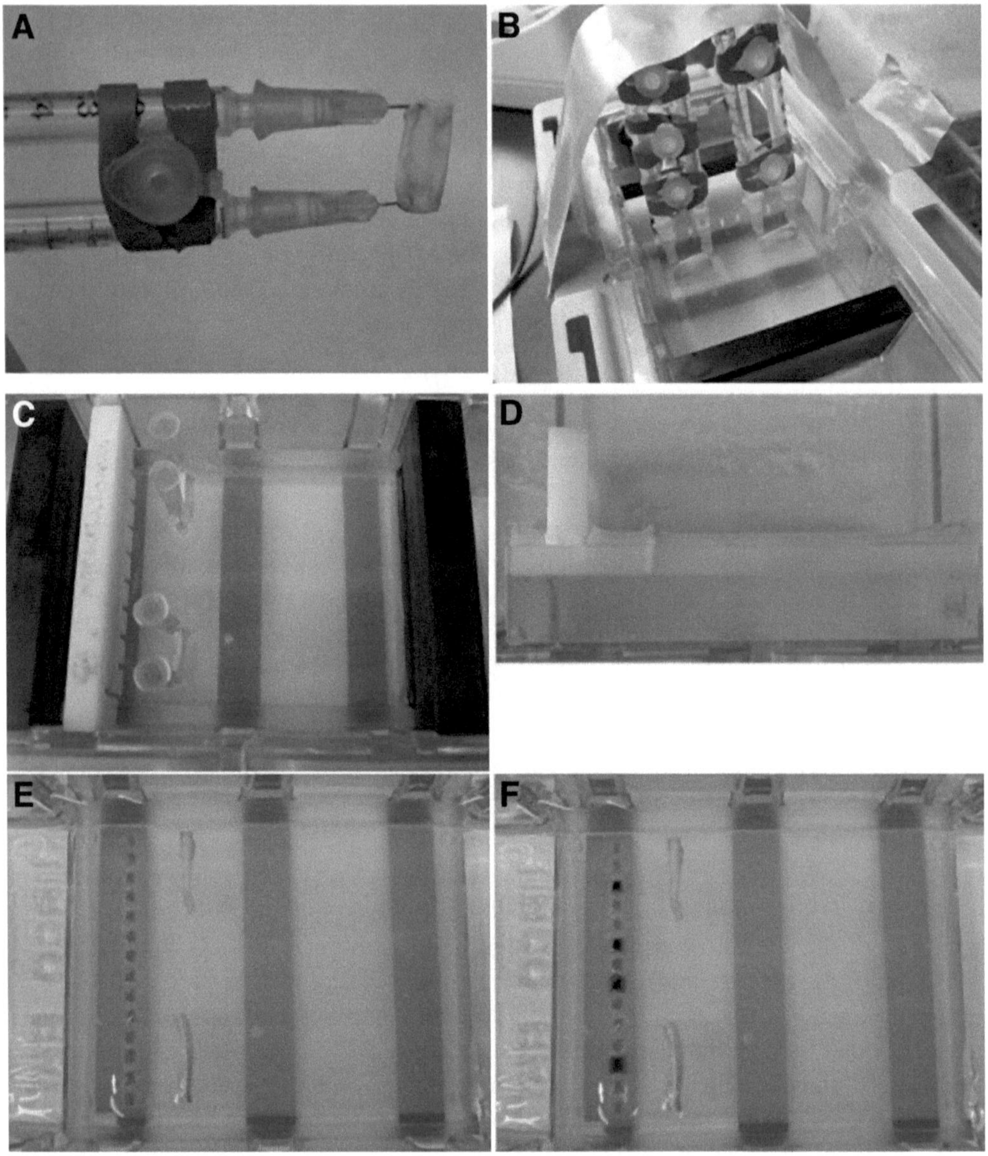

Fig. 1. Transscleral electrophoresis (TSE) experimental apparatus. The arrangement and assembly of human cadaveric scleral fragments in an agarose gel apparatus is shown in **A** through **F**. (**A**) Mounting the scleral fragments on syringe needles before embedding in agarose. (**B**) Securing the mounted scleral fragments during agarose gel solidification. (**C**) Removal of the syringe supports. (**D**) Side view of the embedded scleral fragments. Note the plastic boosts elevating the gel comb. (**E**) Top view of the embedded scleral fragments. (**F**) Loaded DNA and dyes prior to electrophoresis. (Reproduced with permission from ref. *1*.) *See* color version on companion CD.

DNAs (ranging from ~50 bp to 12 kb long) passed through the sclera in the electric field (Fig. 3). The DNAs were recovered after passage through the sclera nearly quantitatively. The mobility of the smaller double-stranded DNA fragments is largely unaffected. In larger fragments, from about 400 bp and higher, mobility is reduced in

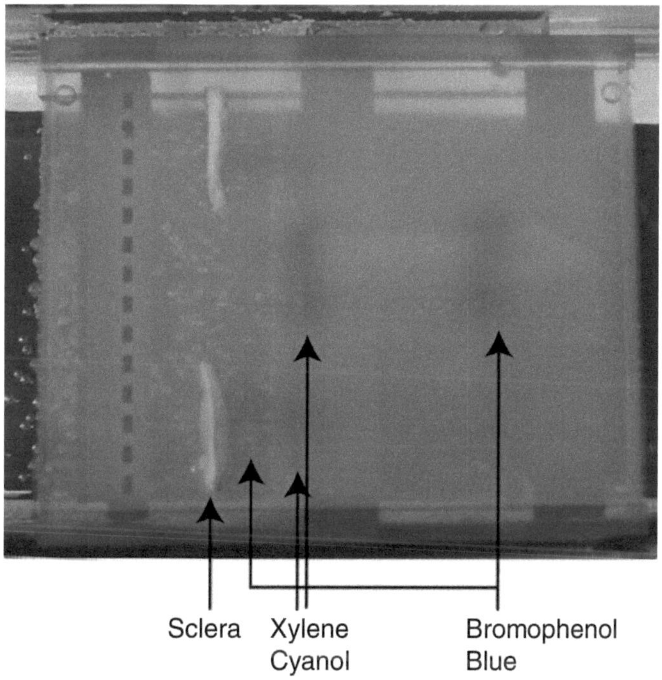

Fig. 2. Electrophoresis of charged dyes through human sclera. Rectangular fragments of human cadaveric sclera were mounted vertically in a horizontal gel electrophoresis chamber. The tissue samples were oriented with the outside eye surface facing and closest to the gel wells. Two percent agarose was poured into the gel chamber and allowed to solidify, which embedded the sclera and formed wells. The agarose contained 1X TAE buffer (40 m*M* Tris-acetate, 1 m*M* EDTA, pH 8.0). Bromophenol blue and xylene cyanol in 1X TAE buffer and 10% glycerol were loaded into well positions 3, 6, 8, and 12. Two samples (lanes 6 and 8 from the top down) were unimpeded by sclera, and two other wells (lanes 3 and 12) were completely occluded by human scleral fragments. The samples were subjected to an electric field of 3.3 V/cm for 114 min, and digital photographs were taken every 3 min during electrophoresis. The final picture of the series is shown (**A**). The 39 pictures of the run are shown in sequence as a movie (**B**). Lanes 6 and 8 show that bromophenol blue migrated roughly twice as quickly (about 4 cm/h) as xylene cyanol (about 2 cm/h) when unimpeded by sclera. Lanes 3 and 12 show that bromophenol blue ran into the sclera first, but its passage was slowed or delayed in this encounter while xylene cyanol met the sclera second. Xylene cyanol in lanes 3 and 12 appeared to pass through the sclera relatively unimpeded except for some band spreading when compared to the movement of xylene cyanol in control lanes 6 and 8 that lacked the scleral obstacle. After the xylene cyanol passed through the sclera, bromophenol blue was observed slowly appearing in agarose on the inner side of the scleral face. The movie (**B**) illustrates that the dyes were not migrating around the sclera. Bromophenol blue was retained and slowly passed through human sclera while a different dye, xylene cyanol, simultaneously passed through the same scleral fragments with minor band spreading and nearly the same migration rate as xylene cyanol through agarose alone. (Reproduced with permission from ref. *1*.) *See* color version on companion CD.

proportion to the size of the DNA. Figure 2 illustrates that the DNAs were not migrating around the sclera: Bromophenol blue was retained in the sclera and slowly passed through, whereas xylene cyanol simultaneously passed through the same scleral fragment with minor band spreading and nearly the same migration rate as xylene cyanol

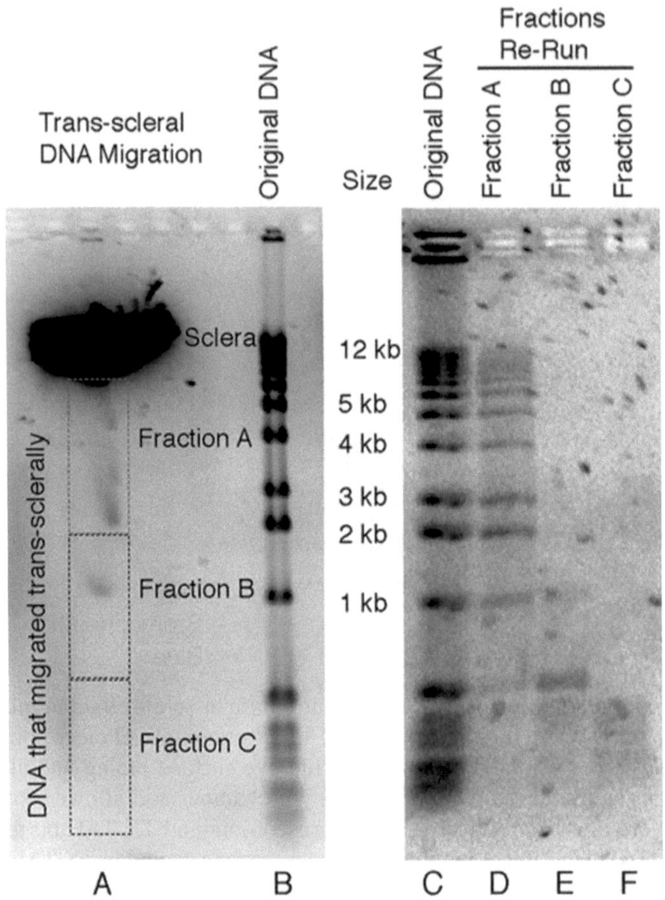

Fig. 3. Electrophoresis of linear double-stranded DNA fragments through the sclera. Typical results from the electrophoresis of DNA of differing sizes through human sclera. DNA (ranging from approx 50 bp to 12 kb long) passed through the sclera in the electric field. This experiment was repeated five times; data shown are representative. Lane A shows a DNA ladder (1 kb ladder; Invitrogen, Carlsbad, CA) that passed through the sclera. Lane B shows the same DNA ladder unimpeded by sclera. The lane A material that had passed through the sclera was retrieved in three fractions labeled fractions A, B, and C, as illustrated by the dotted lines (the fraction A box is in red to indicate the upper boundary of the excised gel, which was about 2 mm downstream of the scleral fragment). The DNA from each agarose gel fragment was recovered and analyzed on a second gel. Wells D, E, and F were loaded with DNA extracted from fractions A, B, and C, respectively. The original DNA ladder is shown in lane C. There was no scleral tissue in fraction A. Fraction A (lane D) shows that DNA as large as 12 kbp migrated through the sclera. The mobility of the smaller double-stranded DNA fragments is largely unaffected. In larger fragments, from about 400 bp and greater, mobility is reduced in proportion to the size of the DNA. (Reproduced with permission from ref. *1*.) *See* color version on companion CD.

through agarose. In other experiments *(1)* we demonstrated the passage of single-stranded DNAs of 43 to 51 nucleotides in length, RNA–DNA double-hairpin oligonucleotides, and a plasmid 3 kb in length. The essential point is that therapeutic-sized DNAs passed through the human sclera quickly and near-quantitatively (Fig. 3).

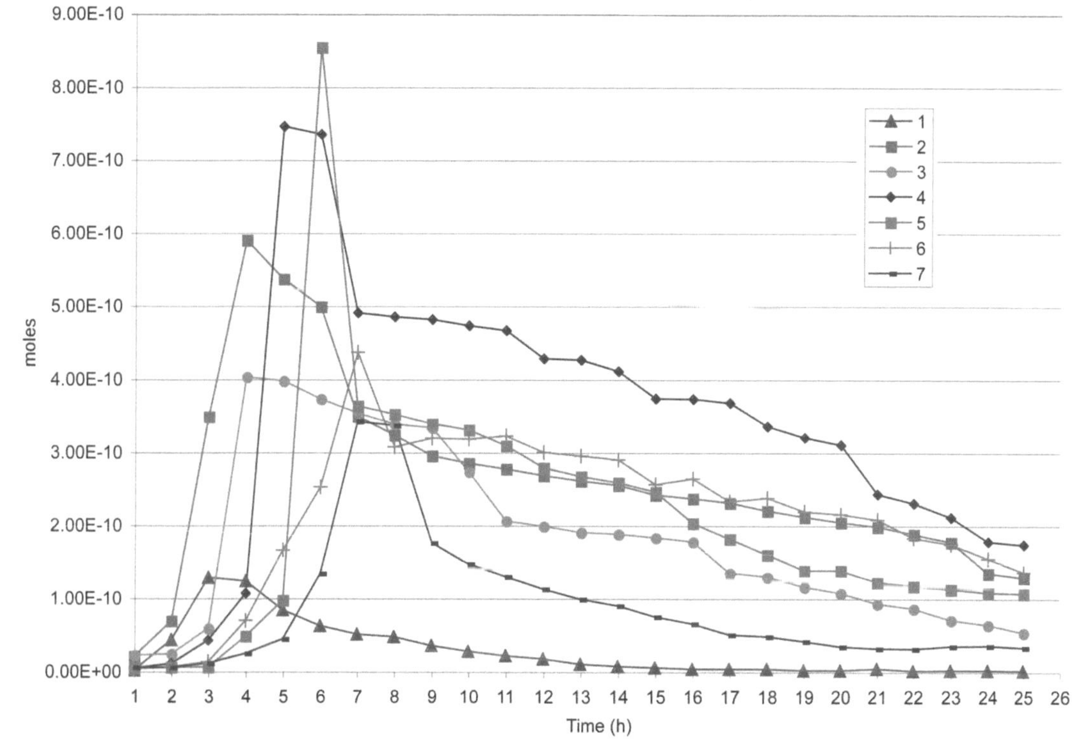

Fig. 4. Transscleral diffusion of a fluorescently end-labeled oligonucleotide. An oligonucleotide was end-labeled with fluorescein The DNA was placed on the external surface of a scleral fragment from which the conjunctiva, choroid, retinal pigment epithelium, and sensory retina had been removed. Care was taken to avoid sclera having vortex veins or the posterior pole. The DNA diffused through the sclera and was collected on the choroidal side of the sclera. Samples were collected hourly for 24 h. Fluorescence measurements were used to determine the amount of DNA in each fraction. This figure illustrates the oligonucleotide diffusion versus time. A maximum was reached at about 5 h after initiating diffusion. The data suggest that the DNA passively diffused a small but significant distance through a porous scleral matrix of fibers. The means of seven independent determinations are shown. The error bars represent the standard error of the mean. *See* color version on companion CD.

Experiment 2: Permeability of Sclera to Oligonucleotides

Shuler et al. *(2)* conducted permeability studies of oligonucleotides traversing the sclera by diffusional processes. In these experiments, sclera was clamped between two Silgard rings in a two-chamber apparatus. DNA solution was placed in the upper chamber and the fluid in the lower chamber was periodically collected and assayed for DNA that had diffused through the sclera. The results indicate that there is a continuum of pores allowing a small single-stranded DNA to pass through the sclera. The permeability, albeit low, is clearly measurable and consistent with the Stoke's radius of the DNA. This suggests that the collagen fibers making up the sclera do not bind DNA or have limited binding capacity. The diffusible nature suggests that the pores are large in comparison to the molecular radius of the oligonucleotide. Figure 4, from ref. *(2)*, shows the transscleral diffusion of the naked, single-stranded, fluorescein-labeled oligonucleotide as a function of time. The permeability constant or K_{trans} for the transscleral diffusion of the naked, single-stranded, fluorescein-labeled oligonucleotide was $7.67 \pm 1.8 \times 10^{-7}$ cm/s (mean ± SEM, $N = 7$). After 24 h, 21.93 ± 5.44% of the total amount of oligonucleotide had diffused across the sclera, leaving approximately 3.35 ± 1.18% in the sclera itself and 12.94 ± 4.31% in the donor chamber (mean ± SEM).

Experiment 3: Electrophoresis of Intact Mouse Globe

Figure 5 shows an apparatus containing a freshly harvested mouse eye. Xylene cyanol was electrophoresed into and through the eye. The eye is mounted with the cornea facing forward and the fundus is observed until xylene cyanol is carried into the cornea. At that point, the entire eye is seen to contain blue color by dissection and by examination of unstained frozen sections (Fig. 6), which show blue color though the entire eye, suggesting that most of the eye can be electrophoretically filled with a charged molecule such as this dye. We expect that DNA and RNA, because they are highly charged, will migrate into the same interstitial spaces as well.

Experiment 4: Transscleral Iontophoresis In Vivo

We have gained some experience with transscleral iontophoresis in living mice. In Fig. 7A, a pipet tip with a platinum wire running its length is filled with buffer containing DNA. This is placed against the posterior sclera and a current is applied through the wire. As shown in Fig. 7B, the DNA sequesters in the retina, including all the layers, and the plasmid, p70-EGFP, is expressed in all these neuronal layers as fluoresecence is detected in these locations. Because this eye was from a pigmented mouse, it was not possible to assess whether the plasmid is within the RPE.

DISCUSSION

These reports *(1–3)* and additional data that are summarized here establish that charged dyes and nucleic acids pass through human sclera when driven by an electric field. Transscleral mobility in the electric field was monitored in simple apparatuses. The voltage and current used in these experiments are probably higher than what would be possible in human treatment, but here the emphasis was to show that an electrical field could, in principle, be used to transport charged molecules through the sclera. Future experiments are planned at more physiological conditions.

It seems remarkable that large molecules can readily pass through the sclera. Many investigators have delivered small drugs (<1,000 Daltons) through the cornea or sclera. With succeeding reports, investigators have considered the behavior of larger molecules. Ambati et al. *(54,60)* delivered molecules of about 150,000 Daltons. In our studies *(1–3)*, we delivered DNA up to about 8 million Daltons.

Several approaches have been used to drive materials across the sclera. For example, Ambati et al. *(63)* implanted an osmotic pump to provide a long-term high concentration source of material for diffusion across the sclera. This technique, however, is invasive (requiring surgical implantation) and carries the potential for infection. Many other approaches have been considered elsewhere *(61,64–66)*.

Our studies *(1–3)* support the hypothesis that the sclera has many microscopic to molecular-scale, water-filled pores *(67)*. The pores allow the sclera to behave as a

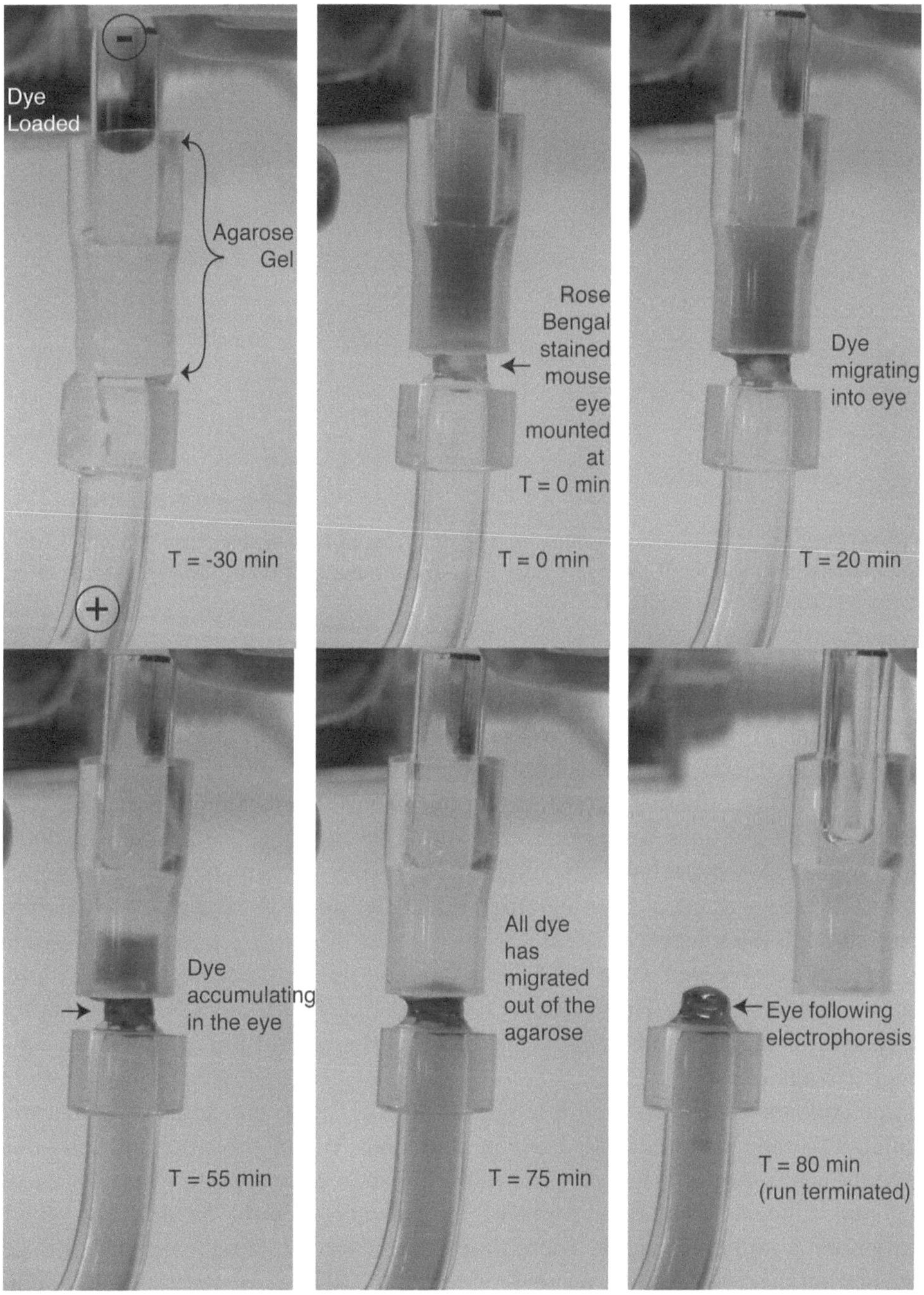

Fig. 5. Transscleral electrophoresis of xylene cyanol through an intact mouse eye. Xylene cyanol was electrophoresed through about 1 cm of agarose and then through an intact mouse globe. Current flowed through the eye as indicated by the absence of dye in the upper reservior at the 80 min time point when the run was terminated. Dye was found within the eye in all tissues by inspection during gross dissection. Cryosections showed dye throughout the thickness of the sclera, choroid, retinal pigment epithelium, and neural retina. Electrophoretic conditions were similar to those employed in transscleral electrophoresis of human sclera in Figs. 1–3, about 3 V/cm, in 1X TAE buffer. *See* color version on companion CD.

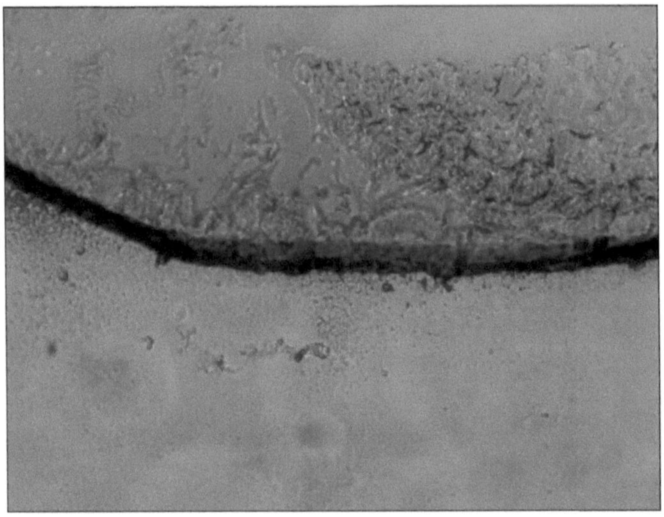

Fig. 6. Cryosection of an unstained mouse eye. The bluish-violet color derives from the transocular electrophoresis of the dye xylene cyanol from the outside of the eye into the interior. *See* color version on companion CD.

hydrophilic network of fibers. In an electric field, DNA easily passes through the sieve that constitutes the majority of the sclera.

Davies et al. *(1)* did not detect any major differences among sclera from different ages or among scleral fragments from different parts of the eye, suggesting that the approach should be effective, robust, and applicable in many patient populations.

Small oligonucleotides were electrotransferred through the sclera. Both the double-hairpin RNA–DNA hybrid and the single-stranded DNA fragment passed through the sclera under the influence of an electric field. The mobility of the oligonucleotides passing through the sclera was slightly slower versus their respective unimpeded counterparts, and we observed extra band spreading and tailing when compared with their unimpeded counterparts. These findings suggest that DNA and RNA have approximately similar electrophoretic mobility through the scleral pores versus migration through 2% agarose.

Large and small DNAs passed through the scleral fragments, suggesting that many potentially therapeutic nucleic acids, even large ones, can be electrophoretically delivered to the interior of human eyes. The relatively short time span for transit is encouraging and suggests that high doses of nucleic acids could be delivered by the electrophoretic route repeatedly. These doses and sizes of fragments suggest that gene augmentation therapy could be achieved through the sclera. This is especially significant for cases in which the packaging size of AAV is exceeded.

Administering an electrical current for 2 h (as occurs in our electrophoresis gel box in Fig. 3) would be very difficult in a patient and may cause significant toxicity *(42,48)*. However, the length of electrophoresis in our present experiments in the agarose gel was much longer than could be used clinically because: (1) The DNAs would travel a fraction of a millimeter before contacting the sclera. Similarly, the length of time after the DNA crossed the sclera would be much less in a patient, and the DNA would need

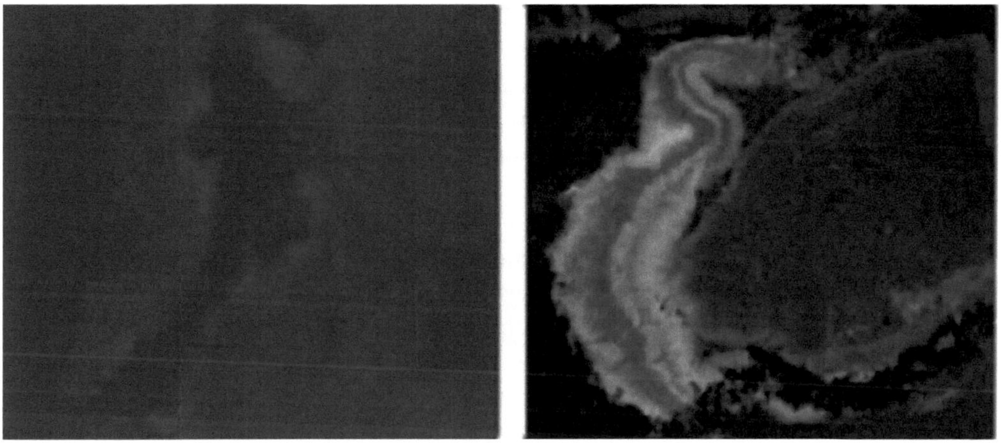

Fig. 7. Transocular iontophoresis. Left panel: A p70-EGFP DNA *(79,80)* was iontophoresed trans-sclerally using a Microphor® Model 6121 (Life-Tech, Inc.) power supply for 20 min at 0.5 mA. A 32-gage silver or platinum wire was used as the cathode, and was placed in the barrel of a non-beveled pipet tip (200 µL) with an inner tip diameter of about 0.5 mm. This pipet was filled with 50 µL of the DNA solution and the wire was introduced about 0.5 cm into the solution. Dual electrodes were also tested. The anode was an alligator clip attached to a BSS-soaked kimwipe wrapped around the tail of an anesthetized mouse (ketamine-xylazine [intramuscular] and a local of 0.5% proparacaine, one drop on the eye). The small end of the pipet tip was placed vertically in direct contact with the conjunctiva just posterior to the pars plana of the mouse eye. The plasmid was dissolved in BSS (Alcon), at a concentration of 1 mg/mL. With the pipet tip and contained cathode in the vertical position, the generated H_2 gas bubbles formed on the cathode wire but mostly would detach, float upward, and pop at the surface before current flow was interrupted. The eyes of the mouse were harvested 4 d after treatment to allow expression of enhanced green fluorescent protein (EGFP) from the plasmid. Left and right panels: Photomicrographs of confocal images of mouse eye cryosections. The left panel is untreated. The right panel is of an eye that was transsclerally iontophoresed with p70-EGFP, a plasmid that should produce EGFP in all neuronal cells of the retina *(79,80)*. All retina cell layers fluoresce much more than untreated. The confocal microscope and imaging settings are identical across the two photomicrographs. *See* color version on companion CD.

to migrate only 100 to 200 µm to the delivery targets of the RPE or sensory retina. Thus, in a clinical setting, treatment times would be about 5 to 10 min. (2) Also, the current flow is in large part a function of the "buffer strength." By reducing buffer concentration, current flow and heating of tissue are reduced. Such a reduction in current density would reduce the risk of burn damage, fibrosis, and necrosis *(42,48)*.

Supercoiled plasmid DNA can cross the sclera via electrophoresis. No apparent damage to the plasmids occurred because the plasmids had identical mobilities before and after transscleral electrophoresis. The amount of DNA recovered was nearly the same as was applied to the well, as determined from relative fluorescent intensities of the bands.

Our hypothesis predicted that small DNAs would migrate through the sclera. The data from Figs. 2 through 5 indicate that this prediction is valid. Larger DNA exhibited no clear size limit beyond which DNA would no longer pass through the sclera (as shown in Figs. 4 and 5). These results suggest that the sclera functions as a sieve of fibers similar to the more characterized networks in agarose or polyacrylamide.

The absence of a maximum size limit in the scleral sieve may imply that fragments of DNA much larger than we tested may pass through the sclera (or even other tissues or barriers). We speculate that, much as pulsed-field or field inversion gel electrophoresis allows very large DNA fragments to transit agarose pores, DNAs thought too large may pass through pores in the sclera if field inversion pattern and frequency are optimized.

Future Studies

Regarding the evaluation of potential damage to the sclera, we plan in the near future to study hematoxylin and eosin (H&E) sections of the treated sclera for intercellular damage including swelling, increased spacing between collagen bundles, and disruption of collagen bundles. Cuprolinic blue staining of sections would reveal changes among treatment groups and untreated controls as proteoglycans might change in structure and amount following electric field treatments. Intracellular damage will be noted when cytoplasmic fragmentation is evident or if cells have an indefinite outline suggesting electroporation damage to the plasma membrane. Coagulation of proteins within tissue would suggest thermal damage. Because tissue damage can be irregular or scattered, we plan to examine serial sections of the scleral fragments, especially in the thinnest regions.

Success in Gene Therapy With Small DNAs

The most notable success using a single-stranded oligonucleotide for treatment of human chorioretinal disease is Formivirsen (Isis Pharmaceuticals, Carlsbad, CA). Formivirsen is a 21-nucleotide phosphorothioate antisense oligonucleotide for treatment of CMV retinitis *(68,69)*. Intravitreal injection of antisense oligonucleotides targeting vascular endothelial growth factor (VEGF) reduces new blood vessel growth by 25 to 31% in a murine model of neovascularization *(70–73)*. However, despite the effective delivery of oligonucleotides by intravitreal injection, oligonucleotides are rapidly broken down in or cleared from the vitreous making repeated injections necessary to maintain effective therapy. Repeated intravitreal administration of drugs and bioactive molecules increases the risk of endophthalmitis, retinal detachment, vitreous hemorrhage, and possible retinal toxicity *(74)*. Electrophoretic delivery might embed DNA in the sclera, increasing the depot of the DNA drug. In the present review, we compared our DNA electrotransfer method with intra-orbital injection. Electrotransfer moves the DNA across the sclera and adjacent to the RPE with a low continuous voltage via a noninvasive process called electrophoresis. In contrast, other labs inject DNA into the vitreous or subretinal space, an invasive process, and follow with short pulses of a high-voltage field *(46)*. This electric field is not the same electrophoretic field that is intended to transfer DNA a macroscopic distance; instead the field is intense and pulsed to transiently open pores in the plasma membrane of the cells. Diffusion allows the DNA to enter these cells. This process is called electroporation and it should not be mistaken for the electrophoretic fields that we apply to move DNA a significant distance from outside the eye to inside.

Limitations of Transscleral Delivery

Even though transscleral diffusion permits a less invasive method of oligonucleotide delivery, this method has limitations as well. Periocular injections might be too indiscriminant or transient to administer bioactive molecules to the posterior segment of the eye. Large volumes injected into the subconjunctival space may overwhelm the absorption capacity of the sclera leading to dispersion into nonocular, orbital tissues or systemic exposure and not achieve therapeutic levels in the posterior segment by simple diffusion, although Demetriades et al. *(30)* were successful. Therefore, (1) a sustained-release delivery system (i.e., fibrin sealant or biodegradable polymers) may be advantageous by allowing continuous transscleral diffusion, or (2) immediate electro transfer may create an internal depot within the sclera or eye close to the target cell; for example the RPE65 cDNA might be delivered near the RPE. After diffusion across the sclera, the DNA still must traverse the vascular choroid. Washout may be a problem, requiring higher starting concentrations. Systemic expression could result from plasmids captured in blood flowing out of the eye. As mentioned in the introduction section, the sclera represents just one of several barriers to the therapeutic delivery of large or small nucleic acids to the retina and other ocular tissues. However, it is encouraging that the present electrophoretic approach seems to be effective for transscleral delivery of several forms and sizes of nucleic acids. Further work is needed to evaluate strategies to optimize crossing other barriers and transfecting the nucleic acids into the target cells.

SUMMARY

Although many steps and barriers remain to clinical application, other investigators are testing procedures for low current iontophoresis of several classes of drugs across the conjunctiva and cornea *(36–45)*. We suggest that the charged nature of DNA and RNA may make virtually any size nucleic acid an excellent drug for delivery by electric fields through porous tissues.

Speculation

It seems useful at this point to consider a calculation concerning the efficacy of the mass transfer capabilities within the eye and into the RPE cell. Let us consider the situation of the mouse RPE. The mouse eye contains about 54,000 RPE cells *(75,76)*. We speculate that electrotransfer can deliver about 1 μg of DNA into the immediate vicinity of the RPE cell, likely embedding most of the DNA into basolateral infoldings. With further manipulations—including, for example, electroporation—perhaps 10% of the DNA would enter into each RPE cell. Assuming that the delivered DNA is an episomally expressed plasmid of about 3.5 kb, this corresponds to 26 billion copies or the delivery of about half a million copies of the plasmid within each RPE cell. Even with a modest efficiency of delivery across the nuclear pore complex, it seems likely that a large number of plasmids would enter the nucleus. That is, suppose the efficiency of DNA delivery into the nucleus from the cytoplasm is 1 to 10%, then 5000 to 50,000 copies would be delivered into the nucleus. Also, we suggest that if the DNA were delivered when the mouse is young (before the accumulation of binucleate RPE cells, a process requiring fission of the nucleus) DNA might be more readily taken up into nuclei of RPE cells. We can compare this DNA delivery strategy with that of rAAV. AAV is exceedingly well taken up by RPE cells when injected subretinally, but only about 10 billion particles are injected into the eye at any one time *(77,78)*, corresponding to about 200,000 therapeutic gene or cDNA copies per RPE cell. The joint efficiency of AAV delivery into the cell and nucleus is high, but assuming it is 10%, about 20,000 copies would be delivered into the nucleus. Thus, we speculate that the electrophoretic delivery of DNA into the mouse RPE should be on par with rAAV delivery. While the efficacy of rAAV is not in question, the simpler technology of plasmid preparation and the noninvasive delivery of the plasmid by electrophoresis may make it more attractive in the long run.

In conclusion, application of an electric field may in part solve one of the most difficult and important problems in gene therapy for eye diseases—the need to transfer large amounts of therapeutic agents to the interior of the eye without damaging ocular tissues. Electrophoresis or iontophoresis of nucleic acids into the eye may be ideal for gene therapy because RNA and DNA are hydrophilic and charged.

ACKNOWLEDGMENTS

Supported by NEI R03 EY13986, R01 EY000933, T32 EY007092, P30 EY006360, Fight for Sight, the Foundation Fighting Blindness, and an unrestricted grant to the Emory Eye Center from Research to Prevent Blindness.

REFERENCES

1. Davies JB, Ciavatta VT, Boatright JH, Nickerson JM. Delivery of several forms of DNA, DNA–RNA hybrids, and dyes across human sclera by electrical fields. Mol Vis 2003; 9:569–578.
2. Shuler RK Jr, Dioguardi PK, Henjy C, Nickerson JM, Cruysberg LP, Edelhauser HF. Scleral permeability of a small, single-stranded oligonucleotide. J Ocul Pharmacol Ther 2004;20: 159–168.
3. Nickerson JM, Wolchok SM, Ciavatta VT, Boatright JH. Delivery of dyes into intact mouse eyes by electrical field. Invest Ophthalmol Vis Sci 2004;45:ARVO E-Abstract 4761.
4. Borras T. Recent developments in ocular gene therapy. Exp Eye Res 2003;76:643–652.
5. Campochiaro PA. Gene therapy for retinal and choroidal diseases. Expert Opin Biol Ther 2002;2:537–544.
6. Singh VK, Tripathi P. Gene therapy in ocular diseases. Indian J Ophthalmol 2002;50:173–181.
7. Lang JC. Ocular drug delivery conventional ocular formulations. Adv Drug Del Rev 1995;16:39–43.
8. Olsen TW, Aaberg SY, Geroski DH, Edelhauser HF. Human sclera thickness and surface area. Am J Ophthalmol 1998;125:237–241.
9. Rudnick DE, Noonan JS, Geroski DH, Prausnitz MR, Edelhauser HF. The effect of intraocular pressure on human and rabbit scleral permeability. Invest Ophthalmol Vis Sci 1999;40: 3054–3058.
10. Ambati J, Canakis CS, Miller JW, et al. Trans-scleral delivery of bioactive protein to the choroids and retina. Invest Ophthalmol Vis Sci 2000;41:1186–1191.
11. Sanborn GE, Anand R, Torti RE. Sustained-release ganciclovir therapy for treatment of cytomegalovirus retinitis. Arch Ophthalmol 1992;110:188–195.
12. Ganciclovir implants (Vitrasert). Treat Rev. (no 21) 1996;10.
13. Geroski DH, Edelhauser HF. Drug delivery for posterior segment disease. Invest Ophthalmol Vis Sci 2000;41:961–964.
14. Comer RM, King WJ, Ardjomand N, Theoharis S, George AJ, Larkin DF. Effect of administration of CTLA4-Ig as protein or cDNA on corneal allograft survival. Invest Ophthalmol Vis Sci 2002;43:1095–1103.

15. De Kozak Y, Thillaye-Goldenberg B, Naud MC, Da Costa AV, Auriault C, Verwaerde C. Inhibition of experimental autoimmune uveoretinitis by systemic and subconjunctival adenovirus-mediated transfer of the viral IL-10 gene. Clin Exp Immunol 2002;130: 212–223.
16. Zhang Y, Schlachetzki F, Li JY, Boado RJ, Pardridge WM. Organ-specific gene expression in the rhesus monkey eye following intravenous non-viral gene transfer. Mol Vis 2003;9: 465–472.
17. Bennett J. Immune response following intraocular delivery of recombinant viral vectors. Gene Ther 2003;10:977–982.
18. Borras T, Gabelt BT, Klintworth GK, Peterson JC, Kaufman PL. Non-invasive observation of repeated adenoviral GFP gene delivery to the anterior segment of the monkey eye in vivo. J Gene Med 2001;3:437–449.
19. Pollack A. FDA halts 27 gene therapy trials after illness: leukemia-like cases in 2 children in France prompt the action. NY Times (Print) January 15, 2003;A1,A17.
20. Check E. Cancer fears cast doubts on future of gene therapy. Nature 2003;421:678.
21. Lehrman S. Virus treatment questioned after gene therapy death. Nature 1999;401:517, 518.
22. Marshall E. Gene therapy death prompts review of adenovirus vector. Science 1999;286: 2244–2245.
23. Weber M, Rabinowitz J, Provost N, et al. Recombinant adeno-associated virus serotype 4 mediates unique and exclusive long-term transduction of retinal pigmented epithelium in rat, dog, and nonhuman primate after subretinal delivery. Mol Ther 2003;7:774–781.
24. Narfstrom K, Katz ML, Ford M, Redmond TM, Rakoczy E, Bragadottir R. In vivo gene therapy in young and adult RPE65–/– dogs produces long-term visual improvement. J Hered 2003;94:31–37.
25. Narfstrom K, Katz ML, Bragadottir R, et al. Functional and structural recovery of the retina after gene therapy in the RPE65 null mutation dog. Invest Ophthalmol Vis Sci 2003;44: 1663–1172.
26. Acland GM, Aguirre GD, Ray J, et al. Gene therapy restores vision in a canine model of childhood blindness. Nat Genet 2001;28:92–95.
27. Van Hooser JP, Liang Y, Maeda T, et al. Recovery of visual functions in a mouse model of Leber congenital amaurosis. J Biol Chem 277, 2002;19,173–19,182.
28. Huttner NA, Girod A, Schnittger S, Schoch C, Hallek M, Buning H. Analysis of site-specific transgene integration following cotransduction with recombinant adeno-associated virus and a rep encoding plasmid. J Gene Med 2003;5:120–129.
29. Behrens A, Gordon EM, Li L, et al. Retroviral gene therapy vectors for prevention of excimer laser-induced corneal haze. Invest Ophthalmol Vis Sci 2002;43:968–977.
30. Demetriades AM, Lu L, Gehlbach P, et al. Transscleral delivery of proteins by periocular gene transfer. Invest Ophthalmol Vis Sci 2003;44: ARVO E-Abstract 2329.
31. Stechschulte SU, Joussen AM, von Recum HA, et al. Rapid ocular angiogenic control via naked DNA delivery to cornea. Invest Ophthalmol Vis Sci 2001;42:1975–1991.
32. Shen WY, Rakoczy PE. Uptake dynamics and retinal tolerance of phosphorothioate oligonucleotide and its direct delivery into the site of choroidal neovascularization through subretinal administration in the rat. Antisense Nucl Acid Drug Dev 2001;11:257–264.
33. Kren BT, Chen Z, Felsheim R, Roy Chowdhury N, Roy Chowdhury J, Steer CJ. Modification of hepatic genomic DNA using RNA/DNA oligonucleotides. Gene Ther 2002; 9:686–690.
34. Hannon GJ. RNA interference. Nature 2002;418:244–251.
35. Lyngstadaas SP. Synthetic hammerhead ribozymes as tools in gene expression. Crit Rev Oral Biol Med 2001;12:469–478.
36. Burstein NL, Leopold LH, Bernacchi DB. Trans-scleral iontophoresis of gentamicin. J Ocul Pharmacol 1985;1:363–368.

37. Sakamoto T, Oshima Y, Nakagawa K, Ishibashi T, Inomata H, Sueishi K. Target gene transfer of tissue plasminogen activator to cornea by electric pulse inhibits intracameral fibrin formation and corneal cloudiness. Hum Gene Ther 1999;10:2551–2555.
38. Oshima Y, Sakamoto T, Nakamura T, et al. The comparative benefits of glaucoma filtering surgery with an electric-pulse targeted drug delivery system demonstrated in an animal model. Ophthalmology 1999;106:1140–1146.
39. Oshima Y, Sakamoto T, Yamanaka I, Nishi T, Ishibashi T, Inomata H. Targeted gene transfer to corneal endothelium in vivo by electric pulse. Gene Ther 1998;5:1347–1354.
40. Voigt M, de Kozak Y, Halhal M, Courtois Y, Behar-Cohen F. Down-regulation of NOSII gene expression by iontophoresis of anti-sense oligonucleotide in endotoxin-induced uveitis. Biochem Biophys Res Commun 2002;295:336–341.
41. Behar-Cohen FF, Parel JM, Pouliquen Y, et al. Iontophoresis of dexamethasone in the treatment of endotoxin-induced-uveitis in rats. Exp Eye Res 1997;65:533–545.
42. Yoshizumi MO, Lee DA, Sarraf DA, Equi RA, Verdon W. Ocular toxicity of iontophoretic foscarnet in rabbits. J Ocul Pharmacol Ther 1995;11:183–189.
43. Sarraf D, Equi RA, Holland GN, Yoshizumi MO, Lee DA. Transscleral iontophoresis of foscarnet. Am J Ophthalmol 1993;115:748–754.
44. Sarraf D, Lee DA. Iontophoresis of reactive black 5 for pulsed dye laser sclerostomy. J Ocul Pharmacol 1993;9:25–33.
45. Grossman RE, Sarraf D, Lee DA. Iontophoresis of methylene blue for gonioscopic pulsed dye laser sclerostomy. J Ocul Pharmacol 1993;9:277–285.
46. Matsuda T, Cepko CL. Electroporation and RNA interference in the rodent retina in vivo and in vitro. Proc Natl Acad Sci USA 2004;101:16–22.
47. Singh P, Maibach HI. Iontophoresis in drug delivery: basic principles and applications. Crit Rev Ther Drug Carrier Syst 1994;11:161–213.
48. Sarraf D, Lee DA. The role of iontophoresis in ocular drug delivery. J Ocul Pharmacol 1994;10:69–81.
49. Sasaki H, Yamamura K, Mukai T, et al. Enhancement of ocular drug penetration. Crit Rev Ther Drug Carrier Syst 1999;16:85–146.
50. Kurz D, Ciulla TA. Novel approaches for retinal drug delivery. Ophthalmol Clin North Am 2002;15:405–410.
51. Dische Z. Biochemistry of connective tissue of the vertebrate eye. Int Rev Connect Tissue Res 1970;5:209–279.
52. Lee SB, Geroski DH, Prausnitz MR, Edelhauser HF. Drug delivery through the sclera: effects of thickness, hydration, and sustained release systems. Exp Eye Res 2004;78:599–607.
53. Prausnitz MR, Noonan JS. Permeability of cornea, sclera, and conjunctiva: a literature analysis for drug delivery to the eye. J Pharm Sci 1998;87:1479–1488.
54. Ambati J, Adamis AP. Transscleral drug delivery to the retina and choroid. Prog Retin Eye Res 2002;21:145–151.
55. Geroski DH, Edelhauser HF. Transscleral drug delivery for posterior segment disease. Adv Drug Deliv Rev 2001;52:37–48.
56. Maurice DM, Polgar J. Diffusion across the sclera. Exp Eye Res 1977;25:577–582.
57. Barza M, Kane A, Baum J. Intraocular penetration of gentamicin after subconjunctibal and retrobulbar injection. Am J Ophthalmol 1978;85:541–557.
58. Ahmed I, Gokhale RD, Shah MV, Patton TF. Physicochemical determinants of drug diffusion across the conjunctiva, sclera, and cornea. J Pharm Sci 1987;76:583–586.
59. Weinreb RN. Enhancement of scleral macromolecular permeability with prostaglandins. Trans Am Ophthalmol Soc 2001;99:319–343.
60. Ambati J, Canakis CS, Miller JW, et al. Diffusion of high molecular weight compounds through sclera. Invest Ophthalmol Vis Sci 2000;41:1181–1185.

61. Cruysberg LP, Nuijts RM, Geroski DH, Koole LH, Hendrikse F, Edelhauser HF. In vitro human scleral permeability of fluorescein, dexamethasone-fluorescein, methotrexate-fluorescein and rhodamine and the use of a coated coil as a new drug delivery system. J Ocul Pharmacol Ther 2002;18:559–569.
62. Watson PG, Hazleman BL. The Sclera and Systemic Disorders. W.B. Saunders, Philadelphia:1976.
63. Ambati J, Gragoudas ES, Miller JW, et al. Transscleral delivery of bioactive protein to the choroid and retina. Invest Ophthalmol Vis Sci 2000;41:1186–1191.
64. Simpson AE, Gilbert JA, Rudnick DE, Geroski DH, Aaberg TM Jr, Edelhauser HF. Transscleral diffusion of carboplatin: an in vitro and in vivo study. Arch Ophthalmol 2002;120:1069–1074.
65. Gilbert JA, Simpson AE, Rudnick DE, Geroski DH, Aaberg TM Jr, Edelhauser HF. Transscleral permeability and intraocular concentrations of cisplatin from a collagen matrix. J Control Release 2003;89:409–417.
66. Kompella UB, Bandi N, Ayalasomayajula SP. Subconjunctival nano- and microparticles sustain retinal delivery of budesonide, a corticosteroid capable of inhibiting VEGF expression. Invest Ophthalmol Vis Sci 2003;44:1192–1201.
67. Unlu N, Robinson JR. Scleral permeability to hydrocortisone and mannitol in the albino rabbit eye. J Ocul Pharmacol Ther 1998;14:273–281.
68. de Smet MD, Meenken C, van der Horn GJ. Formivirsen a phosphorothioate oligonucleotide for the treatment of CMV retinitis. Ocul Immunol Inflamm 1999;7:189–198.
69. Perry CM, Balfour JAB. Fomivirsen. Drugs 1999;57:375–380.
70. Rakoczy PE, Shen WY, Lai M, Rolling F, Constable IJ. Development of gene therapy-based strategies for the treatment of eye diseases. Drug Dev Res 1999;46:277–285.
71. Leeds JM, Henry SP, Bistner S, Scherrill S, Williams K, Levin AA. Pharacokinetics of an anti-sense oligonucleotide injected intravitreally in monkeys. Drug Metab Dispos 1998;26: 670–675.
72. Ogata N, Otsuji T, Matsushima M, et al. Phosphorothioate oligonucleotides induction into experimental choroidal neovascularization by HVJ-liposome system. Curr Eye Res 1999;18:261–269.
73. Robinson GS, Pierce EA, Rook SL, Foley E, Webb R, Smith LE. Oligodeoxynucleotides inhibit retinal neovascularization in a murine model of proliferative retinopathy. Proc Natl Acad Sci USA 1996;93:4851–4856.
74. Zeng S, Hu C, Wei H, et al. Intravitreal pharmacokinetics of liposome-encapsulated amikacin in a rabbit model. Ophthalmol 1993;100:1640–1644.
75. Bodenstein L, Sidman RL. Growth and development of the mouse retinal pigment epithelium. I. Cell and tissue morphometrics and topography of mitotic activity. Dev Biol 1987;121: 192–204.
76. Sidman R. Histogenesis of mouse retina studies with thymidine3H. In: Smelser G, ed. The Structure of the Eye: Proceedings of the symposium held April 11–13, 1960 during the seventh International Congress of Anatomists, New York, New York. Academic Press, New York: 1961:487–505.
77. Surace EM, Auricchio A, Reich SJ, et al. Delivery of adeno-associated virus vectors to the fetal retina: impact of viral capsid proteins on retinal neuronal progenitor transduction. J Virol 2003;77:7957–7963.
78. Dejneka NS, Surace EM, Aleman TS, et al. In utero gene therapy rescues vision in a murine model of congenital blindness. Mol Ther 2004;9:182–188.
79. Boatright JH, Borst DE, Peoples JW, et al. A major cis activator of the IRBP gene contains CRX-binding and Ret-1/PCE-I elements. Mol Vis 1997;3:15.
80. Boatright JH, Knox BE, Jones KM, et al. Evidence of a tissue-restricting DNA regulatory element in the mouse IRBP promoter. FEBS Lett 2001;504:27–30.

22
Novel Drug Delivery Systems for Posterior Segment Ocular Disease

Heather Sheardown, PhD and W. Mark Saltzman, PhD

CONTENTS

RATIONALE FOR ADVANCED DRUG DELIVERY METHODS

Delivery of drugs to the eye, particularly for the treatment of posterior segment diseases, is a challenging task that requires drug transport across barriers in the eye, which are present for the purpose of limiting the entry of drugs and xenobiotics. The common methods of drug delivery to the eye—eyedrops, direct injection, and systemic administration—all have problems that limit their usefulness, particularly for agents that are high in molecular weight and water-soluble.

At present, most ocular diseases are treated with the topical application of solutions administered as eyedrops for water-soluble drugs and as ointments or aqueous suspensions for water-insoluble drugs *(1,2)*. These dosage forms account for approx 90% of currently marketed formulations. The cornea represents a primary pathway for ocular penetration of topically applied drugs. Annular tight junctions (zonula occludens), which completely surround and effectively seal the superficial epithelial cells, make the cornea an effective barrier to drug penetration. Binding of drug molecules to corneal tissues also appears to hinder transcorneal penetration *(3)*. Conjunctival penetration and uptake of topically applied drugs is typically an order of magnitude higher than corneal uptake *(4)*. In addition, high tear fluid turnover rates and nasolacrimal drainage contribute to rapid and extensive precorneal losses, limiting the effectiveness of conjunctival penetration *(5)*. As a result, after instillation of an eyedrop, less than 5% and as little as 1% of the drug applied penetrates the cornea and reaches the intraocular tissues *(6,7)*. It has been suggested that, after instillation of a drop, the maximum concentration in the vitreous is approximately one hundred-thousandth that of the drop itself *(8)*.

From: *Ophthalmology: Ocular Angiogenesis: Diseases, Mechanisms, and Therapeutics*
Edited by: J. Tombran-Tink and C. J. Barnstable © Humana Press Inc., Totowa, NJ

Furthermore, this is the major route of entry into the circulatory system for topically applied drugs *(9,10)* and has been shown, in rare cases, to result in systemic exposure that is sufficiently high to be toxic *(11)*. Therefore, although simple in terms of formulation development and production, as well as being widely accepted by patients, these conventional dosage forms have numerous deficiencies that make the development of alternative delivery strategies desirable, particularly when delivery to the back of the eye is indicated.

Direct injection of drugs into the vitreous cavity is sometimes used to achieve high drug concentrations in the vitreous and the retina. However, in order to maintain drug concentrations at therapeutic levels for a prolonged period of time, repeated injections are necessary, as the half-life of drugs in the vitreous is generally relatively short *(12)*. Repeated injections result in patient discomfort and can potentially lead to complications such as vitreous hemorrhage, infection, and lens or retinal injury. Furthermore, the low therapeutic index of the majority of the drugs used for treating diseases of the posterior segment may require drug concentrations that are at or near levels toxic to the retina *(13)*. Periocular delivery using subconjuctival or retrobulbar injections provides an alternative to intravitreal injections that is safer and less invasive; this area has been targeted as a potential site for controlled drug delivery *(14)*.

Systemic delivery of ophthalmic drugs, while sometimes used in the treatment of vitreoretinal diseases, is not an effective alternative due to the high efficiency of the blood–ocular barrier *(15)*. The large systemic dose required to obtain a therapeutic level of drug in the eye severely limits the applicability of this method in most cases; toxicity in tissues outside the eye is a frequent limitation. Furthermore, the blood–retinal barrier, which is located at the level of retinal vascular endothelial cells and in the retinal pigment epithelium, inhibits the entry of certain drugs from the systemic circulation.

Based on these delivery problems it is not surprising that, despite accounting for more than 55% of all ocular diseases, problems related to the posterior segment account for less than 5% of the ophthalmic drug market. Most of the currently available clinical therapies for the treatment of diseases resulting in loss of sight due to neovascularization in the eye—i.e., laser photocoagulation therapy for diabetic retinopathy and photodynamic therapy for age-related macular degeneration *(16)*—use either surgical intervention or systemic delivery of a therapeutic agent as the delivery method. The application of novel angiostatic agents, particularly proteins or protein-like drugs including anti-vascular endothelial growth factor (VEGF) *(17)*, matrix metalloproteinase (MMP) inhibitors *(18,19)*, integrin agonists *(20)*, pigment epithelium-derived factor (PEDF) *(21,22)*, and inhibitors of insulin-like growth factor-1 and growth hormone *(23)*, will require more sophisticated methods of delivery to ensure activity and efficacy of the drug over a prolonged period of time and to minimize drug-induced complications. Novel delivery systems are also needed for therapeutics with a high level of systemic toxicity, such as steroids *(24–26)*.

A number of novel methods are under development or in clinical use. Devices made from both biostable (nondegradable) and from biodegradable polymers have been investigated and studied. Devices made from biodegradable polymers have the advantage that they degrade and therefore disappear from the site of implantation over time. The potential for further development, particularly for protein agents, is significant; this development can take advantage of knowledge obtained in delivery of protein drugs to other sites.

Table 1
Polymeric Materials for Drug Delivery Systems

Polymer	*Properties*
Polydimethylsiloxane, silicone elastomers (PDMS)	Used in implanted medical devices Hydrophobic, rubbery material
Poly(2-hydroxyethylmethacrylate) (pHEMA)	Used in soft contact lenses Hydrophilic, soft material
Poly(ethylene-co-vinyl acetate) (EVAc)	Used in drug delivery devices (Progestasert; Ocusert) Hydrophobic, rubbery material
Poly(L-lactic acid), Poly(glycolic acid), and Poly(lactide-co-glycolide) (PLA, PGA, and PLGA)	Used in drug delivery devices and sutures Hydrophobic material that slowly degrades in water
Polyanhydrides such as poly(carboxyphenoxypropane-co-sebacic acid) (pCPP:SA)	Used in drug delivery devices (Gliadel®) Hydrophobic material that slowly degrades in water

NOVEL DRUG DELIVERY SYSTEMS BASED ON POLYMERS

Biocompatible polymers can be used to build drug delivery systems that provide controlled release of agents. "Controlled" release can refer to control over the rate and duration of drug release or control over the local site of release into the body; both of these are useful attributes for an ocular drug delivery system. Many polymeric materials are available for the development of drug delivery systems; Table 1 provides a partial list.

Reservoir Systems

Nondegradable, hydrophobic polymers have been used the most extensively in drug delivery systems. Reservoir drug delivery devices, in which a liquid reservoir of drug is enclosed in a silicone elastomer tube, were first demonstrated to provide controlled release of small molecules several decades ago *(27)*. This discovery eventually led to clinically useful devices, including the Norplant® contraceptive delivery system, which provides reliable delivery of levonorgestrel for 5 yr following subcutaneous implantation. Norplant has been available to women in the United States since 1990, after use by millions of women in other countries, and it has been generally well received *(28)*. Other polymers, most notably ethylene vinyl acetate copolymer (EVAc), have been used to control the delivery of contraceptive hormones to the female reproductive tract (Progestasert®) and lipophilic drugs to the eye or the skin (Ocusert®, Estraderm®, and Transderm Nitro®; *see* Fig. 1). The reservoir configuration offers a number of potential advantages, including the possibility of long service life (because large quantities of drug can be stored in the reservoir), excellent control over release kinetics, and nearly constant release rates. Because the rate of agent release depends only on diffusion of the agent through the surrounding polymer membranes, release is reproducible, predictable across a variety of agents, and constant for as long as the drug reservoir remains saturated with drug.

Ocusert was designed to be inserted by patients into the cul-de-sac of the eye. The rate and duration of drug release can be adjusted by changing the properties of the

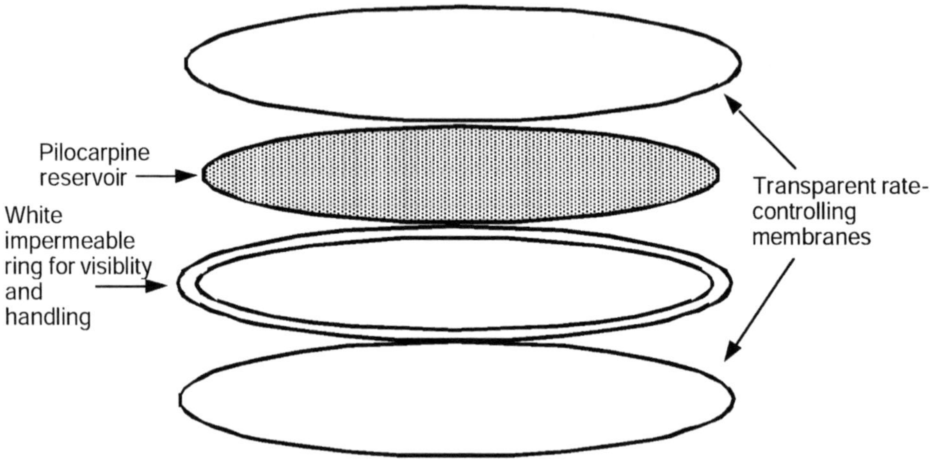

Fig. 1. Schematic diagram of the Ocusert reservoir drug delivery system. The figure shows an exploded view of the system. The rate-controlling membranes are composed of EVAc, a nondegradable, highly biocompatible material.

membrane and the concentration of drug in the reservoir. The clinical versions of the device release pilocarpine at a controlled rate (either 20 or 40 μg/h) for 7 d. The rate of release is higher than the nominal rate during the first 6 h of use, as drug that has saturated the membrane during storage is released and steady-state conditions are established; the rate is approximately three times the nominal rate during the first hour of use. The encapsulated drug is not completely released during the 7-d lifetime. A substantial quantity of drug must be retained to serve as the diffusional source. A device that releases 40 μg/h has an initial loading of 11 mg of pilocarpine; approx 40% of that amount is left in the device at the end of its 7-d use.

Vitrasert® is an intravitreal device for controlled release of ganciclovir to treat cytomegalovirus retinitis in immunocompromised patients *(29–33)*. The tablet-shaped ganciclovir core (4.5 mg of agent) has a coating of EVAc and poly(vinyl alcohol) (PVA); the coating controls the rate of ganciclovir diffusion into the vitreous. These devices can deliver controlled amounts of drug for a prolonged period of time (release occurs over a period of 5 to 8 mo at a rate of 1 to 2 μg/h) and are highly efficacious. In one study, the median time to progression of cytomegalovirus (CMV) retinitis increased from 15 d in the deferred treatment group to 226 d in the implant group *(30)*. In another study, which compared two different-concentration ganciclovir implants but used intravenous (iv) administration of the drug as a control *(29)*, the ganciclovir implant was more effective than iv administration of the drug for the treatment of the CMV infection; in fact, due to the marked improvement observed in study patients receiving the implants, many of the iv-treated patients were offered implants after early progression. However, patients treated with the implant were at greater risk of developing CMV in the contralateral eye and elsewhere in the body, compared to those receiving iv drug. No differences were observed between the implants loaded with different amounts of the drug.

The Vitrasert® device is not biodegradable; hence retrieval may be necessary. The need for a surgical removal procedure is offset by the greater reproducibility of the release rates compared with degradable devices. Techniques have been developed to aid with implant removal *(34)*. If the patient's immune system remains seriously compromised, a second device may be implanted. This procedure is well tolerated *(35)*, although multiple sclerotomies can weaken the wall of the eye and multiple implants can impede vision. A small number of patients (0.46%) develop endophthalmitis associated with placement of the ganciclovir implant, with the majority of cases occurring in the early postoperative period *(36)*.

The Retisert® intravitreal device, which provides long-term delivery of fluocinolone acetonide (a synthetic corticosteroid) for the treatment of severe uveitis and diabetic macular edema, is also being tested. The system, consisting of pure drug pellets coated in a PVA/silicone laminate and affixed to a PVA suture strut, releases drug at a rate of approx 2 μg/d *(37)*. More recently, release rates as low as 0.1 μg/d were shown efficacious in a rabbit model *(38)*. Constant intraocular drug levels were observed for extended periods in a normal rabbit eye *(39)*, with indications that devices might release drug at a constant rate for periods as long as 18 yr. Reduced intraocular inflammation and maintenance of useful vision was observed in all patients for an extended time period with minimal additional topical therapy, including in patients with simultaneous intraocular lens implantation *(40,41)*. The device was also effective in the treatment of proliferative vitreoretinopathy *(41)* and diabetic macular edema *(42)*.

The sclera has a large surface area and substantial permeability to drugs with a wide range of molecular weights, including drugs with a molecular weight up to 70,000 Daltons *(43–45)* and higher *(46)*. These factors make it amenable for the delivery of drugs to the back of the eye *(47,48)*. Ideally, a transscleral delivery device would provide controlled, long-term drug release and specific scleral site delivery, targeting the thinner areas of the tissue.

The high permeability of the sclera has been exploited in the development of a depot delivery system for anecortave acetate for the treatment of age-related macular degeneration (AMD) *(49–51)*. The device, fabricated from medical-grade silicone, is curved to conform to the eye. The inner core contains a cylindrical 25-mg tablet. The device is inserted into a surgically created sub-Tenon tunnel at the superotemperal quadrant. Although injection of the drug results in therapeutic drug concentrations for approx 6 mo, levels of drug in the choroid and retina of rabbits treated with the device remained at between 0.1 and 0.2 m*M* for approx 2 yr, suggesting that the device could be used to safely treat AMD continuously for long periods of time. Implantation of the device did not affect corneal thickness or endothelial integrity and did not produce signs of ocular toxicity. A new-generation device may provide even longer delivery *(52)*.

Matrix Systems

For some therapeutic agents, it is not possible to find membrane materials that provide adequate drug permeability to permit release from a reservoir device. Proteins, for example, do not diffuse readily through any of the hydrophobic, biocompatible polymers that are commonly used for implantable reservoir systems (Table 1), or they diffuse very slowly ($D < 10^{-13}$ cm^2/s). In addition, reservoir devices are structurally complex, requiring several manufacturing steps, with resulting additional expense. For this combination of reasons, matrix systems for the delivery of agents (particularly protein or large molecular weight drugs) have been examined in considerable detail.

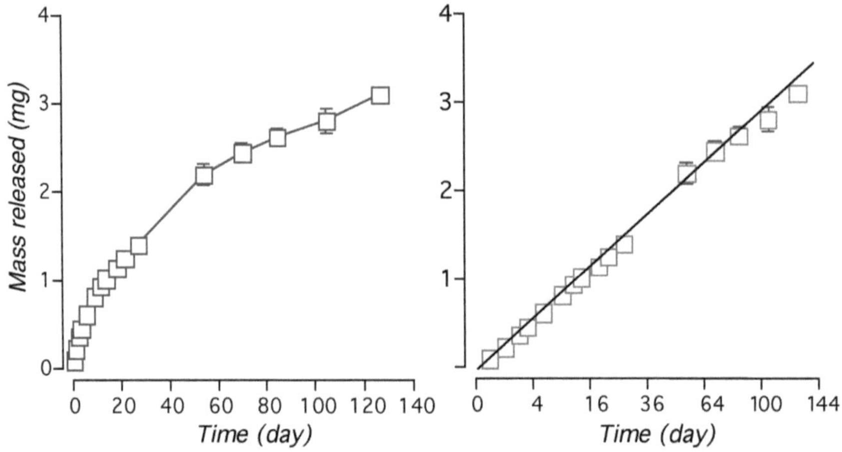

Fig. 2. Release of dexamethasone from a small EVAc matrix (~1 mm^3). (Data from ref. *117*.) *See* color version on companion CD.

In a matrix system, the drug molecules are dissolved or dispersed throughout a solid polymer phase. In many cases, the polymer materials are the same as those used for the rate-limiting membrane in reservoir devices, nondegradable materials such as EVAc. In a matrix drug delivery system, molecules of drug are dissolved in a biocompatible polymer, producing a homogeneous device with drug molecules uniformly dispersed throughout the material; if the drug is not soluble in the polymer, a matrix composite is produced by dispersing small particles of solid drug within a continuous polymer scaffold. In this case, the drug molecules are released by diffusing through the polymer to the surface of the device from which they are released into the external environment. For dissolved drugs, the polymer matrix provides the diffusion pathway; for dispersed particles, diffusion pathways are created by water entry into the composite and dissolution of the solid particles (*see* ref. *53* for details). For many agents, biocompatible polymers such as EVAc can be used to prepare long-lasting delivery systems that are approx 1 mm in size (Fig. 2). Biodegradable polymers—such as poly(lactide-co-glycolide) (PLGA), poly(ortho esters), and polyanhydrides (*see* Table 1)—can also be used to make matrix systems. In most drug delivery systems fabricated from degradable polymers, diffusion is responsible for release, which is often complete long before substantial degradation has occurred. The use of degradable polymers can complicate device design (these materials often are more difficult to process and the local reaction to the device may be more complex due to the long-lasting release of polymer degradation products), but the implanted matrix will eventually disappear, so surgical removal is unnecessary.

Matrix systems have been used to deliver various drugs via device implantation into the sclera. For example, PLGA scleral implants containing betamethasone released the drug for a period of approx 1 mo into the eyes of rabbits; the local drug concentration suppressed inflammatory responses for more than 1 mo without substantial toxic reactions in the retina *(54,55)*. A similar device containing ganciclovir maintained drug concentration within an effective range for a period of 6 mo *(56)*, and was effective at treating experimentally induced human cytomegalovirus infections in rabbits *(57)*. Another matrix device, which released tacrolimus, was effective in treating experimental uveitis

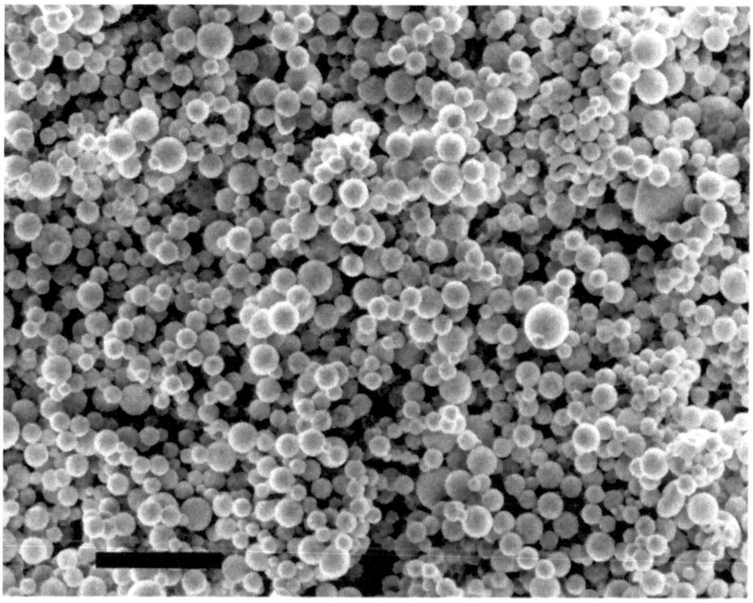

Fig. 3. Scanning electron micrograph of poly(d,l-lactic acid-*co*-glycolic acid) 50:50 microspheres containing iodomelatonin (original magnification ×1500, the scale bar is 10 μm). The mean diameter of the spheres is ~1 μm. (From Gemeinhart and Saltzman [submitted].)

in rabbits *(58)*. Other materials have also been used in this setting; Ciulla et al. used PVA matrices loaded with triamcinolone acetonide (TAAC), as well as a combination PVA device containing a solid reservoir of TAAC surrounded by the TAAC/PVA matrix, to treat the eyes of rats that had been previously laser-treated *(59)*. Delivery rates were found to be significantly different between the matrix-only and matrix/reservoir devices; the reservoir device delivered the drug for a significantly longer time period (7 wk vs 30 d). The results revealed no difference in efficacy between the two devices, but both devices produced significant improvements relative to implants containing no drug.

Microparticle Carriers for Drug Delivery to Back of Eye

Reservoir and matrix devices are generally large and therefore must either be implanted through a potentially large surgical incision or a smaller tissue perforation. For example, the Norplant system for long-term contraception, six 2.4-mm-diameter cylinders, is inserted subcutaneously using a trochar. Surgical insertion into the eye is possible, as illustrated by some of the examples in the previous sections, but is not optimal. As an alternative, injectable microparticles (>1 μm in size) and nanoparticles (<1 μm), consisting of drug entrapped within a polymer, have been developed and applied to the delivery of drugs to the posterior segment of the eye *(60–63)* (Fig. 3). These particles are generally classified as either microspheres, in which the drug is dispersed within a homogeneous polymer matrix, or microcapsules, in which a drug core is surrounded by a thin polymeric film *(64)* (in many senses, microparticles are miniaturized versions of matrix systems, whereas microcapsules are miniaturized reservoirs). Because micro- and nanoparticulates cannot be easily recovered after administration, they are generally fabricated from biodegradable polymers. A variety of polymers have been investigated, including gelatin, albumin, polyorthoesters, and polyanhydrides, but the family of polyesters synthesized from D,L lactic acid [poly(lactic acid), PLA], and glycolic acid [poly(glycolic acid), PGA] as well as their copolymers (PGLA) are the most widely studied. Under physiological conditions, these polymers degrade to lactic acid and glycolic acid respectively. Poly(ortho esters) (POE), a family of hydrophobic, biocompatible and bioerodible polymers, which have been shown compatible with the tissues at the back of the eye *(65,66)*, have also been used in the preparation of microcapsules for ophthalmic drug delivery *(67)*.

A variety of techniques can be used to prepare microspheres, but the most common preparation method involves evaporation of a solvent from an oil-in-water or an water-in-oil-in-water emulsion, depending on the properties of the drug to be delivered *(62)*. Encapsulation efficiency (drug content in the microparticulate compared with theoretical drug loading) is dependent on the properties of the drug and the polymer as well as the preparation technique used *(68)* and the rate of solvent evaporation *(69)*. Efficiency of encapsulation varies with properties of the agent and the encapsulation technique, but is often low (<10%) with water-soluble agents.

Drug release from particulates usually occurs by a combination of mechanisms including diffusion through either the polymer network or through fluid-filled pores in the network, physical erosion after degradation of the polymer matrix, and ion exchange. The nature of the polymer matrix significantly affects drug release characteristics. For example, in one study of particles prepared for intravitreal delivery, approx 70% of 5-fluorouracil (5-FU) was released from PLA microspheres (MW 3400) over a 7-d period; using PGLA with a similar molecular weight, 98% of the encapsulated drug was released in only 2 d *(70)*. In general, the half-life of degradation of PLGA is shorter than that of PLA because the copolymers have lower crystallinity and, therefore, imbibe water more readily *(71)*; lower molecular weight polymers and copolymers have shorter half-lifes than polymers with higher molecular weights *(72)*. Poly(ortho ester) materials, because of the nature of the degradation process, have release kinetics that are often constant and linear, usually with no burst, and that can be controlled by such factors as the polymer molecular weight or the physiochemical characteristics of the substances that are incorporated within the polymer matrix. Polyanhydride microparticles exhibit surface erosion (particularly when used with hydrophobic agents); this form of degradation can also lead to good control over drug release kinetics from microparticles *(73)*.

Microspheres are generally injected as a suspension using either phosphate-buffered saline (PBS) or balanced salt solution as the vehicle. Viscous vehicles including hyaluronic acid (HA) and hydroxypropylmethyl cellulose (HPMC) have also been used to improve delivery and may be particularly appropriate for intravitreal delivery *(74)*.

PGLA microspheres have been used for the delivery of various ophthalmic drugs and in various ophthalmic applications for periods of between 2 and 8 wk. Microspheres loaded with adriamycin *(75)*, 5-FU *(76,77)*, and retinoic acid *(78)* have been examined in animal models for the treatment of proliferative vitreoretinopathy (PVR). Adriamycin-loaded spheres were reported to significantly decrease the rate of retinal detachment in a rabbit model of PVR at 4 wk by 10 to 50%. A direct injection of 10 μg of the drug was found to be toxic to the retina, while delivery of the same dose in microspheres inhibited PVR and did not cause histological abnormalities in the eye. Administration of microspheres containing retinoic acid produced a similar effect, reducing the incidence of tractional retinal detachment in a rabbit eye model in comparison with blank microspheres. Microspheres loaded with dexamethasone have also been used for the treatment of uveitis *(79,80)*. Acyclovir-loaded microspheres, designed for the treatment of acute retinal necrosis, resulted in measurable drug in the vitreous for 14 d after administration of microspheres *(81)*. A number of in vitro and in vivo studies in rabbits have been performed with ganciclovir-loaded microspheres for the treatment of cytomegalovirus retinitis *(82–85)*. In summary, the release rates of lipophilic compounds were almost uniform, whereas the more hydrophilic compounds exhibited substantial short-term release (or a "burst" of initial release). A mild foreign-body response to the particles was observed after injection, with macrophages and multinucleated giant cells surrounding fragments of degraded particles *(78)*. This response disappeared after degradation of the particles and there were no other adverse responses noted. A recent study suggests that intravitreally injected PLA nanoparticles can accumulate in cells of the retinal pigment epithelium, persist in the cells for many months, and release encapsulated agent into the cells *(86)*.

Despite the above results, which show the promise of microspheres and microcapsules for delivery of pharmaceutical agents to the back of the eye, there are no current clinical applications using micro- or nanoparticulates. Several factors may be responsible for this slow progress. Although less frequent injections are needed with particulate delivery systems, repeat injections into the back of the eye might still be needed. In addition, the extent and duration of inflammation produced by the degrading particles is still not completely understood. Finally, microparticles, in general, exhibit less reproducible release kinetics than the implantable systems *(87)*.

DELIVERY SYSTEMS FOR PROTEINS AND OTHER MACROMOLECULAR DRUGS

Because proteins diffuse very slowly through films of silicone and EVAc, many early investigators believed that it was impossible to develop matrix delivery systems capable of releasing proteins *(88)*. In the late 1970s, however, a method for achieving controlled release of proteins from nondegradable polymers was described *(89)*. These polymers provide sustained release of biologically active molecules for extended periods of time, up to several years in some cases *(90)*. One particular hydrophobic polymer, EVAc, has been investigated extensively as a matrix system for protein delivery. Other classes of hydrophobic polymers, such as silicone elastomers and polyurethanes, may also be useful for controlled protein delivery, although there are fewer examples available in the literature. Nondegradable, hydrophilic polymers, such as poly(2-hydroxyethyl methacrylate) (which is frequently used in soft contact lenses and other biomaterials), are also biocompatible, but usually release proteins over a relatively short period of several hours and so may be useful for protein delivery in cases in which prolonged release is not needed.

In general, proteins are loaded into a polymer matrix by dispersing solid particles of protein throughout the polymer. When protein-loaded matrices are immersed in water, the proteins are released slowly. The initial rate of release from the matrix is higher for matrices with higher loading (initial mass fraction of protein particles within the matrix). This release is frequently linear with respect to the square root of time, consistent with a diffusive release mechanism (Fig. 4). To account for the complex structure of the composite matrix material, the diffusion equation incorporates an effective diffusion coefficient for the protein in the polymer matrix. This effective diffusion coefficient, which is typically much lower than the diffusion coefficient of the protein in water, provides a quantitative measure of the rate of protein release, decreasing as the rate of protein release from the matrix decreases.

EVAc matrix systems have been used to release a variety of macromolecules, such as polypeptide and protein hormones *(91,92)*, heparin *(93)*, growth factors *(94–97)*, inhibitors of tumor angiogenesis *(98)*, polyclonal antibodies *(90)*, monoclonal antibodies (MAb) *(99–103)*, antigens *(104,105)*, and DNA *(106)*. Macromolecules retain their biological activity after release from EVAc. For example, MAbs against human chorionic gonadatropin (hCG) retained its ability to bind to hCG after release from an EVAc matrix *(100,101)* and MAbs that neutralize herpesvirus were effective after long-term delivery in animals *(107)*. In addition, when released from EVAc matrices, nerve growth factor (NGF) stimulated neurite outgrowth in cultured cells *(94)*, NGF enhanced choline acetyltransferase activity in neurons in the brain *(108)*, insulin altered the blood glucose levels in diabetic rats *(91)*, and angiogenesis inhibitors blocked new blood vessel growth *(98)*.

EVAc matrices, usually prepared by solvent evaporation *(109)*, consist of protein particles dispersed throughout a continuous polymer phase. When matrices are placed in an aqueous environment, particles at the surface of the matrix can dissolve. Because water-soluble molecules diffuse very slowly through the continuous polymer phase, and because the polymer is hydrophobic and does not swell appreciably in water, protein release must occur through pores in the polymer, which form as the dispersed protein particles dissolve. In fact, microscopic observations of the matrix structure reveal a network of interconnected pores in which large pores (diameters of 100–400 μm) are connected by smaller pores or channels (1–10 μm in diameter) *(109–111)*. Connected clusters of pores that contact the matrix boundary can release protein to the surrounding environment. At loadings higher than 35%, most protein particles are found in clusters that reach the matrix surface, whereas at lower loadings most particles are disconnected and, therefore, not releasable. This behavior can be seen in the protein release data in Fig. 4.

Biodegradable polymers can also be used for protein delivery; often this can be achieved by adapting one of the methods developed for fabrication of EVAc protein delivery systems for use with a degradable polymer such as PLGA *(101)*. Micro- and nanoparticulate systems from biodegradable polymers are particularly attractive for long-term protein delivery to the posterior segments of the eye. A variety of approaches have been used to encapsulate proteins into degradable polymer microparticles. The encapsulation technique must usually be tailored to the specific protein of interest, but some general principles are emerging *(112)*. A variety of examples of systems are now available, including PLGA systems for the controlled release of nerve growth factor *(113)*, human growth hormone *(114)*, interleukin-2 *(115)*, and HIV vaccine proteins *(116)*.

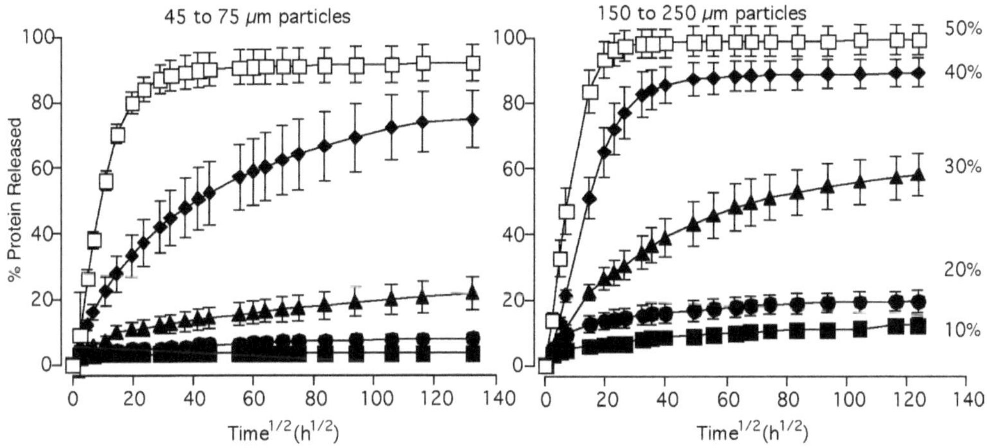

Fig. 4. Release of albumin from an EVAc polymer matrix. Details are provided in ref. *90*. Solid particles of albumin (either 45–75 μm or 150–250 μm in size) were dispersed in a 1-mm-thick EVAc matrix at a total protein loading of 10, 20, 30, 40, or 50%. The cumulative mass of protein released is plotted versus the square root of time (40 $h^{1/2}$ is equal to 67 d; 80 $h^{1/2}$ is 270 d; 120 $h^{1/2}$ is 600 d).

CONCLUSION

Alternate delivery systems are needed for treating disease in the posterior segment of the eye, particularly given the inherent difficulties in the delivery of agents to this site and the desire to reduce the frequency of administration. Reservoir, matrix, and particulate delivery systems are well established as safe and effective approaches for the delivery of agents to the eye. Protein-based agents—which account for a large fraction of the agents now being considered for treatment of angiogenic diseases in the eye—can be delivered reliably from controlled-release systems, but more work is needed to translate this technology into devices that are reliable for delivery to the posterior segment.

REFERENCES

1. LeBourlais C, Acar L, Zia H, Sado P, Needham T, Leverge R. Ophthalmic drug delivery systems—recent advances. Prog Retinal Eye Res 1998;17:33–58.
2. Ding S. Recent developments in ophthalmic drug delivery. PSTT 1998;1:328–335.
3. Romanelli L, Valeri P, Morrone LA, Pimpinella G, Graziani G, Tita B. Ocular absorption and distribution of bendazac after topical administration to rabbits with different vehicles. Life Sci 1994;54:877–885.
4. Ahmed I, Patton TF. Importance of noncorneal absorption route in topical ophthalmic drug delivery. Invest Ophthalmol Vis Sci 1985;26:584–587.
5. Lang JC. Ocular drug delivery conventional ocular formulations. Adv Drug Delivery Rev 1995;16:39–43.
6. Lee VHL, Robinson JR. Topical ocular drug delivery: recent developments and future challenges. J Ocul Pharmacol Ther 1986;2:67–108.
7. Mezei M, Meisner D. Liposomes and nano-particles as ocular drug delivery systems. In: Edman P, ed. Biopharmaceutics in Ocular Drug Delivery. CRC Press, Boca Raton, FL:1993:91–104.
8. Maurice DM. Drug delivery to the posterior segment from drops. Surv Ophthalmol 2002;37:S41–S52.

9. Urtti A, Salminen L. Minimizing systemic absorption of topically administered ophthalmlic drugs. Surv Ophthalmol 1993;37:435–456.
10. Chang SC, Lee VHL. Nasal and conjunctival contributions to the systemic absorption of topical timolol in the pigmented rabbit: implications in the design of strategies to maximize the ratio of ocular to systemic absorption. J Ocular Pharmacol Ther 1987;3:159–169.
11. McMahon CD, Shaffer RN, Hoskins HDJ, Hetherington JJ. Adverse effects experienced by patients taking timolol. Am J Ophthalmol 1979;88:736–738.
12. Ogura Y. Drug delivery to the posterior segments of the eye. Adv Drug Deliv Rev 2001; 52:1–3.
13. Herrero-Vanrell R, Refojo MF. Biodegradable microspheres for vitreoretinal drug delivery. Adv Drug Deliv Rev 2001;52:5–16.
14. Geroski DH, Edelhauser HF. Drug delivery for posterior segment eye disease. Invest Ophthalmol Vis Sci 2000;41:961–964.
15. Peyman GA, Ganiban GJ. Delivery systems for intraocular routes. Adv Drug Deliv Rev 1995;16:107–123.
16. Clark AF, Yorio T. Ophthalmic drug discovery. Nat Rev Drug Discov 2003;2:448–459.
17. Krzystolik MG, Afshari MA, Adamis AP, et al. Prevention of experimental choroidal neovascularization with intravitreal anti-vascular endothelial growth factor antibody fragment. Arch Ophthalmol 2002;120:338–346.
18. Garcia C, Bartsch DU, Rivero ME, et al. Efficacy of Prinomastat (AG3340), a matrix metalloproteinase inhibitor in treatment of retinal neovascularization. Curr Eye Res 2002; 24:33–38.
19. Das A, McLamore A, Song W, McGuire PG. Retinal neovascularization is suppressed with a matrix metalloproteinase inhibitor. Arch Ophthalmol 1999;117:498–503.
20. Friedlander M, Theesfeld CL, Sugita M, et al. Involvement of integrins avb3 and avb5 in ocular neovascular diseases. Proc Natl Acad Sci USA 1996;93:9764–9769.
21. Bouck N. PEDF: anti-angiogenic guardian of ocular function. Trends Mol Med 2002; 8:330–334.
22. Tombran-Tink J, Barnstable CJ. PEDF: A multifaceted neurotrophic factor. Nat Rev Neurosci 2003;4:628–636.
23. Smith LEH, Kopchick JJ, Chen W, et al. Essential role of growth hormone in ischemia-induced retinal neovascularization. Science 1997;276:1706–1709.
24. Clark AF, Bingaman DP, Ma K. Ocular angiostatic agents. Exp Opin Ther Patents 2000;10:427–448.
25. Clark AF. AL-3789: a novel ophthalmic angiostatic steroid. Exp Opin Invest Drugs 1997; 6:1867–1877.
26. Penn JS, Rajaratnam VS, Collier RJ, Clark AF. The effect of an angiostatic steroid on neovascularization in a rat model of retinopathy of prematurity. Invest Ophthalmol Vis Sci 2001;42:283–290.
27. Folkman J, Long D. The use of silicone rubber as a carrier for prolonged drug therapy. J Surg Res 1964;4:139–142.
28. Frank ML, Poindexter AN, Johnson ML, Bateman L. Characteristics and attitudes of early contraceptive implant acceptors. Family Planning Perspect 1992;24:208.
29. Musch MC, Martin DF, Gordon JF, Davis MD, Kupperman BD. The gancyclovir implant study group. Treatment of cytomegalovirus retinitis with a sustained-release gancyclovir implant. N Engl J Med 1997;337:83–90.
30. Martin DF, Parks DJ, Mellow SD, et al. Treatment of cytomegalovirus retinitis with an intraocular sustained release gancyclovir implant—a randomized controlled clinical-trial. Arch Ophthalmol 1994;112:1531–1539.
31. Sanborn GE, Anand R, Torti RE, et al. Sustained release gancyclovir therapy for treatment of cytomegalovirus retinitis. Arch Ophthalmol 1992;110:188–195.

32. Smith TJ, Pearson PA, Blandford DL, et al. Intravitreal sustained release gancyclovir. Arch Ophthalmol 1992;110:255–258.
33. Marx JL, Kapustra MA, Patel SS, et al. Use of the gancyclovir implant in the treatment of recurrent cytomegalovirus retinitis. Arch Ophthalmol 1996;114:815–820.
34. MacCumber M, Sadeghi S, Cohen JA, Deutsch TA. Suture loop to aid in ganciclovir implant removal. Arch Ophthalmol 1999;117:1250–1254.
35. Morley MG, Duker JS, Ashton P, Robinson MR. Replacing ganciclovir implants. Ophthalmology 1995;102:388–392.
36. Shane TS, Martin DF. Endophthalmitis after ganclyclovir implant in patients with AIDS and cytomegalovirus retinitis. Am J Ophthalmol 2003;136:649–654.
37. Jaffe GJ, Ben-nun J, Guo H, Dunn JP, Ashton P. Fluocinolone acetonide sustained drug delivery device to treat severe uveitis. Ophthalmology 2000;107:2024–2033.
38. Mruthyunjaya P, Khalatbari D, Yang P, Stinnett S, Hanes M, Jaffe GJ. An intravitreal sustained release fluocinolone acetonide device to treat severe experimental uveitis. Invest Ophthalmol Vis Sci 2003;44:4215.
39. Hainsworth DP, Pearson PA, Conklin JD, Ashton P. Sustained release intravitreal dexamethasone. J Ocular Pharmacol Ther 1996;12:57–63.
40. Denny JP, Carlson A, McCallum R, Ashton P, Branchaud B, Jaffe GJ. Combined fluocinolone acetonide sustained drug delivery system implantation and phacoemulsification / intraocular lens implantation in patients with severe uveitis. Invest Ophthalmol Vis Sci 2003;44:2410.
41. Mruthyunjaya P, Tseng W, Stinnett S, Ashton P, Jaffe GJ. Fluocinolone acetonide sustained drug delivery system in the treatment of experimental proliferative vitreoretinopathy. Invest Ophthalmol Vis Sci 2002;43:3003.
42. Pearson P, Baker CW, Eliott D, Ip MS, Morse LS, Callanan D. Fluocinolone acetonide intravitreal implant in patients with diabetic macular edema: 12 month results. Invest Ophthalmol Vis Sci 2003;44:4288.
43. Maurice DM, Polgar K. Diffusion across the sclera. Exp Eye Res 1977;25:577–582.
44. Edelhauser HF, Maren TH. Permeability of human cornea and sclera to sulfonamide carbonic anhydrase inhibitors. Arch Ophthalmol 1988;106:1110–1115.
45. Olsen TW, Edelhauser HF, Lim JI, Geroski DH. Human scleral permeability: effects of age, cryotherapy, transscleral diode laser and surgical thinning. Invest Ophthalmol Vis Sci 1995;36:1893–1903.
46. Ambati J, Canakis CS, Miller JW, et al. Diffusion of high molecular weight compounds through the sclera. Invest Ophthalmol Vis Sci 2000;41:1181–1185.
47. Ahmed I, Patton TF. Importance of the non-corneal absorption route in topical ophthalmic drug delivery. Invest Ophthalmol Vis Sci 1985;26:584–587.
48. Geroski DH, Edelhauser HF. Transscleral drug delivery for posterior segment disease. Adv Drug Deliv Rev 2001;52:37–48.
49. Yaacobi Y. Drug delivery device. US Patent #6,413,540;2002.
50. Yaacobi Y, Chastain J, Lowseth L, et al. In vivo studies with trans scleral anecortave acetate delivery device designed to treat choroidal neovascularization in AMD. Invest Ophthalmol Vis Sci 2003;44:4210.
51. Yaacobi Y. Ophthalmic drug delivery device. US Patent #6,416,777;2002.
52. Yaacobi Y. Drug delivery device. US Patent #6,669,950;2003.
53. Saltzman WM. Drug Delivery: Engineering Principles for Drug Therapy. Oxford University Press, New York:2001.
54. Kunou N, Ogura Y, Honda Y, Hyon SH, Ikada Y. Biodegradable scleral implant for controlled intraocular delivery of betamethasone phosphate. J Biomed Mater Res 2000;51:635–641.
55. Kato A, Kimura H, Okabe K, Okabe J, Kunou N, Ogura Y. Feasibility of drug delivery to the posterior pole of the rabbit eye with an episcleral implant. Invest Ophthalmol Vis Sci 2004;45:238–244.

56. Kunou N, Ogura Y, Yasukawa T, et al. Long-term sustained release of ganciclovir from biodegradable scleral implant for the treatment of cytomegalovirus retinitis. J Controlled Rel 2000;68:263–271.
57. Sakurai E, Matsuda Y, Ozeki H, Kunou N, Nakajima K, Ogura Y. Scleral plug of biodegradable polymers containing ganciclovir for experimental cytomegalovirus retinitis. Invest Ophthalmol Vis Sci 2001;42:2043–2048.
58. Sakuri E, Nozaki M, Okabe K, Kunou N, Kimura H, Ogura Y. Scleral plug of biodegradable polymers containing tacrolimus (FK506) for experimental uveitis. Invest Ophthalmol Vis Sci 2003;44:4845–4852.
59. Ciulla TA, Criswell MH, Danis RP, et al. Choroidal neovascular membrane inhibition in a laser treated rat model with intraocular sustained release triamcinolone acetonide microimplants. Br J Ophthalmol 2003;87:1032–1037.
60. Joshi A. Microparticulates for ophthalmic delivery. J Ocul Pharmacol 1994;10:29–45.
61. Zimmer A, Kreuter J. Microspheres and nanoparticles used in ocular delivery systems. Adv Drug Deliv Rev 1995;16:61–73.
62. Herrero-Vanrell R, Refojo MF. Intravitreal microsphere drug delivery and method of preparation. US Patent #5,718,922;1998.
63. Wong GB. Biodegradable ocular implants. US Patent #4,997,652;1991.
64. Ross ML, Yuan P, Robinson MR. Intraocular drug delivery implants. Rev Ophthalmol 2000;7:95.
65. Einmahl S, Ponsart S, Bejjani RA, et al. Ocular biocompatibility of a poly(ortho ester) characterized by autocatalyzed degradation. J Biomed Mater Res 2003;67A:44–53.
66. Einmahl S, Savoldelli M, D'Hermies F, Tabatabay C, Gurny R, Behar-Cohen F. Evaluation of a novel biomaterial in the suprachoroidal space of the rabbit eye. Invest Ophthalmol Vis Sci 2002;43:1533–1539.
67. Lin YHE, Vasavada RC. Studies on microencapsulation of 5-fluorouracil with poly(ortho ester) polymers. J Microencapsul 2000;17:1–11.
68. Jalil R, Nixon JR. Biodegradable poly(lactic acid) and poly(lactide-co-glycolide) microcapsules—problems associated with preparative techniques and release properties J Microencapsul 1990;7:297–325.
69. Torres AI, Boisdron-Celle M, Benoit JP. Formulation of BCNU-loaded microspheres: Influence of drug stability and solubility on the design of the microencapsulation procedure. J Microencapsul 1996;13:41–51.
70. Giordano G, Chevez-Barrios P, Refojo MF, Garcia CA. Biodedegradation and tissue reaction to intravitreous biodegradable poly(D,L-lactic-co-glycolic) acid microspheres. Curr Eye Res 1995;14:761–768.
71. Li SM. Hydrolytic degradation characteristics of aliphatic polyesters derived from lactic and glycolic acids. J Biomed Mater Res 1999;48:342–353.
72. Grizzi I, Garreau H, Li S, Vert M. Hydrolytic degradation of devices based on poly(D,L-lactic acid) size dependence. Biomaterials 1995;16:305–311.
73. Mathiowitz E, Saltzman WM, Domb A, Dor P, Langer R. Polyanhydride microspheres as drug carriers. II. Microencapsulation by solvent removal. J Appl Polymer Sci 1988;35: 755–774.
74. Chan IM, Tolentino FI, Refojo MF, Fournier G, Albert DM. Vitreous substitute—experimental studies and review. Retina 1984;4:51–59.
75. Moritera T, Ogura Y, Yashimura N, et al. Biodegradable microspheres containing adriamycin in the treatment of proliferative vitreoretinopathy. Invest Ophthalmol Vis Sci 1992;33:3125–3130.
76. Moritera T, Ogura Y, Honda Y, Wada R, Hyon SH, Ikada Y. Microspheres of biodegradable polymers as a drug delivery system in the vitreous. Invest Ophthalmol Vis Sci 1991;32: 1785–1790.

77. Peyman GA, Conway M, Khoobehi B, Soike K. Clearance of microsphere entrapped 5-fluorouracil and cytosine-arabinoside from the vitreous of primates. Int Ophthalmol 1992;16:109–113.
78. Giordano GG, Refojo MF, Arroyo MH. Sustained delivery of retinoic acid from microspheres of biodegradable polymer in PVR. Invest Ophthalmol Vis Sci 1993;34:2743–2751.
79. Kwak HW, D'Amico DJ. Evaluation of the retinal toxicity and pharmacokinetics of dexamethasone after intravitreal injection. Arch Ophthalmol 1992;110:259–266.
80. Herrero-Vanrell R, Herradon C, Ramirez L, Refojo MF. Biodegradable microspheres loaded with dexamethasone for intravitreal administration. Invest Ophthalmol Vis Sci 1999;40:444.
81. Conti B, Bucolo C, Giannavola C, Puglisi G, Guinchedi P, Conte U. Biodegradable microspheres for the administration of acyclovir: in vitro in vivo evaluation. Eur J Pharm Sci 1997;5:287–293.
82. Refojo MF, Herrero-Vanrell R. Biodegradable microspheres loaded with ganciclovir sterilized by gamma irradiation. Invest Ophthalmol Vis Sci 2000;41:4110.
83. Herrero-Vanrell R, Herradon C, Ramirez L, Refojo MF. Biodegradable microspheres loaded with ganciclovir influence of tocopherol acetate on drug release. Invest Ophthalmol Vis Sci 1997;38:721.
84. Veloso AAS, Zhu Q, Herrero-Vanrell R, Refojo MF. Ganciclovir loaded polymer microspheres in rabbit eyes inoculated with human cytomegalovirus. Invest Ophthalmol Vis Sci 1997;38:665–675.
85. Merkli A, Heller J, Tabatabay R, R G. Gamma-sterilization of a semisolid poly (ortho ester) designed for controlled drug-delivery—validation and radiation effects. Pharm Res 1994;11:1485–1491.
86. Bourges J, Gautier SE, Delie F, et al. Ocular drug delivery targeting the retina and retinal pigment epithelium using polylactide nanoparticles. Invest Ophthalmol Vis Sci 2003;44: 3562–3569.
87. Colthurst MJ, Williams RL, Hiscott PS, Grierson I. Biomaterials used in the posterior segment of the eye. Biomaterials 2000;21:649–665.
88. Stannett VT, Koros WJ, Paul DR, Lonsdale HK, Baker RW. Recent advances in membrane science and technology. Adv Polymer Sci 1979;32:69–121.
89. Langer R, Folkman J. Polymers for the sustained release of proteins and other macromolecules. Nature 1976;263:797–800.
90. Saltzman WM, Langer R. Transport rates of proteins in porous polymers with known microgeometry. Biophys J 1989;55:163–171.
91. Brown L, Siemer L, Munoz C, Edelman E, Langer R. Controlled release of insulin from polymer matrices: control of diabetes in rats. Diabetes 1986;35:692–697.
92. Fischel-Ghodsian F, Brown L, Mathiowitz E, Brandenburg D, Langer R. Enzymatically controlled drug delivery. Proc Nat Acad Sci USA 1988;85:2403–2406.
93. Edelman E, Adams D, Karnovsky M. Effect of controlled adventitial heparin delivery on smooth muscle cell proliferation following endothelial injury. Proc Nat Acad Sci USA 1990;87:3773–3777.
94. Powell EM, Sobarzo MR, Saltzman WM. Controlled release of nerve growth factor from a polymeric implant. Brain Res 1990;515:309–311.
95. Murray J, Brown L, Langer R, Klagsburn M. A micro sustained release system for epidermal growth factor. In Vitro 1983;19:743–748.
96. Beaty CE, Saltzman WM. Controlled growth factor delivery induces differental neurite outgrowth in three-dimensional cell cultures. J Controlled Rel 1993;24:15–23.
97. Hoffman D, Wahlberg L, Aebischer P. NGF released from a polymer matrix prevents loss of ChAT expression in basal forebrain neurons following a fimbria-fornix lesion. Exper Neurol 1990;110:39–44.

98. Lee A, Langer R. Shark cartilage contains inhibitors of tumor angiogenesis. Science 1983; 221:1185–1187.
99. Radomsky ML, Whaley KJ, Cone RA, Saltzman WM. Macromolecules released from polymers: diffusion into unstirred fluids. Biomaterials 1990;11:619–624.
100. Radomsky ML, Whaley KJ, Cone RA, Saltzman WM. Controlled vaginal delivery of antibodies in the mouse. Biol Reprod 1992;47:133–140.
101. Sherwood JK, Dause RB, Saltzman WM. Controlled antibody delivery systems. Bio/ Technology 1992;10:1446–1449.
102. Saltzman WM. Antibodies for treating and preventing disease: the potential role of polymeric controlled release. Crit Rev Ther Drug Carrier Syst 1993;10:111–142.
103. Saltzman WM, Sheppard NF, McHugh MA, Dause RB, Pratt JA, Dodrill AM. Controlled antibody release from a matrix of poly(ethylene-co-vinyl acetate) fractionated with a supercritical fluid. J Appl Polymer Sci 1993;48:1493–1500.
104. Preis I, Langer RS. A single–step immunization by sustained antigen release. Journal of immunological methods 1979;28:193–197.
105. Wyatt TL, Whaley KJ, Cone RA, Saltzman WM. Antigen-releasing polymer rings and microspheres stimulate mucosal immunity in the vagina. J Controlled Rel 1998;50:93–102.
106. Luo D, Woodrow-Mumford K, Belcheva N, Saltzman WM. Controlled DNA delivery systems. Pharmaceutical Research 1999;16:1300–1308.
107. Sherwood JK, Zeitlin L, Whaley KJ, Cone RA, Saltzman WM. Controlled release of antibodies for sustained topical passive immunoprotection of female mice against genital herpes. Nat Biotechnol 1996;14:468–471.
108. Mahoney MJ, Saltzman WM. Millimeter-scale positioning of a nerve-growth-factor source and biological activity in the brain. Proc Nat Acad Sci USA 1999;96:4536–4539.
109. Siegel R, Langer R. Controlled release of polypeptides and other macromolecules. Pharmaceut Res 1984;1:2–10.
110. Saltzman WM, Pasternak SH, Langer R. Quantitative image analysis for developing microstructural descriptions of heterogeneous materials. Chem Eng Sci 1987;42: 1989–2004.
111. Hsu T, Langer R. Polymers for the controlled release of macromolecules: Effect of molecular weight of ethylene-vinyl acetate copolymer. J Biomed Mater Res 1985;19:445–460.
112. Cleland J. Protein delivery from biodegradable microspheres. In:Protein Delivery—Physical Systems, Sanders L, Hendren W, eds. Plenum Press, New York:1997;1–43.
113. Saltzman WM, Mak MW, Mahoney MJ, Duenas ET, Cleland JL. Intracranial delivery of recombinant nerve growth factor: release kinetics and protein distribution for three delive systems. Pharmaceut Res 1999;16:232–240.
114. Johnson OL, Cleland JL, Lee HJ, et al. A month-long effect from a single injection of microencapsulated human growth hormone. Nat Med 1996;2:795–799.
115. Hora MS, Rana RK, Nunberg JH, Tice TR, Gilley RM, Hudson ME. Controlled release of interleukin-2 from biodegradable microspheres. Bio/Technology 1990;8:755–758.
116. Cleland J, Barron L, Berman P, Daugherty A, Gregory T, Lim A. Development of a single-shot subunit vaccine for HIV-1 2. Defining optimal autoboost characteristics to maximize the humoral immune response. J Pharmaceut Sci 1996;85:1346–1348.
117. Reinhard C, Radomsky ML, Saltzman WM, Hilton J, Brem H. Polymeric controlled release of dexamethasone in normal rat brain. J Controlled Rel 1991;16:331–340.

INDEX

MIX
Papier aus verantwortungsvollen Quellen
Paper from responsible sources
FSC® C105338

If you have any concerns about our products,
you can contact us on
ProductSafety@springernature.com

In case Publisher is established outside the EU,
the EU authorized representative is:
Springer Nature Customer Service Center GmbH
Europaplatz 3, 69115 Heidelberg, Germany

Printed by Libri Plureos GmbH
in Hamburg, Germany